Recent Results in Cancer Research 143

Springer
Berlin
Heidelberg
New York
Barcelona
Budapest
Hong Kong
London
Milan
Paris
Santa Clara
Singapore
Tokyo

H.K. Müller-Hermelink
H.-G. Neumann W. Dekant (Eds.)

Risk and Progression Factors in Carcinogenesis

With 129 Figures and 31 Tables

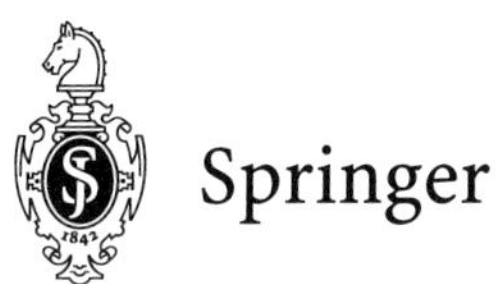

Prof. Dr. med. H.K. Müller-Hermelink
Pathologisches Institut der Universität Würzburg
Josef-Schneider-Straße 2
97080 Würzburg
Germany

Prof. Dr. rer. nat. H.-G. Neumann
Institut für Pharmakologie und Toxikologie
der Universität Würzburg
Versbacher Straße 9
97078 Würzburg
Germany

Prof. Dr. rer. nat. W. Dekant
Institut für Pharmakologie und Toxikologie
der Universität Würzburg
Versbacher Straße 9
97078 Würzburg
Germany

ISBN 3-540-60953-9 Springer-Verlag Berlin Heidelberg New York

Library of Congress Cataloging-in-Publication Data. Risk and progression factors in carcinogenesis/H.K. Müller-Hermelink, H.-G. Neumann, W. Dekant, eds. p. cm. – (Recent results in cancer research: 143) Includes bibliographical references and index. ISBN 3-540-60953-9 (hardcover) 1. Carcinogenesis – Congresses. 2. Cancer cells – Congresses. I. Müller-Hermelink, Hans Konrad. II. Neumann, H.-G. (Hans-Günter) III. Dekant, W. (Wolfgang) IV. Series. [DNLM: 1. Cell Transformation, Neoplastic. 2. Carcinogens. 3. DNA Damage. 4. Risk Factors. W1 RE106P v. 143 1995/QZ 202 R5942 1995] RC261.R35 vol. 143 [RC268.5] 616.99'4071 – dc20 DNLM/DLC for Library of Congress 96-12853

Typesetting: Scientific Publishing Services (P) Ltd, Madras

SPIN: 10498912 19/3133/SPS – 5 4 3 2 1 0 – Printed on acid-free paper

Preface

Cellular transformation and carcinogenesis is a multistep process, starting with initial DNA lesions and progressing through impairment and, finally, loss of cellular growth control and a gain in invasive and metastatic properties. Although the principal features of tumor phenotype among the different cancers may resemble each other, it is well known that at the molecular level various different genes and gene families are involved and altered, depending on the cellular origin as well the state of tumor differentiation and progression. This book demonstrates the important steps in carcinogenesis, ranging from the chemical interaction of carcinogens with cellular DNA in experimental tumors and cell lines to the analysis of selected human tumors. In the first part special emphasis is placed on how the first DNA changes in carcinogenesis are produced and recognized. Chemical carcinogens, UV irradiation, and endogenous oxidative damage and impairment of repair mechanisms and its sequelae are considered. The second part adds new strategies to analyze the relevant cell biological alterations and controlling genes and proteins in established cancer cells. In the final section the relevance of genomic alterations in selected human tumors for cellular transformation and tumor progression is discussed.

Leading scientists met at a SFB 172 International Symposium entitled "Molecular Mechanisms of Primary Carcinogenic Alterations," where in short review articles, the state of the art of specific fields of interest was described, from the chemistry of carcinogens to the cellular biology and clinical course of tumor formation and progression. Given the high specialization in each field, this kind of survey was considered to be especially valuable since it is only seldomly found and should provide the reader with stimulating results and methods in fields related to his own main interest.

Current trends and methodologically oriented scientific approaches for recognizing relevant pathogenetic mechanisms and factors in carcinogenesis are thus brought together.

The editors of this volume are especially grateful that, due to the great cooperative effort of everyone involved in the writing and publishing process, it was possible to hand over this book to the public in the shortest time possible. In particular, we thank B. Hasenmüller and E. Albero for their excellent secretarial help, which made the hard job of collecting manuscripts an easy task. The rapid evaluation process and editorial process at Springer-Verlag is gratefully acknowledged. In particular, Janet Sterritt-Brunner and Lindrun Weber as desk editors and Sherryl Sundell as copy editor helped considerably in putting this volume together. We hope that this timely report will find an interested readership and be worthwhile in this rapidly progressing field.

Würzburg, April 1996

H.K. Müller-Hermelink
H.-G. Neumann
W. Dekant

Contents

List of Contributors[*]

[*]The address of the principal author is given on the first page of each contribution.
[1]Page on which contribution begins.

Kalla, J. *307*
Kämpfe, D. *321*
Katzenberger, T. *307*
Kielbassa, C. *35*
Kim, M.-S. *49*
Klöhn, P.-C. *209*
Koffel-Schwartz, N. *1*
Kovacech, B. *251*
Kreipe, H. *307*
Kunze, J. *321*
Lambert, I. *1*
Lefèvre, J.-F. *1*
Liebetrau, W. *353*
Liechty, M.C. *161*
Lindsley, J.E. *1*
Lobo-Napolitano, R. *1*
Lowe, L.G. *49*
Luo, L.-di. *145*
Maenhaut-Michel, G. *1*
Mielke, K. *21*
Milhé, C. *1*
Möller, K. *337*
Möller, M. *21*
Mullenders, L.H.F. 89
Müller, J.G. *307*
Müller, M. *49*
Müller-Hermelink, H.K. *307*
Naumann, U. *237*
Neumann, H.-G. *209*
Norén, U.G. *275*
Ott, G. *307*
Ott, M.M. *307*
Otteneder, M. *65*
Pagany, M. *225*
Pflaum, M. *35*
Poot, M. *353*
Price, C. *251*
Rapp, U.R. *237, 245*
Richter, H. *195*
Rossoll, W. *251*
Rünger, T.M. *21, 337, 353*
Ruven, H.-J. *89*
Saha-Möller, C.R. *21*
Schartl, A. *225*
Schartl, M. *225*
Schindler, D. *353*
Schmitt, I.M. *101*
Schönberger, A. *21*
Schryen, B. *307*
Schuler, D. *65*
Schulz, W.A. *183*
Schuster, T. *251*
Soussi, T. *369*
Stopper, H. *21, 161, 183*
Sundqvist, K. *275*
Thomas, G. *369*
Troppmair, J. *245*
Valladier-Belguise, P. *1*
Valsamas, S. *321*
Vamvakas, S. *195*
van Hoffen, A. *89*
van Zeeland, A.A. *89*
von Brevern, M.-C. *369*
Vreeswijk, M.P.G. *89*
Vrieling, H. *89*
Wagener, P. *183*
Wirth, P.J. *145*
Zernak, C. *321*
Zheng, X. *275*

I. Interaction of Carcinogens with Cellular DNA

Induction of Frameshift Mutations at Hotspot Sequences by Carcinogen Adducts

D. Burnouf, M. Bichara, C. Dhalluin, A. Garcia, R. Janel-Bintz, N. Koffel-Schwartz, I. Lambert, J.-F. Lefèvre, J.E. Lindsley, G. Maenhaut-Michel, C. Milhé, R. Lobo-Napolitano, P. Valladier-Belguise, and R.P.P. Fuchs

UPR 9003 Centre National de la Recherche Scientifique, Ecole Supérieure de Biotechnologie, Pole API Bld Sébastien Brant, 67400 Illkirch, France

Introduction

Living organisms are exposed to various agents that damage DNA. These agents may be endogeneous, resulting from such normal cell processes as oxidative metabolism (Demple and Harrison 1994), or exogenous, coming from sources as diverse as sunlight, cigarette smoke, foods, or automobile exhaust.

Mutagenic agents can be classified into two categories: those that directly react with DNA, and those that are biochemically activated into forms that react with DNA bases. Alternatively, one could also differentiate between direct miscoding lesions which change the coding properties of the modified base, and noncoding lesions for which conversion of the DNA adduct into a mutation is an active process that requires inducible functions belonging to the so-called SOS system, in the bacterium *Escherichia coli* (Walker 1987). Because of the existence of efficient repair mechanisms (Sancar and Sancar 1988), only a very small proportion of DNA lesions is converted into mutations.

The specificity of the mutagenic effect of genotoxic agents has been studied as a first step toward understanding molecular mechanisms by which mutations arise. We have focused on the aromatic amide *N*-2-acetylaminofluorene (AAF). This potent carcinogen binds primarily to the C8 position of guanine in vivo, forming two major adducts, one acetylated (-AAF) and one deacetylated (-AF) (Miller and Miller 1983). These adducts can also be formed by the in vitro modification of DNA by two ultimate carcinogens: *N*-hydroxy-*N*-2-aminofluorene, which forms the deacetylated adducts (dG-C8-AF), and *N*-acetoxy-*N*-2-acetylaminofluorene, which forms the acetylated adducts (dG-C8-AAF).

Recent Results in Cancer Research, Vol. 143

This review summarizes an ongoing study in our laboratory on the mutagenic specificity of AAF. On the basis of diverse lines of evidence, we propose a model for carcinogen-induced frameshift mutagenesis at specific hotspot sequences.

Determination of AAF-Induced Mutation Spectra in *E. coli*

Strategy

A first step in analyzing the mutagenicity of a given mutagen is to determine the spectrum of the mutations that it induces. We used a forward mutation assay based on the inactivation of the tetracycline resistance gene of the plasmid pBR322 (Fuchs et al. 1981). This assay presents as little bias as possible in mutant selection and can actually detect base substitutions, frameshift mutations, and complex mutations (Koffel-Schwartz et al. 1984; Bichara and Fuchs 1985; Burnouf et al. 1987). We chose the BamHI-SalI restriction fragment (276 bp long), which lies in the part of the tetracycline resistance gene of pBR322 that encodes for the N-terminal part of the protein, as a target sequence because it is short enough to allow a quick analysis of the mutated sequences. The strategy of this assay is summarized in Fig. 1. Briefly, the BamHI-SalI restriction fragment (6S) from a plasmid that has been modified with a mutagen in vitro is purified and ligated to the remainder (16S) of the plasmid that has not been chemically modified. Thus, the reconstructed plasmid bears lesions only in the target sequence. *E. coli* is then transformed with this plasmid. Transformants are selected on plates containing ampicillin, and tetracycline-sensitive mutants are detected by replica plating on medium containing tetracycline. The nature of the mutation is determined by DNA sequencing.

Mutagenesis Is Dependent on SOS Induction and the Number of Carcinogen Adducts

The recovery of -AF- or -AAF-induced mutations depends on the induction of the SOS system of the cells (Koffel-Schwartz et al. 1984; Bichara and Fuchs 1985). The response is dose-dependent in that the mutation frequency increases as a function of the extent of modification. The background mutation frequency due to cryptic lesions on unmodified plasmids is about 6×10^{-4} under optimal conditions of SOS induction (UV irradiation of cells at a dose of 30 J/m^2). The mutation frequency is increased to about 130×10^{-4} when there are 2.8 AAF adducts per 6S fragment and 190×10^{-4} with 7 AF adducts per 6S fragment (Koffel-Schwartz et al. 1984; Bichara and Fuchs 1985). The results indicate that AF- and AAF-induced mutagenesis requires specific inducible functions and is therefore an active process.

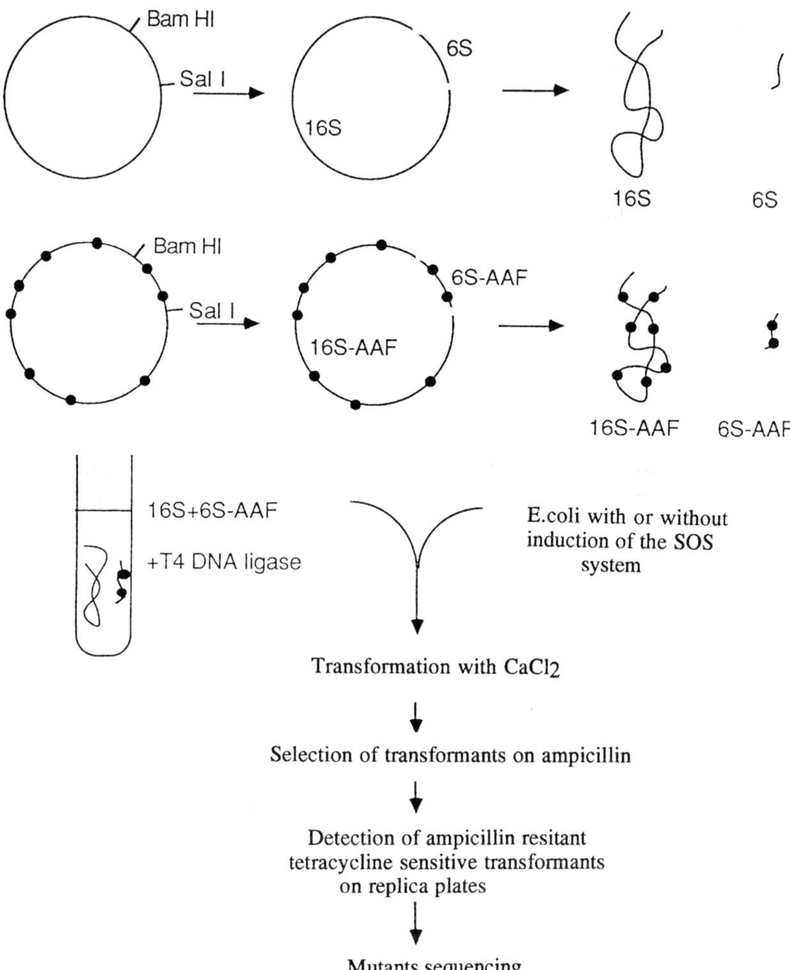

Fig. 1. Strategy for the forward mutation assay in the tetracycline resistance gene of pBR322. *Black dots* represent covalent adducts (dG-C8-AAF)

The Spectrum of Mutations Induced by AAF Reveals Sequences Highly Sensitive to Mutations

The analysis of mutations induced by DNA sequencing reveals a distinctive mutation spectrum for each type of adduct (Fig. 2). AF adducts induce mainly G→T base substitutions that are randomly distributed in the BamHI-SalI fragment.

In contrast, AAF adducts induce primarily frameshift mutations (>90%) that are clustered at two types of sequences: (1) runs of monotonous GC base pairs and (2) the recognition sequence of the NarI restriction enzyme

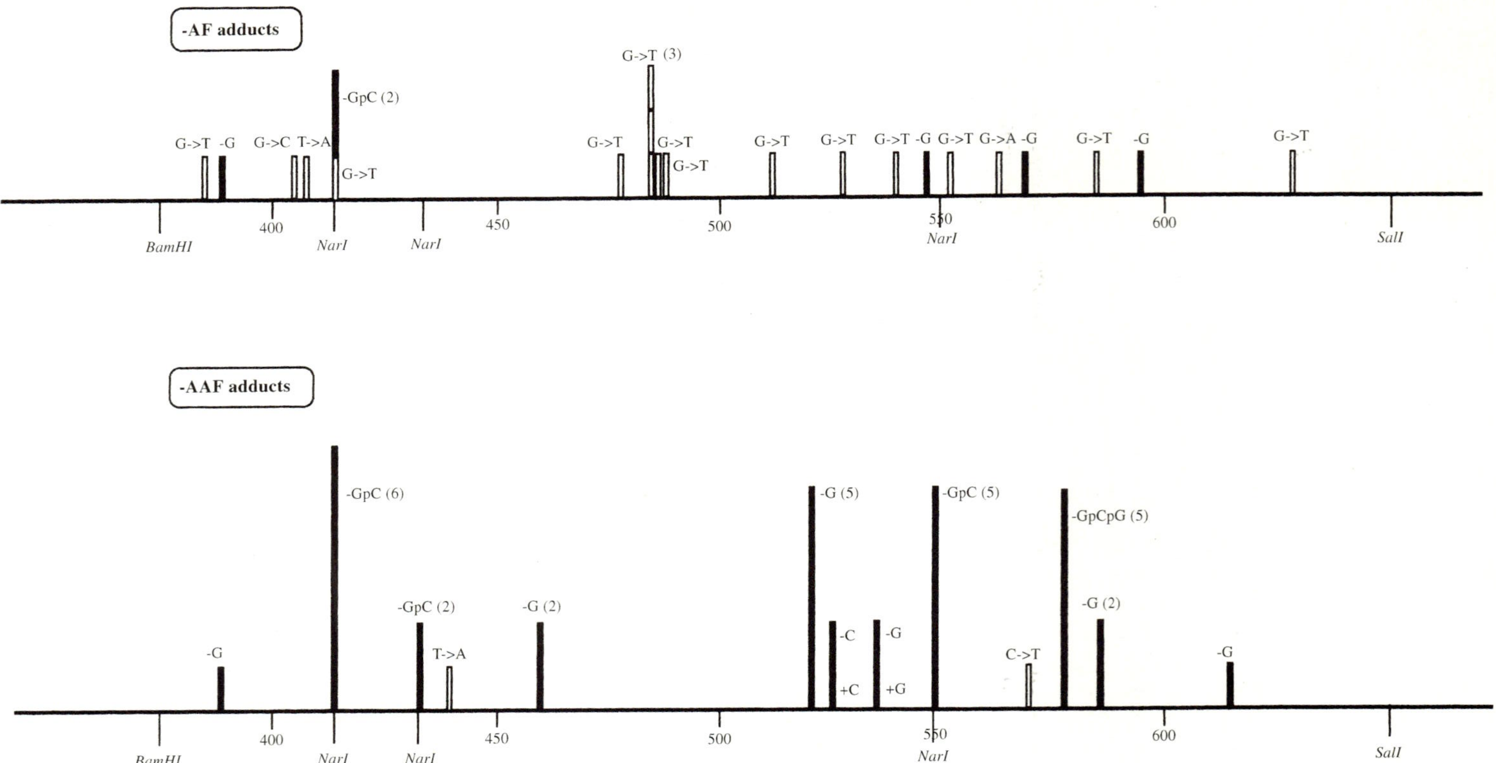

Fig. 2. Mutation spectra induced by -AF and -AAF adducts in the BamHI-SalI restriction fragment of pBR322 in *E. coli*. The AAF spectrum combines data obtained in wild-type and *uvrA* strains. *Open bars*, base substitutions; *solid bars* frameshift mutations. Note that the height of the bars is proportional to the number of occurrences shown in *parentheses*

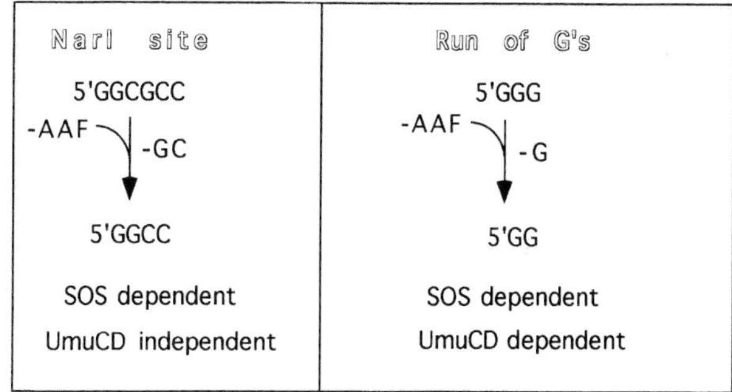

Fig. 3. Specificity of *N*-2-acetylaminofluorene (AAF)-induced mutagenesis at hotspot sequences in *Escherichia coli*. Mutations are primarily (>90%) frameshift

5′GGCGCC. These sites are called mutation hotspots because of their high susceptibility to mutagenesis. The mutations in repetitive sequences (e.g., 5′GGGGG) are usually single base deletions, while those at NarI sites are two base pair deletions (5′GGCGCC→5′GGCC) (Fig. 3). There are three NarI sites in the 6S fragment, making it an especially good target for studying mutagenesis in this sequence.

To ensure that the high responsiveness of the hotspot sequences cannot be ascribed to a bias in lesion formation or mutation detection such as specificity of -AAF modification or preferential repair of -AAF lesions in the other sequences, we established the AAF modification spectrum along the BamHI-SalI sequence (Fuchs 1984). This modification spectrum showed that all guanines in the sequence react with the carcinogen, but the reactivity varies by a factor of about 40. Nevertheless, guanines in the hotspot sequences do not exhibit increased reactivity compared to other positions in the fragment. Thus, preferential binding of the carcinogen cannot explain the existence of the hotspot.

We also determined the -AAF induced mutation spectrum in a *uvrA* strain, which is defective in the major pathway of repair of -AAF lesions (Schmid et al. 1982), and found no difference in mutation spectrum from the wild-type strain (Koffel-Schwartz et al. 1984). The similarity of the mutation spectra indicates that the existence of hotspots cannot be attributed to differential repair of -AAF lesions in repetitive sequences, NarI sites, or other sequence contexts.

The increased frequency of mutation at hotspot sequences is thought to result from specific mutagenic processing of adducts in these sequences. We have been interested in elucidating the molecular mechanisms by which the premutational lesions are processed into mutations.

Genetic Control of Mutagenesis of AAF Hotspots

Mutagenesis by UV and many chemicals in *E. coli* is under the control of SOS functions encoded by the *umuDC* operon (Kato and Shinoura 1977; Murli and

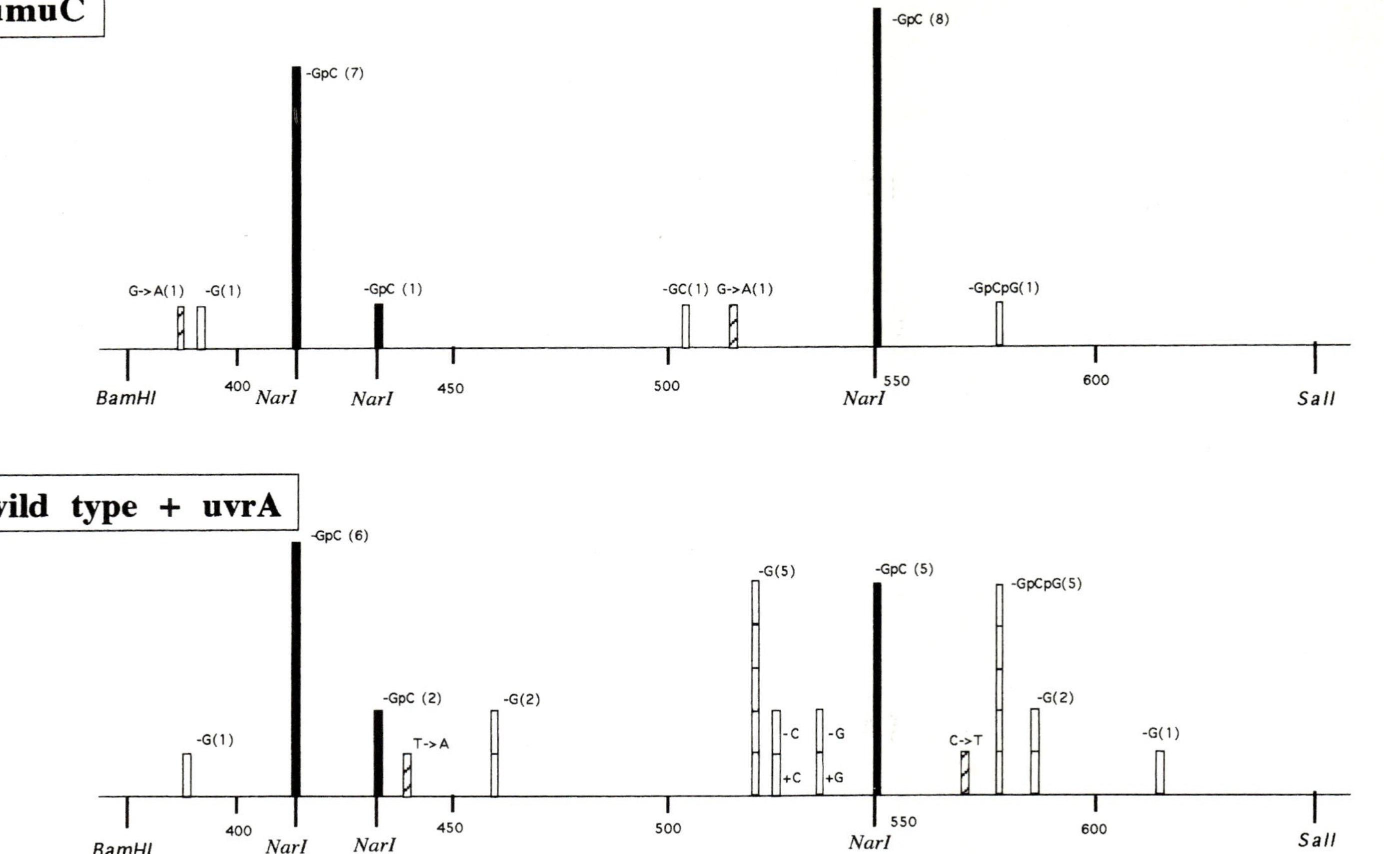

Fig. 4. Mutation spectra induced by AAF in the BamHI-SalI restriction fragment of pBR322 in *umuC*$^{+}$ (wild-type +*uvrA*) or *umuC* strains of *E. coli*. *Dark bars* represent –2 base-pair frameshift mutations at NarI sites; *open bars* represent frameshift mutations at repetitive sequences, and *hatched bars* represent base substitutions

Walker 1993). To define the genetic requirements for the mutagenicity of AAF adducts, we determined the mutation spectrum of AAF in a *umuC* strain (Koffel-Schwartz et al. 1984) (Fig. 4). Unlike the wild-type strain, the *umuC* strain showed few mutations at repetitive sequences, and 80% of the mutations were located in NarI sites. This observation suggests that two pathways of mutagenesis occur in the mutagenic processing of AAF lesions: a *umuDC*-dependent pathway that acts on repetitive sequences and causes deletion of single base pairs, and a *umuDC*-independent, yet SOS-dependent, process (Janel-Bintz et al. 1991) that is responsible for the two-base-pair deletions at NarI sites (Fig. 3).

Our study of AAF-induced mutagenesis in *E. coli* highlights the fact that some DNA sequences, upon modification with carcinogens, are more prone to mutations than surrounding sequences. Streisinger et al. (1966) had shown much earlier that repetitive sequences are hotspot for spontaneous mutagenesis in phage T4, and we suggest that the binding of mutagens in these sequences enhances the frequency of the mutagenic event (see next and Lambert et al. 1992). To gain insight into the mutagenic processes that operate at these AAF-modified hotspot sequences, we performed single adduct mutagenesis studies that enabled us to determine the contribution to mutagenesis of each possible adduct formed in these sequences.

Studies of Mutagenesis by a Single AAF Adduct

A difficulty in interpreting results from experiments in which adducts are formed randomly in DNA is that the hotspot sequences present multiple modification sites whose mutagenic processing may lead to the same mutated sequence. For example, in the NarI sequence 5′$G_1G_2CG_3CC$, deletion of G_2C, CG_3, or G_3C is equivalent at the sequence level, in that all give rise to a mutant whose sequence is 5′GGCC. However, the processing of adducts at these sites may differ mechanistically. We therefore analyzed the fate of individual AAF adducts at each guanine residue in the NarI site. We similarly analyzed the three guanine residues in the SmaI restriction sequence 5′$CCCG_1G_2G_3$ as a model for mutagenesis in repetitive sequences.

General Strategy for Single Adduct Mutagenesis

The details of the procedures have been described elsewhere (Koehl et al. 1989; Lambert et al. 1992). Briefly, we constructed pUC-derived plasmids that we could use to form "gapped-duplex" vectors. These molecules have a short single-stranded region that contains the NarI or SmaI sequence. After in vitro modification, monomodified oligonucleotides bearing a single AAF lesion at each possible site (G_1, G_2, and G_3) were purified on HPLC, and the position of the adduct was biochemically determined. After ligation of these oligonucleotides bearing a single adduct into the gapped-duplex vectors, the closed circular monomodified plasmids were purified on cesium chloride gradients and used to transform *E. coli*.

The Different AAF Adducts of a Hotspot Sequence Are not Equally Efficient in Inducing Mutations

Table 1 summarizes the results obtained in mutagenesis studies with single AAF adducts in two kinds of hotspot sequences. SOS induction was required for optimal mutant recovery in all cases, as it was in studies with random modification of DNA by AAF. These data show that the mutation frequency is strongly influenced by the position of the AAF adduct within the sequence. In the case of the NarI site, only G_3-AAF lesions produced -(GC) mutations (Burnouf et al. 1989). AAF adducts on G_1 or G_2 did not give rise to mutants.

Lesions at all positions in the case of the run of Gs were processed into mutations, but the G_3-AAF adduct was one and two orders of magnitude more efficient in triggering the mutagenic event than G_2-AAF and G_1-AAF, respectively (Lambert et al. 1992). Molecular characterization of the mutations showed that most of them were targeted and result in the deletion of one G in the SmaI site (5′CCCGGG→5′CCCGG). However, 10% of all the mutations result from semitargeted mutagenic events, defined as AAF-induced (-C) deletions occurring in the C run. These mutations were observed only when the AAF lesion is bound to G_1 or G_2, and represent 64% and 76% of the overall mutation frequency for each type of adduct, respectively (Table 1). This finding suggests that G_1 and G_2 adducts are able to alter the replication process locally on their 5′ side, where they promote a specific mutational event with a higher efficiency than AAF-targeted mutagenesis.

Table 1. Mutation frequencies ($\times 10^{-4}$) induced by single AAF adducts at hotspot sequences in *E. coli*

Strain		SmaI 5′CCC$G_1G_2G_3$ JM103*uvrA*				NarI 5′$G_1G_2CG_3CC$ JM103			
		G_0	G_1	G_2	G_3	G_0	G_1	G_2	G_3
– SOS		–	–	–	–	–	< 19	< 9	4
+ SOS	Overall	0.07	1.85	19.1	146	< 1	< 6	< 10	102
	Targeted		0.67	4.6	146				
	Semitargeted		1.18	14.5	< 3.5				

AAF, N-2 acetylaminofluorene; G_0, unmodified vectors.
Induction of the SOS system was achieved by UV irradiation at 60 J/m^2 and 5 J/m^2 for wild-type and *uvrA* strains, respectively.
–, not done.

Mutagenesis Data and Biophysical Studies of Slipped Mutagenic Intermediates Suggest a Model for AAF-Induced Frameshift Mutagenesis

The data summarized in Table 1 support a slippage model for AAF-induced mutagenesis at repetitive sequences. Spontaneous frameshifts in monotonous sequences have long been thought to result from strand slippage (Ripley 1990), the intermediate being stabilized by normal base pairing. We have suggested that in the case of AAF mutagenesis (Lambert et al. 1992), as C is first incorporated opposite the adduct (Fig. 5). This might occur because of the rapid conversion of the modified guanine from the *syn* to the *anti* configuration, which allows pairing between the modified G and the incoming C (Rabkin and Strauss 1984). Moreover, the elongation rate of the polymerase is slowed by the presence of the AAF adduct (Lindsley and Fuchs 1994), due to the denaturation of the 3′ end of the nascent strand. This creates an opportunity for a slippage event to occur, during which the C pairs with the G immediately 5′ to the lesion, thus forming a slipped intermediate with a correct GC base pair at the template-primer terminus, allowing the polymerase to resume elongation (Fig. 5).

To test our hypothesis on the involvement of such a mutagenic intermediate, we studied the melting behavior of several oligonucleotide duplexes bearing the SmaI sequence, or related heteroduplexes (Table 2) (Garcia et al. 1993). We compared the effect of an AAF adduct on the melting temperature of a homoduplex to that of a heteroduplex that mimics a mutagenic intermediate. A decrease in melting temperature (about 10°C) suggests that the heteroduplex, which lacks a cytosine, is destabilized relative to the homoduplex (Fig. 6, Table 2). Introduction of an AAF adduct on any G of the sequence of the homoduplex similarly results in its destabilization. However, the adduct stabilizes the heteroduplex, increasing its melting temperature roughly to that

Table 2. Thermal denaturation of single AAF-modified duplexes bearing the SmaI sequence

	Tm, °C			
	Position of modification			
	Unmodified	G_1	G_2	G_3
Homoduplexes				
5′ATACCCG$_1$G$_2$G$_3$ACATC TATGGGC C C TGTAG 5′	54.5	46	44.5	43
Heteroduplexes				
5′ATACCCG$_1$G$_2$G$_3$ACATC TATGGGC C TGTAG 5′	43.5	54	50	50

Melting experiments were done in 100 mM sodium phosphate buffer at pH 7. The precision of the determination is ± 0.5 °C.

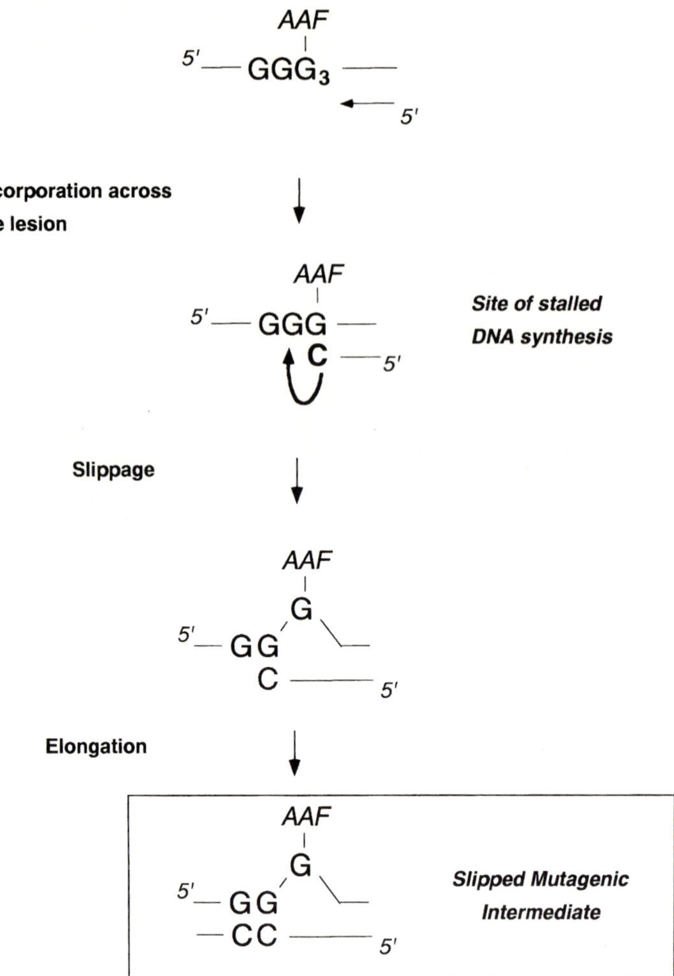

Fig. 5. Model for AAF-induced –1 mutations at repetitive sequences. The AAF-lesion-induced destabilization of the G-AAF::C mispair results in reduced processivity and stalling of the polymerase. Slippage of the modified strand would be favored by correct pairing of the 3′ nucleotide of the growing strand to the G immediately 5′ to the modified base. The AAF adduct stabilizes the slipped mutagenic intermediate, thus facilitating mutagenesis

of the unmodified homoduplex. Chemical probing experiments using the same constructs (Garcia et al. 1993) showed that the presence of an AAF lesion in heteroduplexes reduces the reactivity of the probes at the two cytosines located in the complementary strand opposite the modified base, as compared to the reactivity in AAF-modified homoduplexes. A nuclear magnetic resonance (NMR) study has been conducted on a (11 mer::10mer) heteroduplex containing a bulged guanine, either AAF-modified or not, in order to mimic

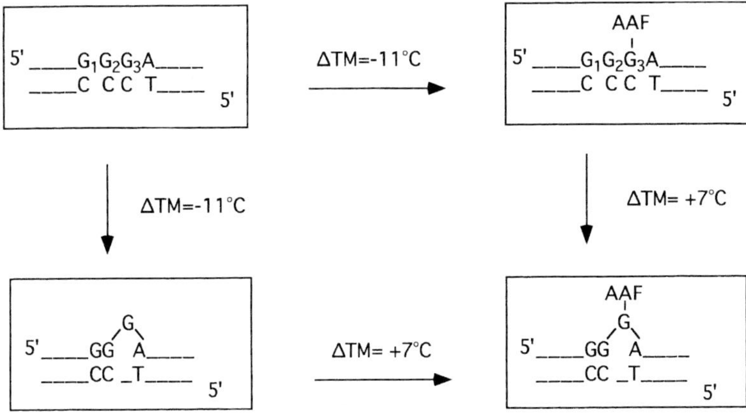

Fig. 6. Effect of AAF modification on thermal stability of a (14::14mer) homoduplex (*above*) containing the SmaI site, and a (14::13mer) heteroduplex (*below*) which mimics a slipped mutagenic intermediate. This figure summarizes the results obtained for the duplexes modified on G_1, G_2, or G_3

a slipped mutagenic intermediate (Milhé et al. 1994). Analysis of the base-pairing of the modified and unmodified heteroduplexes as a function of temperature shows that the pairing of bases 5′ and 3′ to the bulge guanine is disrupted at 25 °C in the unmodified duplex. However, they remain stable at 30 °C in the AAF modified heteroduplex, which explains its higher stability as compared to the unmodified molecule. All these results (Garcia et al. 1993; Milhé et al. 1994) show that AAF adducts have a denaturing effect on homoduplexes but stabilize a structure where the modified G bulges out of the helix, as would occur as a result of slippage.

An important element of this slippage mutagenesis model is the presence of a guanine 5′ to the position of AAF modification. In such a case, one would expect the mutagenic efficiency of each possible adduct (namely G2-AAF and G3-AAF) to be roughly the same, as the 5′ adjacent base is a G residue. The mutagenesis data, however, indicate a strong polarity of the lesion position along the repetitive sequence (Table 1). Moreover, we also detected mutagenic events, referred to as semitargeted mutations, which consist of the loss of one of the three cytosines located 5′ of the modified guanine (Table 1). These events, which are observed only for G1-AAF and G2-AAF lesions, show that an AAF-induced slippage may still occur even when the polymerase replicates sequences located 5′ of the lesion. These results led us to suggest that mutagenic efficiency depends on how many slipped mutagenic intermediates (SMI) may form. Figure 7 shows that the number of possible SMI is greatest when the modified base is at the 3′ extremity of the repetitive sequence, because slippage may occur after the lesion has been bypassed by the polymerase.

In summary, we propose a "correct incorporation-slippage" mechanism as a model for the induction by AAF of frameshift mutations at repetitive

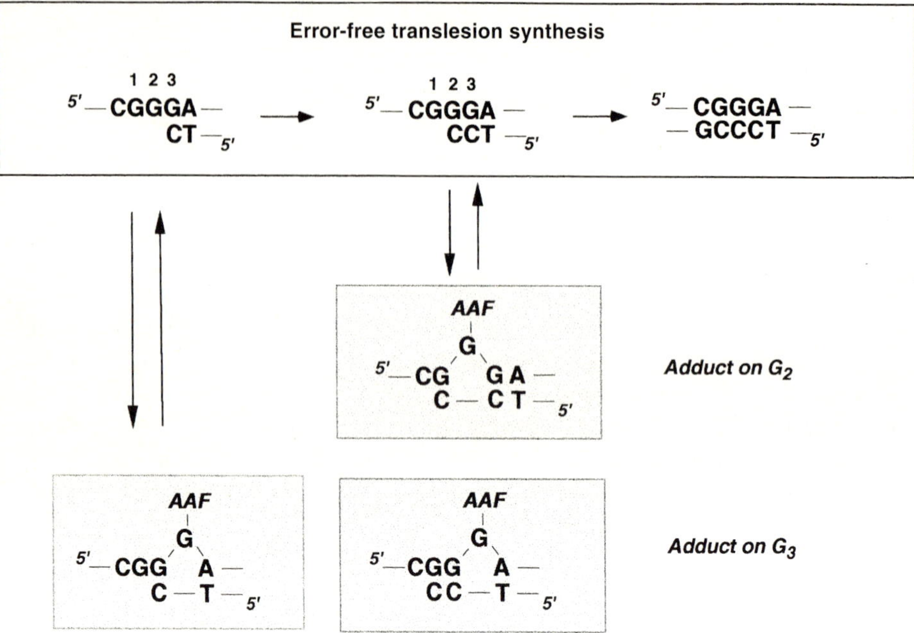

Fig. 7. Potential slipped mutagenic intermediates that may form depending on the position of the -AAF lesion within a repetitive sequence. The *larger upper frame* displays the processive elongation of the primer by the DNA polymerase via an error-free process. The mutagenic process is driven by the incorporation of a cytosine residue opposite the modified guanine residue, followed by the formation of transient slipped mutagenic intermediates. The formation of this intermediate is favored by the fact that the AAF adduct hinders elongation of the primer, destabilizes the 3′ extremity of the nascent strand, and stabilizes the slipped intermediate. The total number of intermediates depends on the number of possible pairing sites 5′ of the position of modification. When -AAF is bound on G_1, no slipped mutagenic intermediate (SMI) is formed: actually, -AAF-G_1-induced mutations are mainly deletions of one base in the adjacent C run (Table 1)

sequences. We suggest that the slipped intermediate that forms through pairing of the 3′ terminal C with the guanine 5′ to the lesion is stabilized by the presence of the AAF moiety. The adduct hinders elongation and increases the time in which slipped intermediates can form (Lindsley and Fuchs 1994). The number and stability of possible slipped intermediates depends on the position of the lesion within the repetitive sequence and influences the efficiency of mutagenesis. These thermodynamic and kinetic properties are responsible for the 10^3–10^4-fold increase in –1 frameshift mutations over the spontaneous frequency (Lambert et al. 1992).

In vitro Structural and Biochemical Studies on AAF-Modified Hotspot Sequences

Conformational Analysis of Distortions in DNA Caused by AAF Adducts

The conformation of AAF-modified B-DNA has been described by the insertion-denaturation (Fuchs and Daune 1972) or the base displacement model (Grunberger et al. 1970). These models propose that the -AAF moiety stacks into the helix, causing a local denaturation in which the modified G rotates from the *anti* to the *syn* conformation and protrudes out of the helix. However, in the case of 5′CpG sequences, AAF modification causes the pyrimidine-purine alternating sequence to undergo a transition from the B to Z conformation (Sage and Leng 1981; Santella et al. 1981). In this case, no denaturation of the helix occurs, and the AAF moiety stays outside the helix.

The AF lesion is less disruptive than the -AAF adduct (Daune et al. 1981). Broyde and Hingerty (1983) suggested a model in which the AF moiety stays outside the helix in the major groove, while the guanine keeps an *anti* configuration. Norman et al. (1989) defined the NMR structure of an AF-modified 11-mer duplex, in which the modified guanine pairs with adenine, thus mimicking a mutagenic intermediate for AF-induced G→T transversions (Bichara and Fuchs 1985). The "wedge model" places the AF moiety in the minor groove of a slightly bent B-DNA. The modified guanine stays inside the helix and eventually shares a hydrogen bond with the opposite adenine.

Mutagenesis experiments and repair studies (Seeberg and Fuchs 1990) have provided evidence that AAF adducts in different positions in hotspot sequences induce structurally different deformations. To investigate these structural alterations at the nucleotide level, we analyzed the conformation of AAF monomodified oligonucleotide duplexes containing the SmaI or NarI site with chemical probes (Garcia et al. 1993; Belguise-Valladier and Fuchs 1991). These probes either sense the geometry of DNA and cut at every nucleotide or react with specific bases in distorted regions of the helix (see Nielsen 1990 for a general review).

AAF modification at any position of the SmaI sequence has a strong denaturing effect on the repetitive tract extending over at least three base pairs (Garcia et al. 1993). However, pronounced differences in DNA structure occur for the AAF adduct on each of the guanine residues in the sequence $5'G_1G_2CG_3CC$ (Belguise-Valladier and Fuchs 1991). The deformation extends over four to six base pairs centered around the lesion. G_2-AAF is the least disturbing lesion and is best described by the insertion-denaturation model. The other two adducts are more disruptive; the deformation seems to affect the 3′ and 5′ neighbouring bases of the modified G_1 residue while that caused by G_3-AAF appears to be confined to the $5'CpG_3$ dinucleotide. We proposed that modification of G_1 or G_3 causes DNA to assume a local Z-like structure with the AAF moiety external to the helix. The structural differences between these adducts may result from modulation of the conformational change by the adjacent sequence. Such an influence has been observed in mutagenesis experiments (Koffel-Schwartz and Fuchs 1995).

Combining the results of the mutagenesis and structural studies is not straightforward, because the DNA structure involved in replication-dependent mutagenic events is a junction between double-stranded and single-stranded DNA covered by the polymerase. Consequently, structural studies of double-stranded oligonucleotides do not exactly represent the actual deformation that the polymerase encounters. In any case, it seems that the strong differences in mutagenesis among adducts are not attributable to specific deformations induced by peculiar adducts but rather to the likelihood of forming mutagenic intermediates. In the case of the SmaI sequence, we have shown that the lesion stabilizes the slipped intermediates, thereby providing better substrates to be elongated by the polymerase, thus fixing the –1 frameshift mutation. As to AAF-induced mutagenesis at the NarI sequence, we have evidence that the mutagenic event also occurs through a slippage mechanism (Lobo-Napolitano and Fuchs, in preparation).

In Vitro Replication of -AAF Monomodified Oligonucleotides

We have used single -AAF modified oligonucleotides as templates for in vitro replication by several DNA polymerases (Belguise-Valladier et al. 1994; Burnouf and Fuchs, unpublished results) to get a better understanding of the molecular events involved in the mutagenic processing of the -AAF lesion. The general strategy is described in Fig. 8. Briefly, oligonucleotides bearing the NarI or SmaI sequence are modified in vitro by *N*-acetoxy-*N*-2-acetylaminofluorene, and site-specific monomodified molecules are purified by HPLC (Koehl et al. 1989). They are primed with a 5′ P^{32} labeled 20-mer that serves as a substrate for elongation by replicative enzymes. Because it is thought to be involved in SOS mutagenesis (Bryan et al. 1990; Hagensee et al. 1987), DNA polymerase III holoenzyme of *E. coli* has been used in these studies, along with its α subunit, which carries out the polymerase activity of this multiprotein complex enzyme (McHenry 1991). Simpler polymerases with different processivities or proofreading activities have also been used, such as DNA polymerase I of *E. coli* (exo+ or –) (Derbyshire et al. 1988; Ollis et al. 1985), and Sequenase 2.0. (Tabor and Richardson 1989). The elongation products are then analyzed on sequencing gels.

Replication of unmodified templates with any polymerase gives full-length products. For both types of AAF modified templates, primer extension using Pol III holoenzyme stops one nucleotide before the lesion, although a weak band reveals some incorporation opposite the G1- and G2-AAF adduct. When the α subunit is used, this weaker band is more intense except for G3-AAF. This pattern is also obtained with polymerases lacking exonuclease activity (e.g., Sequenase 2.0 and Pol I *exo*$^-$), which suggests that the polymerases are

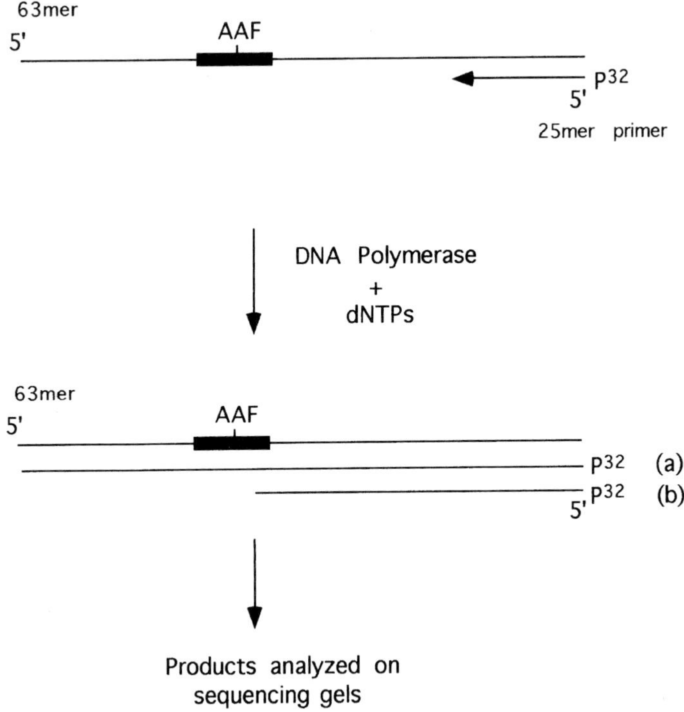

Fig. 8. General strategy for in vitro replication of -AAF modified templates by DNA polymerases. Construction of the 63-mer templates has been described elsewhere (Belguise-Valladier et al. 1994). Termination of polymerization by the lesion results in shorter elongation products (*b*). Full-length elongation products result from polymerization on unmodified template or bypass of the lesion by the DNA polymerase (*a*)

able to incorporate nucleotides opposite the -AAF lesion. The -AAF adduct, however, destabilizes the 3′ end of the duplex and impedes the elongation rate (Lindsley and Fuchs 1994), allowing the proofreading activity of *exo*$^+$ polymerases to remove the 3′ incorporated nucleotide; this is effectively observed in elongation experiments with DNA polymerase I. Some variability in the incorporation of nucleotides opposite the lesion is noted for *exo*$^-$ polymerases and could be related to the fine structure induced by each adduct.

Fast kinetic studies have also been conducted to analyze the influence of the lesion on the polymerase functions (Lindsley and Fuchs 1994). Primed oligonucleotides containing a unique dGuo-C8-AF or dGuo-C8-AAF have been replicated by T7 DNA polymerase (*exo*$^-$) (Patel et al. 1991), using various reaction times from 20 ms to 10 min. Figure 9 shows that unmodified oligonucleotides are replicated in 30 ms, with an overall rate constant of 300 nucleotides/s. When it encounters a dGuo-C8-AF lesion, the polymerase stops one nucleotide before the lesion and stalls for about 5 s. Translesion synthesis then occurs and is complete after 10 s. Unlike the AF adducts, AAF lesions are

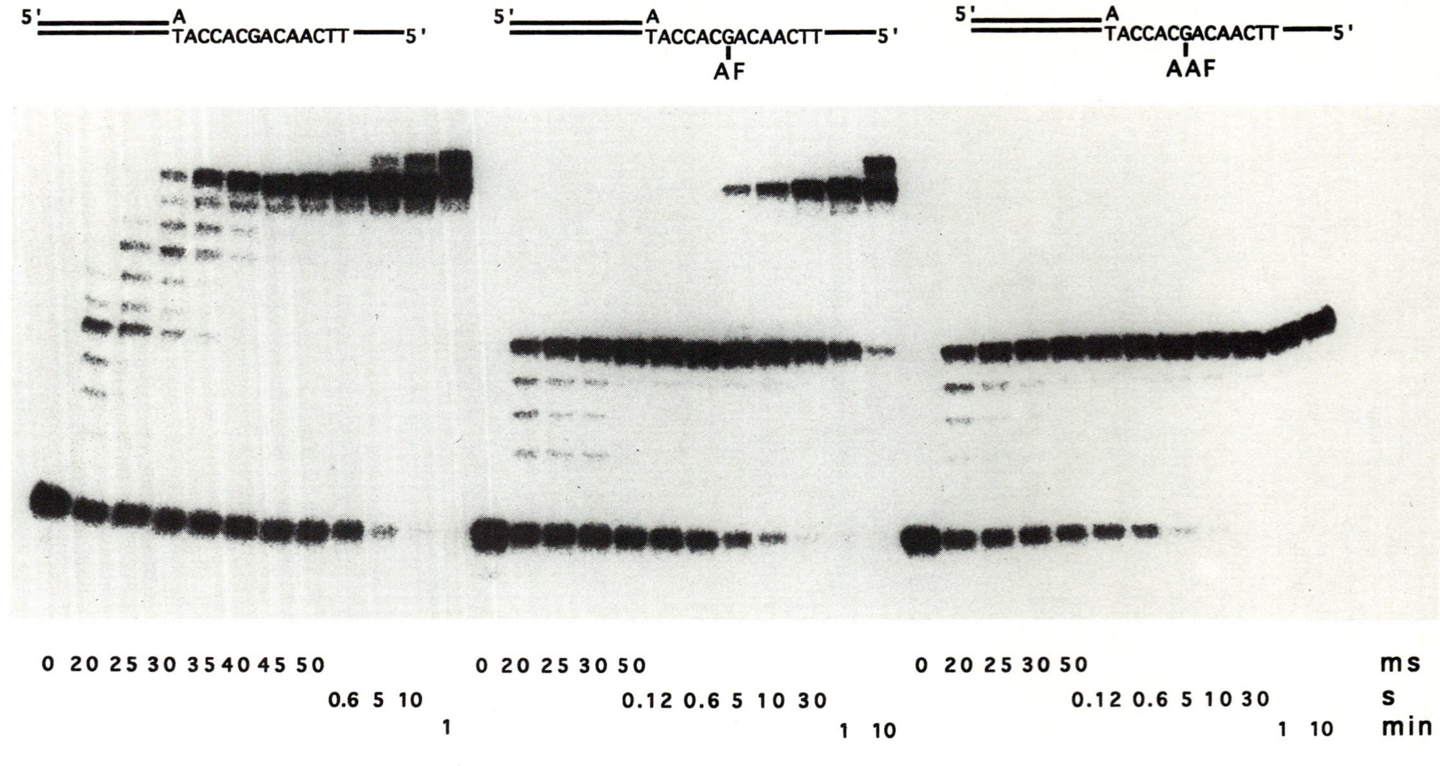

5'
A
TACCACGACAACTT
5'
5'
A
TACCACGACAACTT
AF
5'
5'
A
TACCACGACAACTT
AAF
5'
0 20 25 30 35 40 45 50
0.6 5 10
1
0 20 25 30 50
0.12 0.6 5 10 30
1 10
0 20 25 30 50
0.12 0.6 5 10 30
1 10
ms
s
min
time

not bypassed under these conditions. It should be stressed at this point that the capacity of an adduct to impede translesion synthesis by a polymerase is not solely determined by its chemical structure. In a recent paper (Belguise-Valladier and Fuchs 1995), we described in vitro replication experiments showing that a G_3-AF adduct in the NarI site behaves almost as a G_3-AAF adduct in that it blocks (or in some cases strongly reduces) DNA translesion synthesis, while G_1-AF and G_2-AF adducts in the same sequence context do not block replication. These observations stress the strong influence of the local sequence on the biological impact of an adduct.

Single nucleotide incorporation studies (Lindsley and Fuchs 1994) showed that the adducts strongly affect the rate of incorporation of nucleotides opposite and immediately after the lesion. Incorporation of dCTP opposite the lesion was reduced by four and six orders of magnitude for -AF and -AAF adducts, respectively, as compared to incorporation in the unmodified duplex (Table 3). The rate of incorporation of the first nucleotide past the lesion (Table 3) is reduced to roughly the same extent.

The in vitro replication studies indicate that AF- and AAF-induced lesions block elongation by polymerases (Lindsley and Fuchs 1994; Belguise-Valladier and Fuchs 1991, 1995; Burnouf, unpublished data) to an extent that correlates with the extent of the deformation they cause in the DNA helix (Fuchs and Daune 1972; Daune et al. 1981; Belguise-Valladier and Fuchs 1995). The AAF adduct modifies the kinetics of the polymerase and drastically reduces incorporation rates opposite or after the lesion (Lindsley and Fuchs 1994). However, the toxic effects induced by this lesion, which were noted in the in vitro replication experiments, were not observed in vivo. Actually, the survival of a single AAF-adducted plasmid, measured by assessing its transfection efficiency, is not affected, as compared to the nonmodified vector. This suggests that additional factors are probably involved in vivo. *UmuDC* proteins are likely to play a central role in AF-induced mutagenesis and in AAF- induced frameshift mutagenesis at repetitive sequences (Koffel-Schwartz et al. 1984; Bichara and Fuchs 1985). The SOS-dependence of -AAF induced (–2) frameshift mutagenesis at NarI sites suggests that some unknown genetic

◀

Fig. 9. PAGE analysis of elongation products of $5'P^{32}$ 25-mer primer hybridized on 44-mer, 44-AF, or 44-AAF templates, by T7 (*exo*$^-$) DNA polymerase. Only dCTP, dGTP, and dTTP were added in the extension mix (200 μM each). Reactions were quench at indicated times by addition of EDTA (0.3 M final concentration). Radioactive band at time 0 represent the 25-mer primer. When hybridized with the unmodified template (*left*), it is processively elongated by *exo*$^-$ T7 DNA polymerase to give a 36-mer fragment (the 37-mer fragment results from the nonencoded incorporation of an additional nucleotide by the *exo*$^-$ polymerase). When the primer is hybridized to AF- (*center*) or AAF-modified template (*right*), the polymerase is blocked at position 30, one nucleotide before the lesion. After stalling for 5 s, the enzyme resumes elongation past the AF lesion and gives rise to full-length products. It is, however, totally blocked by the AAF lesion

Table 3. Approximate incorporation times per nucleotide, one nucleotide before, opposite, or one nucleotide after the lesion when the T7 DNA polymerase (*exo*$^-$) encounters an AF- or AAF adduct

Adducts Nucleotide incorporation	AF-dG		AAF-dG	
	Average incorporation time per nucleotide	F	Average incorporation time per nucleotide	F
1 Nucleotide before the lesion	4 ms	1	4 ms	1
Opposite the lesion	20–200 s	$5 \times 10^3 - 5 \times 10^4$	1.7×10^4 s	4.25×10^6
1 Nucleotide after the lesion	5–50 s	$1.25 \times 10^3 - 1.25 \times 10^4$	8×10^3 s	2×10^6

F, reduction factor of the average incorporation time per nucleotide.
Single nucleotide incorporation experiments were done at a dNTP concentration of 100 μM, and the rate constants were calculated from kcat/K_m values.

functions are involved in this mutagenic process. Experiments are in progress to identify these genes, and to elucidate their role in helping the polymerase to cope with the lesion. Alternatively, other mechanisms that allow the replication apparatus to skip the lesion may be envisioned and are presently being investigated in our laboratory.

Acknowledgement. Professor G. Hoffmann (Holy Cross College, Worcester, MA, USA) is gratefully acknowledged for improving the manuscript. This work was supported by grants from ARC, LNFCC, EC, and HFSP.

References

Belguise-Valladier P, Fuchs RPP (1991) Strong sequence-dependent polymorphisms in adduct-induced DNA structure: analysis of single N-2-acetylaminofluorene residues bound within the NarI mutation hot spot. Biochemistry 30: 10091–10100

Belguise-Valladier P, Fuchs RPP (1995) N-2-aminofluorene and N-2-acetylaminofluorene adducts: the local sequence context of an adduct and its chemical structure determine its replication properties. J Mol Biol 249: 903–913

Belguise-Valladier P, Maki H, Sekiguchi M, Fuchs RPP (1994) Effect of a single DNA lesions on in vitro replication with DNA polymerase III holoenzyme: comparison with other DNA polymerases. J Mol Biol 236: 151–164

Bichara M, Fuchs RPP (1985) DNA binding and mutation spectra of the carcinogen N-2-aminofluorene in Escherichia coli. A correlation between the conformation of the premutagenic lesion and the mutation specificity. J Mol Biol 183: 341–351

Broyde S, Hingerty BE (1983) Conformation of 2-aminofluorene-modified DNA. Biopolymers 22: 2423–2441

Bryan SK, Hagensee M, Moses RE (1990) Holoenzyme DNA polymerase III fixes mutations. Mutat Res 242: 313–318

Burnouf D, Daune MP, Fuchs RPP (1987) Spectrum of cisplatin-induced mutations in E. coli. Proc Natl Acad Sci USA 84: 3758–3762
Burnouf D, Koehl P, Fuchs RPP (1989) Single adduct mutagenesis: strong effect of the position of a single acetylamino-fluorene adduct within a mutation hot spot. Proc Natl Acad Sci USA 86: 4147–4151
Daune MP, Fuchs RPP, Leng M (1981) Structural modification and protein recognition of DNA modified by N-2-fluorenylacetamide, its 7-iodo derivative, and by N-2-fluorenamine. J Natl Cancer Inst 58: 201–210
Demple B, Harrison L (1994) Repair of oxidative damage to DNA. Enzymology and biology. Annu Rev Biochem 63: 915–948
Derbyshire V, Fremont PS, Sanderson MR, Beese L, Friedman JM, Joyce CM, Steitz TA (1988). Genetic and cristallographic studies of the $3' \rightarrow 5'$ exonucleolytic site of DNA polymerase I. Science 240: 199–201
Fuchs RPP (1984) DNA binding spectrum of the carcinogen N-acetoxy-N-2-acetylaminofluorene significantly differs from the mutation spectrum. J Mol Biol 177: 173–180
Fuchs RPP, Daune MP (1972) Physical studies on deoxyribonucleic acid after covalent binding of a carcinogen. Biochemistry 11: 2659–2666
Fuchs RPP, Schwartz N, Daune MP (1981) Hot spots of frameshift mutations induced by the ultimate carcinogen N-acetoxy-N-2-acetylaminofluorene. Nature 294: 657–659
Garcia A, Lambert IB, Fuchs RPP (1993) DNA adduct-induced stabilization of slipped frameshift intermediates within repetitive sequences: implications for mutagenesis. Proc Natl Acad Sci USA 90: 5989–5993
Grunberger D, Nelson JH, Cantor CR, Weinstein IB (1970) Coding and conformational properties of oligonucleotides modified with the carcinogen N-2-acetylaminofluorene. Proc Natl Acad Sci USA 66: 488–494
Hagensee M, Timme TL, Bryan SK, Moses RE (1987) DNA polymerase III of Escherichia coli is required UV and ethylmethylsulfonate mutagenesis. Proc Natl Acad Sci USA 84: 4195–4199
Janel-Bintz R, Maenhaut-Michel G, Fuchs RPP (1991) Role of RecA mutant alleles (RecA495) in frameshift mutagenesis. Biochimie 73: 491–495
Kato T, Shinoura Y (1977) Isolation and characterisation of mutants of Escherichia coli deficient in induction of mutation by ultraviolet light. Mol Gen Genet 156: 121–131
Koehl P, Burnouf D, Fuchs RPP (1989) Construction of plasmids containing a unique acetylaminofluorene adduct located within a mutation hot spot. A new probe for frameshift mutagenesis. J Mol Biol 207: 355–364
Koffel-Schwartz N, Fuchs RPP (1995) J Mol Biol (in press)
Koffel-Schwartz N, Verdier JM, Bichara M, Freund AM, Daune MP, Fuchs RPP (1984) Carcinogen induced mutation spectrum in wild-type, uvrA, and umuC strains of E. coli. J Mol Biol 177: 33–51
Lambert IB, Napolitano RL, Fuchs RPP (1992) Carcinogen-induced frameshift mutagenesis in repetitive sequences. Proc Natl Acad Sci USA 89: 1310–1314
Lindsley JE, Fuchs RPP (1994) Use of single-turnover kinetics to study bulky adducts bypass by T7 DNA polymerase. Biochemistry 33: 764–772
McHenry CS (1991) DNA polymerase III holoenzyme. J Biol Chem 266: 19127–19130
Milhé C, Dhalluin C, Fuchs RPP, Lefèvre J-F (1994) NMR evidence of the stabilisation by the carcinogen N-2-acetylaminofluorene of a frameshift mutagenesis intermediate. Nucleic Acid Res 22: 4646–4652
Miller JA, Miller EC (1983) Some historical aspects of N-aryl carcinogens and their metabolic activation. Environ Health Perspect 49: 3–12
Murli S, Walker GC (1993) SOS mutagenesis. Curr Opin Gen Dev 3: 719–725

Nielsen PE (1990) Chemical and photochemical probing of DNA complexes. J Mol Recognit 3: 1–25

Norman D, Abuaf P, Hingerty BE, Live D, Grundberger D, Broyde S, Patel DJ (1989) NMR and computational characterization of the N-(deoxyguanosine-8-yl) aminofluorene adduct ((AF)G) opposite adenosine in DNA: (AF)G (syn). A (anti) pair formation and its pH dependence. Biochemistry 28: 7462–7476

Ollis DL, Brick P, Hamlin R, Xuong NG, Steitz TA (1985) Structure of large fragment of Escherichia coli DNA polymerase I complexed with dTMP. Nature 313: 762–766

Patel SS, Wong I, Johnson KA (1991) Pre-steady-state kinetic analysis of processive DNA replication including complete characterization of an exonuclease-deficient mutant. Biochemistry 30: 511-525

Rabkin SD, Strauss BS (1984) A role for DNA polymerase in the specificity of nucleotide incorporation opposite N-acetyl-2-aminofluorene adducts. J Mol Biol 178: 569–594

Ripley LS (1990) Frameshift mutation: determinants of specificity. Annu Rev Genet 24: 189–213

Sage E, Leng M (1981) Conformationnal changes of poly(dGdC). poly(dG-dC) modified by the carcinogen N-acetoxy-N-acetyl-2-aminofluorene. Nucleic Acids Res 9: 1241–1250

Sancar A, Sancar GB (1988) DNA repair enzymes. Annu Rev Biochem 57: 29–67

Santella RM, Grunberger D, Hingerty BE (1981) Z-DNA conformation of N-2-acetylaminofluorene modified poly(dG-dC). poly(dG-dC) determined by reactivity with anti cytidine antibodies and minimized potential energy calculations. Nucleic Acids Res 9: 5459–5467

Schmid SE, Daune MP, Fuchs RPP (1982) Repair and mutagenesis of plasmid DNA modified by ultraviolet irradiation or N-acetoxy-N-2-acetylaminofluorene. Proc Natl Acad Sci USA 79: 4133–4137

Seeberg E, Fuchs RPP (1990) Acetylaminofluorene bound to different guanines of the sequence -GGCGCC is excised with different efficiencies by the UvrABC excision nuclease in a pattern not correlated to the potency of mutation induction. Proc Natl Acad Sci USA 87: 191–194

Streisinger G, Okada Y, Emrich J, Newton J, Tsugita A, Terzaghi E, Inouye M (1966) Frameshift mutations and the genetic code. Cold Spring Harbor Symp Quant Biol 42: 77–90

Tabor S, Richardson CC (1989) Selective inactivation of the exonuclease activity of bacteriophage T7 DNA polymerase by in vitro mutagenesis. J Bio Chem 264: 6447–6458

Walker GC (1987) The SOS response of Escherichia coli in Escherichia coli and Salmonella typhimurium. Neidhartdt FC (ed) Cellular and molecular biology, vol 2. American Society for Microbiology, Washington, pp 1346–1357

Oxidative DNA Damage Induced by Dioxetanes, Photosensitizing Ketones, and Photo-Fenton Reagents

W. Adam[1], S. Andler[1], D. Ballmaier[2], S. Emmert[3], B. Epe[2], G. Grimm[1], K. Mielke[1], M. Möller[2], T.M. Rünger[3], C.R. Saha-Möller[1], A. Schönberger[1], and H. Stopper[2]

[1]Institute of Organic Chemistry, University of Würzburg, Am Hubland, 97074 Würzburg, Germany
[2]Department of Toxicology, University of Würzburg, Versbacher Str. 9, 97078 Würzburg, Germany
[3]Department of Dermatology, University of Würzburg, Josef-Schneider-Str. 2, 97080 Würzburg, Germany

Introduction

In the last decade, the importance of oxidative DNA damage in mutagenesis, carcinogenesis, aging, and various diseases has prompted intensive investigations of chemical, biochemical, and biological aspects of DNA oxidation caused by reactive species, which are involved in oxidative stress (Sies 1991). Oxidative degradation of DNA causes mutations predominantly at GC base pairs to yield single base substitutions and G to T transversions (Piette 1991). Consequently, the DNA transformation efficiency is diminished and replication is inhibited.

Numerous reagents are reported as DNA oxidizing agents (Cadet 1994a). Photosensitizers cause efficient oxidative modifications in cell-free and cellular DNA (Cadet and Vigny 1990; Epe et al. 1993a; Piette et al. 1986). A wide variety of chromophores, e.g. cellular constituents such as flavins and porphyrins and the simple carbonyl compounds acetone and acetophenone, can act as photosensitizers for DNA oxidation (Kochevar and Dunn 1990).

Among the established biologically relevant DNA-oxidizing reagents, hydroxyl radicals are the most reactive species (von Sonntag 1987; Steenken 1989). While hydroxyl radicals give rise to a variety of base and sugar modifications in DNA, the predominant target of photooxidation is the purine base guanine to form three major oxidation products (Fig. 1).

Because of its high in vitro and in vivo mutagenicity, 7-8-dihydro-8-oxo-2′-deoxyguanosine (8-oxodGuo) is considered as one of the most biologically significant DNA oxidation product (Pavlov et al. 1994; Wood et al. 1990). In addition to being produced by the oxidation of DNA with hydroxyl radicals (HO·), it is efficiently formed in photosensitized oxidation processes, either directly through electron transfer (ET) chemistry (type I photooxidation), or indirectly (energy transfer to triplet oxygen) through singlet oxygen ($^1O_2$) reaction with guanine (type II photooxidation) (Foote 1991). The latter process

Recent Results in Cancer Research, Vol. 143

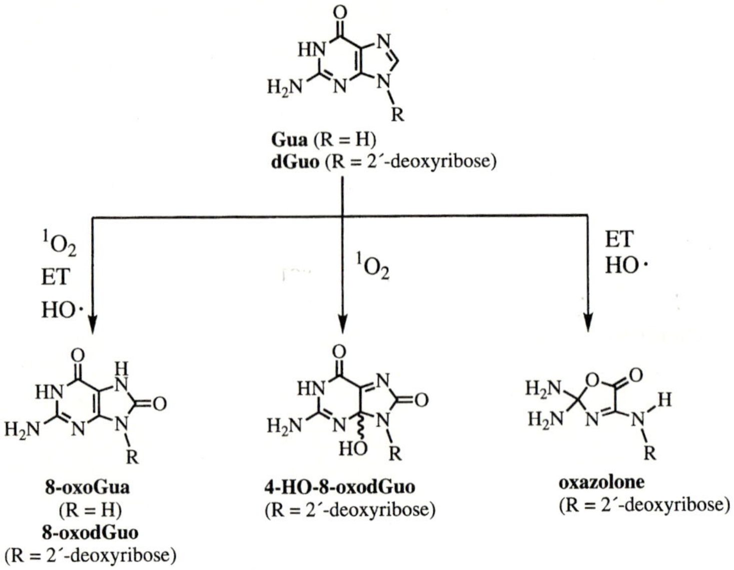

O
HN N
H2N N N
R
Gua (R = H)
dGuo (R = 2´-deoxyribose)

$^1O_2$ ET HO· | $^1O_2$ | ET HO·

8-oxoGua (R = H) **8-oxodGuo** (R = 2´-deoxyribose)

4-HO-8-oxodGuo (R = 2´-deoxyribose)

oxazolone (R = 2´-deoxyribose)

Fig. 1. Oxidation products of guanine (R = H) generated by singlet oxygen ($^1O_2$), electron transfer (ET), and hydroxyl radicals (HO·)

yields specifically the two 4R* and 4S* diastereomers of 4,8-dihydro-4-hydroxy-8-oxo-2′-deoxyguanosine (4-HO-8-oxodGuo) in the photooxidation reaction of 2′-deoxyguanosine (Buchko et al. 1992) (in DNA, however, it yields only traces). 2,2-Diamino-[(2-deoxy-*β*-D-*erythro*-pentofuranosy1)-4-amino]-5(*2H*)-oxazolone (oxazolone) has been isolated as a third guanine oxidation product in the oxidative degradation of DNA, both by type I photooxidation (ET) and by hydroxyl radical attack (Cadet et al. 1994b).

In addition to generally used photosensitizers, e.g. methylene blue, rose bengal (predominantly type II), xanthone or riboflavin (predominantly type I), triplet-excited ketones constitute another class of active oxidants (Epe et al. 1993a; Cilento 1984) which are of biological interest because they may be generated in cells on exposure to UV irradiation or by dark reactions, e.g., lipid peroxidation (Russell mechanism) and enzymatic oxidation reactions (Sies 1991). Alternatively to their conventional photochemical generation, triplet-excited ketones can be conveniently produced by spontaneous thermal decomposition of the high-energy, four-membered, cyclic peroxides, namely the 1,2-dioxetanes (Fig. 2) (Adam and Cilento 1983; Cilento and Adam 1988). For genotoxicity studies, the generation of triplet-excited ketones by the thermal decomposition of dioxetanes is more advantageous than the photochemical method, since the former circumvents the exposure of DNA to UV light during the direct photolysis.

Since hydroxyl radicals constitute the most reactive oxygen species which are involved in oxidative stress, it is of general interest to elucidate their role in

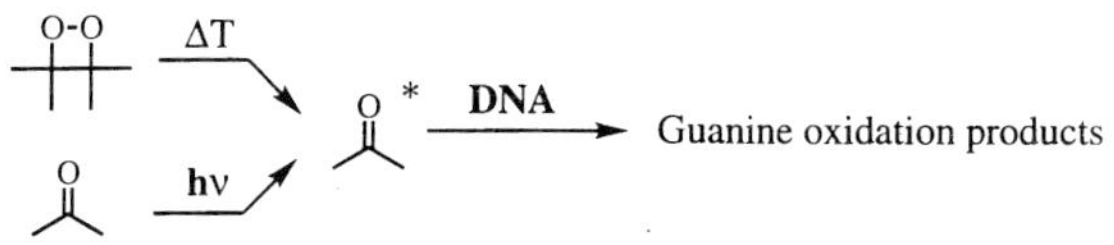

Fig. 2. Oxidation of guanine by triplet-excited ketones generated from the thermal decomposition of 1,2-dioxetanes and photoexcitation of ketones

oxidative cell damage. The conventional chemical sources of hydroxyl radicals, for example H_2O_2/Fe^{2+} (Fenton reaction) or γ irradiation, are not properly suited for biochemical or biological investigations because they generate, besides hydroxyl radicals, other reactive oxygen species (von Sonntag 1987).

In recent years, phthalimide and furocoumarin hydroperoxides were developed as effective photochemical hydroxyl radical sources (photo-Fenton reagents), which circumvent the use of transition metals and γ irradiation in genotoxicity and mutagenicity studies (Saito et al. 1990; Epe et al. 1993b; Adam et al. 1995a). Moreover, *N*-hydroxypyridinethione was reported as a non-peroxidic photochemical source of hydroxyl radicals (Boivin et al. 1990), which (Adam et al. 1995c) was recently shown to serve as an effective DNA oxidant.

To obtain mechanistic insight into the complexities of oxidative DNA damage at the molecular level, we have investigated DNA oxidations during the last few years by using dioxetanes as thermal sources of triplet-excited ketones; more recently we have employed photosensitizers and photo-Fenton reagents. Here, we summarize the results of our chemical, biochemical, and toxicological investigations.

Results and Discussion

Dioxetane-Induced Oxidations of Guanine Base in DNA and 2′-Deoxyguanosine

As a well-established marker for oxidative DNA damage, 8-oxoGua is conveniently detected by the HPLC/electrochemical detection assay (Floyd et al. 1986, 1990). In order to evaluate the oxidative efficacy of 1,2-dioxetanes towards DNA, we monitored the formation of 8-oxoGua in the thermolysis of 1,2-dioxetanes in the presence of isolated *calf thymus* DNA. The reactivity profile is displayed in Fig. 3. The experimental details of the assay have been published elsewhere (Adam et al. 1995b).

We have unequivocally established that 1,2-dioxetanes, in particular the alkyl-substituted ones, efficiently oxidize guanine base in DNA to form 8-oxoGua in high yield on thermal decomposition in the dark. Unfortunately, the distinct reactivities of the various dioxetanes are not reflected by their photophysical data and the thermal properties (Adam et al. 1990; Epe et al.

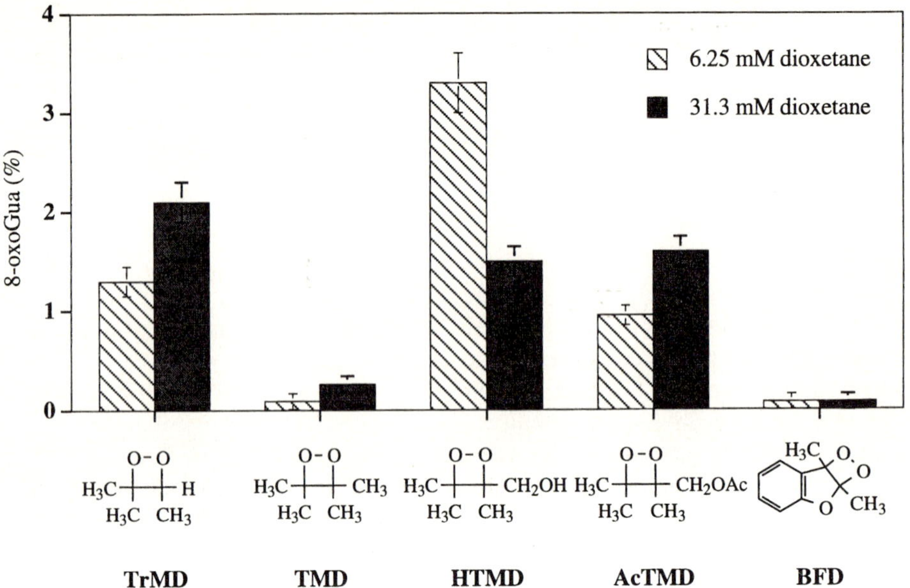

Fig. 3. Effect of dioxetane structure on the yield (%) of 8-oxoGua in the thermally induced oxidation of *calf thymus* DNA. The experiments were carried out at 37 °C for 10 h in 5 m*M* phosphate buffer, pH 7.0 with 0.1 mg/ml *calf thymus* DNA (62.5 μ*M* Gua); dioxetanes were dissolved in acetone (10% final volume). Yield is shown relative to unmodified guanine; mean value of at least three independent experiments

1992). The surprisingly high efficiency of 3-hydroxymethyl-3,4,4-Arimethyl-1,2-dioxetane (HTMD), with yields up to 5% 8-oxoGua, may be due to association of this reagent with DNA through hydrogen bonding, which may facilitate the generation of triplet-excited ketones in closer contact with the particular base target. The lack of oxidative activity in the case of BFD, which is strongly mutagenic in the *Salmonella typhimurium* strain TA 100 (Adam et al. 1991a, 1993), may derive from its complex chemical behavior in the aqueous medium (Adam et al. 1991b), which may explain the inefficient generation of triplet-excited ketones.

Further investigations were carried out exclusively with the most efficient dioxetane HTMD and additionally included the analysis of oxazolone, a characteristic type I photooxidation product. The latter was monitored in the reaction with *calf thymus* DNA by the indirect HPLC/fluorescence labeling assay with 1,2-naphthoquinone sulfonic acid (Ravanat et al. 1992). Some representative results are summarized in Table 1. In addition to 8-oxoGua, significant amounts of oxazolone were detected in the reaction of HTMD with DNA as the result of electron transfer (type I photooxidation) from DNA to the excited triplet ketone. The concentration dependence (entries 1–3) revealed that at higher HTMD concentrations the yield of 8-oxoGua is substantially decreased. This may be explained by further oxidation of 8-oxodGuo and is

Table 1. Yield (%) of 8-oxoGua and oxazolone in the thermal reaction of HTMD with *calf thymus* DNA

Entry	Conditions[b]	Yield(%)[a]	
		8-oxoGua	Oxazolone
1	1.5 m*M* HTMD	1.9 ± 0.1	0.5 ± 0.05
2	5m*M* HTMD	4.8 ± 0.3	2.4 ± 0.1
3	25 m*M* HTMD	2.6 ± 0.2	2.9 ± 0.2
4	5 × 5 m*M* HTMD[c]	1.6 ± 0.1	8.5 ± 0.4
5	5 m*M* HTMD + 1 *M* t-BuOH	4.5 ± 0.2	1.7 ± 0.2
6	5 m*M* HTMD + 0.2 m*M* DBAS	0.62 ± 0.05	0.40 ± 0.04
7	5 m*M* HTMD + 0.1 m*M* DBH	2.8 ± 0.2	0.60 ± 0.05
8	1.5 m*M* HTMD / D_2O[d]	2.8 ± 0.1	0.60 ± 0.07
9	20 *μM* riboflavin / hν, 3 h[e]	3.5 ± 0.5	1.5 ± 0.4
10	10 *μM* methylene blue / hν, 1.5 h[e]	2.0 ± 0.2	1.5 ± 0.1

[a]Yield relative to guanine in DNA (625 pmol/μg).
[b]Carried out with 0.1 mg/ml *calf thymus* DNA in 5 m*M* phosphate buffer (pH 7.0); for entries 1–8, HTMD was dissolved in acetonitrile (10% final volume) and reacted at 37 °C for 15 h.
[c]Added in five batches every 15–20 h at 37 °C.
[d]Reaction in D_2O-phosphate buffer (5 m*M*, pD 7.0).
[e]150-W Na lamp, placed at 10-cm distance, 4 °C.

clearly reflected in the result shown in entry 4, in which repetitive treatment of DNA with HTMD also leads to a significant decrease in the yield of 8-oxoGua. In this case, only guanine is degraded (up to 90%), whereas the other DNA bases remain intact, which confirms that photooxidation occurs when DNA is thermally treated with dioxetanes.

Another proof that triplet-excited states are indeed involved comes from quenching experiments with the triplet quenchers (Catalani et al. 1987; Kavarnos and Turro 1986) such as sodium 9,10-dibromoanthracene-2-sulfonate (DBAS) and 2,3-diazabicyclo[2.2.1]hept-2-ene (DBH), which decrease the yield of 8-oxoGua and oxazolone significantly (Table 1, entries 6, 7). That hydroxyl radicals are not responsible for the observed oxidation of DNA was established by control experiments with the hydroxyl radical scavenger *tert*-butanol (entry 5). Under optimized reaction conditions, a small positive D_2O effect was observed, which implies that singlet oxygen may also be involved (entries 1 and 8). Finally, comparison of the results of the two commonly used photosensitizers riboflavin (type I) and methylene blue (predominantly type II) with those of the dioxetane HTMD show that dioxetanes serve as efficient photooxidants of DNA without the application of light.

To obtain further mechanistic insight into the dioxetane-induced oxidation of nucleic acid derivatives, in particular the oxidation of guanine base, 2′-deoxyguanosine (dGuo) was thermally treated with HTMD. In addition to 8-oxodGuo, which in the nucleoside reaction is only formed by the reaction with singlet oxygen (Cadet et al. 1994b), and the specific type I oxidation product

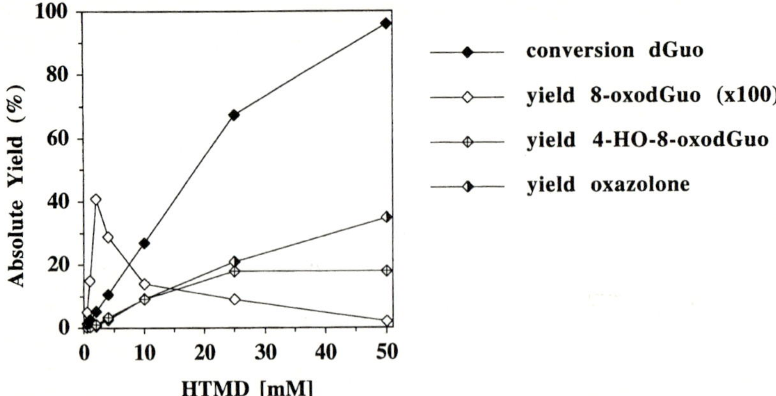

Fig. 4. Oxidation of 2′-deoxyguanosine (dGuo) by the thermal decomposition of HTMD. The experiments were carried out with 0.5 m*M* dGuo in 10 m*M* sodium cacodylate buffer (pH 7.0) at 50 °C for 15 h; HTMD was dissolved in acetonitrile (10% final volume). Mean values of triplicate determinations, error range ± 10%

oxazolone, the oxidation of dGuo may additionally lead to the two 4R* and 4S* diastereomers of 4-HO-8-oxodGuo, as the characteristic singlet oxygen oxidation products of dGuo. The latter are formed either through [2+4] cycloaddition of singlet oxygen with dGuo (Sheu and Foote 1993) or [2+2] cycloaddition with 8-oxodGuo (Sheu and Foote 1995).

Thermally induced oxidation of dGuo by HTMD resulted in concentration-dependent product yields, which are shown in Fig. 4 (details will be published elsewhere). Besides significant amounts of 8-oxodGuo (≤ 1%), up to approximately 20% of 4-HO-8-oxodGuo and approximately similar amounts of oxazolone were observed. From the formation of 8-oxodGuo and 4-HO-8-oxodGuo we conclude that singlet oxygen plays a significant role in these oxidations, which was substantiated by a large positive D_2O effect (200–300%) in the formation of 8-oxodGuo. Interestingly, like in the case of DNA, we found that the 8-oxodGuo formation decreased significantly at a higher excess of HTMD. This result implies that 8-oxodGuo is a good substrate for oxidation by thermal decomposition of HTMD; presumably singlet oxygen is the ultimate oxidant in this case.

Genotoxicity and Mutagenicity of Dioxetanes in Human Cells

Once the formation of guanine oxidation products, in particular 8-oxoGua, was confirmed in the thermal reaction of dioxetane with cell-free *calf thymus* DNA, the genotoxicity and mutagenicity of dioxetanes in human cells were investigated. The plasmid shuttle vector assay was employed to assess the biological consequences of the oxidative DNA damage induced by photosensitization in the dark. For this purpose, the replicating shuttle vector pZ189 was treated in vitro with HTMD or TrMD in phosphate buffer at 50 °C for 2 h and subsequently transfected into normal human lymphoplast cells. The details of this study have been published recently (Emmert et al. 1995). A dose-dependent increase of genotoxicity and mutation frequency was found with both dioxetanes. However, HTMD exhibits a higher mutagenicity at low doses than TrMD at similar genotoxicity. Sequence analysis of the *supF* gene revealed that point mutations prevailed over deletions. Single base substitutions occurred exclusively at G:C sites with G:C to T:A and G:C to C:G transversions. These types of transversions are indicative for 8-oxodGuo formation. In the case of TrMD small amounts of G:C to A:T transitions were also observed, which reflect higher yields of pyrimidine dimers with this dioxetane than with HTMD, a result in harmony with the established higher triplet flux of TrMD (Adam et al. 1990). These findings indicate that dioxetanes efficiently cause mutagenicity in human cells, predominantly through the formation of 8-oxodGuo.

Inhibitory Effect of Fatty Acid Ester Hydroperoxides in Oxidative DNA Damage Induced by Photosensitizers

To investigate the DNA-oxidizing properties of fatty acid ester hydroperoxides under photosensitization conditions, we used xanthone as an efficient type I photosensitizer. The xanthone-photosensitized oxidation of *calf thymus* DNA yielded approximately 1.4% 8-oxoGua as a major oxidation product of guanine in DNA after irradiation at 350 nm for 60 min. By the addition of ethyl oleate hydroperoxide, we surprisingly observed a nearly complete (85%) inhibition of 8-oxoGua formation in DNA. To assess which structural features of the hydroperoxide are important for the observed inhibitory effect, a comparative study with other additives was performed. The results are displayed in Fig. 5. The details were published elsewhere (Adam et al. 1996). On addition of equal amounts of ethyl oleate, the yield of 8-oxoGua in the xanthone-photosensitized oxidation of DNA was decreased insignificantly (up to 15%). In contrast, the ethyl oleate alcohol had nearly the same inhibitory effect on the formation of 8-oxoGua as the corresponding hydroperoxide. Interestingly, the effect of 3-cyclohexenyl hydroperoxide and the structurally simple *tert*-butyl hydroperoxide was even more pronounced than that of the ethyl oleate hydroperoxide (Fig. 5). Only a very small amount of 8-oxoGua was formed in the presence of these hydroperoxides (< 0.1%). However, *tert*-butanol, which efficiently scavenges hydroxyl radicals, did not show any inhibitory effect, while the allylic cyclohexenyl alcohol decreased the yield of 8-oxoGua only to a small extent. The same trend as for 8-oxoGua was also observed for the formation of the characteristic type I photooxidation product oxazolone (data not shown).

To obtain some insights into the mechanism of the inhibitory effect of fatty acid ester hydroperoxides on photosensitized DNA oxidation, the influence of

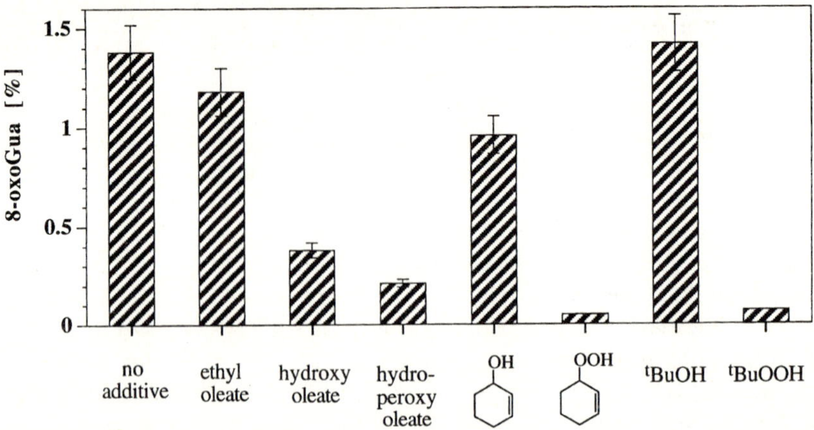

Fig. 5. Inhibitory effect of hydroperoxy and hydroxy fatty esters in the photosensitized oxidation of DNA. The experiments were carried out with *calf thymus* DNA (0.1 mg/ml = 62.5 μM guanine) in 5 mM phosphate buffer (pH 7.0), 62.5 μM xanthone and 6.25 mM additive (both dissolved in acetonitrile, 10 % final volume); irradiation at 350 nm in a Rayonet photochemical reactor at 4 °C for 1 h. Yields are mean values of triplicate determinations

ethyl oleate hydroperoxide and its alcohol on the photooxidation of DNA induced by the sensitizers benzophenone or methylene blue was investigated. The irradiation of *calf thymus* DNA in the presence of methylene blue (predominantly type II photosensitizer) without additive yielded ca. 2.5% of 8-oxoGua and 2.6% of oxazolone. The formation of these oxidation products was not affected by the ethyl oleate hydroperoxide or its alcohol. Benzophenone (predominantly type I photosensitizer) sensitized the photo-oxidation of DNA to afford 1.9% of 8-oxoGua and 0.9% of oxazolone. In this case a significant decrease in the yield of 8-oxoGua and oxazolone was observed when 100 equivalents of the ethyl oleate hydroperoxide were added. These results clearly demonstrate that ethyl oleate hydroperoxide and its alcohol inhibit the type I but not the type II-sensitized photooxidation of guanine in DNA. The inhibitory effect of these additives may be explained by quenching of the type I photosensitization process through hydrogen abstraction.

Intercalating Hydroperoxides and N-Hydroxypyridinethiones as Photochemical Hydroxyl Radical Sources (Photo-Fenton Reagents) for Oxidative DNA Damage

In addition to commonly used methods for the generation of hydroxyl radicals (γ irradiation, Fenton reaction), in recent years some hydroperoxides and also *N*-hydroxypyridinethiones were established as photochemical sources for hy-

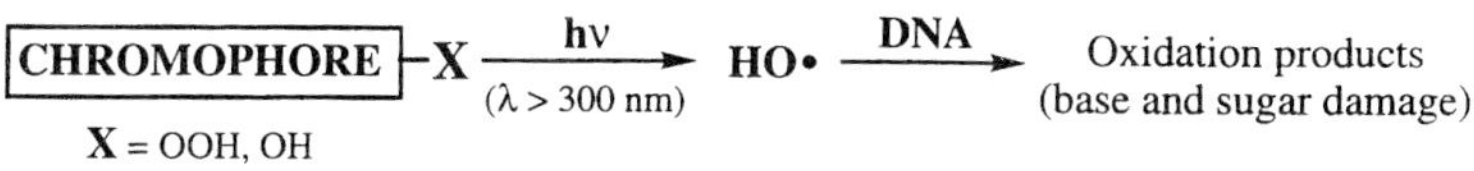

CHROMOPHORE –X $\xrightarrow[(\lambda > 300\ nm)]{h\nu}$ HO• $\xrightarrow{DNA}$ Oxidation products (base and sugar damage)

X = OOH, OH

Fig. 6. Photochemical generation of hydroxyl radicals from photo-Fenton reagents

droxyl radicals (photo-Fenton reagents). In both cases the formation of hydroxyl radicals is induced by energy transfer from the excited chromophore to the N-OH or HOO moiety with subsequent release of HO radicals (Fig. 6).

During the last few years we have investigated the *N*-hydroxypyridinethiones **1a,b** (Adam et al. 1995c), furocoumarin **2** (Epe et al. 1993b; Adam et al. 1995a), and phenanthridine **3** hydroperoxides with respect to their ability to serve as efficient photochemical hydroxyl radical sources. Advantageous properties of these photo-Fenton reagents include the convenience of controlling the amount of hydroxyl radicals formed as a function of the irradiation time. Moreover, in view of their intercalating ability, the hydroxyl radicals are expected to be generated close to the DNA target to facilitate more effective damage.

The formation of hydroxyl radicals from the photo-Fenton reagents was verified by spin trapping experiments with 5,5-dimethylpyrroline-1-oxide (DMPO). The photo-Fenton reagents **1**–**3** gave all the characteristic electron spin resonance (ESR) signals of the hydroxyl radical addition product to DMPO, which was efficiently suppressed by adding ethanol as a hydroxyl radical quencher. Additionally, significant amounts of hydroxyl radical adducts were observed when benzene solutions of the hydroxyl radical sources **1**–**3** or their aqueous solutions in the presence of benzoic acid were irradiated. In all cases appropriate control experiments established that these chromophores without the photoactive hydroxyl radical source were ineffective for the hydroxylation of arenes.

The quantum yields for the decomposition of the photo-Fenton reagents **1**–**3** were determined by potassium ferrioxalate actionometry and are shown in Fig. 7. For the *N*-hydroxypyridinethiones **1** the quantum yields are above 100% since a chain reaction applies, which is in accord with the proposed mechanism for the ortho derivative **1a** (Boivin et al. 1990).

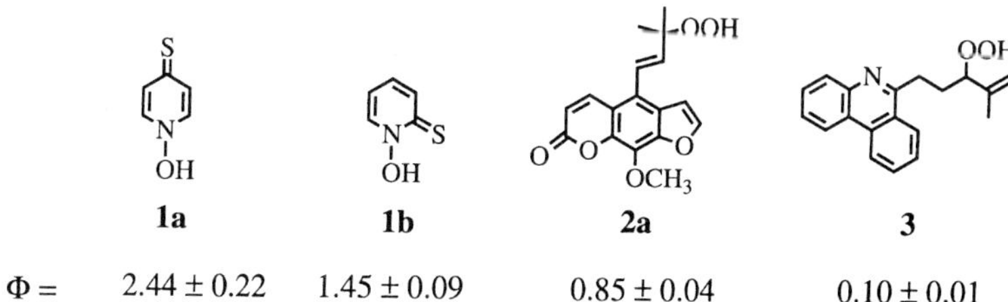

Fig. 7. Quantum yields (Φ) for the photochemical decomposition of the *N*-hydroxypyridinethiones **1** and hydroperoxides **2a** and **3**

Table 2. Photoinduced generation of 8-oxoGua in *calf thymus* DNA by photo-Fenton reagents **1**, **2a**, and **3**; influence of *tert*-butanol and mannitol on the formation of 8-oxoGua

Entry	Structure	Conditions[a]	tert-BuOH (% v/v)	Mannitol (m*M*)	Yield (%)[b] 8-oxoGua
1	**1a**	62.5 μM, 20 min	–	–	0.42 ± 0.09
2	**1a**	62.5 μM, 20 min	2	–	0.26 ± 0.02
3	**1a**	62.5 μM, 20 min	–	40	0.19 ± 0.06
4	**1b**	62.5 μM, 20 min	–	–	0.19 ± 0.03
5	**2a**	20.0 μM, 30 min	–	–	1.16 ± 0.09
6	**2a**	20.0 μM, 30 min	2	–	0.81 ± 0.05
7	**3**	31.2 μM, 30 min	–	–	0.68 ± 0.03
8	**3**	31.2 μM, 30 min	5	–	0.44 ± 0.07
9	**3**	31.2 μM, 30 min	–	5	0.37 ± 0.18

[a]Carried out with *calf thymus* DNA (0.1 mg/ml, 62.5 μM guanine) in 5 m*M* phosphate buffer (pH 7.0) at 10 °C; irradiations were conducted in a Rayonet photochemical reactor (λ, 350 nm), in which samples were placed at approximately 5 cm distance.
[b]Yield relative to guanine content in DNA; consumption of photo-Fenton reagents **1** to **3** was > 98%.

To evaluate the DNA-oxidizing activity of photo-Fenton reagents **1**–**3**, the formation of 8-oxoGua in isolated *calf thymus* DNA was monitored by HPLC/electrochemical detection. Furthermore, the addition of *tert*-butanol and mannitol was conducted to assess whether hydroxyl radicals are indeed the ultimate DNA-oxidizing species. The results are listed in Table 2. Details of these investigations are reported in a recent publication (Adam et al. 1995c). With both photo-Fenton systems **1** and **2** we found efficient generation of 8-oxoGua in DNA, which is significantly reduced by the addition of the hydroxyl radical scavengers *tert*-butanol and mannitol. This substantial reduction points towards the involvement of hydroxyl radicals as tangible DNA-oxidizing species.

For the furocumarin hydroperoxide **2a** we examined the DNA binding properties by the fluorescence titration technique as well as by linear flow dichroism measurements (Adam et al. 1995a). By applying the McGhee and von Hippel analysis for the fluorescence data, we determined a binding constant for the hydroperoxide **2a** to *salmon testes* DNA of $2.39 \times 10^4\ M^{-1}$. Additionally, the negative linear dichroism of an aqueous solution of **2a** with DNA indicates complexation of **2a** parallel to the DNA base pairs (Tjerneld et al. 1979). In order to get better insight into the activity and nature of the ultimate DNA-damaging species, the supercoiled PM2 DNA relaxation assay was employed by using a specific set of DNA repair endonucleases (Epe et al. 1993b; Epe and Hegler 1994). The DNA damage profiles for the photo-Fenton reagents **1**–**3**, compared with conventional hydroxyl radical generation by γ irradiation, are shown in Fig. 8. The characteristic pattern for hydroxyl

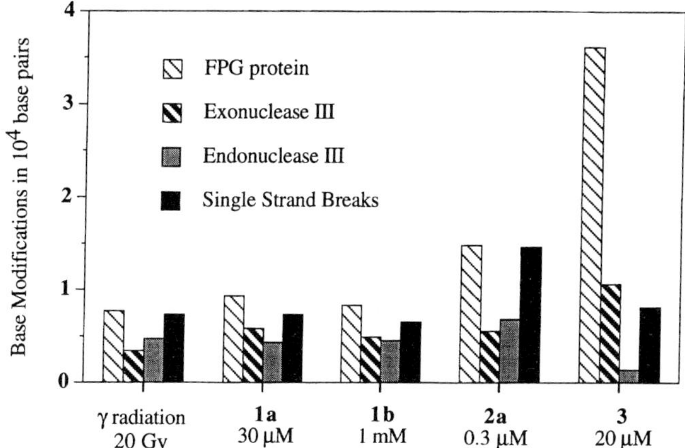

Fig. 8. DNA damage profiles for *N*-hydroxypyridinethiones **1a,b**, hydroperoxides **2a** and **3**, and the γ radiolysis of water. *FPG,* formamidopyrimidine-DNA glycosylase

radical-mediated DNA damage by γ irradiation is indeed also observed for all investigated photo-Fenton reagents, with the exception of **3**, which produces significantly more formamidopyrimidine-DNA glycosylase (FPG protein)-sensitive lesions. In this special case, the DNA damage profile indicates that other DNA-oxidizing processes may additionally be involved, presumably from photooxidation-type reactions.

Genotoxicity of Furocoumarin Hydroperoxides in Cells

Chemical and enzymatic studies of furocoumarin hydroperoxides revealed that these novel intercalating photo-Fenton reagents efficiently cause oxidative DNA damage in cell-free systems. To assess their genotoxicity in cellular systems, the mutagenicity and micronucleus induction by furocoumarin hydroperoxides **2a** and **2b** and, for comparison, their alcohols **2a′** and **2b′** (Fig. 9) were investigated in L5178Y tk$^{+/-}$ mouse lymphoma cells and AS52 Chinese hamster fibroblasts . In both cell systems the furocoumarin hydroperoxides **2a** and **2b** exhibited concentration-dependent mutagenicity under UVA irradiation (360 nm). Under identical conditions, the corresponding alcohol **2a′**

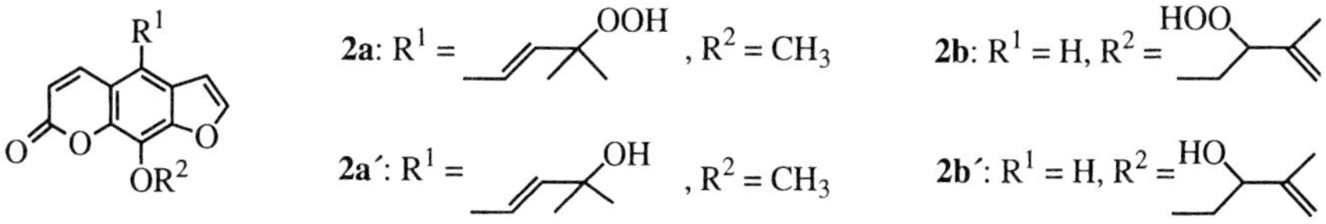

R¹ … OR²

2a: R^1 = [OOH side chain], $R^2 = CH_3$ **2b**: R^1 = H, R^2 = [HOO side chain]

2a′: R^1 = [OH side chain], $R^2 = CH_3$ **2b′**: R^1 = H, R^2 = [HO side chain]

Fig. 9. Structures of furocoumarin hydroperoxides and alcohols

proved to be inactive. However, the alcohol **2b′** was mutagenic in both L5178Y and AS52 cells. In L5178Y cells the hydroperoxide **2b** and its alcohol **2b′** induced a significant number of micronucleus at very low concentrations (2 *μM*), while for the **2a** and **2a′** pair, micronucleus formation was observed only at higher concentrations (15–20 *μM*) and the alcohol **2a′** was less active than the hydroperoxide **2a**. The furocoumarin derivatives **2a**,**b** and **2a′**,**b′** did not show any genotoxicity without UVA (360 nm) irradiation. The details of this genotoxicity study have been published recently (Möller et al. 1995).

Conclusion

We have established that dioxetanes are unique peroxidic oxidants which oxidize predominantly guanine base in DNA by the action of excited triplet states and, consequently, are able to perform "photochemistry in the dark". In this context, we have shown that dioxetanes constitute excellent model systems to study the photooxidation reactions in biological systems without light.

Our investigations on the oxidative DNA damage with fatty acid ester hydroperoxides revealed that lipid hydroperoxides may protect cells against oxidative stress, especially by suppressing type I photooxidation.

Finally, our novel work on the photo-Fenton reagents demonstrates that the readily available furocoumarin **2** and phenanthridine **3** hydroperoxides, as well as *N*-hydroxypyridinethiones **1**, serve as convenient sources for the generation of hydroxyl radicals, which promote significant oxidation of DNA. Because of the conveniently controllable generation of hydroxyl radicals and the intercalating ability of the hydroperoxides **2** and **3**, these photo-Fenton reagents are predestined for the investigation of hydroxyl radical damage of biomolecules such as DNA or proteins.

References

Adam W, Cilento G (1983) Four-membered ring peroxides as excited state equivalents: a new dimension in bioorganic chemistry. Angew Chem Int Ed Engl 22: 529–542

Adam W, Beinhauer A, Mosandl T, Saha-Möller CR, Vargas F, Epe B, Müller E, Schiffmann D, Wild D (1990) Photobiological studies with dioxetanes in isolated DNA, bacteria, and mammalian cells. Environ Health Perspect 88: 89–97

Adam W, Albrecht O, Feineis E, Reuter I, Saha-Möller CR, Seufert-Baumbach P, Wild D (1991a) Benzofuran dioxetanes, a new class of mutagenic agents: synthesis by photooxygenation of benzofuran derivatives. Liebigs Ann Chem: 33–40

Adam W, Hadjiarapoglou L, Mosandl T, Saha-Möller CR, Wild D (1991b) Chemical model studies on the mutagenesis of benzofuran dioxetanes in the Ames test: evidence for the benzofuran epoxide as ultimate mutagen. J Am Chem Soc 113: 8005–8011

Adam W, Ahrweiler M, Saha-Möller CR, Sauter M, Schönberger A, Epe B, Müller E, Schiffmann D, Stopper H, Wild D (1993) Genotoxicity studies of benzofuran dioxetanes and epoxides with isolated DNA, bacteria and mammalian cells. Toxicol Lett 67: 41–55

Adam W, Epe B, Cadet J, Dall'Acqua F, Ramaiah D, Saha-Möller CR (1995a) Photosensitized formation of 8-hydroxy-2'-deoxyguanosine in *salmon testes* DNA by furocoumarin hydroperoxides: a novel intercalating "photo-Fenton" reagent for oxidative DNA damage. Angew Chem Int Ed Engl 34: 107–110

Adam W, Saha-Möller CR, Schönberger A, Berger M, Cadet J (1995b) Formation of 7,8-dihydroxy-8-oxoguanine in the 1,2-dioxetane-induced oxidation of *calf thymus* DNA: evidence for photosensitized DNA damage by thermally generated triplet ketones in the dark. Photochem Photobiol 62: 231–238

Adam W, Ballmeier D, Epe B, Grimm G, Saha-Möller CR (1995c) *N*-Hydroxypyridinethiones as photochemical hydroxyl radical sources for oxidative DNA damage. Angew Chem Int Ed Engl 34: 2156–2158

Adam W, Andler S, Saha-Möller CR, Schönberger A (1996) Inhibitory effect of ethyl oleate hydroperoxide and alcohol in photosensitized oxidative DNA damage. J Photochem Photobiol B Biol (in press)

Boivin J, Crépon E, Zard SZ (1990) *N*-Hydroxy-2-pyridinethione: a mild and convenient source of hydroxyl radicals. Tetrahedron Lett 37: 6869–6872

Buchko GW, Cadet J, Berger M, Ravanat J-L (1992) Photooxidation of d(TpG) by phthalocyanines and riboflavin. Isolation and characterisation of dinucleoside monophosphates containing the 4R* and 4S* diastereomers of 4,8-dihydro-4-hydroxy-8-oxo-2'-deoxyguanosine. Nucleic Acids Res 20: 4847–4851

Cadet J, Vigny P (1990) The photochemistry of nucleic acids. In: Morrison H (ed) Bioorganic photochemistry: photochemistry and the nucleic acids, vol 1. Wiley, New York, pp 1–272

Cadet J (1994a) DNA damage caused by oxidation, deamination, ultraviolet radiation and photoexcited psoralens. In: Hemminki K, Dipple A, Shuker DEG, Kadlubar FF, Segerbäck D, Bartsch H (eds) DNA adducts: identification and biological significance, vol 125. IARC Publications, Lyon, pp 245–276

Cadet J, Berger M, Morin B, Ravanat J-L, Raoul S (1994b) Photooxidation reactions of the guanine moiety of DNA and nucleosides. Spectrum 7: 21–24

Catalani LH, Wilson T, Bechara EJH (1987) Two water-soluble fluorescence probes for chemiexcitation studies: sodium 9,10-dibromo- and 9,10-diphenylanthracene-2-sulfonate. Synthesis, properties and application to triplet acetone and tetramethyl-dioxetane. Photochem Photobiol 45: 273–281

Cilento G (1984) Generation of electronic excited triplet species in biological systems. Pure Appl Chem 56: 1179–1190

Cilento G, Adam W (1988) Photochemistry and photobiology without light. Photochem Photobiol 48: 361–368

Emmert S, Epe B, Saha-Möller CR, Adam W, Rünger TM (1995) Assessment of genotoxicity and mutagenicity of 1,2-dioxetanes in human cells using a plasmid shuttle vector. Photochem Photobiol 61: 136–141

Epe B, Hegler J (1994) Oxidative DNA damage: endonuclease fingerprinting. Methods Enzymol 234: 67–82

Epe B, Müller E, Adam W, Saha-Möller CR (1992) Photochemical DNA modifications induced by 1,2-dioxetanes. Chem Biol Interact 85: 265–281

Epe B, Henzl H, Adam W, Saha-Möller CR (1993a) Endonuclease-sensitive DNA modifications induced by acetone and acetophenone as photosensitizers. Nucleic Acids Res 21: 863–869

Epe B, Häring M, Ramaiah D, Stopper H, Abou-Alzahab MM, Adam W, Saha-Möller CR (1993b) DNA damage induced by furocoumarin hydroperoxides plus UV (360 nm). Carcinogenesis 14: 2271–2276

Floyd RA, Watson JJ, Wong PK, Altmiller DH, Rickard RC (1986) Hydroxyl free radical adduct of deoxyguanosine: sensitive detection and mechanism of formation. Free Radic Res Commun 1: 163–172

Floyd RA, West MS, Eneff KL, Schneider JE, Wong PK, Tingey DT, Hogsett WE (1990) Conditions influencing yield and analysis of 8-hydroxy-2′-deoxyguanosine in oxidatively damaged DNA. Anal Biochem 188: 155–158

Foote CS (1991) Definition of type I and type II photosensitized oxidation. Photochem Photobiol 54: 659

Kavarnos GJ, Turro NJ (1986) Photosensitization by reversible electron transfer: theories, experimental evidence, and examples. Chem Rev 86: 401–449

Kochevar IE, Dunn DA (1990) Photosensitized reactions of DNA: cleavage and addition. In: Morrison H (ed) Bioorganic photochemistry: photochemistry and the nucleic acids, vol 1. Wiley, New York, pp 273–316

Möller M, Stopper H, Häring M, Schleger Y, Epe B, Adam W, Saha-Möller CR (1995) Genotoxicity induced by furocoumarin hydroperoxides in mammalian cells upon UVA irradiation. Biochem Biophy Res Commun 216: 693–701

Pavlov YI, Minnick DT, Izuta S, Kunkel TA (1994) DNA replication fidelity with 8-oxodeoxyguanosine triphosphate. Biochemistry 33: 4695–4701

Piette J (1991) Biological consequences associated with DNA oxidation mediated by singlet oxygen. J Photochem Photobiol B Biol 11: 241–260

Piette J, Merville-Louis MP, Decuyper J (1986) Damage induced in nucleic acids by photosensitization. Photochem Photobiol 44: 793–802

Ravanat J-L, Berger M, Benard F, Langlois R, Ouellet R, van Lier JE, Cadet J (1992) Phthalocyanine and naphthalocyanine photosensitized oxidation of 2′-deoxyguanosine: distinct type I and type II products. Photochem Photobiol 55: 809–814

Saito I, Takayama M, Matsuura T (1990) Phthalimide hydroperoxides as efficient photochemical hydroxyl radical generators. a novel DNA-cleaving agent. J Am Chem Soc 112: 883–884

Sheu C, Foote CS (1993) Endoperoxide formation in a guanosine derivative. J Am Chem Soc 115: 10446–10447

Sheu C, Foote CS (1995) Photosensitized oxygenation of a 7,8-dihydro-8-oxoguanosine derivative. Formation of dioxetane and hydroperoxide intermediates. J Am Chem Soc 117: 474–477

Sies H (1991) Oxidative stress, oxidants and antioxidants. Academic Press, New York

Steenken S (1989) Purine bases, nucleosides, and nucleotides: aqueous solution redox chemistry and transformation reactions of their radical cations and e^- and OH adducts. Chem Rev 89: 503–520

Tjerneld F, Norden B, Ljunggren B (1979) Interaction between DNA and 8-methoxypsoralen studied by linear dichroism. Photochem Photobiol 29: 1115–1118

von Sonntag CV (1987) The chemical basis of radiation biology. Taylor and Francis, London

Wood ML, Dizdaroglu M, Gajewski E, Essigmann JM (1990) Mechanistic studies of ionizing radiation and oxidative mutagenesis: genetic effects of a single 8-hydroxyguanine (7-hydro-8-oxoguanine) residue inserted at a unique site in a viral genome. Biochemistry 29: 7024–7032

Oxidative DNA Damage Profiles in Mammalian Cells

D. Ballmaier, M. Pflaum, C. Kielbassa, and B. Epe

Department of Pharmacy, University of Mainz, Staudinger Weg 5,
55099 Mainz, Germany

Introduction

Reactive oxygen species (ROS) are formed inside cells not only under the influence of exogenous agents (visible light, ionizing radiation, and many oxidants such as peroxides or quinones), but also under normal (physiological) conditions as byproducts of oxygen metabolism and other cellular redox reactions (Pryor 1986; Halliwell and Gutteridge 1986; Sies 1986; Clayson et al. 1994). ROS such as hydroxyl radicals and singlet oxygen are a serious threat to the integrity of the cellular genome, since they efficiently react with DNA to generate many types of DNA modifications, at least some of which are premutagenic (Breimer 1990; Halliwell and Aruoma 1991; Epe 1991; Feig et al. 1994). Steady-state levels of 8-hydroxyguanine (8-oxoG) and other oxidative DNA base modifications observed in untreated cells indicate that the various cellular defense and DNA repair systems (Demple and Harrison 1994) do not completely eliminate the mutagenic risk associated with ROS formation even under normal growth conditions. This led to the assumption that oxidative DNA damage is a causal or ancillary risk factor for the development of cancer and several age-correlated degenerative diseases (Ames 1983; Wallace 1992; Gutteridge 1993). A strategy to verify this hypothesis and to quantify the mutagenic risk associated with oxidative DNA damage could be to determine (a) what type of oxidative DNA damage profile (pattern of DNA modifications) is generated in the cells under the conditions of interest and (b) the mutagenicity associated with this damage profile. Then, the quantification of any suitable marker modification of this damage profile should allow an estimation of the mutagenicity to be expected.

Here we describe several DNA damage profiles measured by means of repair endonucleases after exposure of cells to various types of oxidants. Two different types of damage profiles can be distinguished which result from the reaction of DNA with hydroxyl radicals and "mild" oxidants, respectively. Mutagenicity data for the second type of damage profile are presented.

Recent Results in Cancer Research, Vol. 143

Materials and Methods

Materials

L1210 mouse leukemia cells (Flow Laboratories, Meckenheim, Germany) were cultured in RPMI 1640 medium without phenol red containing 10% fetal calf serum. AS52 Chinese hamster ovary cells (*hprt*$^-$) carrying the *E. coli gpt* gene on an autosome were obtained from W.J. Caspary, Research Triangle Park, NC, USA, and cultured in Ham's F12 medium with 5% fetal calf serum. DNA from bacteriophage PM2 (PM2 DNA) was prepared according to the method of Salditt et al. (1972). *E. coli* formamidopyrimidine-DNA glycosylase (Fpg protein) and endonuclease III were kindly provided by S. Boiteux (Villejuif, France). T4 endonuclease V was partially purified by the method described by Nakabeppu et al. (1982) from the *E. coli* strain A 32480 (*uvrA*, *recA*, F′lac IQ1) carrying the plasmid ptac-den V (kindly provided by L. Mullenders, Leiden, Netherlands) after induction with isopropyl-β-D thiogalactopyranoside. *E. coli* endonuclease IV was kindly provided by B. Demple (Boston, MA, USA). Exonuclease III was purchased from Boehringer, Mannheim, (Germany). All repair endonucleases were tested for their incision at reference modifications under the applied assay conditions to ensure that the correct substrate modifications were fully recognized and no incision at nonsubstrate modifications took place (see Epe and Hegler 1994).

Exposure of Cells and Cell-Free PM2 DNA to Damaging Agents

PM2 DNA was exposed to singlet oxygen (generated by thermal decomposition of $NDPO_2$, the disodium salt of 1,4-etheno-2,3-benzodioxin-1,4-dipropanoic acid in D_2O; see Di Mascio and Sies 1989), ionizing radiation, potassium bromate plus glutathione, acridine orange plus light, and acetone plus UV (333 nm) in phosphate buffer as described previously (Müller et al. 1990; Epe et al. 1993a,b; Ballmaier and Epe 1995). Exposure to *N*-hydroxypyridine-2-thione (2-HPT; Sigma-Aldrich Chemie, Deisenhofen, Germany) plus light (1000-W halogen lamp at a distance of 33 cm) was carried out similarly.

Exposure of L1210 and AS52 cells to H_2O_2 (Epe and Hegler 1994) visible light (Pflaum et al. 1994), acridine orange plus visible light (Epe et al. 1993a), and potassium bromate (Ballmaier and Epe 1995) was carried out in PBSG (140 m*M* NaCl, 3 m*M* KCl, 8 m*M* Na_2HPO_4, 1 m*M* KH_2PO_4, 1 m*M* $CaCl_2$, 0.5 m*M* $MgCl_2$, 0.1% glucose, pH 7.4) on ice (10^6 cells/ml) as described previously. The exposure to 2-HPT plus light was carried out in an analogous way.

All illuminations with visible light were carried out with a 1000-W halogen lamp, which emitted 5.4 kJ/m^2 per min between 400 and 800 nm at a 66-cm distance.

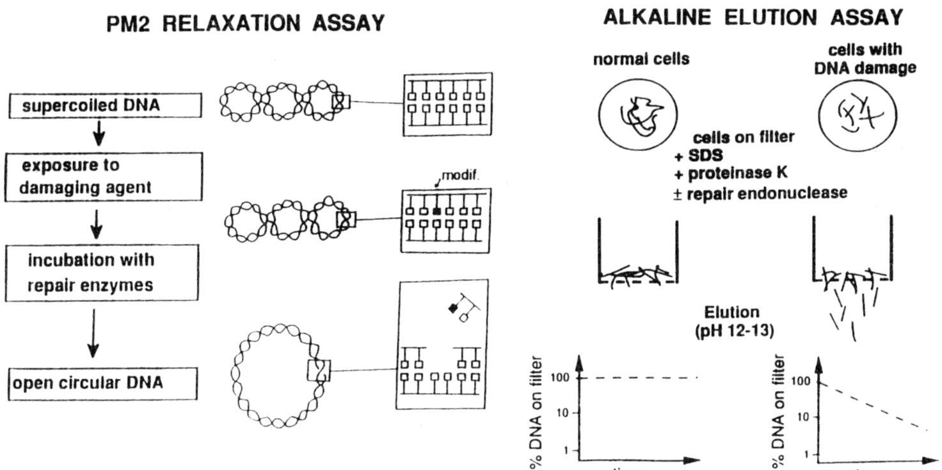

Fig. 1. Principle of damage analysis by means of repair endonucleases in supercoiled PM2 DNA (*left*) and in cultured mammalian cells (*right*). The relaxation assay makes use of the fact that supercoiled DNA is converted by either a single-strand break or the incision of a repair endonuclease into a nicked (open circular) form which migrates separately from the supercoiled form in agarose gel electrophoresis. The number of single-strand breaks (incisions) is calculated from the relative amounts of the two forms of DNA. In the alkaline elution technique, the rate at which cellular DNA is eluted with an alkaline solution from a membrane filter is determined. The rate is increased when the DNA has single-strand breaks or was incised by a repair endonuclease in a preceding incubation. The sum of endonuclease-sensitive modifications and single-strand breaks (generated directly by the damaging agent) is obtained from incubations with repair endonucleases. Incubations without repair endonuclease give the number of single-strand breaks alone, which can be subtracted to obtain the number of endonuclease-sensitive modifications. All values are corrected for the number of sites determined in unmodified PM2 DNA or in control cells. For experimental details, see Epe and Hegler (1994)

DNA Damage Analysis

The quantification of endonuclease-sensitive modifications and direct single-strand breaks was carried out in the case of PM2 DNA by means of a relaxation assay and in the case of cultured cells by means of the alkaline elution technique. Both techniques are outlined in Fig. 1 and have been described in detail elsewhere (Epe and Hegler 1994).

Mutation Analysis and Cytotoxicity

AS52 cells were cultured in a cleansing medium (containing purine and pyrimidine bases and mycophenolic acid) for 1 week to eliminate spontaneous gpt$^-$ mutants. Cells were exposed in PBSG to damaging agents under the same conditions that were used for damage analysis. The subsequent quantification of 6-thioguanine-resistant cells and the determination of cytotoxicity (ratio of the plating efficiencies of treated and untreated cells) was carried out according to the protocol of Tindall et al. (1986).

Results and Discussion

Oxidative DNA Damage Profiles Generated Under Cell-Free Conditions

DNA damage profiles, which give the relative or absolute numbers of various types of DNA modifications, can be obtained by means of a set of repair endonucleases which selectively recognize certain types of DNA modifications (Table 1) (Epe and Hegler 1994). Thus, Fpg protein from *E. coli* recognizes several purine modifications (8-oxoG, formamidopyrimidines) and both regular and 4′-oxidized sites of base loss (AP sites). Endonuclease III recognizes several 5,6-dihydropyrimidines (thymine glycols, cytidine hydrates) in addition to regular and 4′-oxidized AP sites. Exonuclease III and endonuclease IV both recognize exclusively sites of base loss. The two enzymes differ, however, in their recognition of oxidized AP sites (Häring et al. 1994). The repair endonucleases incise the DNA at their substrate modifications, generating single-strand breaks. These can be quantified sensitively, for instance by the alkaline elution technique in the case of nuclear DNA of mammalian cells or by a

Table 1. Recognition of oxidative DNA modifications by repair endonucleases[a]

Repair endonuclease	Recognition spectrum			
	Sites of base loss (AP sites)			Base modifications
	regular[b]	1′ -oxid.[c]	4′ -oxid.[d]	
Fpg protein	+	–	+	8-oxoG[e], Fapy[f]
Endonuclease III	+	–	+	5,6-dihydropyrimidines; hyd[g]
T4 endonuclease V	+	–	+	Py < > Py[h]
Endonuclease IV	+	+	+	—
Exonuclease III	+	+	(+)[i]	—

Fpg, formamidopyrimidine-DNA glycosylase.
[a]See Wallace 1988; Lindahl 1990; Boiteux 1993; Tchou et al. 1994; Häring et al. 1994; Demple and Harrison 1994.
[b]Unmodified desoxyribose moiety.
[c]Desoxyribose oxidized in the 1′ position.
[d]Desoxyribose oxidized in the 4′ position
[e]7,8-Dihydro-8-oxoguanine (8-hydroxyguanine).
[f]Formamidopyrimidines (imidazole ring-opened purines).
[g]5-Hydroxy-5-methylhydantoin.
[h]Cyclobutane pyrimidine photodimers.
[i]Recognition requires high enzyme concentrations (200 U/ml).

relaxation assay in the case of supercoiled plasmids or mitochondrial DNA (Fig. 1). After exposure to a damaging agent (oxidant), the sum of endonuclease sites and direct single-strand breaks (generated by the damaging agent) is obtained in these assays; the number of direct strand breaks are determined in parallel assays without endonucleases and are subtracted.

In Fig. 2, DNA damage profiles are shown which were observed in DNA from bacteriophage PM2 after exposure to various oxidizing agents in phosphate buffer. For these cell-free damaging conditions, the reaction mechanisms and the nature of the species that directly react with the DNA are frequently known from experiments with scavengers or other indications. Thus, the PM2 DNA damage induced by the aromatic endoperoxide $NDPO_2$ is caused mostly by singlet oxygen, which is generated from $NDPO_2$ upon thermal decomposition (Epe et al. 1988; Epe 1991). Both ionizing radiation and the photoinduced decomposition of 2-HPT (*N*-hydroxypyridine-2-thione; see Hess and Dix 1992) modify cell-free DNA exclusively via hydroxyl radicals (see Epe et al. 1993c and unpublished results). The damage induced by acetone upon irradiation at 333 nm with an argon ion laser has been demonstrated to be due to a direct reaction of DNA with the triplet-excited state of the carbonyl

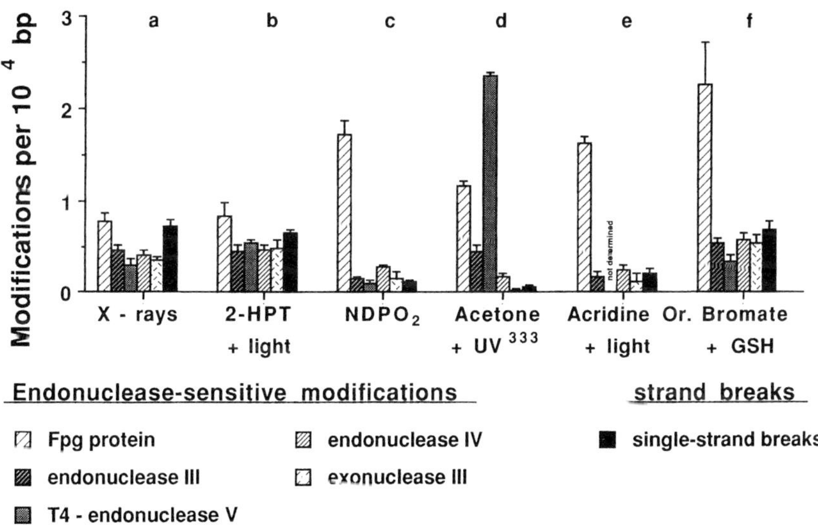

Fig. 2. DNA damage profiles induced under cell-free conditions (phosphate buffer) in PM2 DNA by **a** ionizing radiation, 20 Gy at 0 °C, **b** *N*-hydroxy-pyridine-2-thione (1 m*M*) plus visible light (225 kJ/m^2) at 0 °C, **c** $NDPO_2$ (3.5 m*M* in D_2O) at 37 °C, **d** acetone (2.6 *M*) plus UV^{333} (8.6 J/m^2) at 25 °C **e** acridine orange [7.5 μM plus visible light (2.8 kJ/m^2) at 0 °C], and **f** $KBrO_3$ (1.5 m*M*) plus GSH (2m*M*) at 37 °C. Columns indicate the numbers of single-strand breaks and various endonuclease-sensitive DNA modifications. They represent the means of three or more independent experiments (±SD). The damage profiles **a, c, e** (Epe et al. 1993a), **d** (Epe et al. 1993b), and **f** (Ballmaier and Epe 1995) have been described previously

compound (Epe et al. 1993b). The damage profile observed after treatment with bromate, which is a renal carcinogen (Kurokawa et al. 1990), in the presence of glutathione has been ascribed to a reaction with bromine radicals or related species (Ballmaier and Epe 1995). Acridine orange in the presence of light modifies PM2 DNA predominantly via type I reaction, i.e., the excited photosensitizer mostly reacts directly with the DNA (Epe et al. 1993a).

It is evident from Fig. 2 that two rather different types of DNA damage profiles are induced by the various oxidants: hydroxyl radicals generated by ionizing radiation or photodecomposition of 2-HPT (Fig. 2a,b) give rise to a 2:1 ratio of direct single-strand breaks and AP sites (specifically recognized by endonuclease IV, exonuclease III and – in the absence of pyrimidine dimers – T4 endonuclease V). The sum of AP sites and base modifications recognized by Fpg protein is twice the number of AP sites; therefore, base modifications sensitive to Fpg protein such as 8-oxoG and formamidopyrimidines are as frequent as AP sites. Pyrimidine base modifications recognized by endonuclease III (5,6-dihydropyrimidine derivatives) are less than half as frequent. Agents as different as singlet oxygen (generated from $NDPO_2$) (Fig. 2c), acridine orange plus light (Fig. 2e), and potassium bromate in the presence of glutathione (Fig. 2f) give rise to the second type of damage profile. It is characterized by the fact that base modifications sensitive to Fpg protein are formed in high excess of strand breaks, AP sites, and pyrimidine modifications (sensitive to endonuclease III). Analysis by HPLC and by gas chromatography/mass spectrometry indicated that most of the Fpg-sensitive base modifications in these and similar damage profiles actually are 8-oxoG residues (Boiteux et al. 1992; Ballmaier and Epe 1995); however, the presence of other (unknown) modifications sensitive to Fpg protein and of modifications not recognized by any of the endonucleases is not completely excluded. The damage profile induced by triplet-excited carbonyl compounds (photoexcited acetone) (Fig. 2d) is also similar to the damage profile induced by singlet oxygen except that pyrimidine dimers (recognized by T4 endonuclease V) are generated in even higher yields than Fpg-sensitive base modifications. This is explained by the high triplet energy of the excited carbonyl, which allows energy transfer to the thymine residues of DNA.

Oxidative DNA Damage Profiles in Cellular DNA

DNA damage profiles determined by means of repair endonucleases in L1210 mouse leukemia cells after exposure to various oxidants are shown in Fig. 3. It is apparent that the two types of DNA damage profiles that are observed after treatment with oxidants under cell-free conditions (Fig. 2) are also found in the cellular DNA. Both H_2O_2 at 0 °C and 2-HTP plus light generate similar yields of single-strand breaks and Fpg-sensitive base modifications (Fig. 3a,b). This is consistent with the assumption that a reaction with hydroxyl radicals is directly responsible for the cellular DNA modifications in both cases. The relatively

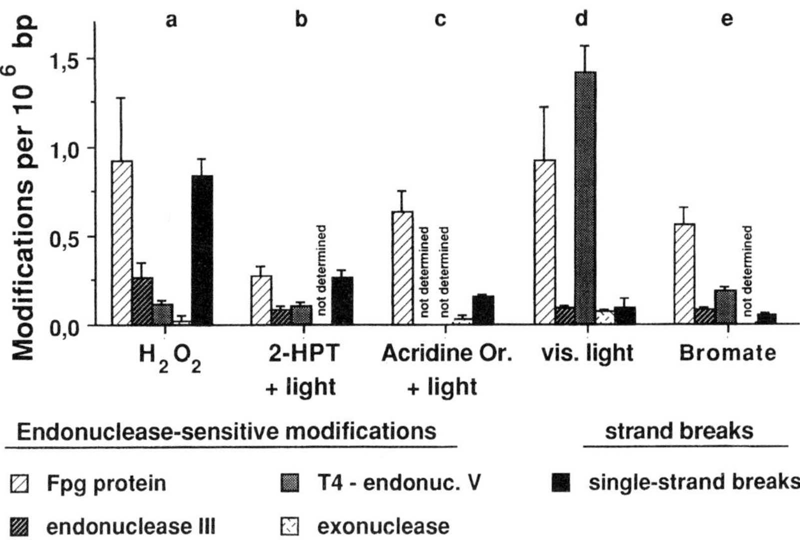

Fig. 3. DNA damage profiles induced in L1210 mouse leukemia cells by **a** H_2O_2 (500 μM at 0 °C), **b** N-hydroxypyridine-2-thione (2-HPT) (40 μM) plus light (225 kJ/m^2) at 0 °C, **c** acridine orange (6.6 μM) plus light (450 J/m^2) at 0 °C, **d** light (450 kJ/m^2) at 0 °C, and **e** potassium bromate (10 mM) at 37 °C. Data in **c** and **e** are taken from Epe et al. 1993a and Ballmaier and Epe 1995, respectively

low number of AP sites (sensitive to exonuclease III) may be explained by the alkaline elution conditions which convert oxidized AP sites into single-strand breaks. In contrast, the illumination of cells with high doses of light (Fig. 3d) generates predominantly pyrimidine dimers (recognized by T4 endonuclease V) and Fpg-sensitive base modifications. The generation of pyrimidine dimers is caused by small doses of UV emitted from the halogen lamp: when wavelengths below 400 nm are eliminated by means of a cutoff filter, generation of the T4 endonuclease V-sensitive base modifications is completely prevented, while the formation of Fpg-sensitive modifications is only slightly reduced (data not shown). The cellular damage profile induced in the visible range of the spectrum (at wavelengths above 400 nm) is therefore similar to that induced under cell-free conditions by singlet oxygen and type I photosensitizers. This indicates that the cellular DNA damage in this case is not induced by hydroxyl radicals, but is caused by a direct reaction of singlet oxygen or excited endogeneous photosensitizers such as porphyrins with the DNA. Treatment of the cells with acridine orange plus low doses of light (Fig. 3c), but also with potassium bromate (Fig. 3e), gives rise to the same type of damage profile. Again, it has to be concluded that the cellular DNA damage is induced by the same species as under the corresponding cell-free conditions (see Fig. 2) and that hydroxyl radicals are not involved. The cellular activation of bromate by glutathione is confirmed by the finding that the extent of the bromate-induced DNA damage is decreased in cells pretreated with diethylmaleate (Ballmaier and Epe 1995).

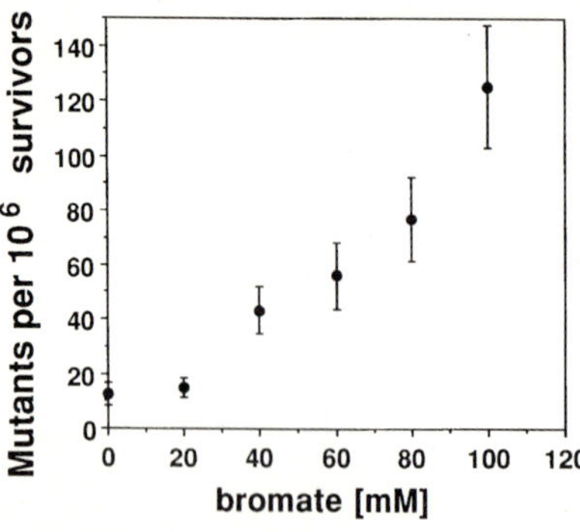

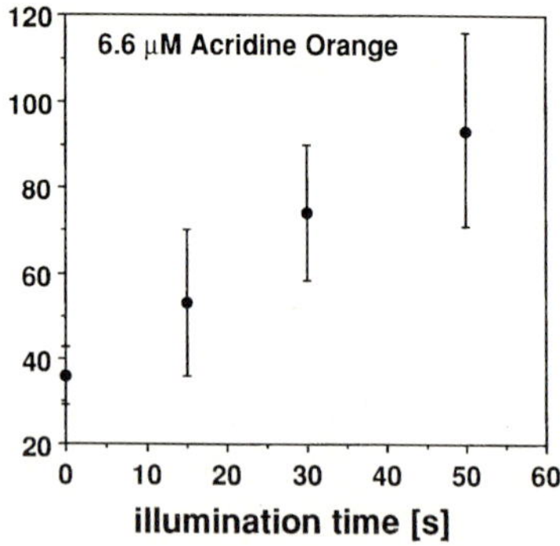

Fig. 4. Mutagenicity observed in the *gpt* locus of AS52 cells treated in a phosphate buffer with various concentrations of potassium bromate (15 min; 37 °C) (*left*) or illuminated in the presence of acridine orange (6.6 μM) with various doses of visible light (halogen lamp; 1 min = 5.4 kJ/m^2) (*right*)

Mutagenicity Associated with Oxidative Damage Profiles

The induction of thioguanine resistance was used to determine the mutagenicity associated with oxidative DNA damage profiles in AS52 Chinese hamster ovary cells, which are deficient in the mammalian hypoxanthine-guanine phosphoribosyl transferase (*hprt*) gene, but carry the bacterial *gpt* (guanine phosphoribosyl transferase) gene on an autosome (Tindall et al. 1986). In Fig. 4, the results of mutagenicity assays are shown for the treatments with bromate and acridine orange plus light. The associated cytotoxicities are shown in Fig. 5. For both damaging agents, the number of mutants increased linearly with dose. Moderate cytotoxicity is observed at doses required to induce significant mutagenicity (Fig. 5).

As bromate and acridine orange plus light generate the same type of DNA damage profile (Fig. 3c,e), they are expected to induce the same mutagenicity at

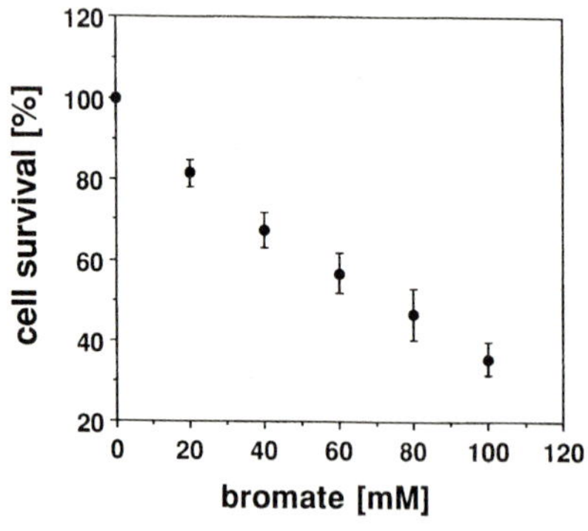

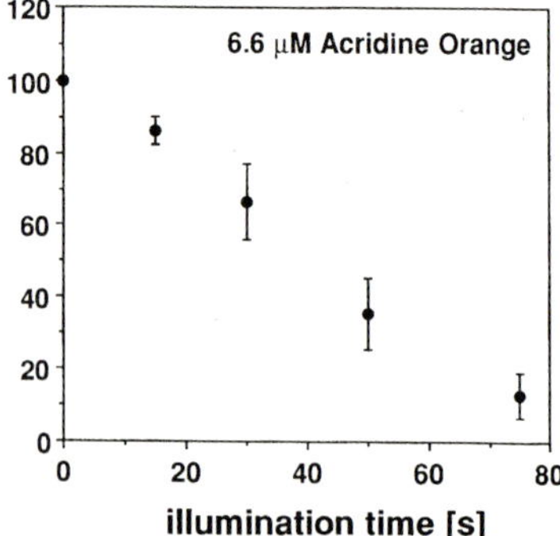

Fig. 5. Cytotoxicity observed in AS52 cells treated with potassium bromate (*left*) or acridine orange in the presence of light (*right*) under the conditions described in Fig. 4

the same extent of DNA damage, provided that there is no significant (or no different) influence of the agents on the processing of the DNA damage. To test this assumption, in Fig. 6 the numbers of *gpt* mutants induced by bromate and acridine orange plus light are plotted against the number of Fpg-sensitive base modifications determined by alkaline elution. Since for both agents the extent of DNA damage at those doses required to induce a significant number of mutants was too high to be determined by alkaline elution directly, low doses (similar to those indicated in Fig. 3) were used for the quantification of the damage, and values for the doses shown in Fig. 6 were calculated by linear extrapolation. The data indicate that the number of mutants/10^6 cells per Fpg-sensitive modification/10^6 bp is only slightly higher for bromate (13.0 ± 1.7) than for acridine orange plus light (9.2 ± 0.9).

Data shown in Fig. 6 are not corrected for background, i.e., the number of Fpg-sensitive modifications and *gpt* mutants present in untreated cells or in cells treated with acridine orange in the dark. These background values are included as data points with open symbols in Fig. 6. If Fpg-sensitive modifications were the cause for both background *gpt* mutations and induced mutations, the regression line should extend through the origin. This is obviously not the case for the data obtained in the presence of acridine orange, most probably because the dye gives rise to some mutations in the dark that may best be explained by its intercalating properties. In the case of bromate, the extrapolation is less clear and more data at low bromate concentrations are required to decide whether the spontaneous mutations can be explained by the steady-state level of Fpg-sensitive sites alone.

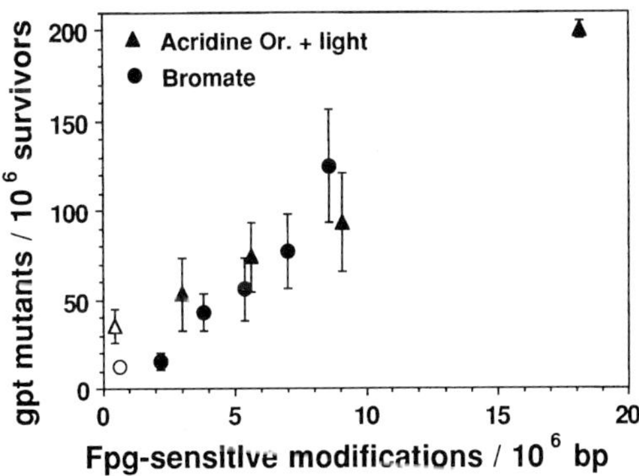

Fig. 6. Numbers of *gpt* mutants induced (1) by various concentrations of potassium bromate and (2) by acridine orange plus various doses of light (see Fig. 4 for reaction conditions) plotted against the number of DNA base modifications sensitive to formamidopyrimidine-DNA glycosylase (Fpg protein) induced under the same conditions. The numbers of modifications were calculated from data determined at lower concentrations/illumination times assuming a linear dose response. Background values, i.e., the numbers of Fpg-sensitive modifications and *gpt* mutants observed (1) in the absence of potassium bromate and (2) with acridine orange in the dark, have not been subtracted and are shown as data points with *open symbols*

Conclusions

The results show that DNA damage profiles obtained by means of repair endonucleases can serve as fingerprints of the agent or species that is ultimately (directly) responsible for the DNA damage and that the comparison of cellular and cell-free damage profiles can help to elucidate the cellular mechanisms that lead to DNA damage formation. Thus, the formation by H_2O_2 of single-strand breaks and Fpg-sensitive modifications in similar yields indicates that hydroxyl radicals are directly responsible, in agreement with earlier suggestions (Meneghini 1988). The generation of single-strand breaks via an activation of cellular nucleases, which is a reasonable alternative or additional mechanism (Cantoni et al. 1989; Halliwell and Aruoma 1991; Weis et al. 1994; Zhivotovsky et al. 1994), can be excluded as a major pathway for the reaction conditions used (0 °C). The cellular DNA damage profile observed in cells treated with high doses of visible light, on the other hand, allows us to rule out that this DNA damage is mediated by H_2O_2 and subsequent Fenton reaction, a mechanism that otherwise might have been expected.

The results further show that oxidants induce two rather different types of DNA damage profile. A great number of different modifications is characteristic for the damage induced by hydroxyl radicals. It reflects the high reactivity and thereby low selectivity of this species. In contrast, the quite selective induction of Fpg-sensitive base modifications, probably mostly 8-oxoG, by oxidants as different as potassium bromate and acridine orange plus light indicates that guanine is the preferential target for mild (less reactive) oxidants, possibly because it has the lowest oxidation potential in DNA (Steenken 1989). Damage formation in these cases may proceed via a common intermediate, possibly a guanine radical.

The damage profile induced by hydroxyl radicals is most probably responsible for the mutagenicity observed in shuttle vectors exposed to H_2O_2 in the presence of transition metals (Moraes et al. 1989; Akman et al. 1991) or to ionizing radiation (Waters et al. 1991). Among the many modifications that may contribute to the mutagenicity, DNA strand breaks and 5-hydroxycytosine residues (Feig et al. 1994) may be particularly important. The data provided here support the assumption that the second type of damage profile, which is generated both by acridine orange plus light and by potassium bromate, is also mutagenic in mammalian cells, since doses of the two agents that generate the same extent of DNA damage give rise to a similar number of mutations. Several observations indicate that the most relevant premutagenic modification in this case is 8-oxoG. Thus, 8-oxoG is the most frequent Fpg-sensitive modification in this type of DNA damage according to HPLC analysis (Ballmaier and Epe 1995). Furthermore, the most frequent type of mutation observed in vectors treated with $NDPO_2$ or methylene blue plus light are G:C→T:A transversions, both in bacteria and in mammalian cells (Decuyper-Debergh et al. 1987; McBride et al. 1992; Costa de Oliveira et al. 1992; Tudek et al. 1993; Retèl et al. 1993), which is in accordance with the known miscoding properties of 8-oxoG (Wood et al. 1990; Shibutani et al. 1991). Sequence analysis of the *gpt* mutations described in this report is in progress and will provide additional information.

The finding that different oxidants induce the same type of oxidative DNA damage profile supports the assumption that the number of different oxidative DNA damage profiles induced in cells under a variety of conditions is much lower than the number of different oxidative DNA modifications generated under the same conditions. Therefore, it seems convenient to correlate oxidative damage profiles rather than individual modifications with the genotoxic consequences.

Acknowledgements. Fpg protein and endonuclease III were kindly provided by S. Boiteux (Villejuif, France). Endonuclease IV was a gift from B. Demple (Boston, USA). The *E. coli* strain A 32480 overproducing T4 endonuclease V was obtained from L. Mullenders (Leiden, Netherlands). W.J. Caspary (Research Triangle Park, NC, USA) provided AS52 cells. This work was supported by the Deutsche Forschungsgemeinschaft (SFB 172).

References

Akman SA, Forrest GP, Doroshow JH, Dizdaroglu M (1991) Mutation of potassium permanganate- and hydrogen peroxide-treated plasmid pZ189 replicating in CV-1 monkey kidney cells. Mutat Res 261: 123–130

Ames BN (1983) Dietary carcinogens and anticarcinogens. Oxygen radicals and degenerative diseases. Science 221: 1256–1264

Ballmaier D, Epe B (1995) Oxidative DNA damage induced by potassium bromate under cell-free conditions and in mammalian cells. Carcinogenesis 16: 335–342

Boiteux S, Gajewski E, Laval J, Dizdaroglu M (1992) Substrate specificity of the *Escherichia coli* Fpg protein (formamidopyrimidine-DNA glycosylase): excision of purine lesions in DNA produced by ionizing radiation or photosensitization. Biochemistry 31: 106–110

Boiteux S (1993) Properties and biological functions of the NTH and FPG proteins of *Escherichia coli*: two DNA glycosylases that repair oxidative damage in DNA. Photochem Photobiol B 19: 87–96

Breimer (1990) Molecular mechanisms of oxygen radical carcinogenesis and mutagenesis: the role of base damage. Molec Carcinogenesis 3: 188–197

Cantoni O, Sestili P, Cattabeni F, Bellomo G, Pou S, Cohen M, Cerutti P (1989) Calcium chelator quin 2 prevents hydrogen-peroxide-induced DNA breakage and cytotoxicity. Eur J Biochem 182: 209–212

Clayson DB, Mehta R, Iverson F (1994) Oxidative DNA damage – the effects of certain genotoxic and operationally non-genotoxic carcinogens. Mutat Res 317: 25–42

Costa de Oliveira R, Ribeiro DT, Nigro RG, Di Mascio P, Menck CFM (1992) Singlet oxygen induced mutation spectrum in mammalian cells. Nucleic Acids Res 20: 4319–4323

Decuyper-Debergh D, Piette J, van de Vorst A (1987) Singlet oxygen-induced mutations in M13 lacZ phage DNA. EMBO J 6: 3155–3161

Demple B, Harrison L (1994) Repair of oxidative damage to DNA: enzymology and biology. Annu Rev Biochem 63: 915–948

Di Mascio P, Sies H (1989) Quantification of singlet oxygen generated by thermolysis of 3,3′-(1,4-naphthylidene)dipropionate. Monomol and dimol photoemission and the effects of 1,4-diazabicyclo[2.2.2]octane. J Am Chem Soc 111: 2909–2914

Epe B (1991) Genotoxicity of singlet oxygen. Chem Biol Interact 80: 239–260

Epe B, Hegler J (1994) Oxidative DNA damage: endonuclease fingerprinting. Methods Enzymol 234: 122–131

Epe B, Mützel P, Adam W (1988) DNA damage by oxygen radicals and excited state species: a comparative study using enzymatic probes in vitro. Chem Biol Interact 67: 149–165

Epe B, Pflaum M, Boiteux S (1993a) DNA damage induced by photosensitizers in cellular and cell-free systems. Mutat Res 299: 135–145

Epe B, Henzl H, Adam W, Saha-Möller CR (1993b) Endonuclease-sensitive DNA modifications induced by acetone and acetophenone as photosensitizers. Nucleic Acids Res 21: 863–869

Epe B, Häring M, Ramaiah D, Stopper H, Adam W, Abou-Elzahab MM, Saha-Möller CR (1993c) DNA damage induced by furocoumarin hydroperoxides plus UV (360 nm). Carcinogenesis 14: 2271–2276

Feig DI, Sowers LC, Loeb LA (1994) Reverse chemical mutagenesis: identification of the mutagenic lesions resulting from reactive oxygen species-mediated damage to DNA. Proc Natl Acad Sci USA 91: 6609–6613

Gutteridge JMC (1993) Free radicals in disease processes: a compilation of cause and consequences. Free Radical Res Commun 19: 141–158

Halliwell B, Aruoma OI (1991) DNA damage by oxygen-derived species: Its mechanism and measurement in mammalian cells. FEBS Lett 281: 9–19

Halliwell B, Gutteridge JM (1986) Oxygen free radicals and iron in relation to biology and medicine, some problems and concepts. Arch Biochem Biophys 246: 501–514

Häring M, Rüdiger H, Demple B, Boiteux S, Epe B (1994) Recognition of oxidized abasic sites by repair endonucleases. Nucleic Acids Res 22: 2010–2015

Hess KM, Dix TA (1992) Evaluation of N-hydroxy-2-thiopyridone as a nonmetal dependent source of the hydroxyl radical (HO·) in aqueous systems. Anal Biochem 206: 309–314

Kurokawa Y, Maekawa A, Takahashi M, Hayashi Y (1990) Toxicity and carcinogenicity of potassium bromate – a new renal carcinogen. Environ Health Perspect 87: 309–335

Lindahl T (1990) Repair of intrinsic DNA lesions. Mutat Res 238: 305–311

McBride TJ, Schneider JE, Floyd RA, Loeb LA (1992) Mutations induced by methylene blue plus light in single-stranded M13mp2. Proc Natl Acad Sci USA 89: 6866–6870

Meneghini R (1988) Genotoxicity of active oxygen species in mammalian cells. Mutat Res 195: 215–230 (1988)

Moraes EC, Keyse SM, Pidoux M, Tyrrell RM (1989) The spectrum of mutations generated by passage of a hydrogen peroxide damaged shuttle vector plasmid through a mammalian host. Nucleic Acids Res 17: 8301–8312

Müller E, Boiteux S, Cunningham RP, Epe B (1990) Enzymatic recognition of DNA modifications induced by singlet oxygen and photosensitizers. Nucleic Acids Res 18: 5969–5973

Nakabeppu Y, Yamashita K, Sekiguchi M (1982) Purification and characterization of normal and mutant forms of T4 endonuclease V. Proc Natl Acad Sci USA 257: 2556–2562

Pflaum M, Boiteux S, Epe B (1994) Visible light generates oxidative DNA base modifications in high excess of strand breaks in mammalian cells. Carcinogenesis 15: 297–300

Pryor WA (1986) Oxy-radicals and related species: their formation, lifetimes, and reactions. Annu Rev Physiol 48: 657–667

Retèl J, Hoebee B, Braun JEF, Lutgerink JT, van der Akker E, Wanamarta AH, Joenje H, Lafleur MVM (1993) Mutational specificity of oxidative DNA damage. Mutat Res 299: 165–182

Salditt M, Braunstein SN, Camerini-Otero RD, Franklin RM (1972) Structure and synthesis of a lipid-containing bacteriophage. Virology 48: 259–262

Shibutani S, Takeshita M, Grollman AP (1991) Insertion of specific bases during DNA synthesis past the oxidation-damaged base 8-oxodG. Nature 349: 431–434

Sies H (1986) Biochemistry of oxidative stress. Angew Chem Int Ed Engl 25: 1058–1071

Steenken S (1989) Purine bases, nucleosides, and nucleotides: aqueous solution redox chemistry and transformation reactions of their radical cations and e^- and OH adducts. Chem Rev 89: 503–520

Tchou J, Bodepudi V, Shibutani S, Antoshechkin I, Miller J, Grollman AP, Johnson F (1994) Substrate specificity of Fpg protein. J Biol Chem 269: 15318–15324

Tindall KR, Stankowski LF Jr, Machanoff R, Hsie AW (1986) Analyses of mutation in pSV2*gpt*-transformed CHO cells. Mutat Res 160: 121–131

Tudek B, Laval J, Boiteux S (1993) SOS-independent mutagenesis in lacZ induced by methylene blue plus visible light. Mol Gen Genet 236: 433–439

Wallace SS (1988) AP endonucleases and DNA glycosylases that recognize oxidative DNA damage. Environ Mol Mutagen 12: 431–477

Wallace DG (1992) Mitochondrial genetics: a paradigm for aging and degenerative diseases? Science 256: 628–632

Waters LC, Sikpi MO, Preston RJ, Mitra S, Jaberaboansari A (1991) Mutations induced by ionizing radiation in a plasmid replicated in human cells. Radiat Res 127: 190–201

Weis M, Kass GE, Orrenius S (1994) Further characterization of the events involved in mitochondrial Ca^{2+} release and pore formation by prooxidants. Biochem Pharmacol 47: 2147–2156

Wood ML, Dizdaroglu M, Gajewski E, Essigmann JM (1990) Mechanistic studies of ionizing radiation and oxidative mutagenesis: genetic effects of a single 8-hydroxyguanine (7-hydro-8-oxoguanine) residue inserted at a unique site in a viral genome. Biochemistry 29: 7024–7032

Zhivotovsky B, Wade D, Gahm A, Orrenius S, Nicotera P (1994) Formation of 50 kbp chromatin fragments in isolated liver nuclei is mediated by protease and endonuclease activation. FEBS Lett 351: 150–154

Chemical Mechanisms of Formation of DNA-Carcinogen Adducts, Elucidation of Potential of Adducts for Mutagenicity, and Mechanisms of Polymerase Fidelity and Mutation in the Presence of Adducts

F.P. Guengerich, M.-S. Kim, M. Müller, and L.G. Lowe

Department of Biochemistry and Center in Molecular Toxicology, Vanderbilt University School of Medicine, Nashville, TN 37232-0146, USA

Introduction

There is a long history of epidemiology associating human cancers with exposure to chemicals, dating back more than two centuries (Cartwright 1984). Over 80 years ago, scientists were able to produce tumors in animals with the administration of a single pure chemical. Although the fraction of human cancer related to occupational and incidental exposure to industrial chemicals is debatable, concerns about the development of cancer and birth defects from chemicals in the environment are very great among the public and deserve to be addressed seriously.

Chemical carcinogenesis also provides an excellent experimental model for many kinds of cancers. Historically the paradigm consisted of the events shown in Fig. 1A and was considered to follow a linear path. However, findings in recent years suggest that a scheme such as that presented in Fig. 1B may be more appropriate. "Endogenous events" include things such as aberrant methylation and the generation of oxygen species that damage DNA. Indeed, levels of DNA modifications generated by these events may be higher than those resulting from exogenous chemicals. The group of events designated collectively as "mutation, transduction, disruption of (normal) signaling, and cell proliferation" does not necessarily follow a specific order in all cases. For instance, mutation may be a late event in some cancers. Also, DNA repair may not always be a protective process and there is some limited evidence of error-prone repair in human cells.

With this introduction, we will focus on the "earlier" events in the pathway that we study in our laboratory, i.e., metabolism, formation of adducts, and mutagenesis.

Recent Results in Cancer Research, Vol. 143

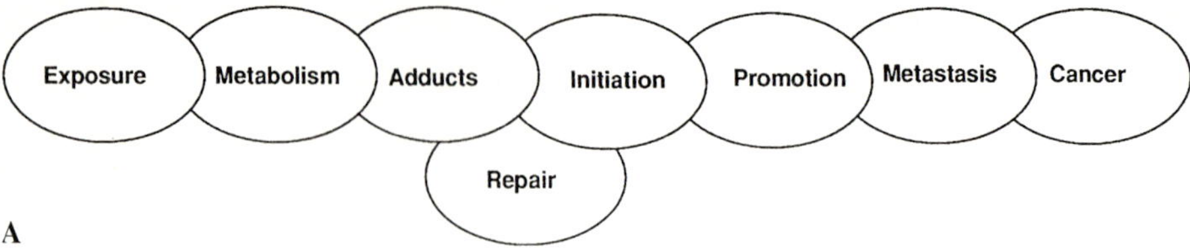

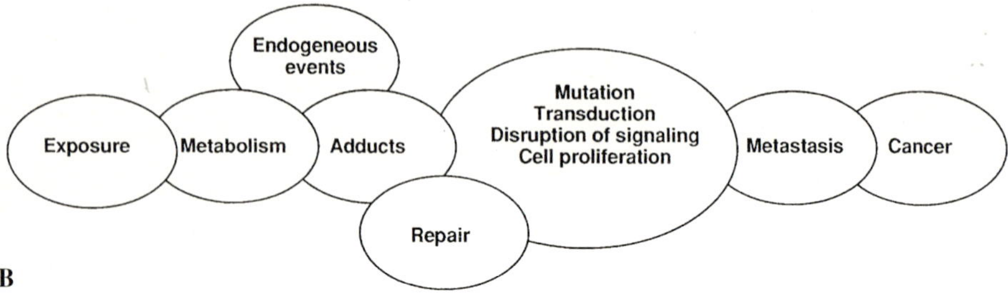

Fig. 1. Paradigms for chemical carcinogenesis: **A** Classical. **B** Revised

Mechanisms of Formation of DNA Adducts

Aflatoxin B_1 (AFB_1)

AFB_1 (Fig. 2) is one of the most potent hepatocarcinogens known and poses a serious health hazard in parts of the world where people ingest large quantities of moldy grain. The events involved in mutagenicity are still unclear, with several frameshifts and base substitutions. The major adduct is an N^7-guanyl derivative of the *exo*-8,9-epoxide, the imidazole ring of which is prone to base-catalyzed opening. Evidence for small amounts of N^7-adenyl adduct has been presented recently (Iyer et al. 1994b).

Human cytochrome P450 (P450) 3A4 forms both aflatoxin Q_1 (AFQ_1) and the *exo*-8,9-epoxide (Raney et al. 1992b; Ueng et al. 1995). Other P450s can form the epoxide to varying extents (Shimada and Guengerich 1989), plus other products. It is of interest that a single P450 can form both activated (8,9-epoxide) and detoxicated (AFQ_1) products, depending upon how AFB_1 interacts with the enzyme. The balance between the two routes can be influenced by the presence of flavonoids (Raney et al. 1992b) or even by alteration of the reduction system used with the P450. Human P450 1A2 forms both the *exo* and *endo* AFB_1-8,9-epoxides, plus the detoxication products aflatoxin M_1 and AFQ_1 (Ueng et al. 1995). The distinction between the *exo* and *endo* epoxides is very important, because the genotoxicity of the former is ~10^3 × the latter (Iyer et al. 1994a). The rationale for the difference involves the short $t_{1/2}$ of the AFB_1-8,9-oxides in H_2O, the intercalation of the AFB_1 ring

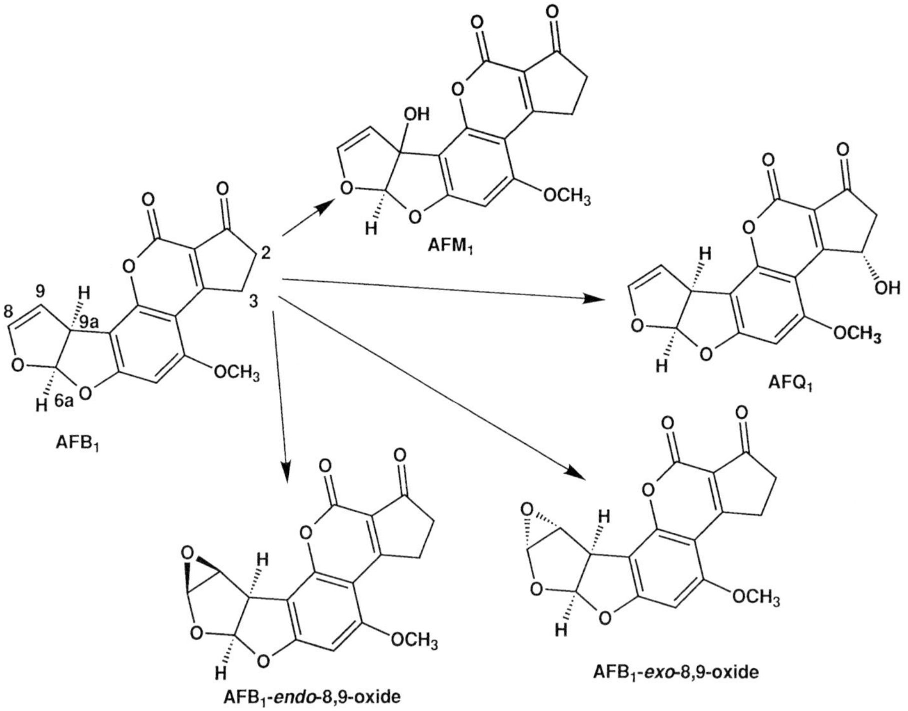

Fig. 2. Major oxidations of aflatoxin B_1 (AFB_1) in human liver microsomes (Ueng et al. 1995)

system between DNA bases, and the essentially obligatory requirement for S_N2 reaction of the (*exo*) epoxide with the purine N7 atom (Iyer et al. 1994a). These factors preclude reaction of the *endo* epoxide with DNA, and it can be considered essentially a detoxication product, formed by P450 1A2. AFQ_1 is not readily epoxidized by P450, and the synthetic epoxide also fails to react well with DNA because of the disruption of intercalation by the 3α-hydroxyl group (Raney et al. 1992b).

The subject of AFB_1 metabolism is quite complex; not only are P450 differences important but glutathione (GSH) S-transferases conjugate both epoxide isomers (Raney et al. 1992a) and can influence the toxicity of AFB_1.

N-Hydroxyl Aryl Amines

The major type of DNA adduct formed from the carcinogenic aryl and heterocyclic amines involves reaction at the C8 atom of guanine (Kadlubar and Hammons 1987). The mechanisms of this reaction has not been clear. The C8 atom of guanine is not a particularly reactive site, except for radical reactions. However, there is no strong evidence that radicals play a significant role in

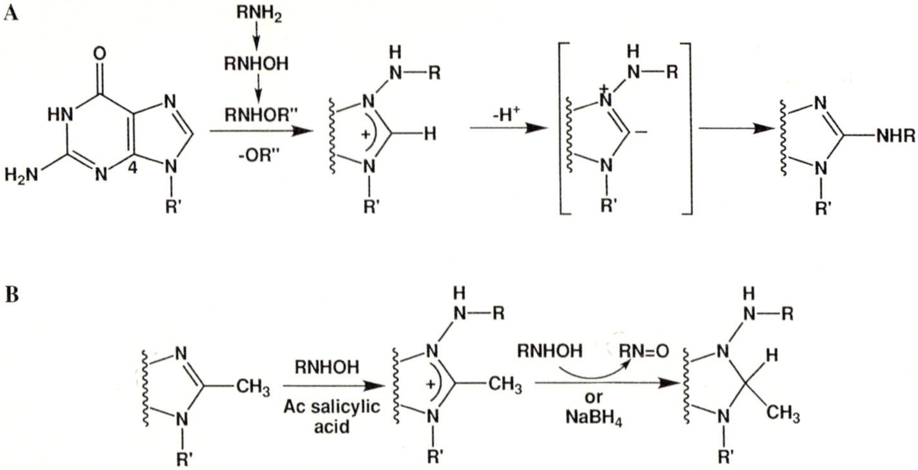

Fig. 3. A Postulated mechanism of Gua C^8-aryl amine adduct formation. **B** Reaction products from 8,9-dimethylGua Characterized in a model reaction system (Humphreys et al. 1992)

adduct formation by activated aryl amines; indeed, nitrenium ion equivalents are more likely (Scribner et al. 1970).

One possible mechanism involves the reaction of a formal nitrenium ion with the nucleophilic guanine (Gua) N7 atom to form a transient adduct that rearranges in a Stevens migration (Fig. 3A). We used guanosine models in which the C8 atom was modified with a small entity to prevent migration. When a methyl was present, we were able to isolate the final product shown in Fig. 3B in high yield (Humphreys et al. 1992). The excess of hydroxyl aryl amine had reduced the intermediate. We also used an 8-bromo derivative of guanosine and were able to rationalize formation of the product with this general mechanism (Humphreys et al. 1992). Attempts are being made to trap or detect Gua-N^7 aryl amine adducts in reactions with unmodified guanosine.

Etheno Adducts

1,N^6-Ethenoadenine (εAde), 3,N^4-ethenocytosine (εCyt), N^2,3-ethenoguanine (N^2 3-εGua), and 1,N^2-ethenoguanine (1,N^2-εGua) can be formed in the reaction of DNA with 2-chlorooxirane, the epoxide of the carcinogen vinyl chloride formed by P450 2E1 (Guengerich et al. 1991). They are also formed with several functional equivalents and the former three etheno adducts have been detected in liver DNA of untreated animals, where they are presumably formed in lipid peroxidation (Fedtke et al. 1990; Barbin et al. 1993). 2-Chlorooxirane rearranges spontaneously to 2-chloroacetaldehyde, which can also react to form all of these etheno adducts. However, evidence has been presented that the epoxide is more important in etheno adduct formation (Guengerich et al. 1981; Guenegerich 1992).

The mechanisms of formation of the etheno adducts from 2-halooxiranes and 2-haloacetaldehyde have been elucidated in this laboratory and serve as a paradigm for some other potentially bifunctional reagents (Fig. 4) (Guengerich and Raney 1992; Guengerich et al. 1993; Guengerich and Persmark 1994). With 2- haloacetaldehydes the initial reaction generally seems to be Schiff base

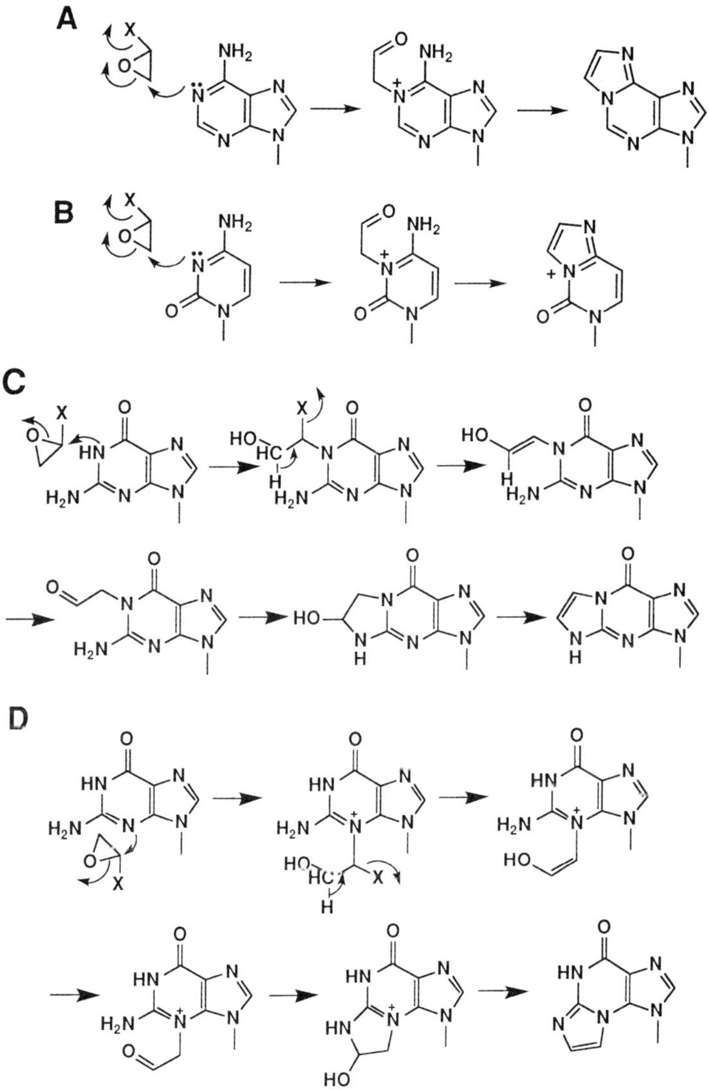

Fig. 4A–D. Pathways of etheno adduct formation from 2-halooxiranes (Guengerich and Raney 1992; Guengerich et al. 1993)

formation between the aldehyde and an exocyclic amine (Guengerich and Persmark 1994). A dominant reaction with the 2-halooxiranes is the attack of a ring nitrogen on the unsubstituted methylene. This reaction explains the formation of εAde and εCyt (Guengerich and Raney 1992). However, labeling studies indicate that 1,N^2-and N^2,3-εGua are formed in a mechanism involving attack of a ring nitrogen (N1 or N3) on the halo-substituted carbon of 2-halooxiranes (Guengerich et al. 1993). This is a less preferred reaction than attack of the N7 or N2 atom on the methylene, but the εGua adducts are minor.

The attack of the guanine N2 atom on the unsubstituted methylene of 2-halooxiranes yields 5,6,7,9-tetrahydro-7-hydroxy-9-oxoimidazo[1,2-*a*]purine, the ring-closed form of N^2-(2-oxoethyl)Gua (Guengerich et al. 1993). This adduct is stable and does not readily dehydrate to from 1,N^2-εGua.

1,2-Dihaloalkanes

In general, enzymatic conjugation of electrophiles with GSH renders them less dangerous. For instance, the AFB_1 epoxides discussed above are conjugated and eliminated, rendering them unable to damage DNA (Raney et al. 1992a). However, sometimes conjugation with GSH is an activation process (Anders et al. 1992).

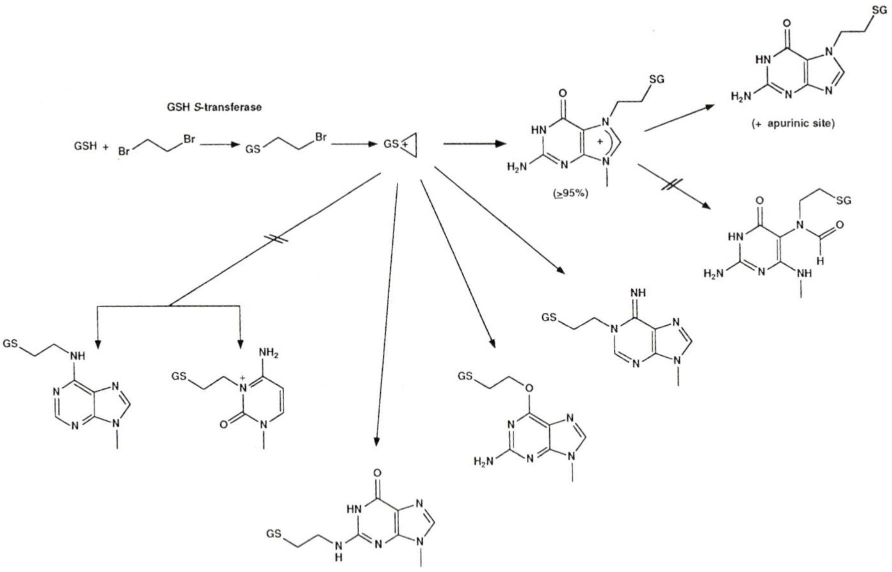

Fig. 5. Activation of 1,2-dibromoethane by glutathione (GSH) conjugation and characterized DNA adducts. *Double lines through an arrow* indicate lack of detection of the product shown (Cmarik et al. 1992)

Rannug et al. (1978) reported that 1,2-dichloroethane was activated by cytosolic enzymes and GSH but not by microsomal oxidation. We found that equal levels of radioactive label from 1,2-dibromoethane and GSH became covalently attached to DNA after reaction with GSH S-transferase (Ozawa and Guengerich 1983). Subsequently we identified *S*-[2-(N^7-guanyl)ethyl] GSH as the major DNA adduct formed in vitro and in vivo (Koga et al. 1986; Inskeep et al. 1986). The reaction is rationalized in terms of a half-mustard and an episulfonium ion, which was implicated in kinetic and stereochemical labeling studies (Peterson et al. 1998). Other adducts that have been identified are shown in Fig. 5 (Kim et al. 1990; Cmarik et al. 1992). There appears to be little tendency for the N^7-guanyl adduct to undergo opening of the imidazole ring (Cmarik et al. 1992), in contrast to some other adducts of this type.

This general type of activation also extends to 1,2,3-trihaloalkanes, such as the nematocide 1,2-dibromo-3-chloropropane (Humphreys et al. 1991). However, a combination of both P450 oxidation and GSH appears to be most effective in forming genotoxic products (Thier et al. 1995).

Dihalomethanes

The above scheme for 1,2-dihaloalkanes also appears to be relevant to dihalomethanes, which are also subject to both oxidation and GSH conjugation (Fig. 6). A clear role of GSH conjugation in genotoxicity had been difficult to demonstrate because of the endogenous levels of GSH and GSH S-transferase activity in test bacteria. We were able to express rat GSH S-transferase directly in *Salmonella typhimurium* TA1535 and show the role of GSH conjugation in the genotoxicity of CH_2Br_2, CH_2BrCl, and CH_2Cl_2, as well as 1,2-dibromoethane (Thier et al. 1993). A model for the GSH-dihalomethane conjugates, *S*-(1-acetoxymethyl)GSH, was prepared and reacted with guanosine to yield *S*-[1-(N^2-guanyl)methyl]GSH as the major adduct (Their et al. 1993). *S*-(1-Acetoxymethyl)GSH was not genotoxic when added directly to bacteria, presumably because of its considerably lesser stability compared to the GSH half-mustards (Böhme et al. 1949; Thier et al. 1993). Minor adducts resulting from modifications with *S*-(1-acetoxymethyl) GSH have not yet been identi-

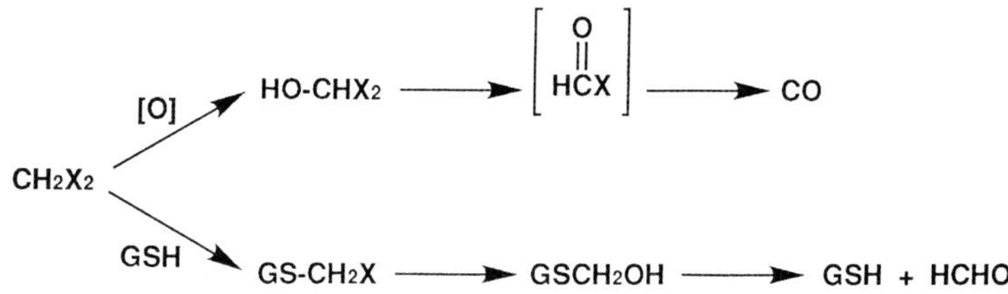

Fig. 6. Transformation of dihalomethanes by oxidation (P450) and conjugation (GSH S- transferase) (Thier et al. 1993)

fied, and current efforts in this laboratory are being directed towards assays of levels of *S*-[1-(N^2-guanyl)methyl]GSH in DNA.

Characterization of Roles of Individual DNA Adducts in Mutations Resulting from Chemicals

Ethylene Dihalides

With most chemicals and even a single activated form of a chemical, a variety of DNA adducts are produced. This is certainly the case with the half-mustards (Fig. 5). The major adduct may not necessarily be the most mutagenic, or may not even be mutagenic at all. Since the role of the half-mustard *S*-(2-haloethyl)-GSH in 1,2-dihaloethane-mediated mutagenicity has been adequately demonstrated, we used such a reagent to do studies on the mutation spectrum seen with bacterophage M13 (RF) DNA in *Escherichia coli*. The mutants were essentially all base pair substitutions and were dominated by GC to AT transitions (Cmarik et al. 1992). No cytosine adducts have ever been found, so we work with the tentative view that guanine adducts are mutagenic. A similar dominance of putative G to A transitions has also been observed by others in *S. typhimurium* (Foster et al. 1988) and *Drosophila melanogaster* (Ballering et al. 1994).

A number of physcial studies have been done with the major adduct *S*-[2-(N^7-gunayl)ethyl]GSH in oligonucleotides (Oida et al. 1991; Kim and Guengerich 1993; Persmark and Guengerich 1994). The results collectively show that the basic B-DNA helical structure is unperturbed (Oida et al. 1991) but that some interactions between the GSH side chain and the DNA bases can be inferred on the basis of comparison with analogs (Kim and Guengerich 1993). The adduct disrupts oligonucleotide pairing to a complement, but we found that the basis of this was in the ΔS; the ΔH for pairing was actually more favorable when the adduct was present (Persmark and Guengerich 1994).

These and other considerations lead us to the view that a proper understanding of mechanism of mutagenesis cannot be obtained solely from comparisons of physical studies of oligonucleotides with mutation data. We are currently using site-specific mutagenesis to examine the mutagenicity of the N^7-, N^2-, and O^6-ethyl-GSH derivatives of guanine in a sequence shown to contain mutations in our earlier M13 experiments. Oligonucleotides containing the N^7-and N^2-guanyl adducts at a specific site (TGCTG*CAAG) have been prepared. In the former case postoligomerization modification was done and the desired adduct was separated by chromatography (Persmark and Guengerich 1994). With the latter, the oligomer was prepared with 2-flurodeoxyinosine at the derived position and reaction with *S*-(2-aminoethyl)GSH gave the desired product. Synthesis of the O^6-guanyl adduct is currently in progress. Interestingly, a recent report suggests a positive effect of O^6-Gua alkyltransferase in the mutagenicity of dibromoalkanes (Abril et al. 1995), but the relevance of such an adduct in this phenomenon is not clear.

Vinyl Halides

The major DNA adduct derived from vinyl halides is N^7-(2-oxoethyl)Gua, but a strong case for its mutagenicity has never been made (Laib et al. 1981). Most of the attention has centered on the etheno adducts, particularly εAde, εCyt, and N^2,3-εGua, all of which are known to be formed. εCyt and N^2,3-εGua have been shown to be mutagenic in site-specific mutagenesis assays (Basu et al. 1993; Cheng et al. 1991). However, some questions about the relevance to vinyl chloride-mediated cancers have been raised with the finding of relatively high levels of these adducts in livers of untreated rats and humans (Fedtke et al. 1990; Barbin et al. 1993).

We discovered that 2-chlorooxirane led to the formation of the stable adduct 5,6,7,9-tetrahydro-7-hydroxy-9-oxoimidazao [1,2-*a*]purine in DNA (4, Fig. 7). An online HPLC/electrospray mass spectrometric assay was developed using a standard adduct synthesized with three ^{13}C atoms, which is added to sample at a level of 5 ng (Müller et al. 1995). Our initial experiments show that the levels of this adduct present in DNA treated in vitro with 2-chlorooxirane is similar to levels of the 1,N^2-εGua adduct detected in DNA under similar conditions, which is an order of magnitude greater than N^2,3-εGua (Guengerich et al. 1993). Further studies indicate that this adduct does not seem to be present in untreated DNA and it appears to be a specific adduct related to exposure to vinyl halides; in vivo studies are in progress.

Other studies are being done to evaluate the mutagenic potential of this adduct and 1,N^2-εGua. The synthesis of oligonucleotides containing 5,6,7,9-tetrahydro-7-hydroxy-9-oxoimidazo[1,2-*a*]purine has not been trivial because of unexpected problems related to the need to close the imidazo ring under acid conditions, to block the 7-hydroxyl group, and to attach the deoxyribose. We have not developed a method involving (1) conversion to Gua to 2-fluorohypoxanthine, (2) condensation with 2-aminoacetaldehyde dimethylacetal, (3) HCl treatment to close the ring, (4) acetylation of the 7-hydroxyl, (5) enzymatic attachment of deoxyribose with *Lactobacillus trans-N*-deoxyribosylase, (6) dimethyltrityl and phosphoramidite modification of the sugar

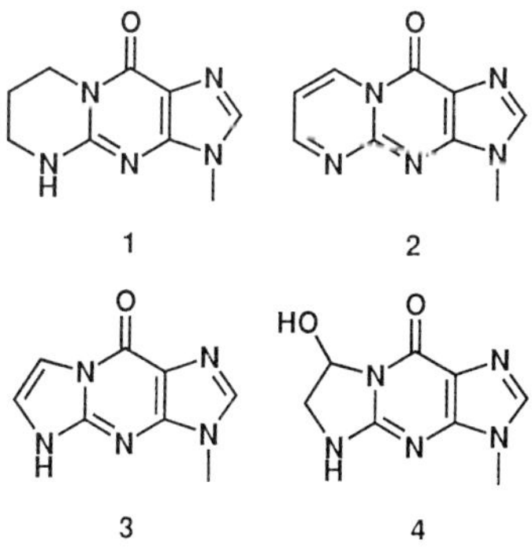

Fig. 7. Structures of **1** propanoGua, **2** the malondialdehyde:Gua adduct, **3** 1,N^2-εGua, and **4** 5,6,7,9-tetrahydro-7-hydroxy-9-oxoimidazo[1,2-*a*]-purine

hydroxyls, (7) oligonucleotide synthesis, and (8) mild base deprotection of the oligomer. The similarity of this adduct and $1,N^2$-εGua to the mutagenic homologs (Basu et al. 1993; Cheng et al. 1991) invites comparison (Fig. 7).

Molecular Mechanisms of Mutation at DNA Adduct Sites by Polymerases

The above brief discussion of two adduct projects shows some of the difficulties in understanding the relationship between DNA adducts and mutations. In many projects of this type there is a real risk in directing experiments towards those that will be merely descriptive. Many physical studies tend to ignore the relevant biology, or assume no role of the polymerases. Also, mutation frequencies can be influenced by the nature of the cellular system and repair backgrounds, which may be interesting in themselves but confounding the study of the mechanism of mutagenesis. Most mammalian polymerases are very complex, and bacterial and viral enzymes have been exploited as models.

We feel that a better understanding of the enzymology of DNA polymerases, as they encounter DNA adducts, is essential to understanding why mutations occur. Alternatively, one can pose the question as one of why so few errors occur when the polymerases copy past some very complex adducts. Some steady-state kinetic approaches to studying replication have been published (e.g., Boosalis et al. 1987). However, the polymerase catalytic cycle is complex (Fig. 8) and a proper understanding of an enzyme's mechanism cannot often be achieved only with the application of steady-state kinetics

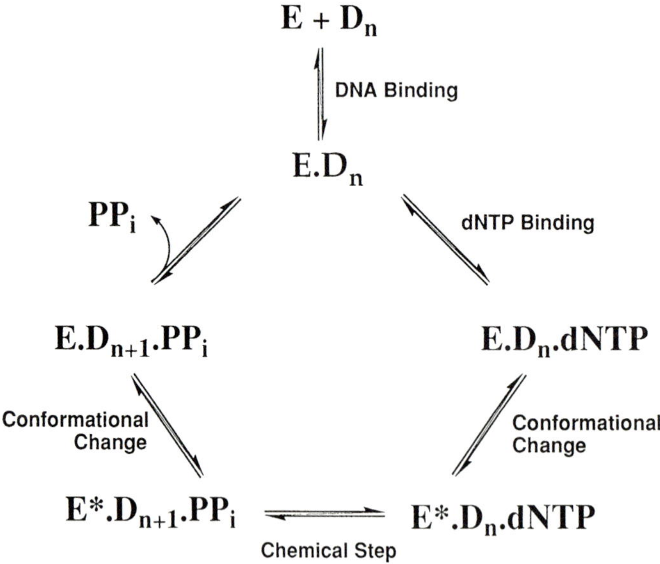

Fig. 8. Kinetic scheme for stepwise polymerization (Johnson 1993)

5' C C G C A G A C G C A G 3'
3' G G C G T C T G C G T C *G**C T C 5'

Fig. 9. Oligonucleotide system used for X-ray crystallography and single turnover kinetic studies with polymerases. *G** represents O^6-MeG

(Kuby 1991). We have prepared several polymerases devoid of exonuclease activity and began to use these to study a series of DNA adducts that appear to vary in their mutagenicity.

Crystallography with Escherichia coli pol II

Recently *E. coli* pol II *exo*$^-$, homologous to the eukaryotic α class polymerases, has been crystallized (Anderson et al. 1994). We feel that high resolution structures of a polymerase incorporating normal and "mutagenic" nucleotides across from a lesion would be valuable. However, biophysical studies of this sort would be hampered by the low mutation frequencies associated with most adducts. To this end, we prepared an oligonucleotide containing O^6-methyl-Gua and showed that a T was incorporated across from it instead of a C, in this sequence context (Fig. 9). One type of analysis used yielded $(V_{max}/K_m)_T/(V_{max}/K_m)_C \cong 5$ (Boosalis et al. 1987), suggesting that ~80% of the time the polymerase will make a mutation. To focus events in the crystal towards binding of the nucleotide, we used an oligomer containing a ribose at the terminus to prevent elongation. An *exo*$^-$ mutant of pol II was used to direct the oligomer into the polymerase site and prevent any nuclease action. The crystal work is now in progress.

Single-Turnover Kinetics

As pointed out in Fig. 8, the kinetics of polymerization are very complex. In this scheme there are 12 individual rate constants. The situation is also complicated in that many of the polymerases are highly processive with DNA but in vitro experiments with defined oligomers require that the enzyme bind and release the oligomer in each cycle. These steps can limit the rates, and it is desirable to obtain rates of individual reactions with the use of pre-steady-state kinetic methods. Such an approach has been used to study the mechanisms of how pol I, pol 7, and HIV reverse transcriptase copy normal DNA and RNA (Mizrahi et al. 1986; Johnson 1993; Hsieh et al. 1993; Spence et al. 1995). These studies indicate that K_m values (for nucleotides) are complex expressions and do not reflect nucleotide affinity (Johnson 1993). In replication of normal DNA bases, conformational steps [apparently induced by nucleotide binding (Johnson 1993)] are often rate-limiting, while in mispairing among the four natural bases the formation of phosphodiester bonds – a chemical step – limits the rates (Eger and Benkovic 1992; Johnson 1993). Values of most of the individual rate constants have been obtained.

This approach requires the use of rapid mixing/quenching systems and has been applied to the study of carcinogen-DNA adducts in two cases, one involving O^6-methylGua and *E. coli* pol I (Klenow fragment) (Tan et al. 1994) and the other pol 7 and the C^8-guanyl1:2-acetylaminofluorenyl adduct (Lindsley and Fuchs 1994). We have studied the incorporation of C and T opposite O^6-metyhlGua with *E. coli* pol I *exo*$^-$ and pol II *exo*$^-$ in the oligonucleotide system shown in Fig. 9. The same oligomer in which 8-oxo-7,8-dihydroGua [synthesized according to (Bodepudi et al. 1992)] has been substituted for O^6-methylGua has also been studied with the same enzymes. The latter adduct is a major one derived from the reaction of oxygen radicals (especially OH·) with DNA. It has been shown to be miscoding in several prokaryotic and eukaryotic systems; in our system the parameters $(V_{max}/K_m)_A/(V_{max}/K_m)_C$ indicate incorporation of A about 10%–20% the time by either pol I *exo*$^-$ or pol II *exo*$^-$.

Pre-steady-state kinetics with the unmodified ("wild-type") oligomer (Fig. 9) show a rapid "burst" of activity consistent with a rapid cycle followed by a steady-state velocity corresponding to release and binding of oligomers. This burst is lost with the adducted oligomers and the rates of the reactions are even slower than the release/rebinding step seen with the normal oligomer. When 8-oxo-7,8-dihydroGua is present, both the incorporation of the normal (C) and abnormal (A) bases are slowed. This is considered to be an effect on the rate constant for the chemical step (phosphodiester bond formation) and not conformation change, although we have not yet measured individual rate constants. In support of this view, there are very large elemental effects (10- to 50-fold decreases) when phosphorothioate dNTP analogs are used in place of the normal ones. It should be possible to further define the changes in rates of individual steps affected by this DNA modification and also to elucidate the mechanisms of "polymerase" stalling/idling suggested qualitatively by others for various adducts (Sambamurti et al. 1988) using these methods.

References

Abril N, Luqueromero FL, Prietoalamo MJ, Margison GP, Pueyo C (1995) ogt Alkyltransferase enhances dibromoalkane mutagenicity in excision repair-deficient *Escherichia coli* K-12. Mol Carcinogen 12: 110–117

Anders MW, Dekant W, Vamvakas S (1992) Glutathione-dependent toxicity. Xenobiotica 22: 1135–1145

Anderson WF, Prince DB, Yu H, McEntee K, Goodman MF (1994) Crystallization of DNA polymerase II from *Escherichia coli*. J Mol Biol 238: 120–122

Ballering LAP, Nivard MJM, Vogel EW (1994) Mutation spectra of 1,2-dibromoethane, 1,2-dichloroethane and 1-bromo-2-chloroethane in excision repair proficient and repair deficient strains of *Drosophila melanogaster*. Carcinogenesis 15: 869–875

Barbin A, El Ghissassi F, Nair J, Bartsch H (1993) Lipid peroxidation leads to formation of 1,N^6-ethenoadenine and 3,N^4-ethenocytosine in DNA bases. Proc Am Assoc Cancer Res 34: 130–136

Basu AK, Wood ML, Niedernhofer LJ, Ramos LA, Essigmann JM (1993) Mutagenic and genotoxic effects of three vinyl chloride-induced DNA lesions: 1,N^6-ethenoadenine, 3,N^4-ethenocytosine, and 4-amino-5-(imidazol-2-yl)imidazole. Biochemistry 32: 12793–12801

Bodepudi V, Shibutani S, Johnson F (1992) Synthesis of 2′-deoxy-7,8-dihydro-8-oxoguanosine and 2′-deoxy-7,8-dihydro-8-oxoadenosine and their incorporation into oligomeric DNA. Chem Res Toxicol 5: 608–617

Boosalis MS, Petruska J, Goodman MF (1987) DNA polymerase insertion fidelity: gel assay for site-specific kinetics. J Biol Chem 262: 14689–14696

Böhme VH, Fischer H, Frank R (1949) Darstellung und Eigenschaften der α-halogenierten Thioäther. Ann Chemie 563: 54–72

Cartwright RA (1984) Cancer epidemiology. In: Searle CE (ed) Chemical carcinogens. American Chemical Society, Washington DC, pp 1–39

Cheng KC, Preston BD, Cahill DS, Dosanjh MK, Singer B, Loeb LA (1991) The vinyl chloride DNA derivative, N^2,3-ethenoguanine, produces G→A transition in *E. coli.* Proc Natl Acad Sci USA 88: 9974–9978

Cmarik JL, Humphreys WG, Bruner KL, Llyod RS, Tibbetts C, Guengerich FP (1992) Mutation spectrum and sequence alkylation selectivity resulting from modification of bacteriophage M13mp18 with *S*-(2-chloroethyl)gluathione. Evidence for a role of *S*-[2-(N^7-guanyl)ethyl]glutathione as a mutagenic lesion formed from ethylene dibromide. J Biol Chem 267: 6672–6679

Eger BT, Benkovic SJ (1992) Minimal kinetic mechanism for misincorporation by DNA polymerase I (Klenow fragment). Biochemistry 31: 9227–9236

Fedtke N, Boucheron JA, Walker VE, Swenberg JA (1990) Vinyl chloride-induced DNA adducts. II. Formation and persistence of 7-(2′-oxoethyl)guanine and N^2,3-ethenoguanine in rat tissue DNA. Carcinogenesis 11: 1287–1292

Foster PL, Wilkinson WG, Miller JK, Sullivan AD, Barnes WM (1988) An analysis of the mutagenicity of 1,2-dibromoethane to *Escherichia coli*: influence of DNA repair activities and metabolic pathways. Mutat Res 194: 171–181

Guengerich FP (1992) Roles of the vinyl chloride oxidation products 2-chlorooxirane and 2-chloroacetaldehyde in the in vitro formation of etheno adducts of DNA bases. Chem Res Toxicol 5: 2–5

Guengerich FP, Persmark M (1994) Mechanism of formation of ethenoguanine adducts from 2-haloacetaldehydes: ^{13}C labeling patterns of 2-bromoacetaldehyde. Chem Res Toxicol 7: 205–208

Guengerich FP, Raney VM (1992) Formation of etheno adducts of adenosine and cytidine from 1-halooxiranes. Evidence for a mechanism involving initial reaction with the endocyclic nitrogens. J Am Chem Soc 114: 1074–1080

Guengerich FP, Mason PS, Stott WT, Fox TR, Watanabe PG (1981) Roles of 2-haloethylene oxides and 2-haloacetaldehydes derived from vinyl bromide and vinyl chloride in irreversible binding to protein and DNA. Cancer Res 41: 4391–4398

Guengerich FP, Kim D-H, Iwasaki M (1991) Role of human cytochrome P-450 IIE1 in the oxidation of several low molecular weight cancer suspects. Chem Res Toxicol 4: 168–179

Guengerich FP, Persmark M, Humphreys WG (1993) Formation of 1,N^2 - and N^2,3-ethenoguanine derivatives from 2-halooxiranes: isotopic labeling studies and formation of a hemiaminal derivative of N^2-(-oxoethyl)guanine. Chem Res Toxicol 6: 635–648

Hsieh J-C, Zinnen S, Modrich P (1993) Kinetic mechanism of the DNA-dependent DNA polymerase activity of human immunodeficiency of virus reverse transcriptase. J Biol Chem 268: 24607–24613

Humphreys WG, Kim DH, Guengerich FP (1991) Isolation and characterization of N^7-

guanyl adducts derived from 1,2-dbromo-3-chloropropane. Chem Res Toxicol 4: 445–453

Humphreys WG, Kadlubar FF, Guengerich FP (1992) Mechanism of C8 alkylation of guanyl residues by activated arylamines: evidence for a role of initial attack at the N7 atom. Proc Natl Acad Sci USA 89: 8278–8282

Inskeep PB, Koga N, Cmarik JL, Guengerich FP (1986) Covalent binding of 1,2-dihaloalkanes to DNA and stability of the major DNA adduct, *S*-[2-(N^7-guanyl)ethyl]glutathione. Cancer Res 46: 2839–2844

Iyer R, Coles B, Raney KD, Thier R, Guengerich FP, Harris TM (1994a) DNA adduction by the potent carcinogen aflatoxin B_1: mechanistic studies. J Am Chem Soc 116: 1603–1609

Iyer RS, Voehler MW, Harris TM (1994b) Adenine adduct of aflatoxin B_1: epoxide. J Am Chem Soc 116: 8863–8869

Johnson KA (1993) Conformational coupling in DNA polymerase fidelity. Annu Rev Biochem 62: 685–713

Kadlubar FF, Hammons GJ (1987) The role of ctyochrome P-450 in the metabolism of chemical carcinogens. In: Guengerich FP (ed) Mammalian cytochromes P-450, vol 2. CRC, Boca Raton, pp 81–130

Kim D-H, Humphreys WG, Guengerich FP (1990) Characterization of *S*-[2-(N^1-adenyl)ethyl]glutathione formed in DNA and RNA from 1,2-dibromoethane. Chem Res Toxicol 3: 587–594

Kim M-S, Guengerich FP (1993) Interactions of N^7-guanyl methyl- and thioethersubstituted d(CATGCCT) derivatives with d(AGGNATC). Chem Res Toxicol 6: 900–905

Koga N, Inskeep PB, Harris TM, Guengerich FP (1986) *S*-[2-(N^7-Guanyl)ethyl]glutathione, the major DNA adduct formed from 1,2-dibromoethane. Biochemistry 25: 2192–2198

Kuby SA (1991) A study of enzymes. Enzyme catalysis, kinetics and substrate binding, vol I. CRC, Boca Raton

Laib RJ, Gwinner LM, Bolt HM (1981) DNA alkylation by vinyl chloride metabolites: etheno derivatives or 7-alkylation of guanine? Chem Biol Interact 37: 219–231

Lindsley JE, Fuchs RPP (1994) Use of single-turnover kinetics to study bulky adduct bypass by T7 polymerase. Biochemistry 33: 764–772

Mizrahi V, Benkovic P, Benkovic SJ (1986) Mechanism of DNA polymerase I: exonuclease/polymerase activity switch and DNA sequence dependence of pyrophosphorolysis and misincorporation reactions. Proc Natl Acad Sci USA 83: 5769–5773

Müller M, Belas F, Ueno H, Guengerich FP (1995) Development of a mass spectrometric assay for 5,6,7,9-tetrahydro-7-hydroxy-9-oxoimidazo [1,2-*a*]pyrine in DNA modified by 2-chlorooxirane. In: Proceedings of the 5th interanational symposium on biological reactive intermediates. 4–8 Jan, Munich (in press)

Oida T, Humphreys WG, Guengerich FP (1991) Preparation and characterization of oligonucleotides containing *S*-[2-(N^7-guanyl)ethyl]glutathione. Biochemistry 30: 10513–10522

Ozawa N, Guengerich FP (1983) Evidence for formation of an *S*-[2-(N^7-guanyl)-ethyl]glutathione adduct in glutathione-mediated binding of 1,2-dibromoethane to DNA. Proc Natl Acad Sci USA 80: 5266–5270

Persmark M, Guengerich FP (1994) Spectroscopic and thermodynamic characterization of the interaction of N^7-guanyl thioether derivatives of d(TGCTG*CAAG) with potential complements. Biochemistry 33: 8662–8672

Peterson LA, Harris TM, Guengerich FP (1988) Evidence for an episulfonium ion intermediate in the formation of *S*-[2-(N^7-guanyl)ehtyl]glutathione in DNA. J Am Chem Soc 110: 3284–3291

Raney KD, Meyer DJ, Ketterer B, Harris TM, Guengerich FP (1992a) Glutathione conjugation of aflatoxin B_1 *exo* and *endo* epoxides by rat and human glutathione S-transferases. Chem Res Toxicol 5: 470–478

Raney KD, Shimada T, Kim D-H, Groopman JD, Harris TM, Guengerich FP (1992b) Oxidation of aflatoxins and sterigmatocystin by human liver microsomes: significance of aflatoxin Q_1 as a detoxication product of aflatoxin B_1. Chem Res Toxicol 5: 202–210

Rannug U, Sundvall A, Ramel C (1978) The mutagenic effect of 1,2-dichloroethane on *Salmonella typhimurium*. I. Activation through conjugation with glutathione in vitro. Chem Biol Interactions 20: 1–16

Sambamurti K, Callahan J, Luo X, Perkins CP, Jacobsen JS, Humayun MZ (1988) Mechanisms of mutagenesis by a bulky DNA lesion at the guanine N7 position. Genetics 120: 863–873

Scribner JD, Miller JA, Miller EC (1970) Nucleophilic substitution on carcinogenic *N*-acetoxy-*N*-arylacetamides. Cancer Res 30: 1570–1579

Shimada T, Guengerich FP (1989) Evidence for cytochrome P-450_{NF}, the nifedipine oxidase, being the prinicpal enzyme involved in the bioactivation of aflatoxins in human liver. Proc Natl Acad Sci USA 86: 462–465

Spence RA, Katti WM, Anderson KS, Johnson KA (1995) Mechanism of inhibition of HIV-1 reverse transcriptase by nonnucleoside inhibitors. Science 267: 988–993

Tan HB, Swann PF, Chance EM (1994) Kinetic analysis of the coding properties of O^6-methylguanine in DNA: the crucial role of the conformation of the phosphodiester bond. Biochemistry 33: 5335–5346

Thier R, Pemble SE, Taylor JB, Humphreys WG, Persmark M, Ketterer B, Guengerich FP (1993) Expression of mammalian glutathione *S*-transferase 5–5 in *Salmonella typhimurium* TA1535 leads to base-pair mutations upon exposure to dihalomethanes. Proc Natl Acad Sci USA 90: 8576–8580

Thier R, Müller M, Taylor JB, Pemble SE, Ketterer B, Guengerich FP (1995) Enhancement of bacterial mutagenicity of bifunctional alkylating agents by expression of mammalian glutathione *S*-transferase. Chem Res Toxicol 8: 465–472

Ueng Y-F, Shimada T, Yamazaki H, Guengerich FP (1995) Oxidation of aflatoxin B_1 by bacterial recombinant human cytochrome P450 enzymes. Chem Res Toxicol 8: 218–225

Assessment of the Tumor-Initiating Potential of α,β-Unsaturated Carbonyl Compounds by ³²P Postlabeling Quantification of DNA Adducts In Vivo

E. Eder, Budiawan, D. Schuler, and M. Otteneder

Department of Toxicology, University of Würzburg, Versbacher Str. 9, 97078 Würzburg, Germany

Introduction

α,β-Unsaturated carbonyl compounds are reactive bifunctional substances which react readily with biological macromolecules, e.g., proteins and DNA. They are important industrial chemicals and environmental pollutants, formed by combustion; they are also, however, biologically formed by microorganisms during wood lignin degradation, formation of humic and fulvic acid, and by plants and animals. These compounds are present in fruit juices and in other nonalcoholic and alcoholic beverages and even in drinking water (Eder et al. 1993). The endogenous formation of these compounds during lipid peroxidation but also by other physiological and pathophysiological processes is of high significance (Witz 1989). Benedetti et al. (1984) found concentrations of 4-hydroxynonenal of about 100 μM in tissues near peroxidating membranes and Koster et al. (1986) calculated concentrations of 4.5 mM in the lipid double layer during lipid peroxidation. Furthermore, these compounds can diffuse within the endoplasmatic reticulum where they are formed associated with the lipid core to the nucleus without cytosolic detoxication (Brambilla et al. 1986). But even cytosolic conjugation with glutathione or similar compounds does not necessarily lead to detoxication since this aldehyde thiol conjugation is reversible and the adducts can dissociate and regenerate the respective α,β-unsaturated carbonyl compounds at the target site (Witz 1989).

Several different DNA adducts are formed with these compounds. We investigated the reaction of about 20 α,β-unsaturated carbonyl compounds with nucleosides and nucleotides and identified and characterized different 1,N^2-cyclic propanodeoxyguanosine adducts, 7,8-cyclic adducts, bis cyclic adducts, and other adducts (Eder et al. 1990, 1993; Eder and Hoffmann 1993, 1994). The 1,N^2-cyclic propanodeoxyguanosine adducts are promutagenic DNA lesions (Marinelli et al. 1990), which lead to G→T transversion (Moriya et al. 1989) but also to frameshift mutation (Benamira et al. 1992). We found strand-breaking activity (Eder et al. 1993) and induction of deletions (Czerny et al., unpublished results). Thymidine adducts lead to DNA-protein-crosslinking (van Beerendonk et al. 1992).

α,β-Unsaturated carbonyl compounds possess a clear mutagenic potential (Eder et al. 1990, 1993, 1994a,b), and many of these compounds have meanwhile been shown to be carcinogenic (see references in Eder et al. 1993).

All data available to date suggest that this group of substances plays a significant role in human carcinogenicity due to the high exposure of humans and the genotoxic, mutagenic, and carcinogenic activities just described. Nevertheless the data base does not allow a clear risk assessment. Detection of DNA adducts of these compounds in animal and human tissue would allow a better evaluation of the role of this group of substances in human cancer. Therefore, we developed a sensitive ^{32}P postlabeling detection method for such adducts.

Methods

The DNA adduct standards were synthesized, isolated, and characterized, and the structures elucidated as described recently (Eder and Hoffman 1994).

The HPLC and thin-layer chromatography (TLC) methods for optimal separation of the adducts were worked out and the chromatographic conditions are shown in the legends to the respective figures in "Results."

The enzyme kinetics of the stability of adducts as well as those of the nonmodified nucleotides towards nuclease P1 were performed according to Reddy and Randerath (1986).

DNA digestion was carried out according to a modification of the method of Vaca et al. (1992): 10 μg DNA were incubated with 1.6 U micrococcal nuclease (Sigma, Deisenhofen, Germany), 5.4 μg spleen phosphodiesterase (Boehringer, Mannheim, Germany) in 25 mM $CaCl_2$ and 50 mM succinate buffer pH 6.0 in a volume of 12 μl for 3 h at 37 °C.

Nuclease P1 enrichment was carried out according to Reddy and Randerath (1986): 30 nmol of nucleotides (or 10 μg DNA) in 3 μl 250 mM sodium acetate buffer pH 5.0, 1.8 μl 0.3 mM ZnCl and 1.5 μl (0.5 μg) nuclease P1 from penicillium citrinum (Boehringer) were incubated for 40 min at 37 °C. The reaction was terminated by addition of 1.5 μl 0.5 M "Tris-base."

When checking the stability of adducts against nuclease P1, 6 nmol of adducts was incubated with nuclease P1 for 120 min as just described.

^{32}P Postlabeling Reaction

Either adduct standards (fmol-pmol) dissolved in 10 μl water or 18.3 μl (10 μg) of DNA digest were mixed with a solution of 4.2 μl kinase buffer (5 mM spermidine, Serva, Heidelberg, Germany; 100 mM dithiothreitol, Merck, Darmstadt, Germany; 25 mM $MgCl_2$, Merck; 200 mM bicin, Merck, pH 7.8),

5 μl ^{32}P-γ-ATP (60 μCi, 3500 Ci/mmol, Amersham, Braunschweig, Germany) and 3–5 units of T4-polynucleotide kinase (Promega, Madison, WI, USA) and incubated for 55 min at 37 °C. Then 4 μl (40 mU) of potato apyrase (Sigma, St. Louis, MO, USA) were added and the mixture was incubated for a further 30 min at 37 °C.

Animal Studies

Eight-week-old female F 344 rats (weighing 200–230 g each) were purchased from Harlan Winkelmann, Borchem, Germany. The animals were housed in polycarbonate cages and had free access to food and drinking water.

Groups of four rats were given 300 mg/kg body weight of crotonaldehyde dissolved in 1 ml corn oil. The rats were killed after 20 h and liver, lung, kidney, and large intestine were excised for analysis of DNA adducts.

DNA isolation (phenol extraction) was performed according to a modification of the method of Marmur (1961). The purity of DNA was checked by the ratio of UV absorptions at 260 nm and 280 nm.

In a second experiment rats received 10 mg/kg body weight of crotonaldehyde for 4 weeks, 5 days a week, and the animals were killed 1 day, 1 week, and 2 weeks after the last gavage.

Results

Synthesis, Separation, and Stability of Adduct Standards

Figure 1a shows the HPLC of the synthesized adduct standards of hexenal (1a,b, two diastereomers of 1, N^2-propanodeoxyguanosine-3′-monophosphate) and the respective UV spectra (Fig. 1b). Similar HPLC data were obtained with deoxyguanosine monophosphate adducts of crotonaldehyde (2a,b) (Fig. 2). The UV, magnetic resonance imaging (MRI), and mass spectra of the respective 1,N^2 propanodeoxyguanosine-3′-monophosphate adducts of 2-hexenal and crotonaldehyde (not shown here) are consistent with those of the respective 1,N^2-propanodeoxyguanosine adducts (Eder and Hoffman 1992, 1993). The adducts were revealed to be stable at pH values between 4 and 11 for 120 h at 37 °C (Fig. 3).

Nuclease P1 Enrichment

The respective adducts were also relatively stable towards nuclease P1. Figure 4a shows the Michaelis-Menten kinetics of the degradation of deoxythymidine-3′-monophosphate (3′-dTMP) by nuclease P1, and Fig. 4b, the kinetics of the degradation of the respective hexenal adducts. 3′-dTMP was the

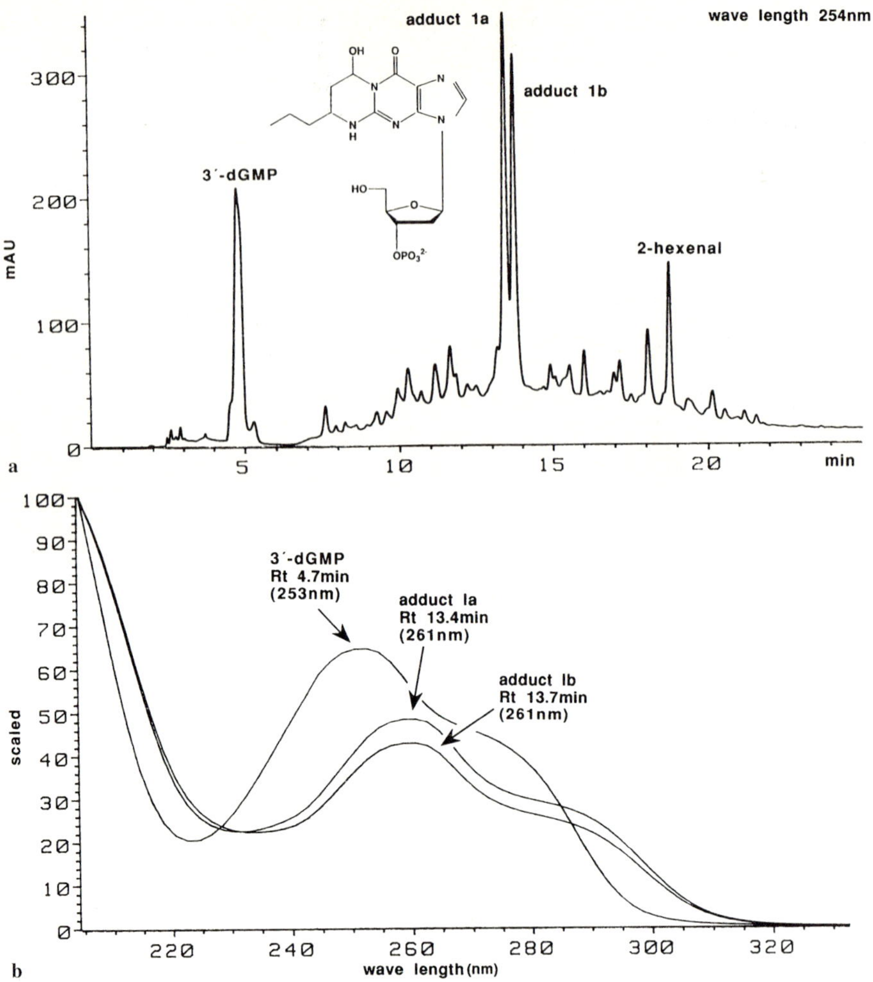

Fig. 1. a HPLC of the two diastereomers 1a and 1b, i.e., the 1,N^2-propanodeoxyguanosine-3′-monophosphate (*trans*) of 2-hexenal. Column: Knauer Eurosphere RP18, 5 μm, 250 × 4 mm. Gradient: 0%–100% B in 20 min; **A** 10 mM ammonium formate buffer pH 4.7, **B** methanol. **b** UV-spectra of 3′ dGMP and the adduct diastereomers 1a, 1b (diode array detector, HP)

most stable among all DNA mononucleotides. In the case of 3′-dTMP, a K_m of 4.7 mM and v_{max} of 8.5 nmol/min per μg enzyme and with the respective hexenal adduct a $K_m = 3.9$ mM and $v_{max} = 6.5$ pmol/min per μg enzyme were determined. From this data a rate constant of $k = 0.10$ min^{-1}/μg enzyme for 3′-dTMP and a rate constant of $k = 0.000077$ min^{-1}/μg enzyme for the adduct can be calculated in case of low substrate concentrations. This means that according to $[X_t] = [X_0] \cdot e^{kt}$ an enrichment factor of 7×10^7 is obtained after 3 h of incubation. Similar results for the nuclease P1 enrichment were found with the

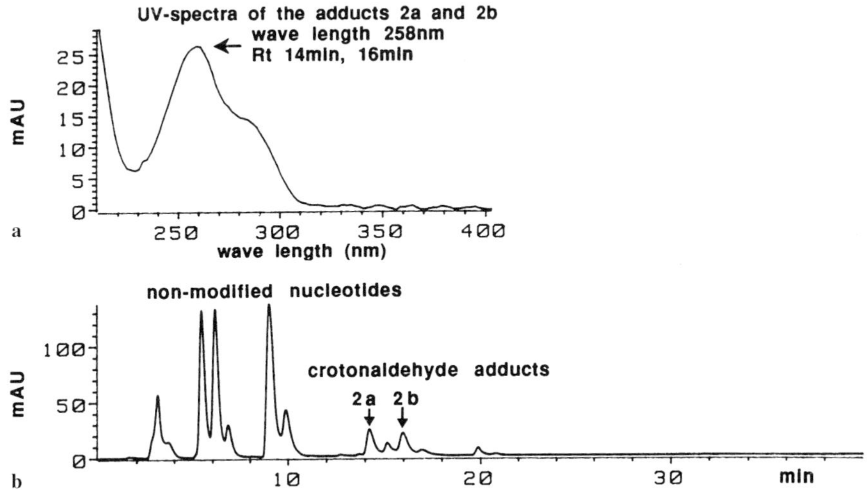

Fig. 2. HPLC of the DNA digest after incubation with crotonaldehyde. Gradient: 0%–60% B in 45 min; **a** 4 m*M* Tris buffer pH 5.7; **b** methanol: water (4:6). Column: Knauer Lichrosphere RP18, 5 μm, 250 × 4 mm

adducts of crotonaldehyde. Figure 5a shows the ^{32}P postlabeling results after incubation of DNA with crotonaldehyde and digestion of the modified DNA without nuclease P1 enrichment, and Fig. 5b, the labeling results of the modified DNA after nuclease P1 enrichment. All nonmodified labeled mononucleotides of the digested DNA found as spots in Fig. 5a are not visible in

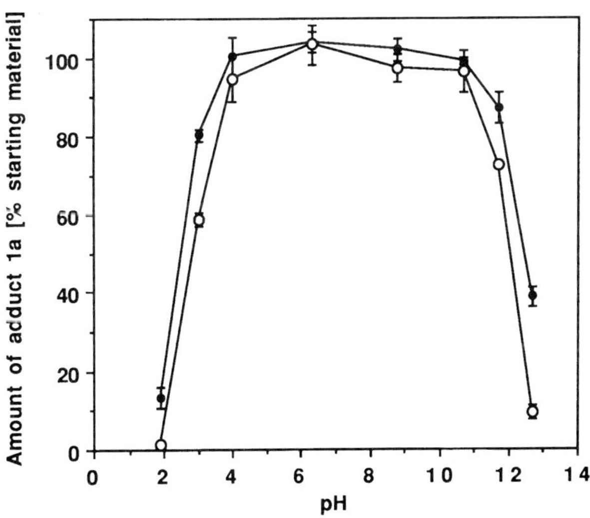

Fig. 3. Stability of the 2-hexenal adduct 1a depending on the pH value. *Solid circles*, after 48 h; *Open circles*, after 120 h

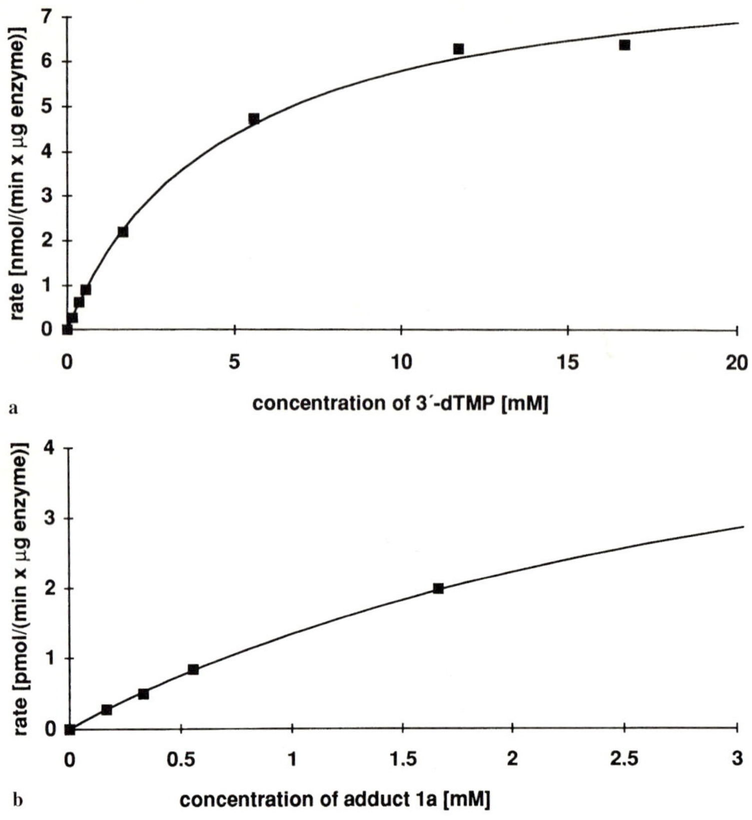

Fig. 4. a Nuclease P1 degradation of 3′-dTMP. **b** Nuclease P1 degradation of adduct 1a

Fig. 5b, where only the spots of the labeled adducts 2a,b can be seen. This demonstrates that practically all unmodified nucleobases are decomposed by nuclease P1, whereas the adducts are not degraded.

Postlabeling

All adduct standards of α,β-unsaturated carbonyl compounds investigated so far in our group (acrolein, crotonaldehyde, 2-hexenal, 4-hydroxy-2-nonenal) can be well labeled with [γ-^{32}P] ATP using the method just described. In all cases labeling efficiencies of more than 30% were found. Fig. 6a shows the dependence of labeling efficiency (LE) of the crotonaldehyde adducts on incubation time. Figure 6b shows the LE at different pH values and Fig. 6c the dependence of the LE on the amount of T4-polynucleotide kinase (PNK). Fig. 6d demonstrates that the LE of crotonaldehyde adducts is very high (80%–90%) at low adduct amounts, i.e., in the range of 1–100 fmol.

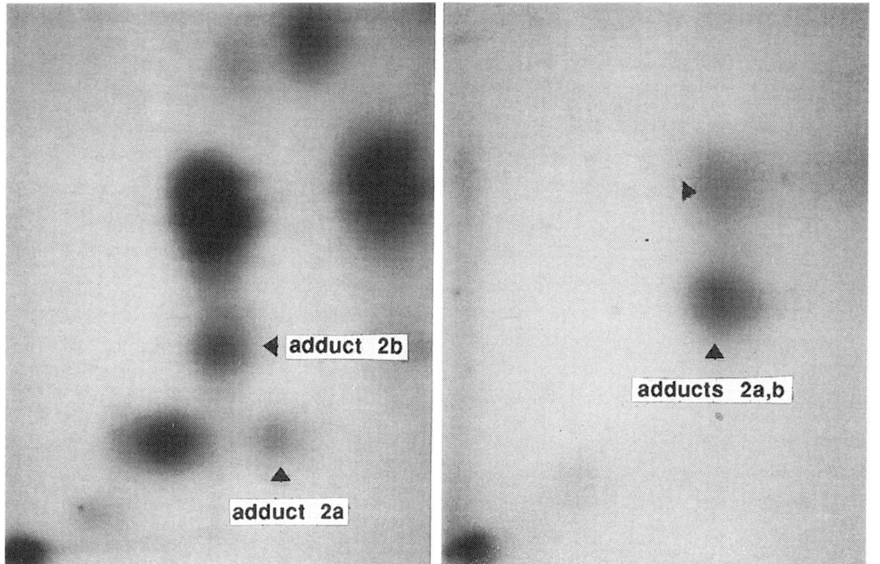

Fig. 5. ^{32}P Postlabeling results of digested DNA after incubation with crotonaldehyde **a** without nuclease P1 treatment, **b** after nuclease P1 treatment. D1: ammonium formate buffer 0.7 *M*, pH 3.5. D2: ammonium sulphate buffer 0.3 *M*, 10 m*M* sodium phosphate buffer, pH 7.5

With both the crotonaldehyde adducts and the hexenal adducts, relative adduct labeling (RAL) of 10^{-9} was achieved with the nuclease P1 procedure. The detection limit is presently 1 fmol adduct per 11.1 μmol of nucleobases or 1 adduct per 10^{10} bases if using [γ-^{32}P] ATP with a specific activity of 5000 Ci/mmol and the nuclease P1 enrichment.

Results of the Animal Studies

After gavage of 300 mg/kg crotonaldehyde, adducts could be detected in all organs examined. The highest amounts of adducts were found in the liver and the lowest, in the small intestine (Fig. 7). No adducts could be found in the respective organs of untreated rats.

In another series of experiments we are presently investigating the persistence of DNA adducts of crotonaldehyde after repeated gavage of low doses (see "Methods"). Figure 8 demonstrates that 1 week (5 weeks after start of the gavage) after the last application of crotonaldehyde, 66% of the original amount of adducts as measured 1 day after the last gavage are still present, and that after 2 weeks (6 weeks after the start) 17% of adducts are still present in the liver. Further experiments with other organs are not yet finished.

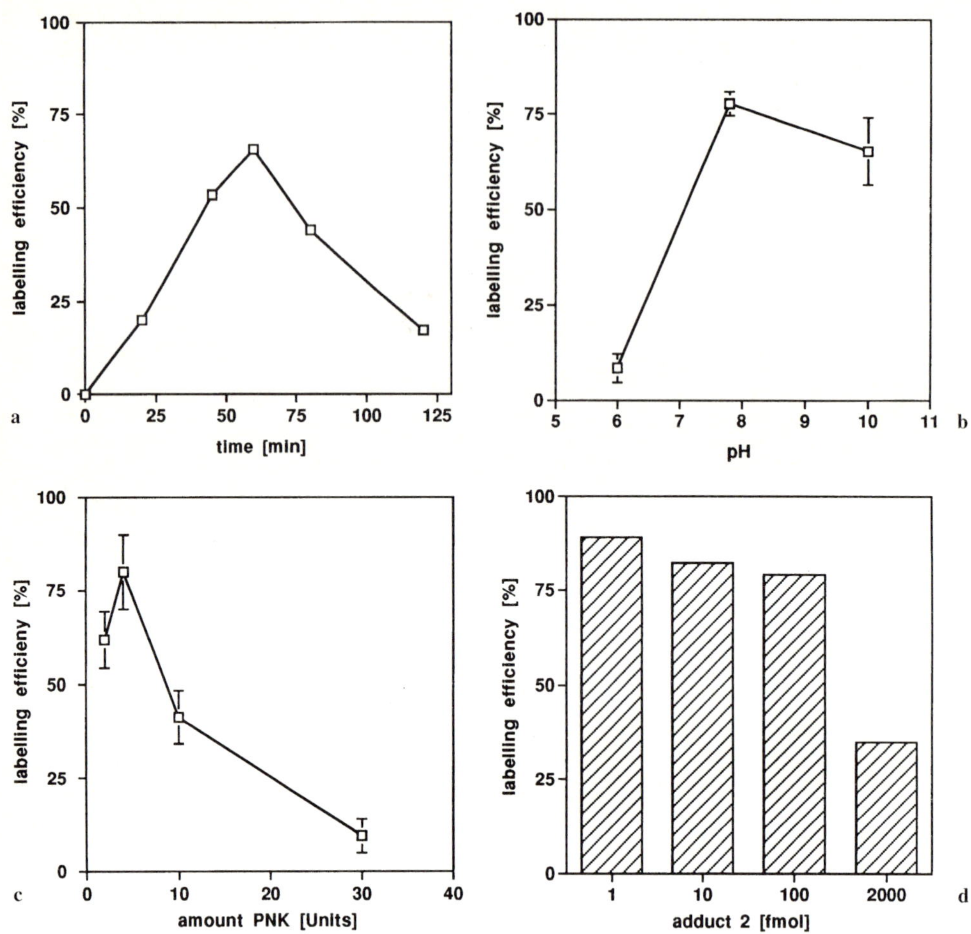

Fig. 6. Dependence of labeling efficiency on **a** incubation time, **b** pH value, **c** amount of T4-polynucleotide kinase enzyme (PNK), **d** amount of adducts

Discussion

Humans are ubiquitously and extensively exposed to α,β-unsaturated carbonyl compounds, and these compounds are formed endogenously. These substances are genotoxic, mutagenic, and some were shown to be carcinogens (see "Introduction"). Therefore, this group of substances is considered to play an important role in human cancer. This role, in particular the significance of the different kinds of exposure as well as that of endogenous formation, cannot yet be evaluated with the present data base. A better risk assessment is, however, required to develop measures to reduce exposure against these compounds or to scavenge those α,β-unsaturated carbonyl compounds already taken up by humans or formed endogenously. Determination of the respective DNA ad-

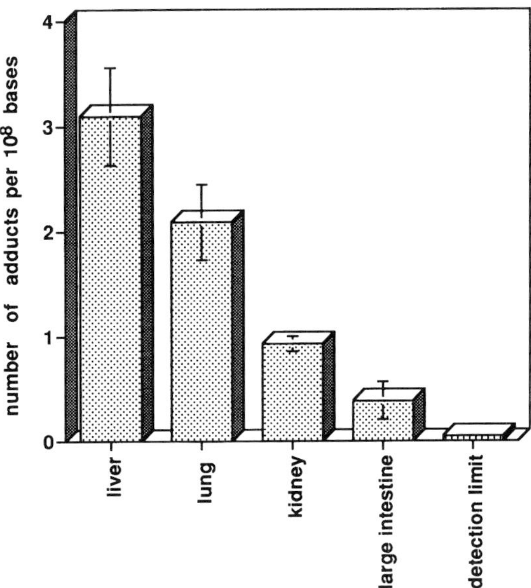

Fig. 7. Adducts 2a,b found in organs of F344 rats after gavage of 300 mg/kg crotonaldehyde

ducts in animal tissue or human tissue would improve risk assessment and lead to a better differentiation of the role of various kinds of exposure in carcinogenesis. Furthermore, adduct monitoring can also be used to examine the effectivity of measures to reduce exposure or to scavenge endogenously formed α,β-unsaturated carbonyl compounds.

Our results demonstrate that ^{32}P postlabeling is suitable for the sensitive detection of such DNA adducts. The sensitivity is in the range of 1 adduct per 10^9 bases. We adapted and developed the procedure and obtained high labeling efficiencies. In particular the nuclease P1 enrichment was shown to be very

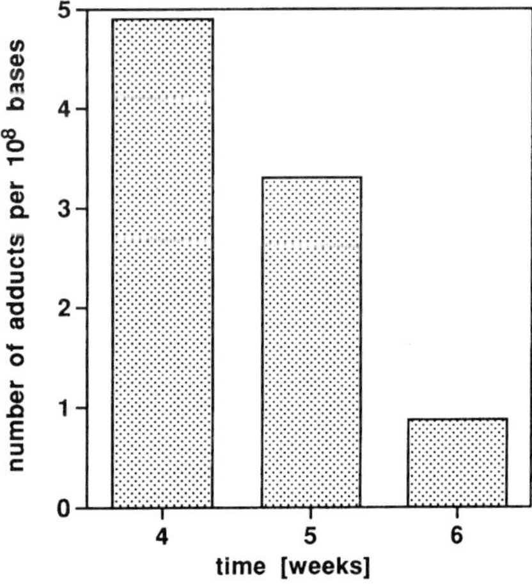

Fig. 8. Persistence of adducts 2a,b in the liver of F344 rats after repeated gavage of small doses of crotonaldehyde. Treatment 4 weeks. Adduct level after 4 weeks of the start of gavage (1 day after the end of treatment), after 5 weeks (1 week after the last gavage), and after 6 weeks after start (2 weeks after last gavage)

appropriate for this type of adduct. Furthermore we have worked out HPLC methods which allow a clear separation of the modified mononucleotides from the other unmodified mononucleotides of the DNA digest so that the detection sensitivity could be increased even more, if necessary.

The adducts of crotonaldehyde are clearly formed in vivo after exposure and they are persistent to a certain extent. We could, however, not find crotonaldehyde adducts in untreated F 344 rats. Raghu and Chung (1994) found the respective adducts even in untreated animals and explained the results by the high environmental exposure or by endogenous formation of crotonaldehyde. It may well be that in our case the rats are not exposed to such a high extent via air, food, drinking water, disinfectants, etc. The endogenous formation of crotonaldehyde is considered very low compared with malondialdehyde, 4-hydroxynonenal, or some other 3-alkyl-substituted 4-hydroxyenals. The endogenous formation of crotonaldehyde may nevertheless be genetically determined and may be different in various animal species or races. In any case, methods are now available to answer these questions and assess the role of α,β-unsaturated carbonyl compounds in human cancer.

References

Benamira M, Singh U, Marnett LJ (1992) Site-specific frameshift mutagenesis by a propanodeoxyguanosine adduct positioned in the (CpG)4 hot-spot of *Salmonella typhimurium* his D 3052 carried on an M13 vector. J Biol Chem 267: 392–400

Benedetti A, Comporti M, Fulceri R, Esterbauer H (1984) Cytotoxic aldehydes originating from the peroxidation of liver microsomal lipids. Identification of 4,5-dihydroxydecenal. Biochim Biophys Acta 792: 172–181

Brambilla G, Sciaba L, Faggin P, Maura A, Marinari UM, Ferro M, Esterbauer H (1986) Cytotoxicity, DNA fragmentation and sister-chromatid exchange in Chinese hamster ovary cells exposed to the lipid peroxydation product 4-hydroxynonenal and homologous aldehydes. Mutat Res 171: 169–176

Eder E, Hoffman C (1992) Identification and characterization of deoxyguanosine crotonaldehyde adducts. Formation of 7,8 cyclic adducts and $1,N^2$, 7,8-bis-cyclic adducts. Chem Res Toxicol 5: 802–808

Eder E, Hoffman C (1993) Identification and characterization of deoxyguanosine adducts of mutagenic β-alkyl substituted acrolein congeners. Chem Res Toxicol 6: 486–494

Eder E, Hoffman C (1994) $1,N^2$-Cyclic deoxyguanosine adducts and guanine adducts of 2-haloacroleins. Isolation, characterization, isomerization and stability. Arch Toxicol 68: 471–479

Eder E, Hoffman C, Bastian H, Deininger C, Scheckenbach S (1990) Molecular mechanisms of DNA damage initiated by α,β-unsaturated carbonyl compounds as criteria for genotoxicity and mutagenicity. Environ Health Perspect 88: 99–106

Eder E, Scheckenbach S, Deininger C, Hoffman C (1993) The possible role of α,β-unsaturated carbonyl compounds in mutagenesis and carcinogenesis. Toxicol Lett 67: 87–103

Eder E, Deininger C, Deininger D, Weinfurtner E (1994a) Genotoxicity of 2-halocinnamaldehydes in two bacterial assays. Induction of SOS repair and frameshift mutation. Mutagenesis 9: 473–476

Eder E, Deininger C, Deininger D, Weinfurtner E (1994b) Genotoxicity of 2-halo-substituted enals and 2-chloroacrylonitrile in the Ames test and the SOS Chromotest. Mutat Res 322: 321–328

Koster JF, Slee RG, Montfoort A, Lang J, Esterbauer H (1986) Comparison of the inactivation of microsomal glucose-6-phosphatase by in situ lipid peroxidation-derived 4-hydroxynonenal and exogenous 4-hydroxynonenal. Free Radic Commun 1: 273–287

Marinelli ER, Johnson F, Iden CR, Yu PL (1990) Synthesis of 1,N^2 (1,3-propano)-2′ deoxyguanosine and incorporation into oligodeoxynucleotides – a model for exocyclic acrolein-DNA adducts. Chem Res Toxicol 3: 49–58

Marmur J (1961) A procedure for the isolation of deoxyribonucleic acid from microorganisms. J Mol Biol 3: 208–218

Moriya M, Marinelli ER, Shibutani S, Joseph J (1989) Site-specific mutagenesis using model exocyclic DNA-adduct 1,N^2-propanodeoxyguanosine. Proc Am Assoc Cancer Res 30 (Carc 555): 140

Raghu GN, Chung FL (1994) Detection of exocyclic 1,N^2-propanodeoxyguanosine adducts as common DNA lesions in rodents and humans. Proc Natl Acad Sci USA 91: 7491–7495

Reddy V, Randerath K (1986) Nuclease P1-mediated enrichment of sensitivity of ^{32}P-postlabeling test for structurally diverse DNA adducts. Carcinogenesis 9: 1543–1551

Vaca CE, Vodicka P, Hemminki K (1992) Determination of malonaldehyde-modified 2′-deoxyguanosine-3′-monophosphate and DNA by ^{32}P-postlabeling. Carcinogenesis 13: 593–599

Van Beerendonk GJM, Nivard JM, Vogel EW, Nelson SD, Meerman JHN (1992) Formation of thymidine adducts and cross-linking potential of 2-bromoacrolein, a reactive metabolite of tris (2,3-dibromopropyl) phosphate. Mutagenesis 7: 19–24

Witz GC (1989) Biological interactions of α,β-unsaturated aldehydes. Free Radic Biol Med 7: 333–349

Glutathione-Dependent Bioactivation and Renal Toxicity of Xenobiotics

W. Dekant

Department of Toxicology, University of Würzburg, Versbacher Str. 9, 97078 Würzburg, Germany

Introduction

Glutathione (γ-glutamyl-cysteinylglycine) is a major low molecular weight peptide in mammalian cells and participates in a variety of cellular reactions (Meister 1988, 1992). Due to the nucleophilicity of the sulfur atom and the antioxidant properties of glutathione, this tripeptide is an important factor in the detoxication of xenobiotics and oxidants (Boyland and Chasseaud 1969). The formation of glutathione *S*-conjugates from xenobiotics and their electrophilic metabolites has long been associated with detoxication. Recent evidence, however, indicated that this generalization is not always true and that some glutathione *S*-conjugates may be toxic (Anders et al. 1988; Dekant et al. 1989; Monks and Lau 1989; Anders 1991). At least four types of toxic glutathione *S*-conjugates have been identified. The objective of this review is to summarize current knowledge on the biosynthesis of toxic glutathione *S*-conjugates from polyhalogenated alkenes and aminophenols, the reactions of these *S*-conjugates in cellular systems, and their association with renal toxicity. Several recent reviews on this topic have appeared (Monks and Lau 1987, 1989; Lock 1988, 1989; Dekant et al. 1990a,b; Koob and Dekant 1991; Dekant and Vamvakas 1992).

Biosynthesis and Cellular Reactions of Toxic Glutathione *S*-Conjugates

Toxic glutathione *S*-conjugates are biosynthesized from three different types of compounds: haloalkanes, haloalkenes, and hydroquinones and aminophenol. Due to their high reactivity, glutathione *S*-conjugates formed from haloalkanes are less likely to be translocated to the kidney to cause renal toxicity. Thus, their biosynthesis and their cellular interactions will not be described here; for information, the reader is referred to a recent monograph (Anders and Dekant 1994).

Halogenated Alkenes

The halogenated alkenes hexachlorobutadiene, perfluoropropene, chlorotrifluoroethene, and the alkyne dichloroacetylene, are selectively nephrotoxic in rats and induce proximal tubular damage (Reichert et al. 1975; Potter et al. 1981; Ishmael et al. 1982). Moreover, the widely used solvents trichloroethene (NCI 1986a) and tetrachloroethene, as well as dichloroacetylene (NCI 1986b) and hexachlorobutadiene (Kociba et al. 1977), induced carcinomas of the proximal tubules in rats after administration of high doses. Glutathione-dependent pathways have been implicated in the renal toxicity of these compounds.

Biosynthesis of Toxic Glutathione *S*-Conjugates from Chloroalkenes. Nephrotoxic haloalkenes are metabolized to glutathione *S*-conjugates by microsomal and cytosolic glutathione *S*-transferases; substantial nonenzymic reaction has been observed only with dichloroacetylene (Kanhai et al. 1989). The microsomal fraction of rat liver generally exhibits a two to ten fold higher activity toward haloalkenes than does the cytosolic fraction.

Hexachlorobutadiene (Wolf et al. 1984; Dekant et al. 1988a,b), 1,1,2-trichloro-3,3,3-trifluoropropene (Vamvakas et al. 1989a), trichloroethene (Dekant et al. 1986a, 1990c), and tetrachloroethene (Dekant et al. 1986a, 1987a) are metabolized by glutathione *S*-transferases from rat liver by an addition-elimination reaction to give exclusively *S*-(haloalkenyl)glutathione conjugates (Fig. 1). Formation of these glutathione *S*-conjugates has also been observed in bile obtained in isolated rat livers perfused with the haloalkenes. Glutathione conjugate formation from hexachlorobutadiene has been detected in mouse liver (Dekant et al. 1988a) and in human liver subcellular fractions; it has been calculated that glutathione-dependent metabolism of hexachlorobutadiene in intact liver cells is mainly catalyzed by microsomal glutathione *S*-transferase (Wallin et al. 1988; Oesch and Wolf 1989). In rats, metabolites indicative of glutathione conjugation reactions were also found in vivo: the bile of rats given hexachlorobutadiene (Nash et al. 1984), 1,1,2-trichloro-3,3,3-trifluoropropene (Vamvakas et al. 1989a), trichloroethene (Dekant et al. 1990c), or tetrachloroethene (Vamvakas et al. 1989b) contains glutathione *S*-conjugates identical to those formed in liver microsomes, and the corresponding mercapturic acids are urinary metabolites (Dekant et al. 1986a,b, 1990c; Reichert and Schuetz 1986; Vamvakas et al. 1989a). Hexachlorobutadiene seems to be metabolized in vivo exclusively by glutathione conjugate formation (Wallin et al. 1988); in contrast, both trichloroethene and tetrachloroethene are mainly metabolized by cytochrome P450 (Dekant et al. 1984). Metabolites whose formation may be explained by *S*-conjugate formation and processing are only minor excretory products.

The highly nephrotoxic alkyne dichloroacetylene (Reichert et al. 1975) is metabolized by addition of glutathione to give *S*-(1,2-dichlorovinyl)-glu-

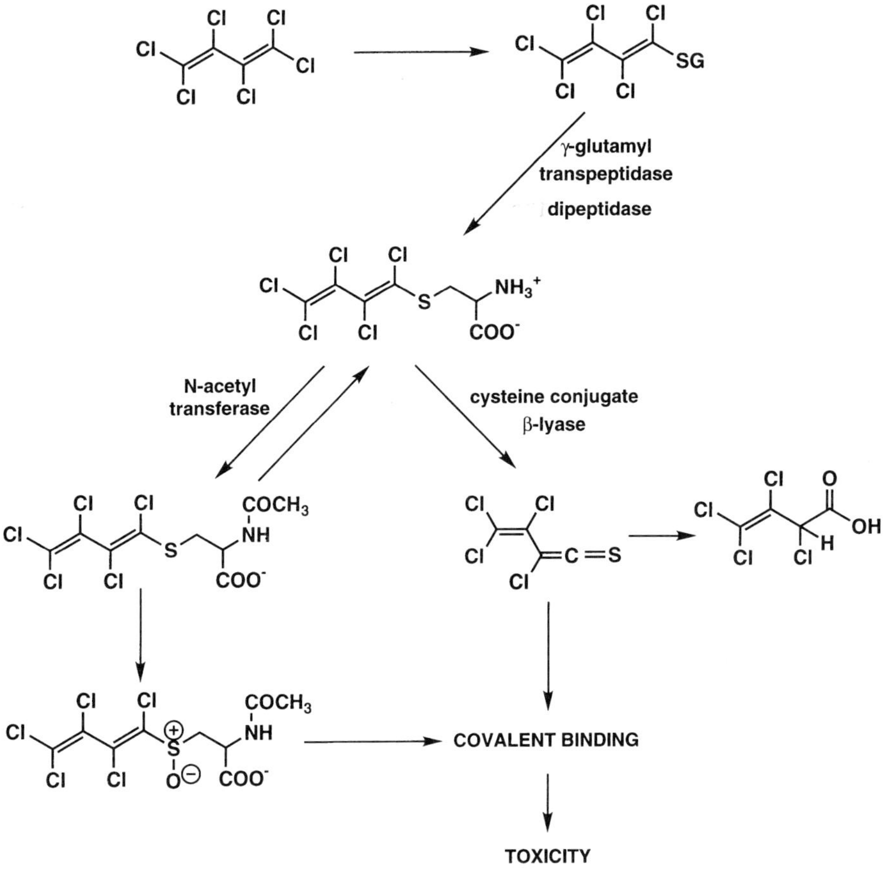

Fig. 1. Biosynthesis of glutathione conjugates from hexachlorobutadiene as a representative compound for polyhalogenated alkenes, renal processing, and bioactivation of cysteine *S*-conjugates by cysteine conjugate *β*-lyase or cytochrome P450

tathione; in rats, *N*-acetyl-*S*-(1,2-dichlorovinyl)-L-cysteine is a major urinary metabolite of dichloroacetylene (Kanhai et al. 1989, 1991).

Biosynthesis of Toxic *S*-Conjugates from Fluoroalkenes. In contrast to the vinylic *S*-conjugates formed from chloroalkenes, fluoroalkenes are generally metabolized by glutathione *S*-transferases to *S*-(fluoroalkyl)glutathione conjugates. For example, chlorotrifluoroethene and tetrafluoroethene are metabolized by the glutathione *S*-transferases to *S*-(1-chloro-1,1,2-trifluoroethyl) glutathione (Dohn and Anders 1982) and *S*-(1,1,2,2-tetrafluoroethyl) glutathione (Odum and Green 1984), respectively.

The enzymic reaction of glutathione with perfluoropropene yields both *S*-(1,1,2,3,3,3-hexafluoropropyl)glutathione and *S*-(1,2,3,3,3-pentafluoropropenyl)glutathione as products (Koob and Dekant 1990). The nephrotoxic chlorofluoroalkene 1,1-dichloro-2,2-difluoroethene is metabolized to *N*-acetyl-*S*-(1,1-dichloro-2,2-difluoroethyl)-L-cysteine in vivo (Commandeur et al. 1987).

Toxicity of Halovinyl *S*-Conjugates. The *S*-conjugates formed are toxic metabolites of the parent haloalkenes, which are accumulated in the kidney. Many studies have been performed to investigate the nephrotoxicity, cytotoxicity, and genotoxicity of synthetic halovinyl *S*-conjugates (Lock 1988, 1989). For detailed reviews, see (Anders et al. 1988; Dekant et al. 1989; Koob and Dekant 1991). The halovinyl *S*-conjugates *S*-(1,2-dichlorovinyl)-L-cysteine, *S*-(1,2,2-trichlorovinyl)-L-cysteine, and *S*-(1,2,3,4,4-pentachlorobutadienyl)-L-cysteine are mutagenic in *Salmonella typhimurium* with (Green and Odum 1985; Commandeur et al. 1991) and without the addition of exogenous activating systems (Dekant et al. 1986c; Vamvakas et al. 1988a,b). Incubation of these *S*-conjugates with *Salmonella typhimurium* homogenates results in time- and dose-dependent production of pyruvate, which is formed by β-lyase-catalyzed cleavage of the *S*-conjugates in equimolar amounts with the presumed mutagenic intermediates. Both the mutagenicity and the pyruvate production are decreased in the presence of aminooxyacetic acid, an inhibitor of the β-lyase. Haloalkyl *S*-conjugates from fluoroalkenes are also cleaved to pyruvate by *Salmonella typhimurium* homogenates; however, they are not mutagenic in the Ames preincubation assay (Vamvakas et al. 1988b).

Halovinyl *S*-conjugates also induce β-lyase-dependent DNA repair in LLC-PK_1 cells, a porcine kidney cell line (Vamvakas et al. 1989c, d). The extent of genotoxicity observed is very low and the concentration range over which DNA repair occurs in the absence of cytotoxicity and cell death is very small. Studies with fluorescence digital imaging microscopy have shown that *S*-(1,2-dichlorovinyl)-L-cysteine increases cytosolic Ca^{2+}-concentrations prior to the onset of cell death. The increase is associated with impaired ability of the mitochondria to sequester cytosolic Ca^{2+} and precedes the collapse of the mitochondrial membrane potential (Vamvakas et al. 1990). This effect is common to some tumor promotors, such as hydroperoxides, that induce oxidative stress (Cerutti 1985). *S*-(1,2-Dichlorovinyl)-L-cysteine also promotes dimethyl-nitrosamine-initiated renal tubule carcinomas in rats (Meadows et al. 1988; Vamvakas et al. 1992). The increased Ca^{2+} concentrations activate Ca^{2+}-and Mg^{2+}-dependent endonucleases. This results in increased formation of DNA-double-strand breaks followed by enhanced poly(ADP-ribosyl)ation of nuclear proteins in LLC-PK_1 cells treated with *S*-(1,2-dichlorovinyl)-L-cysteine. Finally, *S*-(1,2-dichlorovinyl)-L-cysteine induces the expression of the protooncogenes c-*fos* and c-*myc* in LLC-PK_1 cells (Vamvakas and Köster 1993). Both the direct interaction of *S*-(1,2-dichlorovinyl)-L-cysteine-derived reactive intermediates with DNA and the modification of DNA structure by increased poly(ADP-ribosyl)ation, may be involved in the effects of *S*-(1,2-dichlorovinyl)-L-cysteine on c-*fos* and c-*myc* expression.

Reactive Intermediates Formed from Haloalkyl and Halovinyl *S*-Conjugates. Recently, the structures of the final reactive metabolites have been elucidated. Processing of the biosynthetic glutathione *S*-conjugates to the cysteine *S*-conjugates is required for toxicity. Fluoroalkyl and chloroalkenyl cysteine *S*-conjugates are metabolized by the pyridoxal phosphate-dependent β-lyase to unstable thiols that yield reactive electrophiles (Dekant et al. 1987b, 1988c, d). Thioketenes are formed from the enethiols produced by β-lyase-mediated cleavage of halovinyl cysteine *S*-conjugates (Dekant et al. 1991); fluoroalkyl cysteine *S*-conjugates are transformed to reactive thioacyl halides. Both thionoacyl fluorides and thioketenes are potent acylating agents and react with nucleophiles. The role of thioacylating agents in *S*-conjugate-induced toxicity and mutagenicity has been confirmed by structure-activity studies: Only *S*-conjugates that form acylating agents are mutagenic in bacteria and cytotoxic in kidney cells (Vamvakas et al. 1988b, 1989e).

Sulfoxidation of Halovinylmercapturic Acids. Cytochrome P450 enzymes catalyze the sulfoxidation of *N*-acetyl-*S*-(1,2,3,4,4-pentachlorobutadienyl)-L-cysteine, *S*-(1,2,2-trichlorovinyl)-L-cysteine and both isomers of *S*-(dichloro vinyl)-L-cysteine. In vitro studies have elucidated that cytochrome P450 3A is a major catalyst of this sulfoxidation reaction. The sulfoxidation of these mercapturic acids has to be regarded as a bioactivation reaction since the formed sulfoxides are considerably more toxic than their precursor mercapturic acids. These vinyl sulfoxides represent α,β-unsaturated carbonyl analogues which are direct electrophiles and do not require bioactivation by cysteine conjugate β-lyase. Since sulfoxidation of halovinyl mercapturates is only observed in male rats, the formation of these electrophiles may contribute to sex differences in the toxic effects of mercapturic acids and their precursor chloroalkenes in rodent kidney (Lash et al. 1994; Birner et al. 1995; Werner et al. 1995).

Hydroquinones and Aminophenol

Bromohydroquinone is a major toxic metabolite of bromobenzene and is easily converted to bromoquinone (Lau et al. 1984). Bromobenzene-derived covalently bound radioactivity is mainly due to bromohydroquinone (Zheng and Hanzlik 1992). Glutathione-dependent reactions have been implicated in bromohydroquinone-induced nephrotoxicity. Bromohydroquinone is oxidized to bromoquinone which reacts with glutathione (Monks et al. 1985). In microsomes and in rats in vivo, several isomeric mono- and bisglutathione-substituted derivatives of bromohydroquinone have been identified as metabolites (Monks et al. 1985; Lau and Monks 1990). These glutathione *S*-conjugates are nephrotoxic in rats and cytotoxic to renal cells (Lau et al. 1988a). These results indicate that bromohydroquinone nephrotoxicity is probably due to the biosynthetic formation of glutathione conjugates derived from bromohydroquinone (Fig. 2).

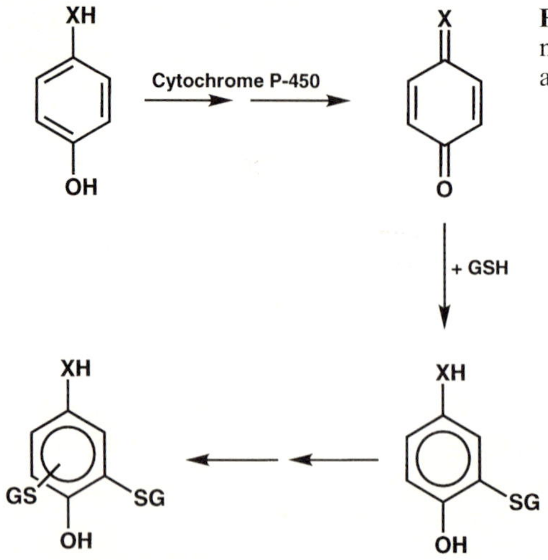

Fig. 2. Glutathione conjugates as toxic metabolites of hydroquinones and aminophenols

Glutathione *S*-conjugates derived from benzoquinone, menadione, and chloroquinones are also nephrotoxic in rats and toxic to kidney cells and renal mitochondria (Mertens et al. 1991; Redegeld et al. 1991; Hill et al. 1992). The biosynthetic glutathione *S*-conjugates (Kleiner et al. 1992) are accumulated by the kidney in a γ-glutamyltranspeptidase-dependent pathway; their toxicity is diminished or increased by inhibition of γ-glutamyltranspeptidase but not by inhibition of β-lyase (Monks et al. 1988; Monks and Lau 1990). These experiments suggest that β-lyase-mediated cleavage does not play a role in the toxicity of these hydroquinone *S*-conjugates. The glutathione conjugates of hydroquinones and quinones may serve as transport forms to γ-glutamyltranspeptidase-rich organs to be accumulated there. In the rat, γ-glutamyltranspeptidase is almost exclusively present in the kidney. Moreover, substitution of bromohydroquinones with cysteine lowers the redox potential and makes these bromohydroquinones more prone to oxidation to toxic quinones (Lau et al. 1988a,b, 1990; Monks and Lau 1990). The reduction of nephrotoxicity of bromohydroquinone glutathione *S*-conjugates by simultaneous administration of ascorbic acid suggests that processes involving oxidation to a reactive quinone and, presumably, peroxidative mechanisms are involved in the nephrotoxicity of these compounds.

p-Aminophenol is an acute nephrotoxin causing necrosis of the pars recta of the proximal tubules in rats (Gartland et al. 1989a,b). p-Aminophenol is oxidized enzymically to the benzoquinone imine which is a reactive α,β-unsaturated compound (Crowe et al. 1979; Newton et al. 1982; Josephy et al. 1983). Its interaction with cellular macromolecules when formed in the kidney may cause renal toxicity. However, several recent experimental findings support the assumption that p-aminophenol toxicity is mediated by glutathione-dependent mechanisms (Fig. 2). Synthetic quinoneimine reacts nonenzymically with glutathione (Eckert et al. 1990). Both direct and indirect evidence for the involvement of glutathione conjugates as a transport form for p-aminophenol metabolites has been obtained. Depletion of glutathione by buthioninsulfoximine, which inhibits glutathione synthesis, completely protected rats against p-aminophenol-induced nephrotoxicity (Gartland et al. 1990). Moreover, biliary cannulation partially protected rats from p-aminophenol-induced nephrotoxicity. These results suggest that nephrotoxins are formed by glutathione conjugation of p-aminophenol metabolites in the liver and are translocated to the kidney. Recent studies identified the formation of toxic glutathione conjugates in p-aminophenol metabolism. Bile of rats given p-aminophenol i.p. contained several glutathione *S*-conjugates, including 1-amino-3-(glutathione-*S*-yl)-4-hydroxybenzene and 1-amino-2-(glutathione-*S*-yl)-4-hydroxybenzene. These metabolites are nephrotoxic in rats and cytotoxic in rat renal epithelial cells. Their toxicity is dependent on γ-glutamyltranspeptidase, but not on β-lyase, which is in line with the effects of hydroquinone *S*-conjugates (Fowler et al. 1991; Klos et al. 1992).

References

Anders MW (1991) Glutathione-dependent bioactivation of xenobiotics. FASEB J 4: 87–92

Anders MW, Dekant W (1994) Conjugation-dependent carcinogenicity and toxicity of foreign compounds. Academic, San Diego (Advances in pharmacology, vol 27)

Anders MW, Lash LH, Dekant W, Elfarra AA, Dohn DR (1988) Biosynthesis and biotransformation of glutathione *S*-conjugates to toxic metabolites. Crit Rev Toxicol 18: 311–342

Birner G, Werner M, Ott MM, Dekant W (1995) Sex-differences in hexachlorobutadiene biotransformation and nephrotoxicity. Toxicol Appl Pharmacol 132: 203–212

Boyland E, Chasseaud LF (1969) Role of glutathione and glutathione *S*-transferases in mercapturic acid biosynthesis. Adv Enzymol 32: 173–177

Cerutti PA (1985) Prooxidant states and tumor promotion. Science 227: 375–381

Commandeur JNM, Oostendorp RAJ, Schoofs PR, Xu B, Vermeulen NPE (1987) Nephrotoxicity and hepatotoxicity of 1,1-dichloro-2,2-difluoroethylene in the rat. Biochem Pharmacol 36: 4229–4237

Commandeur JNM, Boogard PJ, Mulder GJ, Vermeulen NPE (1991) Mutagenicity and cytotoxicity of two regioisomeric mercapturic acids and cysteine *S*-conjugates of trichloroethylene. Arch Toxicol 65: 373–380

Crowe CA, Yong AC, Calder IC, Ham KN, Tange JD (1979) The nephrotoxicity of p-aminophenol. I. The effect on microsomal cytochromes, glutathione and covalent binding in kidney and liver. Chem Biol Interact 27: 235–243

Dekant W, Vamvakas S (1992) Mechanisms of xenobiotic-induced renal carcinogenicity. Adv Pharmacol 23: 297–337

Dekant W, Metzler M, Henschler D (1984) Novel metabolites of trichloroethylene through dechlorination reactions in rats, mice and humans. Biochem Pharmacol 33: 2021–2027

Dekant W, Metzler M, Henschler D (1986a) Identification of *S*-1,2,2-trichlorovinyl-N-acetylcysteine as a urinary metabolite of tetrachloroethylene: bioactivation through glutathione conjugation as a possible explanation of its nephrocarcinogenicity. J Biochem Toxicol 1: 57–72

Dekant W, Metzler M, Henschler D (1986b) Identification of *S*-1,2-dichlorovinyl-*N*-acetyl-cysteine as a urinary metabolite of trichloroethylene: a possible explanation for its nephrocarcinogenicity in male rats. Biochem Pharmacol 35: 2455–2458

Dekant W, Vamvakas S, Berthold K, Schmidt S, Wild Henschler D (1986c) Bacterial *β*-lyase mediated cleavage and mutagenicity of cysteine conjugates derived from the nephrocarcinogenic alkenes trichloroethylene, tetrachloroethylene and hexachlorobutadiene. Chem Biol Interact 60: 31–45

Dekant W, Martens G, Vamvakas S, Metzler M, Henschler D (1987a) Bioactivation of tetrachloroethylene — role of glutathione *S*-transferase-catalyzed conjugation versus cytochrome P-450-dependent phospholipid alkylation. Drug Metab Dispos 15: 702–709

Dekant W, Lash LH, Anders MW (1987b) Bioactivation mechanism of the cytotoxic and nephrotoxic *S*-conjugate *S*-(2-chloro-1,1,2-trifluoroethyl)-L-cysteine. Proc Natl Acad Sci USA 84: 7443–7447

Dekant W, Schrenk D, Vamvakas S, Henschler D (1988a) Metabolism of hexachloro-1,3-butadiene in mice: in vivo and in vitro evidence for activation by glutathione conjugation. Xenobiotica 18: 803–816

Dekant W, Vamvakas S, Henschler D, Anders MW (1988b) Enzymatic conjugation of hexachloro-1,3-butadiene with glutathione: formation of 1-(glutathion-*S*-yl)-1,2,3,4,4-pentachlorobuta-1,3-diene and 1,4-bis(glutathion-*S*-yl)-1,2,3,4-tetrachlorobuta-1,3-diene. Drug Metab Dispos 16: 701–706

Dekant W, Berthold K, Vamvakas S, Henschler D (1988c) Thioacylating agents as ultimate intermediates in the *β*-lyase catalyzed metabolism of *S*-(pentachlorobutadienyl)-L-cysteine. Chem Biol Interact 67: 139–148

Dekant W, Berthold K, Vamvakas S, Henschler D, Anders MW (1988d) Thioacylating intermediates as metabolites of *S*-(1,2-dichlorovinyl)-L-cysteine and *S*-(1,2,2-trichlorovinyl)-L-cysteine formed by cysteine conjugate *β*-lyase. Chem Res Toxicol 1: 175–178

Dekant W, Vamvakas S, Anders MW (1989) Bioactivation of nephrotoxic haloalkenes by glutathione conjugation: formation of toxic and mutagenic intermediates by cysteine conjugate *β*-lyase. Drug Metab Rev 20: 43–83

Dekant W, Vamvakas S, Anders MW (1990a) Biosynthesis, bioactivation, and mutagenicity of *S*-conjugates. Toxicol Lett 53: 53–58

Dekant W, Vamvakas S, Koob M, Köchling A, Kanhai W, Müller D, Henschler D (1990b) A mechanism of haloalkene-induced renal carcinogenesis. Environ Health Perspect 88: 107–110

Dekant W, Koob M, Henschler D (1990c) Metabolism of trichloroethene — in vivo and in vitro evidence for activation by glutathione conjugation. Chem Biol Interact 73: 89–101

Dekant W, Urban G, Görsman C, Anders MW (1991) Thioketene formation from *α*-haloalkenyl 2-nitrophenyl disulfides: models for biological reactive intermediates of cytotoxic *S*-conjugates. J Am Chem Soc 113: 5120–5122

Dohn DR, Anders MW (1982) The enzymatic reaction of chlorotrifluoroethylene with glutathione. Biochem Biophys Res Commun 109: 1339–1345

Eckert K-G, Eyer P, Sonnenbichler J, Zetl I (1990) Activation and detoxication of aminophenols. II. Synthesis and structural elucidation of various thiol addition products of 1,4-benzoquinoneimine and *N*-acetyl-1,4-benzoquinoneimine. Xenobiotica 20: 333–350

Fowler LM, Moore RB, Foster JR, Lock EA (1991) Nephrotoxicity of 4-aminophenol glutathione conjugate. Hum Exp Toxicol 10: 451–459

Gartland KPR, Bonner FW, Nicholson JK (1989a) Investigations into the biochemical effects of region-specific nephrotoxins. Mol Pharmacol 35: 242–250

Gartland KPR, Bonner FW, Timbrell JA, Nicholson JK (1989b) Biochemical characterisation of *para*-aminophenol-induced nephrotoxic lesions in the F334 rat. Arch Toxicol 63: 97–106

Gartland KPR, Eason CT, Bonner FW, Nicholson JK (1990) Effects of biliary cannulation and buthionine sulphoximine pretreatment on the nephrotoxicity of *para*-aminophenol in the Fisher 334 rat. Arch Toxicol 64: 14–25

Green T, Odum J (1985) Structure/activity studies of the nephrotoxic and mutagenic action of cysteine conjugates of chloro- and fluoroalkenes. Chem Biol Interact 54: 15–31

Hill BA, Monks TJ, Lau SS (1992) The effects of 2,3,5-(triglutathion-*S*-yl)hydroquinone on renal mitochondrial respiratory function in vivo and in vitro: possible role in cytotoxicity. Toxicol Appl Pharmacol 117: 165–171

Ishmael J, Pratt I, Lock EA (1982) Necrosis of the pars recta (S3 segment) of the rat kidney produced by hexachloro-1:3-butadiene. J Pathol 138: 99–113

Josephy PD, Eling TE, Mason RP (1983) Oxidation of p-aminophenol catalyzed by horseradish peroxidase and prostaglandin synthase. Mol Pharmacol 23: 461–466

Kanhai W, Dekant W, Henschler D (1989) Metabolism of the nephrotoxin dichloroacetylene by glutathione conjugation. Chem Res Toxicol 2: 51–56

Kanhai W, Koob M, Dekant W, Henschler D (1991) Metabolism of ^{14}C-dichloroethyne in rats. Xenobiotica 21: 905–916

Kleiner HE, Hill BA, Monks TJ, Lau SS (1992) In vivo and in vitro formation of several *S*-conjugates of hydroquinone. Toxicologist 12: 1350

Klos C, Koob M, Kramer C, Dekant W (1992) p-Aminophenol nephrotoxicity: biosynthesis of toxic glutathione conjugates. Toxicol Appl Pharmacol 115: 98–106

Kociba RJ, Keyes DG, Jersey GC, Ballard JJ, Dittenber DA, Quast JF, Wade LE, Humiston CG, Schwetz BA (1977) Results of a two-year chronic toxicity study with hexachlorobutadiene in rats. Am Ind Hyg Assoc J 38: 589–602

Koob M, Dekant W (1990) Metabolism of hexafluoropropene — evidence for bioactivation by glutathione conjugate formation in the kidney. Drug Metab Dispos 18: 911–916

Koob M, Dekant W (1991) Bioactivation of xenobiotics by formation of toxic glutathione conjugates. Chem Biol Interact 77: 107–136

Lash LH, Sausen PJ, Duescher AJ, Elfarra AA (1994) Roles of cysteine conjugate *β*-lyase and *S*-oxidase in nephrotoxicity: studies with *S*-(1,2-dichlorovinyl)-L-cysteine and *S*-(1,2-dichlorovinyl)-L-cysteine sulfoxide. J Pharmacol Exp Ther 269: 374–383

Lau SS, Monks TJ (1990) The in vivo disposition of 2-bromo-[^{14}C]hydroquinone and the effect of *γ*-glutamyl transpeptidase inhibition. Toxicol Appl Pharmacol 103: 121–132

Lau SS, Monks TJ, Gillette JR (1984) Identification of 2-bromohydroquinone as a metabolite of bromobenzene and o-bromophenol: implications for bromobenzene-induced nephrotoxicity. J Pharmacol Exp Ther 230: 360–366

Lau SS, McMenamin MG, Monks TJ (1988a) Differential uptake of isomeric 2-bromohydroquinone-glutathione conjugates into kidney slices. Biochem Biophys Res Commun 152: 223–230

Lau SS, Hill BA, Highet RJ, Monks TJ (1988b) Sequential oxidation and glutathione addition to 1,4-benzoquinone: correlation of toxicity with increased glutathione substitution. Mol Pharmacol 34: 829–836

Lau SS, Jones TW, Highet RJ, Hill B, Monks TJ (1990) Differences in the localization and extent of the renal proximal tubular necrosis caused by mercapturic acid and glutathione conjugates of 1,4-naphthoquinone and menadione. Toxicol Appl Pharmacol 104: 334–350

Lock EA (1988) Studies on the mechanism of nephrotoxicity and nephrocarcinogenicity of halogenated alkenes. Crit Rev Toxicol 19: 23–42

Lock EA (1989) Mechanism of nephrotoxic action due to organohalogenated compounds. Toxicol Lett 46: 93–106

Meadows SD, Gandolfi AJ, Nagle RB, Shively JW (1988) Enhancement of DMN-induced kidney tumors by 1,2-dichlorovinylcysteine in Swiss-Webster mice. Drug Chem Toxicol 11: 307–318

Meister A (1988) Glutathione metabolism and its selective modification. J Biol Chem 263: 17205–17208

Meister A (1992) Commentary: on the antioxidant effects of ascorbic acid and glutathione. Biochem Pharmacol 44: 1905–1915

Mertens JJ, Temmink JH, Bladeren PJ, Jones TW, Lo HH, Lau SS, Monks TJ (1991) Inhibition of γ-glutamyl transpeptidase potentiates the nephrotoxicity of glutathione-conjugated chlorohydroquinones. Toxicol Appl Pharmacol 110: 45–60

Monks TJ, Lau SS (1987) Commentary: renal transport processes and glutathione conjugate-mediated nephrotoxicity. Drug Metab Dispos 15: 437–441

Monks TJ, Lau SS (1989) Sulphur conjugate-mediated toxicity. Rev Biochem Toxicol 10: 41–90

Monks TJ, Lau SS (1990) Glutathione, γ-glutamyl transpeptidase, and the mercapturic acid pathway as modulators of 2-bromohydroquinone oxidation. Toxicol Appl Pharmacol 103: 557–563

Monks TJ, Lau SS, Highet RJ, Gillette JR (1985) Glutathione conjugates of 2-bromohydroquinone are nephrotoxic. Drug Metab Dispos 13: 553–559

Monks TJ, Highet RJ, Lau SS (1988) 2-Bromo-(diglutathion-*S*-yl)hydroquinone nephrotoxicity: physiological, biochemical, and electrochemical determinants. Mol Pharmacol 34: 492–500

Nash JA, King LJ, Lock EA, Green T (1984) The metabolism and disposition of hexachloro-1:3-butadiene in the rat and its relevance to nephrotoxicity. Toxicol Appl Pharmacol 73: 124–137

National Cancer Institute (NCI) (1986a) Carcinogenesis bioassay of trichloroethylene. National toxicology program technical report 311

National Cancer Institute (NCI) (1986b) Carcinogenesis bioassay of tetrachloroethylene. National toxicology program technical report 232

Newton JF, Kuo C-H, Gemborys MW, Mudge GH, Hook JB (1982) Nephrotoxicity of p-aminophenol, a metabolite of acetaminophen, in the Fischer 344 rat. Toxicol Appl Pharmacol 65: 336–344

Odum J, Green T (1984) The metabolism and nephrotoxicity of tetrafluoroethylene in the rat. Toxicol Appl Pharmacol 76: 306–318

Oesch F, Wolf CR (1989) Properties of the microsomal and cytosolic glutathione transferases involved in hexachloro-1:3-butadiene conjugation. Biochem Pharmacol 38: 353–359

Potter CL, Gandolfi AJ, Nagle R, Clayton JW (1981) Effects of inhaled chlorotrifluoroethylene and hexafluoropropene on the rat kidney. Toxicol Appl Pharmacol 59: 431–440

Redegeld FAM, Hofman GA, Loo PGF, Koster AS, Noordhoek J (1991) Nephrotoxicity of glutathione conjugate of menadione (2-methyl-1,4-naphthoquinone) in the isolated perfused rat kidney. Role of metabolism by γ-glutamyltranspeptidase and probenecid-sensitive transport. J Pharmacol Exp Ther 256: 665–669

Reichert D, Schuetz S (1986) Mercapturic acid formation is an activation and intermediary step in the metabolism of hexachlorobutadiene. Biochem Pharmacol 35: 1271–1275

Reichert D, Ewald D, Henschler D (1975) Generation and inhalation toxicity of dichloroacetylene. Food Cosmet Toxicol 13: 511–515

Vamvakas S, Köster U (1993) The nephrotoxin dichlorovinylcysteine induces expression of the protooncogenes c-*fos* and c-*myc* in LLC-PK_1 cells – a comparative investigation with growth factors and 12-*O*-tetradecanoylphorbolacetate. Cell Biol Toxicol 9: 1–13

Vamvakas S, Berthold K, Dekant W, Henschler D (1988a) Bacterial cysteine conjugate β-lyase and the metabolism of cysteine *S*-conjugates: structural requirements for the cleavage of *S*-conjugates and the formation of reactive intermediates. Chem Biol Interact 65: 59–71

Vamvakas S, Elfarra AA, Dekant W, Henschler D, Anders MW (1988b) Mutagenicity of amino acid and glutathione *S*-conjugates in the Ames test. Mutat Res 206: 83–90

Vamvakas S, Kremling EWD (1989a) Metabolic activation of the nephrotoxic haloalkene 1,1,2-trichloro-3,3,3-trifluoro-1-propene by glutathione conjugation. Biochem Pharmacol 38: 2297–2304

Vamvakas S, Herkenhoff M, Dekant W, Henschler D (1989b) Mutagenicity of tetrachloroethylene in the Ames-test–metabolic activation by conjugation with glutathione. J Biochem Toxicol 4: 21–27

Vamvakas S, Dekant W, Henschler D (1989c) Assessment of unscheduled DNA synthesis in a cultured line of renal epithelial cells exposed to cysteine *S*-conjugates of haloalkenes and haloalkanes. Mutat Res 222: 329–335

Vamvakas S, Dekant W, Henschler D (1989d) Genotoxicity of haloalkene and haloalkane glutathione *S*-conjugates in porcine kidney cells. Toxicol In Vitro 3: 151–156

Vamvakas S, Köchling A, Berthold K, Dekant W (1989e) Cytotoxicity of cysteine *S*-conjugates: structure-activity relationships. Chem Biol Interact 71: 79–90

Vamvakas S, Sharma VK, Shen S-S, Anders MW (1990) Perturbations of intracellular calcium distribution in kidney cells by nephrotoxic haloalkenyl cysteine *S*-conjugates. Mol Pharmacol 38: 455–461

Vamvakas S, Bittner D, Dekant W, Anders MW (1992) Events that precede and that follow *S*-(1,2-dichlorovinyl)-L-cysteine-induced release of mitochondrial Ca^{2+} and their association with cytotoxicity to renal cells. Biochem Pharmacol 44: 1131–1138

Wallin A, Gerdes RG, Morgenstern R, Jones TW, Ormstad K (1988) Features of microsomal and cytosolic glutathione conjugation of hexachlorobutadiene in rat liver. Chem Biol Interact 68: 1–11

Werner M, Guo Z, Birner G, Dekant W, Guengerich FP (1995) The sulfoxidation of the hexachlorobutadiene metabolite *N*-acetyl-*S*-(1,2,3,4,4-pentachlorobutadienyl)-L-cysteine is catalyzed by human cytochrome P450 3A enzymes. Chem Res Toxicol 8: 917–923

Wolf CR, Berry PN, Nash JA, Green T, Lock EA (1984) Role of microsomal and cytosolic glutathione *S*-transferases in the conjugation of hexachloro-1:3-butadiene and its possible relevance to toxicity. J Pharmacol Exp Ther 228: 202–208

Zheng J, Hanzlik RP (1992) Dihydroxylated mercapturic acid metabolites of bromobenzene. Chem Res Toxicol 5: 561–567

Ultraviolet-Induced Photolesions: Repair and Mutagenesis

L.H.F. Mullenders[1,2], A. van Hoffen[1], M.P.G. Vreeswijk[1], H.-J. Ruven[1], H. Vrieling[1,2], and A.A. van Zeeland[1,2]

[1]MGC-Department of Radiation Genetics and Chemical Mutagenesis, Leiden University, Wassenaarseweg 72, 2333 AL Leiden, The Netherlands
[2]J.A. Cohen Institute, Interuniversity Research Institute for Radiopathology and Radiation Protection, 2333 AL Leiden, The Netherlands

Introduction

There is convincing evidence that the structure of chromatin may influence both the induction and processing of DNA damage within various parts of the genome that exhibit diverse molecular structures and activities. For a variety of lesions it has been shown that nucleotide excision repair (NER) takes place preferentially in transcriptionally active DNA (Mullenders and Smith 1994). Cyclobutane pyrimidine dimers (CPD) induced by ultraviolet (UV) light as well as DNA adducts induced by chemical carcinogens such as benzo(a)pyrene diol epoxide, aflatoxin B_1 and psoralen are more rapidly repaired in transcriptionally active housekeeping genes than in inactive tissue specific genes, ribosomal genes, regions of noncoding DNA, or the genome overall (Bohr et al. 1985; Mellon et al. 1986; Venema et al. 1990; Ruven et al. 1993). However, from the analysis of repair of other bulky lesions in specific sequences in both rodent and human cells it has become clear that not all bulky lesions are preferentially repaired in active genes and that there are no simple rules predicting whether a given lesion is repaired preferentially or not (Mullenders and Smith 1994).

Several mechanisms may be involved in the process of preferential repair. It is obvious that the more open configuration of chromatin engaged in transcription could underlie the accelerated repair of lesions in transcriptionally active regions of the genome. From this point of view the preferential repair of active genes is seen as a consequence of differential accessibility of chromatin for repair factors. Another possibility would be that the transcription process itself plays an active role in the accelerated repair of active genes. The experimental data obtained so far suggest a role for both chromatin structure and transcription in the process of preferential repair.

From a biological point of view, DNA repair serves to alleviate the lethal, mutagenic, and carcinogenic consequences of DNA damage. Therefore, intragenomic heterogeneity of repair could have major implications for

Recent Results in Cancer Research, Vol. 143

DNA damage frequencies in various genomic regions. As a consequence, poorly repaired nonexpressed DNA sequences might accumulate DNA damage and mutations. However, with the current technology it is difficult to measure mutations in silent sequences, and therefore effects of heterogeneous repair on mutation induction can only be deduced for some expressed genes for which mutant selection systems exist.

In this paper we will focus on the repair of UV-induced photolesions and their role in mutagenesis. The major lesions induced by UVC irradiation are CPD and pyrimidine 6-4 pyrimidone photoproducts (6-4PP). We will briefly review the current knowledge on heterogeneity of repair of these two types of photolesions, propose a model describing the existence of hierarchies of DNA repair, and discuss the ultimate consequences of heterogeneous repair for mutagenesis in mammalian cells.

Repair of CPD in Mammalian Cells

Rodent Cells

At the gene level, intragenomic heterogeneity of repair of UV-induced CPD was first observed in rodent cells (Bohr et al. 1985). The methodology for measuring repair of CPD in defined sequences was initially developed and described for Chinese hamster ovary (CHO) cells containing amplified dihydrofolate reductase (DHFR) sequences. Within the amplified domain, CPD were removed faster and more efficiently from the active DHFR gene than from inactive flanking sequences or the genome overall (Bohr et al. 1985). Further analysis of repair of CPD in various rodent cell lines and genomic sequences (Madhani et al. 1986; Vrieling et al. 1991; Vreeswijk et al. 1994) has revealed that preferential repair of transcriptionally active genes is a general feature of rodent cells. In fact all these studies showed that inactive sequences are repaired as poorly as the genome overall and that efficient removal of CPD is restricted to RNA polymerase II transcribed genes.

An important question relates to which factors and mechanisms account for the rapid repair of active genes. An obvious possibility would be that the transcription process itself plays an active role in the accelerated repair of active genes. A number of observations are consistent with this hypothesis. Insight into the role of transcription in DNA repair was provided by the discovery that the rapid repair of CPD in the DHFR gene in CHO cells was confined to the transcribed strand only (Mellon et al. 1987). This is also the case for other genes in rodent cell lines as shown for the HPRT gene in V79 cells (Vrieling et al. 1991) (Fig. 1a). The nontranscribed strand of active genes in rodent cells is repaired with similar slow kinetics as repair of CPD in the genome overall. This suggests that chromatin configuration alone cannot account for the preferential repair of CPD and implies a role for the transcription process itself in the removal of CPD in rodent cells. Direct

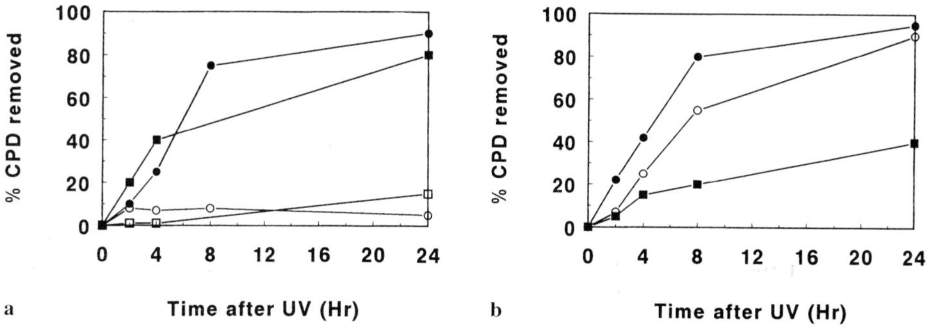

Fig. 1a,b. Removal of cyclobutane pyrimidine dimers (*CPD*) from active and inactive genes in mammalian cells exposed to 10 J/m^2 UV light. **a** Rodent cells. Hamster V79 cells: *Solid circles*, HPRT, ts; *open circles*, HPRT, nts. Mouse epidermis cells: *solid squares*, HPRT, ts; *open squares*, HPRT, nts. *ts*, transcribed strand; *nts*, nontranscribed strand. **b** Human cells. *Solid circles*, adenosine deaminase (ADA), ts; *open circles*, ADA, nts; *solid squares*, factor IX (inactive)

evidence for the participation of transcription in repair of CPD in active genes is given by the fact that inhibition of transcription by the RNA polymerase II inhibitor alpha-amanitin abolishes the removal of CPD from the transcribed strand in CHO cells (Christians and Hanawalt 1992; Leadon and Lawrence 1991). Consequently, the repair pathway which removes lesions from the transcribed strand of active genes and which involves a close coupling of repair to RNA polymerase II-driven transcription has been termed transcription-coupled repair.

It is important to know whether the results obtained with cultured cells actually reflect the situation in whole organisms. It is now clear that the heterogeneity of CPD repair as observed in cultured rodent cells indeed mimics the situation in vivo (Fig. 1a). Ruven et al. (1993, 1994) have demonstrated that in the epidermis of UVB-irradiated hairless mice, CPD are efficiently removed from active genes, but very slowly from inactive sequences. Importantly, the efficient repair of CPD in the p53 and HPRT gene in the mouse epidermis was confined to the transcribed strand only.

Human Cells

Preferential and strand-specific repair of CPD in transcriptionally active genes has also been reported for primary and immortalized human cells (Mellon et al. 1986, 1987; Venema et al. 1990, 1991; Kantor et al. 1990). In that case preferential repair concerns differences in the rate of repair, since human cells are capable of performing complete removal of CPD from their genome. Also in human cells, repair of the transcribed strand of an active gene is more rapid when compared to the nontranscribed strand. The kinetics and extent of repair in the nontranscribed strand of active genes is similar to that of the genome overall, suggesting the absence of gross variations in repair among the different genomic regions (Mellon et al. 1987). However, direct comparison of genomic sequences reveals distinct differences in rate and extent of repair between expressed housekeeping genes, ribosomal genes, and nonexpressed X-chromosomal genes (Fig. 1b). Both the ribosomal and inactive X-chromosomal genes are repaired with significantly slower kinetics than the active genes. Nevertheless, differences in repair efficiencies may exist among inactive sequences as well since the autosomal inactive δ-globin gene is repaired almost as fast as the active DHFR gene in human fibroblasts (Evans et al. 1993). The question whether the different levels of repair efficiencies in active and inactive genes in human cells are mediated by the transcription process was addressed by investigating repair of the adenosine deaminase (ADA) housekeeping gene in a cell strain in which transcription of the gene was shut off by a deletion of the promoter region (Venema et al. 1992). A profound difference in repair efficiency of the ADA and 754 gene is still observed in the absence of ADA transcription, implying that in addition to the transcription other factors contribute to the efficient repair of housekeeping genes. Obviously, in human cells two pathways are involved in the mechanism of preferential repair of CPD in active genes. One pathway concerns the targeting or concentration of global repair activity towards (potentially) active DNA (Venema et al. 1992). A second pathway involves a close coupling of repair to RNA polymerase II driven transcription. This transcription-coupled repair pathway specifically acts on the transcribed strand and appears to be superimposed on the preferential repair of active genes. Thus, rodent cells differ from human cells in the sense that CPD in active genes in rodents are predominantly removed by transcription-coupled repair.

Further experiments with human cells have revealed that the significance of transcription-coupled repair for removal of CPD depends on the dose employed (van Hoffen et al. 1995). Most of the above-mentioned results are obtained with cells exposed to a moderate UV dose of 10 J/m^2. When CPD repair is determined at a dose of 30 J/m^2 (a dose used to study 6-4PP repair), the relative rate of repair of CPD is much slower than at the dose of 10 J/m^2. Moreover, at 30 J/m^2 no significant differences in repair kinetics are found between the transcribed strand and the nontranscribed strand of ADA gene, whereas after 10 J/m^2, repair of the transcribed strand was much more rapid than that of the nontranscribed strand.

Repair of 6-4PP

6-4PP are induced at a lower frequency than CPD and are removed much more rapidly from the genome overall than CPD, as shown by approaches using specific antibodies (Mitchell 1988). However, in spite of the lower frequency of induction, these lesions may play a key role in UV-induced cytotoxicity and mutagenesis (Zdzienicka et al. 1992). Progress in quantification of 6-4PP at the gene level has been hampered for a long time mainly due to the lack of a specific endonuclease to cut the DNA at the site of 6-4PP. To overcome this problem Thomas et al. (1989) developed an alternative approach exploring the property of *E. coli* excinuclease complex UvrABC to cut at sites of DNA damage. However, the UvrABC complex is capable of incising the DNA at a variety of lesions including CPD and 6-4PP. To determine 6-4PP specifically, CPD are first removed from the DNA by in vitro photoreactivation prior to cutting with UvrABC. It is known from immunochemical studies that heterogeneity in induction of 6-4PP exists at the nucleosome level, as 6-4PP are predominantly induced in linker DNA (Mitchell et al. 1990). In spite of this heterogeneity no clear differences in induction of 6-4PP are found between transcribed and nontranscribed sequences in human, hamster, and *Drosophila* cells (Thomas et al. 1989; De Cock et al. 1992; van Hoffen et al. 1995). Following UVC irradiation (predominantly 254 nm) the frequency of 6-4PP is approximately 30% of the CPD frequency. In order to obtain the desirable induction of approximately one 6-4PP per fragment of 15–20 kb which is needed to perform proper estimates of lesion frequencies at the gene level, repair studies of 6-4PP are generally carried out at doses of 30 J/m^2 or higher.

Rodent Cells

In rodent cells (CHO and V79) studies have been focused on the repair of 6-4PP in transcriptionally active housekeeping genes and in inactive sequences or in noncoding DNA (Thomas et al. 1989; Vreeswijk et al. 1994). The general outcome of these experiments is a fast repair of 6-4PP in both active and inactive genes and the absence of clear differences in kinetics of 6-4PP repair between the two types of genes. When considering the repair of 6-4PP and CPD in active genes, i.e., the HPRT and APRT gene, it is obvious that the relative number of 6-4PP removed exceeds the number of CPD during the first 24 h after UV (Fig. 2a). Also, the absolute number of 6-4PP removed exceeds the number of CPD during the first 4 h (Vreeswijk et al. 1994). No differences are found in removal of 6-4PP between the transcribed and nontranscribed strand of the active HPRT and APRT gene, suggesting that the contribution of transcription coupled repair to the repair of 6-4PP in active genes in cells exposed to 30 J/m^2 is very low (Vreeswijk et al. 1994).

Human Cells

Induction and removal of 6-4PP has been studied in primary human fibroblasts irradiated with a UV dose of 30 J/m^2 (van Hoffen et al. 1995). Repair of 6-4PP in the ADA housekeeping gene is very rapid: 50% of the lesions were removed

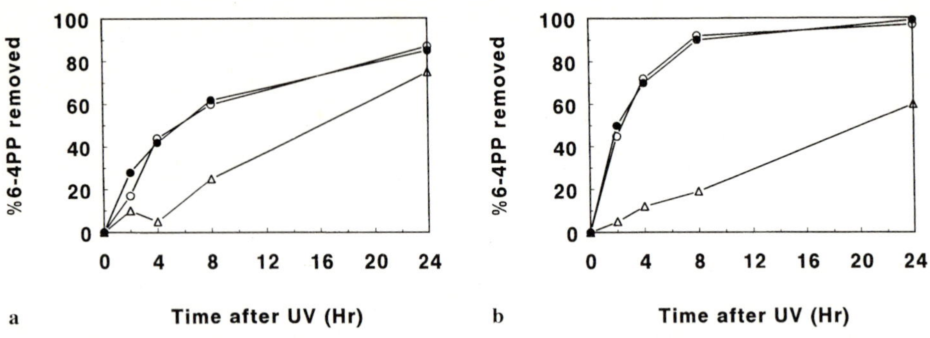

Fig. 2a,b. Removal of 6-4 PP from active and inactive genes in mammalian cells exposed to 30 J/m^2 UV light. **a** Hamster V79 cells. *Solid circles,* HPRT, ts; *open circles,* HPRT, nts; **b** Human cells. *Solid squares*, ADA, ts; *open squares,* ADA, nts. For comparison the repair of CPD in cells exposed to 30 J/m^2 is also shown (*triangles*)

within 2 h (Fig. 2). After 8 h the repair is complete. In these experiments the initial rate of repair of the inactive 754 locus appears to be lower than that of the ADA gene, indicating that intragenomic heterogeneity of 6-4PP repair exists. There is a large difference in the rate of repair between CPD and 6-4PP, the latter being repaired about fivefold more rapidly than CPD when measured at the same dose (30 J/m^2).

Just like in the rodent cells, no significant differences in the rate of repair of 6-4PP are detected between the transcribed strand and the nontranscribed strand of an active gene. So far, no clear evidence for transcription-coupled repair of 6-4PP in repair-proficient mammalian cells exists. However, experiments with repair-deficient human cells definitely demonstrated that 6-4PP really form a target for transcription-coupled repair. Cells from patients suffering from the human UV-sensitive disorder xeroderma pigmentosum and belonging to complementation group C (XP-C), are only capable of performing transcription-coupled repair even at the high UV dose of 30 J/m^2. In these cells CPD as well as 6-4PP are removed selectively and with similar kinetics from the transcribed strand of the ADA gene (van Hoffen et al. 1995). The nontranscribed strand of the ADA gene as well as the inactive 754 gene are hardly repaired. These results strongly suggest that normal cells exposed to 30 J/m^2 lack strand-specific repair of 6-4PP and CPD, because of the fact that transcription-coupled repair is overruled by a general repair system (also designated as global genome repair pathway), probably due to severe inhibition of transcription at this high UV dose. The much more rapid repair of 6-4PP compared to CPD in normal cells is most likely related to higher affinity of the global genome repair system for the former lesion. The similarity of the rate of repair of both 6-4PP and CPD in the transcribed strand as observed in XP-C cells indicates that transcription-coupled repair of photolesions takes place in a processive way.

Hierarchies of DNA Repair

The currently available data for repair of UV-induced photolesions suggest the existence of several hierarchies of DNA repair:

1. Slow repair of transcriptionally inactive (X-chromosomal) chromatin as well as ribosomal genes
2. Rapid repair of transcriptionally poised or active chromatin
3. Accelerated repair of the transcribed strand of transcriptionally active genes

Several factors might contribute to the differences in repair kinetics between active and inactive genes. In the case of CPD it is obvious that transcription itself contributes to the accelerated repair of the transcribed strand. However, in the absence of transcription, repair of CPD in an inactive tissue-specific gene is still less than in a nontranscribed housekeeping gene (Venema et al. 1992). In the case of 6-4PP, the nontranscribed strand of an active gene is repaired as rapidly as the transcribed strand and thus transcription itself cannot contribute to the preferential repair of this lesion in active genes when compared to inactive X-chromosomal genes. Therefore, it is likely that chromatin configuration influences repair efficiency as well. Transcriptional activity is usually accompanied by hyperacetylation of nucleosome core histones, a process which is known to stimulate repair (Ramanathan and Smerdon 1989), and by a reduced level of methylation of DNA (Adams 1990). In CHO cells, reduction of the level of methylation mediated by 5-azacytidine treatment was accompanied by increased UV-induced excision repair measured in the genome overall and in specific genes (Ho et al. 1989). DNA of inactive X-chromosomal loci is known to be heavily methylated (Adams 1990) which may lead to less efficient repair in these regions of the genome. Another factor that could play a role in the preferential repair of lesions in active genes is the positioning of active genes proximal to the nuclear matrix. Recently the transcription factor TFIIH was shown to include proteins playing a role in the global repair pathway (Schaeffer et al. 1993; Drapkin et al. 1994). Given the fact that transcription complexes have been shown to be located at the nuclear matrix (Jackson et al. 1993), it becomes likely that compartmentalization of these complexes facilitates both transcription and repair. As a consequence, genes that are located proximal to the nuclear matrix tend to be repaired more rapidly.

Consequences of Preferential Repair for Mutagenesis

Heterogeneity of DNA repair could have major implications for induction of mutations as the frequency of mutations primarily depends on the extent of repair of mutagenic lesions which can occur before fixation during DNA replication. It is conceivable that the selective removal of CPD from the transcribed strand of active genes in rodent cells, and the accelerated repair of CPD in this strand in human cells, will be reflected in UV light-induced mutations. The molecular nature of mutations induced by UV light has been investigated in HPRT mutants from various Chinese hamster cell lines with different repair capacities (Vrieling et al. 1989, 1991; Menichini et al. 1991) and in APRT mutants of CHO cells (Drobetsky et al. 1987). Among the HPRT mutants analyzed from repair-proficient cells (two cell lines, i.e., V79 and CHO) all possible classes of base pair changes were present, the majority being transversions. This is in contrast to the mutations in the APRT gene, which predominantly consist of GC→AT transitions. Since almost all HPRT and APRT mutations occur at dipyrimidine sites, it is likely that they are caused by UV-induced photoproducts (CPD and/or (6-4) photoproducts) at these sites. In repair-proficient cells, after UV irradiation with 2 J/m^2, over 85% of the HPRT mutations could be attributed to lesions in the non-transcribed strand of the HPRT gene (Vrieling et al. 1991). In the APRT gene the mutations are much more evenly distributed over both strands. It is important to note that in the APRT gene of V79 cells CPD are removed from both strands of the gene, suggesting that the APRT template strand and the nontemplate strand are transcribed (Vreeswijk et al. 1994). Thus the data on the strand distribution of mutations in both genes are consistent with the hypothesis that strand-specific repair of CPD in expressed mammalian genes is associated with strand specificity for mutation induction: the selective removal of CPD from the transcribed strand of the HPRT gene and the efficient repair of both strands of the APRT gene would account for the presence and the absence of a strand bias in mutations, respectively. In vivo the selective repair of CPD in the transcribed strand of the p53 gene in UVB-irradiated hairless mice is in accordance with the notion that the majority of p53 mutations in skin tumors is caused by photolesions in the poorly repaired non-transcribed strand.

Also, in human cells an effect of preferential removal of photoproducts from the transcribed strand of the HPRT gene on mutation induction has been observed (McGregor et al. 1991). In synchronized primary human fibroblasts irradiated in the G1 phase of the cell cycle (6 h before the S-phase), the majority of HPRT mutations were due to photolesions in the nontranscribed strand, suggesting that photoproducts are preferentially removed from the transcribed strand in the time period between G1 and S. However, mutations in cells irradiated in the S-phase were mainly caused by lesions in the transcribed strand, indicating that fixation of mutations quickly happened after UV irradiation, leaving too little time for repair effects on mutagenesis.

The absence of repair results in a dramatic change in the HPRT mutation spectrum compared to repair-proficient conditions, as mutations consist almost solely of GC → AT transitions (Vrieling et al. 1989). The majority of the base pair changes in repair-deficient cells are caused by photoproducts in the transcribed strand of the HPRT gene. Thus the absence of DNA repair affects the mutation spectrum in two ways: it alters the types of UV-induced mutations as well as the strand distribution of mutations. These observations are best explained by assuming that under repair-proficient conditions CPD are the major contributors to mutagenesis, whereas under repair-deficient conditions, mutations are mainly caused by 6-4PP which are known to be highly mutagenic (Zdzienicka et al. 1992; Wood 1985).

Nevertheless, it is still possible that the strand bias in HPRT mutations seen in repair-proficient rodent cells is actually due to strand-specific repair of 6-4PP at the low UV dose used for mutation induction experiments. Although in rodent and human cells repair of 6-4PP occurs without strand preference, it is obvious that the significance of transcription-coupled repair for removal of photolesions in active genes depends on the UV dose employed. Generally speaking, the lower the UV dose, the larger the contribution of transcription-coupled repair to repair of active genes. Consequently, it cannot be ruled out that in cells exposed to a low UV dose (e.g., 2-12 J/m^2, used for mutation induction experiments) 6-4PP repair in active genes may be dominated by transcription-coupled repair. Mutation studies in hamster cells suggest that a UV dose effect on transcription-coupled repair of DNA photolesions might exist. As mentioned above, at a low UV dose (2 J/m^2), a strong bias for mutation induction in the HPRT gene towards the nontranscribed strand is observed, consistent with the preferential repair of UV-induced lesions in the transcribed strand. However, at a higher UV dose (12 J/m^2) at which CPD are still preferentially repaired, the strand bias is much less pronounced (Vrieling et al. 1991). A possible explanation for this phenomenon is that at 12 J/m^2, transcription-coupled repair of 6-4PP is less efficient than at 2 J/m^2 and is overruled by the global repair pathway.

Acknowledgements. This study was supported by the association of Leiden University with Euratom (contract F13P-CT92-0007), the Dutch Cancer Society (contract IKW 92-32), and the Environment Program of the European Community (contract EV5V-CT91-0030).

References

Adams RLP (1990) DNA methylation. Biochem J 265: 309–320

Bohr VA, Smith CA, Okumoto DS, Hanawalt PC (1985) DNA repair in an active gene: removal of pyrimidine dimers from the DHFR gene of CHO cells is much more efficient than in the genome overall. Cell 40: 359–369

Christians FC, Hanawalt PC (1992) Inhibition of transcription and strand-specific DNA repair by α-amanitin in Chinese hamster ovary cells. Mutat Res 274: 93–101

De Cock JGR, van Hoffen A, Wijnands J, Molenaar G, Lohman PHM, Eeken JCJ (1992) Repair of UV-induced 6–4 photoproducts measured in individual genes in the Drosophila embryonic Kc cell line. Nucleic Acids Res 20: 4789–4793

Drapkin R, Sancar A, Reinberg D (1994) Where transcription meets repair. Cell 77: 9–12

Drobetsky EA, Grosovsky AJ, Glickman BW (1987) The specificity of UV-induced mutations at an endogenous locus in mammalian cells. Proc Natl Acad Sci USA 84; 9103–9107

Evans MK, Robbins JH, Ganges MB, Tarone RE, Nairn RS, Bohr VA (1993) Gene-specific DNA repair in xeroderma pigmentosum complementation groups A,C,D and F. J Biol Chem 268: 4839–4847

Ho L, Bohr VA, Hanawalt PC (1989) Demethylation enhances removal of pyrimidine dimers from the genome overall and from specific sequences in Chinese hamster ovary cells. Mol Cell Biol 1594–1603

Jackson DA, Hassan AB, Errington RJ, Cook PR (1993) Visualization of focal sites of transcription within human nuclei. EMBO J 12: 1059–1065

Kantor GJ, Barsalou LS, Hanawalt PC (1990) Selective repair of specific chromatin domains in UV-irradiated cells from xeroderma pigmentosum complementation group C. Mutat Res 235: 171–180

Leadon SA, Lawrence DA (1991) Preferential repair of DNA damage on the transcribed strand of the human metallothionein gene requires RNA polymerase II. Mutat Res 255: 67–78

Madhani HD, Bohr VA, Hanawalt PC (1986) Differential DNA repair in the transcriptionally active and inactive proto-oncogenes c-able and c-mos. Cell 45: 417–423

McGregor WG, Chen RH, Lukash L, Maher VM, McCormick JJ (1991) Cell cycle-dependent strand bias for UV-induced mutations in the transcribed strand of excision repair-proficient human fibroblasts but not in repair-deficient cells. Mol Cell Biol 11: 1927–1934

Mellon I, Bohr VA, Smith CA, Hanawalt PC (1986) Preferential DNA repair of an active gene in human cells. Proc Natl Acad Sci USA 83: 8878–8882

Mellon I, Spivak G, Hanawalt PC (1987) Selective removal of transcription blocking DNA damage from the transcribed strand of the mammalian DHFR gene. Cell 51: 241–249

Menichini P, Vrieling H, van Zeeland AA (1991) Strand specific mutation spectra in repair proficient and repair deficient hamster cells. Mutat Res 251: 143–155

Mitchell DL (1988) The biology of the 6-4 photoproduct. Photochem Photobiol 49: 805–819

Mitchell DL, Nguyen TD, Cleaver JE (1990) Nonrandom induction of pyrimidine-pyrimidone 6–4 photoproducts in ultraviolet-irradiated human chromatin. J Biol Chem 265: 5353–5356

Mullenders LHF, Smith CA (1994) DNA repair in specific sequences and genomic regions. In: Tardiff RG, Lohman PHM, Wogan GN (eds) Methods to assess DNA damage and repair. Interspecies comparisons. Scientific Group on Methodologies for the Safety Evaluation of Chemicals (SGOMSEC). Wiley, Chicester, pp 141–156

Ramanathan B, Smerdon MJ (1989) Enhanced DNA repair synthesis in hyper-acetylated nucleosomes. J Biol Chem 264 (19): 11026–11034

Ruven HJT, Berg RJW, Seelen CMJ, Dekkers JAJ, Lohman PHM, Mullenders LHF, van Zeeland AA (1993) Ultraviolet-induced cyclobutane pyrimidine dimers are selectively removed from transcriptionally active genes in the epidermis of the hairless mouse. Cancer Res 53: 1642–1645

Ruven HJT, Seelen CMJ, Lohman PHM, van Kranen H, van Zeeland AA, Mullenders LHF (1994) Strand-specific removal of cyclobutane pyrimidine dimers from the p53 gene in the epidermis of UV-B irradiated hairless mice. Oncogene 9: 3427–3432

Schaeffer L, Roy R, Humbert S, Moncollin V, Vermeulen W, Hoeijmakers JHJ, Chambon P, Egly JM (1993) DNA repair helicase: a component of BTF2 (TFIIH) basic transcription factor. Science 260: 58–63

Thomas DC, Okumoto DS, Sancar A, Bohr VA (1989) Preferential repair of 6-4 photoproducts in the dihydrofolate reductase gene of the Chinese hamster ovary cells. J Biol Chem 264: 18005–18010

van Hoffen A, Venema J, Meschini R, van Zeeland AA, Mullenders LHF (1995) Transcription coupled repair removes both cyclobutane pyrimidine dimers and 6-4 photoproducts with equal efficiency and in a sequential way from transcribed DNA in xeroderma pigmentosum group C fibroblasts. EMBO J 14: 360–367

Venema J, van Hoffen A, Natarajan AT, van Zeeland AA, Mullenders LHF (1990) The residual repair capacity of xeroderma pigmentosum group C fibroblasts is highly specific for transcriptionally active DNA. Nucleic Acids Res 18: 443–448

Venema J, van Hoffen A, Karcagi V, Natarajan AT, van Zeeland AA, Mullenders LHF (1991) Xeroderma pigmentosum complementation group C cells remove pyrimidine dimers selectively from the transcribed strand of active genes. Mol Cell Biol 4128–4134

Venema J, Bartosova Z, Natarajan AT, van Zeeland AA, Mullenders LHF (1992) Transcription affects the rate but not the extent of repair of cyclobutane pyrimidine dimers in the human adenosine deaminase gene. J Biol Chem 267: 8852–8856

Vreeswijk MPG, van Hoffen A, Westland BE, Vrieling H, van Zeeland AA, Mullenders LHF (1994) Analysis of repair of cyclobutane pyrimidine dimers and pyrimidine (6-4) pyrimidone photoproducts in transcriptionally active and inactive genes in Chinese hamster cells. J Biol Chem 16: 31858–31863

Vrieling H, van Rooyen M-L, Groen NA, Zdzienicka MZ, Simons JWIM, Lohman PHM, van Zeeland AA (1989) DNA strand specificity for UV-induced mutations in mammalian cells. Mol Cell Biol 9: 1277–1283

Vrieling H, Venema J, van Rooijen Ml, van Hoffen A, Menichini P, Zdzienicka MZ, Simons JWIM, Mullenders LHF, van Zeeland AA (1991) Strand specificity for UV-induced DNA repair and mutations in the Chinese hamster HPRT gene. Nucleic Acids Res 19: 2411–2415

Wood RD (1985) Pyrimidine dimers are not the principal premutagenic lesions induced in lambda phage DNA by ultraviolet light. J Mol Biol 184: 577–585

Zdzienicka MZ, Venema J, Mitchell DL, van Hoffen A, van Zeeland AA, Vrieling H, Mullenders LHF, Lohman PHM, Simons JWIM (1992) 6-4 Photoproducts and not cyclobutane pyrimidine dimers are the main UV-induced mutagenic lesions in Chinese hamster cells. Mutat Res 273: 73–83

Psoralen Photobiology: The Relationship Between DNA Damage, Chromatin Structure, Transcription, and Immunogenic Effects

F.P. Gasparro[1], A. Felli[2], and I.M. Schmitt[2]

[1]Photobiology Laboratory, Department of Surgery, Yale University, New Haven, CT 06510, USA
[2]Department of Dermatology, University of L'Aquila, L'Aquila, Italy

Introduction

Background

Cutaneous T-cell lymphoma is a disease characterized by uncontrolled proliferation of a malignant clone of the T helper cell lineage (Edelson 1975). In early stages the disease is localized to the skin (patch stage) and may last for months or even years before progressing to plaques and/or tumors with involvement of the internal organs. Treatment regimens for the early stage have included a variety of topical substances including steroids, local and/or systemic immunochemotherapy and multiple established and experimental combinations (X-rays, electron beam radiation, and chemotherapy such as topical nitrogen mustard) (Kaye et al. 1988). Photochemotherapy using 8-methoxypsoralen (8-MOP) and UVA radiation is considered an important first-line treatment and often induces dramatic responses which can be confirmed histologically by the observed reduction of pathological lymphocytic infiltrates in skin biopsies (Gilchrest 1979). In the later stages, malignant cells appear to further disseminate into lymph nodes and internal organs with characteristic clinical features (e.g., adenopathy). In this case, the effects of psoralen ultraviolet A (PUVA) can be short-lived, thereby necessitating the implementation of adjunctive therapies (Rook et al. 1991). The development of extracorporeal photochemotherapy (or photopheresis) led to improved treatment for both early and late stages of CTCL with an apparent high degree of efficacy (Edelson et al. 1987) and enhanced long-term survival (Heald et al. 1992).

In photopheresis, the oral ingestion of 8-methoxypsoralen is used to achieve a therapeutic level of 8-methoxypsoralen (8-MOP). Heparinized venous blood is centrifuged, separating the red blood cell, white blood cell, and plasma fractions. The red blood cells are returned to the patient immediately while the latter two fractions are combined with the normal saline used to prime the system. A total volume of 740 ml is recirculated through an irradiation chamber (as a 1.4-mm film). At any given instant approximately 100 ml is exposed to UVA radiation. It is essential to remove a significant fraction of the red blood cells (>95%) because they shield the psoralen-containing lymphocytes from the UVA radiation. This process is performed for approximately 3 h during which the leukocytes complete 10–15 excursions through the UVA field. In a single session approximately 10% of the patient's circulating lymphocytes are treated. However, it should be noted that for most patients only a fraction of these are malignant cells. When the irradiation phase is completed the entire treated volume is returned to the patient. Because the UVA activation of 8-MOP occurs extracorporeally, only the target cells are affected by the photoactivated 8-MOP and the vast majority of the patient's cells are spared the cytotoxic effects of the activated drug. Typically, a patient is treated on 2 consecutive days at monthly intervals. The best response rate has been observed in patients with a near-normal population of $CD8^+$ T cells (Heald et al. 1989). Comparison of survival rates of photopheresis patients to historical controls indicated a doubling of mean survival from 32 months to 66 (Heald et al. 1992).

New Perspectives

Although psoralen plus UVA is known to induce modification of DNA (nuclear and cell membrane), lipids, and proteins (Gasparro 1994), the mechanism underlying clinical responses in diseases treated with photopheresis has been elusive. It appears that changes at the cell surface, induced directly or indirectly by 8-MOP and UVA, enhance cellular immunogenicity, leading to the eventual elimination of both treated and untreated cells. In addition, changes in cytokine secretion patterns and antigen presentation due to altered processing of cellular proteins (Schmitt and Gasparro 1995) or to enhanced expression of class I MHC (Schmitt et al. 1995; Moor et al. 1995) could also contribute to therapeutic responses. Thus, photopheresis, in addition to being a new modality, also appears to derive its efficacy from events distinct from those operative in PUVA (Vallat et al. 1994). In this review the molecular basis for these novel events is described in a model derived from the well-characterized repressive effects of chromatin structure on transcription (Grunstein 1992). In this regard, 8-MOP photochemistry can be viewed as a form of nonspecific genetic therapy. It is reasonable to expect that the modification of the genetic program of the treated cells (normal and/or malignant) must have a significant impact on the disease state. Furthermore, the additional effects on molecules other than DNA play a role which is auxiliary but perhaps essential. As we will see in the following pages the low outright cytotoxicity of photopheresis treatment may bring the genetic reprogramming effects to the forefront. Before proceeding, we review the phenomenological data that led to the development of this new paradigm.

8-MOP Photochemistry In Vitro and In Vivo: Brief Review

The structure of 8-MOP and its corresponding numbering system are shown in Fig. 1 (inset). The extended aromaticity of the tricyclic aromatic compound, in which the 2,3 furan bond is fused to the 6,7 bond of the aromatic coumarin moiety (hence, the name furocoumarin), is responsible for its ability to absorb ultraviolet radiation. 8-MOP has strong absorption bands near 250 and 300 nm and a low but finite absorbance reaching into the visible region of the spectrum (Fig. 1). Its planar structure facilitates its intercalation between DNA base pairs (Fig. 2). The extent of intercalation can be related to spectroscopic changes (e.g., an increase or decrease in fluorescence emission or a shift in the wavelength of emission) and hence can be used to calculate the binding constant (770 M^{-1} cm^{-1} for 8-MOP, Dall'Acqua et al. 1979). A comprehensive list of binding constants has been published (Gasparro 1994).

The absorption of a photon by 8-MOP in its ground state (S_0, the singlet state in which electron spins are antiparallel) can lead to several subsequent events. The primary photophysical process is the promotion of an electron to the manifold of excited singlet states (S_1, S_2, etc., in which the spins remain antiparallel or paired). From this excited state, the electron may return to the ground state by the emission of a photon (fluorescence) or by radiationless collisional deactivation (i.e., the release of energy in the form of heat). Because nonradiative relaxation within an excited state manifold is an efficient process, fluorescence emission occurs from the lowest-lying state.

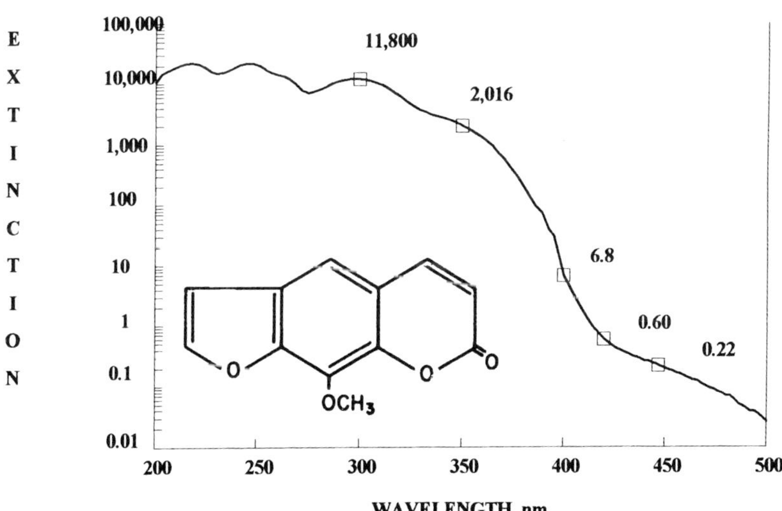

Fig. 1. Structure and UV spectrum for 8-MOP. The log of the extinction coefficient is plotted versus wavelength to illustrate the finite, albeit low, extinction in the short wavelength region of the visible spectrum (400–450 nm). 8-MOP fluorescence occurs at 495 nm, while phosphorescence occurs at even longer wavelengths (Gasparro 1994)

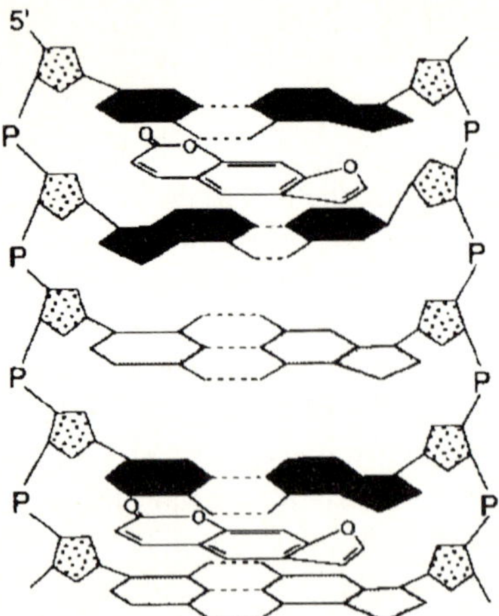

Fig. 2. An 8-MOP molecule is shown intercalated in a short segment of a DNA double helix at a 5′TpA sequence. In this site, the 8-MOP molecule is posed for photoreaction with the thymine

Intersystem crossing (spin inversion – or "flipping" – by the electron in the excited singlet state) leads to the population of the triplet state (T_1, T_2, etc., electron spins now parallel). This is sometimes called a forbidden process (quantum mechanically speaking); however, it occurs with a low but potentially important frequency. Relaxation from the triplet state to the ground state can occur by the emission of radiation (phosphorescence, nominally a forbidden process) or collisional deactivation (heat loss). The triplet state with a lifetime in the range of microseconds to seconds is much longer-lived than the singlet state, which has a lifetime in the nanosecond range.

Photochemical processes for 8-MOP originate from either of these excited states. Photoadditions, -dimerization and/or -oxidations of nearby moieties (nucleic acids, proteins, or membranes) can lead to direct effects on cellular functions. Alternatively, energy from the excited triplet state may be transferred to dioxygen (molecular oxygen, normally in a ground triplet state), leading to the formation of highly reactive oxygen species, such as singlet oxygen and superoxide, which are also capable of modifying biological moieties and thus can disrupt biological processes. These latter effects are referred to as photodynamic effects (type II) The direct generation of reactive free radicals by 8-MOP after absorbing a photon, an example of a type I photodynamic effect, has not been observed. Thus, a sequence of events initiated by a photophysical process, the absorption of a photon and the promotion of an electron to an excited state, can lead to the modification of biomolecules and subsequent effects at the cellular level, e.g., the inhibition of macromolecular synthesis or the induction of specific genes in an SOS-like response, and ultimately to a clinical effect. Although solutions of psoralen alone can undergo photochemical modification (e.g., dimerization and oxidation), it appears that only when psoralen is associated with a biological substance can the resultant photochemistry have cellular consequences with ensuing clinical benefits.

The photochemical reactions of psoralens with nucleic acids are the most well-characterized, having been studied since 1965 (Musajo et al. 1965). After 8-MOP intercalates with DNA hydrogen-bonded base pairs, its reactive sites, located at the carbon-carbon double bonds in the furan (4′,5′) and pyrone rings (3,4), can be activated by exposure to a range of wavelengths (UV or short wavelength visible radiation). The photoadducts formed at these bonds have cyclobutyl bonds involving the 5,6-double bond of a pyrimidine. The extent of photoadduct formation depends on the suitability (base sequence) and base accessibility (affected by chromatin structure and other protein contacts which may occlude some sites and/or induce DNA winding and bending) of intercalation sites between DNA base pairs (Inadomi and Ross 1989).

If the initial photoreaction occurs at a 5′-TpA site, the 4′,5′ monoadduct (Fig. 3) can absorb a second UVA photon and form an interstrand crosslink between two thymines from the adjacent base pairs (Fig. 4). These photoreactions have been completely characterized in vitro using either calf thymus DNA or various synthetic polynucleotides (Olack et al. 1993). Boyer et al. (1988) used short segments of natural DNA to demonstrate conclusively that repetitive runs of adenine and thymine were the most suitable sites for 8-MOP photoadduct formation in vitro. While photoadduct characterization in cells (in vitro and in vivo) was initially hindered by the lack of techniques with sufficient sensitivity to detect the photoadducts at the parts per million level,

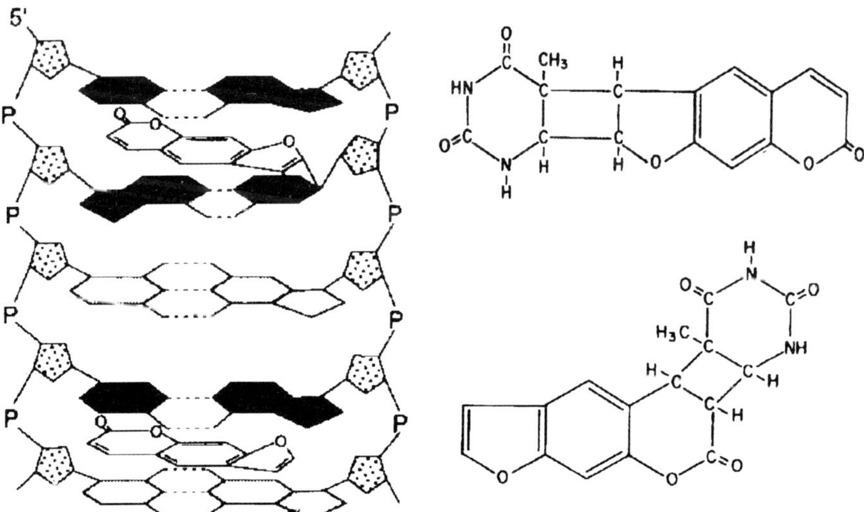

Fig. 3. The primary photoadduct, a 4′,5′-monoadduct, is shown at the 5′TpA site. A two-dimensional representation of the structures of the monoadducts is shown on the *right*

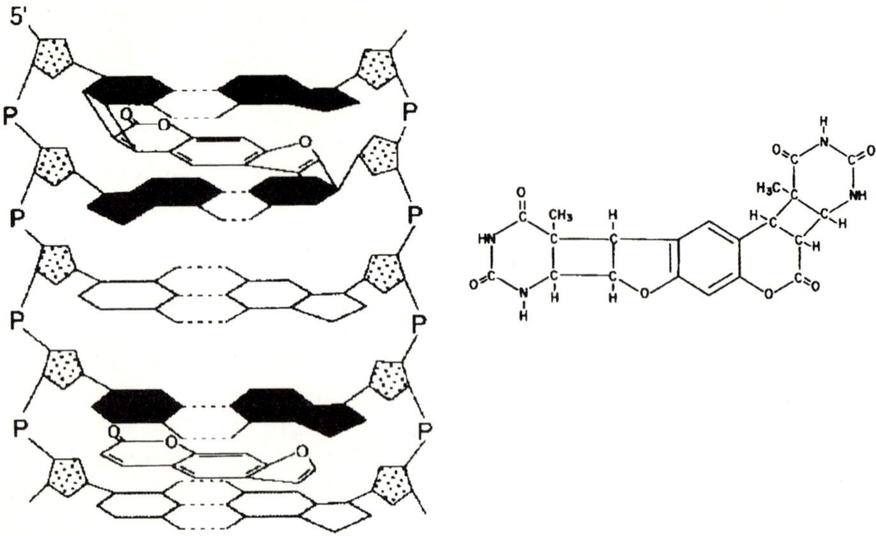

Fig. 4. The absorption of another photon by the 4′,5′-monoadduct leads to an interstrand crosslink

the commercial availability of highly radioactive psoralens has led to the analysis of adduct formation in cells treated with physiological doses of psoralens and UVA (Bevilacqua et al. 1991) or visible radiation (Gasparro et al. 1993a). Thus, thymidine adducts for 8-MOP have been characterized. Cytosine photoadducts, which also form, but more than ten times less efficiently, have similar cyclobutyl ring structures. A psoralen-adenine photoadduct has also been characterized after in vitro photoreactions with adenine but it has not been shown to occur in DNA isolated from cells treated with psoralens and UVA (Yun et al. 1992). Although psoralens also react with uracil in RNA, the extent of reaction in cells and the types of photoadducts formed have not been described as completely as the DNA photoadducts. Another cellular target for 8-MOP, mitochondrial nucleic acid, remains unexamined. Another goal for future studies should be the characterization of 8-MOP photoadduct formation and repair in specific genes and critical binding sequences for transcription factors.

The Fate of Adducts in Cells

Adduct Formation, Repair, and Mutagenesis

Experiments in which various cell types (e.g., human lymphocytes and keratinocytes; murine keratinocytes, lymphoma cells, and fibroblasts; and bovine aorta smooth muscle cells) as well as synthetic DNA have been treated with

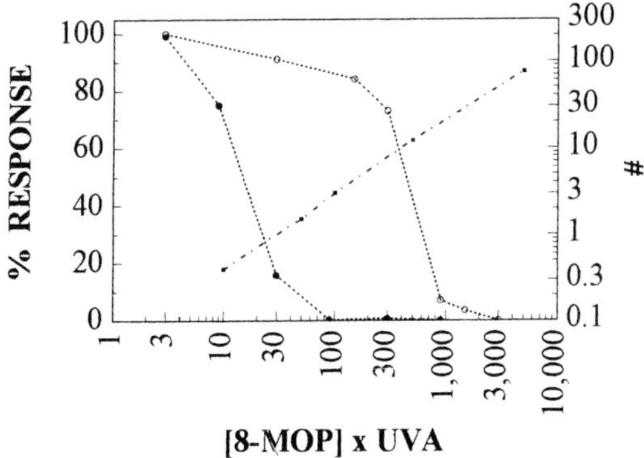

Fig. 5. Dose dependence for photoadduct formation (*solid squares*). Higher doses of 8-MOP and UVA lead to increased yields of photoadducts (correlation coefficient, 1.0). Thus, the number of photoadducts formed can be directly related to the product of 8-MOP concentration in ng/ml and the UVA dose in J/cm^2 (8-MOP concentrations over the range 10–20 000 ng/ml and UVA doses over the range 1–10 J/cm^2). At 10 ng/ml and 1 J/cm^2, 0.4 adducts/mbp are formed, and with 100 ng/ml 8-MOP and 1 J/cm^2, ~4 adducts/mbp. Dose dependence for other phenomena is superimposed on that for adduct formation PHA response (*solid circles*) and viability (*open circles*)

[^{3}H]8-MOP/UVA and have permitted the determination of the photoadduct formation and their distribution. Figure 5 shows that photoadduct formation in 8-MOP/UVA-treated cells (human and murine) is independent of cell type. The extent of photoadduct formation is plotted as the number of photoadducts per million base pairs (mbp) versus the combined dose of 8-MOP (ng/ml) and UVA (J/cm^2). Thus, the amount of 8-MOP present and the UVA dose have a direct effect on the adduct. It is not known what amount of adducts is required for therapeutic efficacy, nor if the latter is affected by the relative numbers of monoadducts and crosslinks.

Extensive repair studies have been carried out in bacterial systems as well as in mammalian cells. Several repair pathways have been described and include excision repair and postreplication recombination repair. 8-MOP photoadducts are known to be repaired, although studies on the repair of discrete adducts in specific genes has been limited. It has often been assumed that crosslinks would not be repaired. However, an excision-recombination mechanism has been proposed to account for crosslink repair in bacteria. Whether such a mechanism is operative in mammalian cells is not known at this time. In cell-free studies of repair, crosslink removal has been observed. Furthermore, it has been suggested that an intermediate product in the repair of crosslink may be a short single-strand segment (~10 base) "dangling" from the repaired site (van Houten et al. 1986).

Under in vitro conditions, freshly isolated human lymphocytes treated with 100 ng/ml 8-MOP and 1 J/cm^2 UVA show no repair after 48 h. However, cells treated with lower 8-MOP doses (10–20 ng/ml) are capable of removing

Table 1. Repair in human and murine cells treated with 8-MOP/UVA

Cell type	8-MOP/UVA[a]	Adducts/mbp	% Repaired (24 h)
Human lymphocytes			
Resting	10/1	0.40	25
PHA-stimulated	10/1	0.80	52
Murine			
Keratinocytes	9/1	0.30	25
Fibroblasts	100/1	2.9	66
Lymphoma cells	100/1	0.42	54
Bovine SMC	1000/12[b]	13.5	25

PHA, phytohemagglutinin; SMC, smooth muscle cells.
[a]8-MOP in ng/ml; UVA in J/cm^2.
[b]J/cm^2 419 nm light.

photoadducts. The removal rate is 25% in 48 h for cells treated with 10 ng/ml of 8-MOP and 1 J/cm^2 UVA (Table 1). The removal of these adducts is also associated with recovery of the proliferative activity as evidenced by the increased levels of tritiated thymidine incorporation after varying repair periods (see above) (Gasparro et al. 1991). In PHA-stimulated lymphocytes it was found that a greater number of photoadducts was formed. In addition there was a greater extent of photoadduct removal. There are two caveats to keep in mind when this repair data is considered. First, these are in vitro studies. The additional stress of being cultured may affect the natural repair of the induced photoadducts. Second, these assays represent the average repair of damage distributed over the entire genome. Since much of the information in DNA is never expressed, this extra damage may not have a direct impact on transcription and replication. Thus, studies designed to measure repair in specific genes will be of great interest. Alternatively, an important effect of DNA damage may be to loosen the chromatin structure (see below).

The effects of monoadducts on cell survival have been examined in more detail in bovine aorta smooth muscle cells (SMC) by using visible light to photoactivate 8-MOP (Sumpio et al. 1994). Although studies in SMC do not have a direct relevance to photopheresis, these data are described here because they are the most detailed studies on 8-MOP monoadducts. We have shown that the survival of SMC cells is proportional to the combined product of 8-MOP concentration, dose of radiation, and the ability to absorb the radiation. Comparable effects can be derived from UVA, 419 nm or 447 nm radiation, despite the progressively lower extinction coefficients at longer wavelengths (see Fig. 1), by increasing the amount of 8-MOP present. The ability of the cells to repair the DNA damage induced by 8-MOP (1 μg/ml) and 12 J/cm^2 419 nm light was measured (including the rate of removal of each type of photoadduct – 3,4-monoadduct, 4′,5′-monoadduct, and crosslink). The doses of 8-MOP and 419 nm light used in this study were selected because it had been shown that they were minimally cytotoxic. Overall adduct removal reached a plateau at ~55% on day 5 following phototreatment. The removal of the monoadducts followed a similar trend while the low level of crosslinks (~10%) appeared to persist over several days.

Depending on the extent of photoadduct formation, a cell may be sublethally or lethally damaged. In the former case, the cellular repair machinery may process the damage faithfully; alternatively the repair may be error-prone which can lead to mutations. We recently reported the correlation between adduct numbers and type with mutations in a transgenic murine system (transgene *supF*) (Gunther et al. 1995). Although psoralen mutagenesis has been studied for nearly 30 years, there have been serious shortcomings. Often the studies have been performed under conditions which differ significantly from those used therapeutically. Furthermore, although certain mutagenic events have been attributed to specific photoadducts (monoadducts or crosslinks) the profiles of these adducts in the treated cells have not been determined in similarly treated cells.

The base substitution mutations detected in *supF* genes rescued from murine fibroblasts (LN12) treated with several different psoralen regimens are shown in Table 2. As expected from the well-characterized photochemistry of 8-MOP, the mutations over background occur mostly at Ts. For 8-MOP/UVA (PUVA) treatments, whether single (column 1) or repetitive (column 3), there is a vast preponderance of transversions (T → A and T → G). Similar results were obtained for repetitive angelicin treatments labeled 5-MeA (3x) in column 4. Also shown is data from Sage and Bredberg (1991) for a split-dose (s-d) regimen (column 5). We have also observed some deletion mutations after 8-MOP/UVA treatments. Our preliminary interpretation is that psoralen crosslinks may lead to deletion mutations perhaps via double strand breaks which might occur during excision repair. More definitive results are pending the further analysis of mutations in additional sets of mutants induced with split-dose regimens which results in a higher proportion of crosslinks.

Table 2. Base substitution mutations in mouse cells

	(1) 8-MOP	(2) Split-dose	(3) 8MOP (3x)	(4) 5-MeA (3x)	(5) Sage (s-d)	(6) Untreated
C:G→T:A	12	4	2	4	10	17
T:A→C:G	3	1	0	3	3	2
C:G→A:T	2	0	6	1	4	7
C:G→G:C	3	0	1	1	4	1
T:A→A:T	16	1	12	4	3	0
T:A→G:C	6	0	2	4	0	1
Deletion < 200	3	0	0	0	–	1
Deletion > 200	4	0	0	0	–	–
Total	49	6	23	17	24	29

The base changes (and the flanking sequences) observed after treatment with either 8-MOP or 5-MeA are summarized in Fig. 6. A hotspot for 8-MOP mutations is seen in the vicinity of base pair 160. Mutations in this region predominate regardless of the regimen (8-MOP, 1x or 3x; 5-MeA), even though it does not contain a photoadduct hotspot (5′TA) (Gunther et al. 1995). In contrast, when Sage employed a split-dose regimen, hotspots for photoadduct formation and mutation were observed at position 45–47 in the promoter region which does contain a 5′TA site. However, it is important to note that while we treated fibroblasts with 5 *μM* 8-MOP and 0.1 J/cm^2 UVA, Sage treated isolated pZ189 DNA with 93 *μM* 8-MOP and consecutive UVA doses of 0.055 and 3.3 J/cm^2 prior to transfection into cells to elaborate the mutations. Clearly, these different treatment regimens would be expected to yield different levels of photoadduct formation and distributions and hence different mutation spectra would result. The latter are not conditions encountered in human photochemotherapy. This comparison highlights the need to perform experiments under conditions that at least approximate the clinical setting. Extracellular and intracellular PUVA treatments of DNA can lead to vastly different numbers of psoralen DNA photoadducts, perhaps with different photoadduct distributions, and hence could have a strong effect on mutation frequencies and spectra.

40	A	A	A	C	T	**A**	T	A	C	T	T		
40	A	A	A	C	T	A	**T**	A	C	T	A	A	
41	A	A	C	T	A	T	**A**	C	T	A	T		
47	A	C	T	A	C	**G**	C	G	G	G	A	A	
47	A	C	T	A	C	G	**C**	G	G	G	T		
81	C	A	T	**T**	T	T	C	G	T	A	A		
83	T	T	T	T	**C**	G	T	A	A	T	T		
88	G	T	A	A	**T**	G	G	A	C	A	A	A	
96	C	A	C	C	**A**	C	C	C	C	A	C	G	
101	C	C	C	C	**A**	A	G	G	G	C	C	C	
123	C	T	C	G	T	**C**	T	G	A	G	T		
128	C	T	G	A	G	**A**	T	T	T	A	T	T	T
132	G	A	T	T	**T**	A	G	A	**C**	G	G	A	
133	A	T	T	T	**A**	G	A	**C**	G	C	T		
136	T	A	G	A	**C**	G	G	C	A	G	G	A	
138	G	A	C	G	G	**C**	A	G	T	A	G	T	
149	C	T	G	A	A	**G**	C	T	T	C	A	A	A
156	T	T	C	C	**A**	A	G	C	T	T	C	G	
157	T	C	C	A	**A**	G	C	T	T	A	C	T	T
158	C	C	A	A	**G**	C	T	T	A	G	A	A	A
161	A	G	C	T	**T**	A	G	G	A	A	C		
163	C	T	T	A	**G**	G	A	A	G	G	T		
171	G	G	G	G	G	**T**	G	G	T	G	A	A	

Fig. 6a

40	A	A	C	T	**A**	T	A	C	T	A	T	C	
40	A	A	C	T	A	**T**	A	C	T	A	G	G	A
82	C	A	**T**	T	T	T	T	C	G	T	A		
84	T	T	T	T	**C**	G	T	A	A	T	T	T	
88	C	G	T	A	**A**	T	G	G	A	C	T	T	T
88	C	G	T	A	A	**T**	G	G	A	C	C		
96	C	A	C	C	**A**	C	C	C	C	A	G		
101	C	C	C	C	**A**	A	G	G	G	C	C	T	
127	T	C	T	G	**A**	G	**A**	T	T	T	T		
129	T	G	A	**G**	A	**T**	T	T	A	G	T		
129	T	G	A	**G**	**A**	T	T	T	A	G	C	G	G
145	C	T	A	G	**C**	T	G	A	A	G	T	T	
145	C	T	A	G	C	**T**	G	A	A	G	G		
147	A	G	C	T	G	**A**	A	G	C	T	G		
149	C	T	G	A	A	**G**	C	T	G	C	A	A	
150	T	G	A	A	G	**C**	T	G	C	A	T		
156	T	T	C	C	**A**	A	G	C	T	T	C		
157	T	C	C	A	A	**G**	C	T	T	A	T	T	
159	C	A	A	G	C	**T**	T	A	G	G	G		
160	A	A	G	C	T	**T**	A	G	G	A	A		
163	C	T	T	A	G	**G**	A	A	G	G	T		**b**

Fig. 6a,b. Mutation spectra in supF DNA. **a** 8-MOP/UVA. **b** 5-MeA/UVA. The flanking sequence around each mutated base (*bold*) is shown on the *left*. On the *right* are the respective base substitutions. In both cases the psoralen concentration was 1050 ng/ml and the UV-dose 0.1 J/cm^2

Gunther et al. (1995) also determined the mutation spectrum for 5-methylangelicin. Mutations produced by both 8-MOP and 5-MeA occurred mostly at 5′TA and 5′AT sites. A slightly higher proportion of mutations was observed at 5′TA sites with the angelicin as opposed to 8-MOP, but the mutation spectra for each were similar in that each exhibited a predominance of transversions at T:A base pairs. Because of its angular structure 5-MeA cannot form crosslinks and under the conditions used in these studies, 8-MOP formed only 20% crosslinks. Hence our data would implicate monoadducts as well as crosslinks as significant premutagenic lesions. Thus, it appears that the similar site-specificity of the mutations induced by these two compounds is governed by their dark binding tendencies (preference for 5′TA and 5′AT sites) and not necessarily by the formation of crosslinks at those sites. *The fact that mutations occur at crosslinkable sites does not necessarily mean that crosslinks were responsible for them.*

Do Mutagenic Events Occur During Photopheresis?

Recently Petersheim et al. (1991) attempted to characterize the mutagenic risks associated with photopheresis by quantitating chromosome aberrations and sister chromatid exchanges in lymphocytes obtained from patients before and after photopheresis. They concluded that there was no evidence for mutagenicity. However, a close inspection of their data indicates that all of the measured parameters (gaps, breaks, exchanges) were significantly increased after photopheresis. Although these manifestations were repaired in 72 h, no molecular information was presented to demonstrate the accuracy of the repair process. Almost certainly sequence analysis of any selected gene (e.g. hprt) would have indicated some level of mutation. The implications of these data for photopheresis are unclear because the level of damage and the relative infrequency of treatment may enable the repair of damaged cells. It has been well documented that PUVA-induced mutagenic events may be responsible for the squamous cell carcinomas that develop in many PUVA patients. It should be noted that after more than a decade of use, there have been no reports of secondary cancers in photopheresis patients. However, there is another aspect to mutagenic events. Briegel et al. (1991) showed that a single base change in the binding site for a transcription factor in the interleukin (IL)-2 gene converted a weakly binding site into a stronger binding site and abolished the T cell restriction on the expression of IL-2. It is conceivable that similar events could result from 8-MOP/UVA mutations.

Additional Effects of Photoadducts in Cells

Several other parameters have been shown to correlate with the product of 8-MOP and UVA doses (Fig. 7). This correlation, first observed for membrane integrity (measured by trypan blue exclusion) and tritiated thymidine incorporation after phytohemagglutinin (PHA) stimulation, has now been extended. For example, apoptosis has been the focus of new interest among researchers in diverse areas of biological research (Raff 1992). In this process, enzymes are produced that lead to chromatin condensation, the inhibition of cell-cell interactions, and cytoskeleton disruption. Apoptosis culminates in the phagocytosis of the apoptotic cells by neighboring cells. A hallmark of this process is the production of a repetitive 180-base-pair banding pattern. In Fig. 7 we show the results of recent studies in which the extent of apoptosis was measured in human lymphocytes (Yoo et al. 1995). In earlier studies, Marks and Fox (1991) showed that the treatment of normal human lymphocytes with 300 ng/ml 8-MOP and 10 J/cm^2 UVA induced the formation of apoptotic cells ($\sim$30%) and the classic DNA ladder pattern (Vowels et al. 1996). As noted above, we showed that the doses of 8-MOP and UVA Marks and Fox (1991) employed (a combined dose of 3000) were highly cytotoxic and we observed a similar level of apoptosis at much lower combined dose (300). The induction of

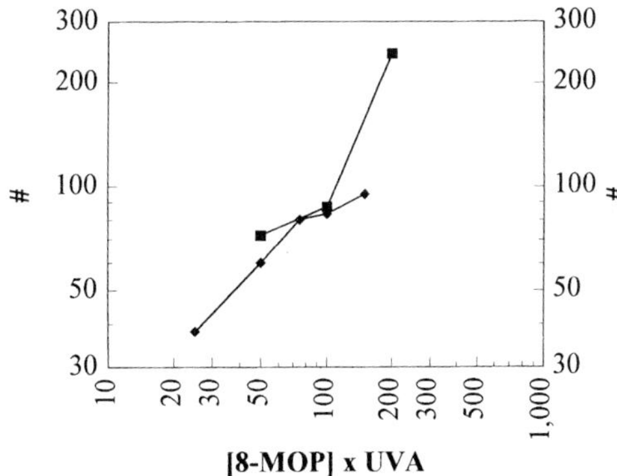

Fig. 7. Dose dependence for apoptosis (*diamonds*) and the induction of class I MHC (*squares*)

apoptosis by cells treated with 8-MOP and UVA could lead to the death of a selected subset of cells which in the process of disassembling could release partially degraded (and perhaps photomodified) proteins. These proteins could be a source of new oligopeptide fragments which may be displayed in surface MHC molecules of surviving cells, resulting in a higher level of antigenicity of these cells. A specific process which may occur during photopheresis is that macrophages may engulf apoptotic cells (see below).

Effect of Temperature on Cell Survival

Recently we examined the survival of murine lymphoma cells after the exposure to several 8-MOP/UVA doses (I.M. Schmitt, unpublished data). When the cells were treated with 8-MOP/UVA and cultured at 37 °C, their decreased viability and their capacity to resume growth was dose-dependent. Cells exposed to 300 ng/ml 8-MOP and 1 J/cm^2 were reduced to 25% viability 1 day later; at 100 ng/ml the viability was 50%, at 30, 76%, and at 10 ng/ml there was no difference compared to sham irradiated controls. By day 2 following treatment, all of the groups showed increases in cell numbers with control levels obtained in all cases by day 5. These data were in striking contrast to those obtained when the cells were treated with the same doses of 8-MOP/UVA but cultured at a subphysiological temperature (~26 °C) instead of 37 °C. Although the phototreatments were still toxic in a dose-dependent fashion, the extent of the effect was significantly reduced, such that at 300 ng/ml and 1 J/cm^2, viability fell by only 25% on day 1 following phototreatment. At the lower doses, the effect was similarly attenuated. Since apoptosis is a process that requires the synthesis of several proteins, what we may have observed at 26 °C is the suppression of the metabolically driven apoptosis process. It is interesting to note that during the 3- to 4-h photopheresis process the cells only spend about 10% of that time in the UVA irradiation chamber. Due to the thermal output of the UVA lamps, the temperature in this chamber is close to

37 °C. However, the cells that are not being irradiated are held in an externally mounted reservoir bag that is exposed to ambient room temperature. The dynamics of blood flow between these two sites (plate and bag) results in a bag temperature of approximately 5 °C higher than room temperature (K. Lee, personal communication). Most hospitals provide an air-conditioned environment at ~70 °F (21 °C). Thus the cells not being irradiated during photopheresis are at about 26 °C. The temporary staging of cells at this subphysiological temperature may contribute to the efficacy of photopheresis by reducing the outright cytotoxicity of the phototreatment.

Another factor that may also contribute to efficacy is the dynamic ex vivo processing of cells. For example, changing the environment and shape of cells is known to inhibit mRNA and protein synthesis (Folkman and Moscona 1978). The centrifugation and manipulation of cells during photopheresis changes cell shape and may induce similar phenomena and predispose cells in a unique way to the subsequent treatment with 8-MOP/UVA.

Class I MHC Expression on 8-MOP/UVA-Treated Murine Cells

The integral role of class I MHC expression is suggested by the observation that patients with a normal ratio of $CD8^+$ to $CD4^+$ cells is critical for a favorable response (Heald et al. 1989). Other studies have shown that reduced class I expression contributes to metastasis (Nava et al. 1992) and that the tumorigenicity of metastatic cells can be reversed by the transfection genes for class I MHC (Nouri et al. 1995). Furthermore, it has been suggested that it might only be necessary to "correct" the defect on a minority of cancer cells. Such limited changes could be associated with disease regression by the induction of bystander immunity against other "uncorrected" tumor cells. In both short-term (Moor et al. 1995) and long-term assays (Schmitt et al. 1995) we have shown that 8-MOP/UVA treatment of murine cells leads to the upregulation of class I MHC molecules on the cell surface. We assessed the rate of synthesis of MHC class I proteins in murine T-cell lymphoma cells (RMA) after treatment with 8-MOP and UVA. RMA cells were treated with 8-MOP (50–200 ng/ml) and UVA (1 J/cm^2) and metabolically labeled with ^{35}S-methionine 4 and 24 h after treatment. MHC class I synthesis was determined by immunoprecipitation of the cell lysates with an anti-K^b monoclonal antibody, Y-3. After 4 h, treated and untreated cells demonstrated no differences in the rate of MHC class I synthesis. However, after 24 h, a dose-dependent increase in MHC class I synthesis was observed (see Fig. 7). Thus, a similar induced increase in class I MHC expresssion could be responsible, at least in part, for the responses observed in patients treated with photopheresis. In earlier studies we showed that the xenogenization of mastocytoma cells with 8-MOP/UVA led to clones that were nontumorigenic (Gasparrao et al. 1993). Recently Schmitt et al. (1995b) found that these latter cells had a much greater level of class I MHC on their surface than untreated control cells.

We have also examined a generation of "empty" class I molecules that are known to be loadable with exogenously added peptide. Ljunggren et al. (1990) showed that *empty* class I MHC molecules are susceptible to rapid disintegration at physiological temperatures. The addition of a peptide with high affinity for the MHC class I haplotype and culturing at subphysiological temperatures (26 °–28 °C) stabilizes the complex. We have shown that the in vitro treatment of murine T lymphoma cell line (RMA) with 8-MOP/UVA generated a significant increase in MHC class I expression on the surface of treated cells compared to untreated cells. In a dose-response study, 300 ng/ml 8-MOP and 1 J/cm^2 of UVA light induced an increase of 35% of empty class I MHC molecules after 24 h, whereas a smaller or higher concentration of 8-MOP/UVA either did not have same effect on MHC class I induction, or killed the cells, respectively (Gasparro et al. 1994). Furthermore, the addition of a nine-amino-acid peptide specific for the haplotype H-2K^b also rendered the complex stable at 37 °C. In a further study performed in the same cell, a 35% increase in fluorescence intensity on the surface of treated cells (300 ng/ml 8-MOP and 1 J/cm^2 UVA) was observed, corresponding to ~300 000 induced class I MHC molecules (Schmitt et al. 1995a). Whereas these assays were performed in vitro with the addition of exogenous oligopeptides, it is conceivable that lethally damaged photopheresed cells may release oligopeptides with the correct class I MHC motif. Similar data have yet to be obtained in human cells. If the kinetics of induction are similar (optimal at ~24 h), it is unlikely that this phenomenon is a contributing factor to the efficacy of photopheresis since we have shown that the time frame for the disruption of cells is 24–48 h (see above) and by that time any photopheresis-induced *empty* class I MHC on the reinfused cells would have been melted by the exposure to physiological temperatures. On the other hand, this highlights the importance of directing future studies towards the analysis of cells obtained from photopheresis patients so that the events induced under those conditions can be better characterized.

Whereas a mutation is an event that occurs at a specific base, a general response to DNA damage may be the induction of genes. This phenomenon has been studied extensively in bacteria and yeast; however, much less is known about the response of mammalian genes (Holbrook and Fornace 1991). In *E. Coli*, these induced effects are known as the "SOS response". In yeast, as many as 80 genes are activated by DNA damage. In mammalian cells, more than 40 genes whose mRNA expression is upregulated by DNA damage have been characterized. Among the induced genes are general transcription regulators that fall in the class of "immediate early" genes (c.*fos*, c-*jun*, jun-B, c-*myc*, and Egr-1) which are induced rapidly (1–4 h) and directly by DNA damage, do not require de novo protein synthesis, and correspond to the time frame over which cells are treated during the photopheresis procedure.

Although direct measurements (i.e., mRNA levels) of genes induced by 8-MOP/UVA have not yet been reported, a significant number of phenomenological observations suggest that gene induction is occurring. In vivo studies have employed monoclonal antibodies to demonstrate the extent of photoadduct formation in human lymphocytes. It has also been demonstrated that UVA-activated psoralens can induce DNA strand breaks, reactive oxygen species, and photoadducts with proteins and lipids. Some combination of these photomodifications (or perhaps all in concert) must be involved in the cascade of events leading to enhanced immunogenicity. The dermatological experience with 8-MOP/UVA photochemotherapy (PUVA) has oriented the mechanistic paradigm in an antiprolilferative direction. In the animal studies purporting to explain photopheresis and in clinical reports describing its efficacy, the authors refer to photoinactivated cells. It has been conclusively demonstrated that other agents (e.g., UVC (Gorelick et al. 1991), X-rays (Hauser et al. 1993), and azacytidine (Chen et al. 1986) induce a similar enhancement of immunogenicity in tumor cells. Hauser et al. (1993), in studying the effects of nonionizing radiation on tumor cells, observed an upregulation of the expression of class I MHC (H-2D^{b}) molecules and concluded that the usual goal of chemotherapy, clonogenic purification, may not be the sole therapeutic goal in cancer therapy. The remainder of this review describes the three ways DNA damage (in concert with damage at other sites) induced by photopheresis could affect the immune status of patients.

Gene Induction and Evidence for the Role of DNA Damage

Direct Evidence: Activation of HIV and Elastin Promoters

Zmudzka et al. (1993) have shown that 8-MOP and UVA treatment of HeLa cells enhanced human immunodeficiency virus (HIV) promoter activity. Although they have yet to determine the cumulative impact of repeated incremental doses of 8-MOP and UVA, these results indicate that events other than inhibition may occur. In fact their data can be interpreted in terms of the DNA damage-induced upregulation of selected genes. The HIV promoter contains an NF-κB binding site. Thus the upregulation of HIV may occur as a result of the induction of NF-κB by 8-MOP/UVA damage. Further support for these effects arising from DNA damage comes from their observation that the induction HIV promoter activity can be correlated with the K_{DNA} of the psoralen employed. In a series of angelicins (4,5′-dimethylangelicin, 1450 M^{-1}; 6,4′-dimethylangelicin, 6300 M^{-1}; and 6,4,4′-trimethylangelicin, 10 100 M^{-1}) an inverse, linear correlation of the efficiency of HIV promoter activation with K_{DNA} was observed. Thus, the greater extent of interaction with DNA was correlated with greater HIV promoter activity. When 8-MOP was tested at the same concentration, the efficiency of HIV induction was anomalously higher than expected on the basis of its K_{DNA} (770 M^{-1}). Based on the characterization of 8-MOP photoadducts in other cells (see Fig. 5) it would be expected that the conditions employed in these HIV induction experiments would have led to 6 adducts/mbp and approximately equal numbers of monoadducts and crosslinks. Thus, the presence of crosslinks appears to enhance the induction of HIV promoter activity. The direct relationship of these effects to damage-induced upregulation of one or more transcription factors is the focus of current studies.

In more recent studies Bernstein et al. (1996) have shown that 8-MOP/UVA treatment of transgenic murine cells containing a human elastin promoter/CAT construct led to the dose-dependent induction of chloramphenicol acetyltransferase (CAT) activity under both in vitro and in vivo conditions. In vitro, the combination of 1 J/cm^2 UVA and 0.3, 1.0, and 3.0 μg/ml of 8-MOP led to 2.6-, 13.2-, and 2.0- fold increases in CAT activity, respectively. The fall-off in activity at the highest 8-MOP dose was due to the excessive toxicity of 3.0 μg/ml 8-MOP. In vivo the skin of mice treated with 8-MOP/UVA showed a 3.1-fold increase in CAT activity. In an earlier study it was shown that a 13-fold increase in CAT activity was induced by a dose of UVB (2.7 mJ/cm^2) capable of causing the formation of $\sim$300 photoproducts/mbp. In the 8-MOP study the combined dose of 8-MOP (1 μg/ml) and UVA (1 J/cm^2) capable of inducing 40 adducts/mbp caused a 13.2-fold increase. UVA alone at the doses employed in these studies would be expected to induce less than 1 photoproduct/mbp and produced no measurable changes in CAT activity (Smith and Paterson 1982).

Elaboration of DNA Damage: Chromatin Remodeling and the Activation of Transcription

The key to the therapeutic effects derived from photopheresis may be related to a coincidence of induced molecular events. The DNA damage recruits the cellular repair machinery which gains access to chromatin-bound DNA to restore the correct base. During this damage-induced process, another set of adventitious molecular interactions may occur. Specifically, cellular transcription factors gain access to sites previously occluded by the native chromatin structure.

A series of DNA representations is shown in Fig. 8. Complementary primary sequences form base pairs which lead to the classical double helical structure (panel A). In the nucleus, the double helix is wrapped twice around a histone core, forming a nucleosome ($\sim$200 bp at a time). Eventually the repeated array of nucleosomes forms a 30-nm chromatin fiber (Grunstein 1992). This folding paradigm results in a tremendous compaction of the DNA and leads to an interesting question. How is the information stored in the DNA primary sequence accessed (for replication, transcription, and repair)? Studies of the nuclear matrix have revealed that nucleosomes are not static structures. Rather, they appear to oscillate over a 20- to 30-basepair range, permitting potential, albeit fleeting, access of DNA binding proteins which can affect cellular processes. When nuclear proteins are considered, it is common to think of *trans*-acting factors like NF-κB. Such a narrow perspective would ignore the

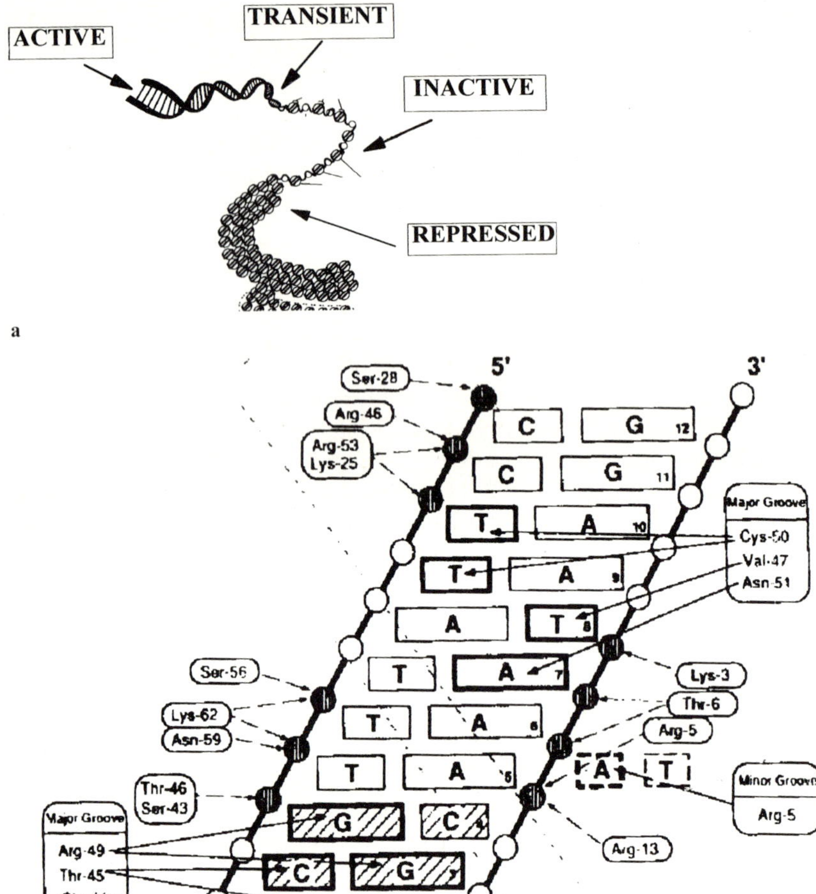

Fig. 8a,b. DNA diagrams. **a** The range of DNA morphology – a two-dimensional representation of DNA chromatin assembly showing the stages of chromatin assembly. Double-helical DNA wraps around histones, forming nucleosomes. The packing of nucleosomes leads to the 30-nm chromatin fiber which eventually forms loops and minibands, leading to a typical chromosome structure. The progression of the dependence of transcriptional activity on the conformation of nucleosomes is indicated. **b** Transcription factor-DNA contacts located at AT-rich sites are shown. In chromatin this site would be occluded by protein contacts. However, as a result of the DNA damage repair process it may become accessible to transcription factor binding

role of nuclear matrix proteins which have functions in addition to maintaining the architecture of the nucleus. Recently it has been shown that the native nucleosomal structure is a natural suppressor of transcriptional activity. Durrin et al. (1992) have shown that the elimination of nucleosomes at tumor-associated transplantation antigen (TATA) boxes leads to a basal level of mRNA synthesis.

McCaffrey and Hamilton (1994) showed that genotoxic chemical carcinogens target inducible genes in vivo. The examined 13 agents (but not 8-MOP), which induced damage ranging from strand breaks to crosslinks, at doses which induced significant levels of DNA damage but without causing cytotoxicity over a 96-h period. Constitutively expressed genes (e.g., β-actin, transferrin, and albumin) were unaffected. In contrast, they detected the induction of five other gene products (aminolevulinate synthetase, two P450 oxigenases, phosphoenolpyruvate carboxykinase, and metallothionein) which was temporally correlated with the induced DNA damage. They attributed these effects to a disruption of DNA-protein interactions in promoter sites. Previously Lambert et al. (1989) showed that several other DNA-damaging agents increased the expression of class I MHC molecules in mammalian cells. While deficiencies in the completeness of our understanding of psoralen photochemical reactions may pose an obstacle to understanding all of the molecular effects that contribute to the efficacy of photopheresis, another possibility is that the dogmatic interpretation of data has overlooked important experimental clues that have been known for a long time. For example, Ross and Yu (1988) showed that heat-shocked cells had a greater tendency to form crosslinks in the induced genes. In independent studies Han and Grunstein (1988) devised a methodology to deplete cells of nucleosomes and showed that the only genes switched on in response to the relaxation of the nucleosome structure were those of the inducible type. On the other hand, housekeeping genes were not unusually active. Furthermore, they showed that the elimination of nucleosomes at TATA boxes led to the synthesis of mRNA.

The well-characterized ability of 8-MOP to photomodify AT-rich sequences may also lead to the disruption of nucleosomes and subsequently enhanced transcription. Distortions induced in the DNA double helical structure by 8-MOP photoadducts (Spielmann et al. 1995) may disrupt the native nucleosome interactions. In addition, the repair process and its byproducts (such as an attached third-strand oligonucleotide fragment) may contribute to the disruption (van Houten et al. 1986). Figure 8 shows a typical contact pattern for DNA-transcription factor binding site. It is a common feature of these sites to contain AT-rich regions (Table 3) which are exactly the regions most susceptible to 8-MOP photomodification. While Fig. 8 depicts the transcription factor interaction at an AT-rich site it should be recognized that this site is ordinarily occluded by the native nucleosomal structure. Although this kind of interaction with a transcription factor alone may not be sufficient to induce therapeutic effects, the induction of transcription factors like NF-κB and proteins like p53 may act synergistically to eliminate nucleosomes at these sites.

Table 3. Transcription factor binding sequences

Transcription factor	Oligonucleotide sequence (5′→3′)
NFκB	AGT TGA GGG GAC TTT CCC AGG C
AP-1	CGC TTG ATG AGT CAG CCG GAA
AP-2	GAT CGA ACT GAC CGC CCG CGG CCC GT
TFIID	GCA GAG CAT ATA AGG TGA GGT AGG A
SP-1	ATT CGA TCG GCG GGG CGG GGC GAG
OCT-1	TGT CGA ATG CAA ATC ACT AGA A

Cell-stressed induced transcription factors may bind to activator sequences and lead to significantly increased rates of transcription. Such a process could be responsible for the observed increases in TNFα, class I MHC, and other immune-regulating molecules (e.g., cytokines). Additional synergy may be derived from the induction of the tumor suppressor protein p53. Of course there are many molecules that could be induced, but there are three important reasons for focusing on p53. First, its induction is a well-characterized response to DNA damage. Second, its proper functioning (arrest of cell cycle progression) may permit cellular energy to be channeled in other directions (synthesis of induced gene products). Finally, oligopeptides potentially derived from its degradation have been shown to fit the class I MHC binding motif (Zeh et al. 1994). Because p53 is not normally expressed by cells, the immune system will not have been previously tolerized to it and hence the presentation of p53-derived oligopeptides in the greater number of class I MHC molecules may stimulate the patient's previously quiescent immune system. The reversible nature of nucleosome repositioning has been described in the mouse mammary tumor virus (MMTV) promoter. Transactivation from its promoter is transient. The transcription factor complex is eventually lost and the TATA box is eventually reincorporated into a nucleosome leading to the repression of transcription.

Synergy: Chromatin Remodeling and Transcription Factor Access

NF-κB

In cellular studies with UV or photoactivatable agents, the activation of NF-κB, probably the most widely studied transcription factor, occurs after its release from an inhibiting factor, IκB (Baeuerle 1991). The events leading to its release appear to be initiated by cellular membrane damage which leads to the phosphorylation of IκB. Although psoralen DNA photoadduct formation is the most well understood aspect of psoralen photobiology, psoralen is distributed throughout the cell (Fig. 9A). Panel B schematically illustrates the range of cell damage induced by 8-MOP/UVA. Photoactivated psoralens have

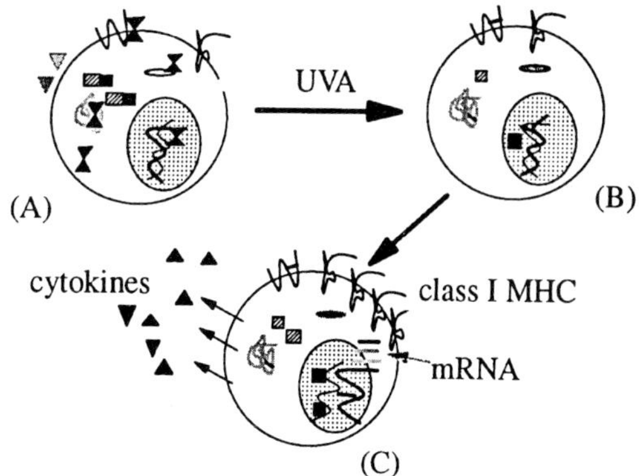

Fig. 9A–C. Repair-induced chromatin remodeling and transcription factor accessibility. For simplicity only one type of cell is shown in this diagram. These effects may be induced to differing extents in the various cells that are treated during photopheresis. **A** 8-MOP, represented by the *hourglass symbol*, is localized throughout the cell. **B** When exposed to UVA, 8-MOP molecules are activated and react with nearby moieties, resulting in their photomodification (*solid bars*). The formation of photoadducts with lipids and proteins induces the release of NF-κB (*solid squares*) from IκB (*hatched squares*) in the cytoplasm (**B**). As a result NF-κB translocates to the nucleus. At the same time the cell has initiated the repair of 8-MOP photoadducts in nuclear DNA. **C** The repair process requires the unwinding of DNA and the loosening of the chromatin structure (Maschek et al. 1989). Hence the newly released NF-κB (as well as other transcription factors) can now gain access to its cognate DNA binding sites (Leiden and Thompson 1994) and upregulate the expression of mRNA for genes containing those sites (e.g., several cytokines and class I MHC). The induction transcription factors occurs in a matter of seconds to minutes (Ronai et al. 1992; Mai et al. 1989) with maximal levels of new transcription peaking in a few hours (Grether-Beck et al. 1994). Hence, when these cells are returned to patients, they may affect other immune cells as a result of an altered cytokine secretion pattern. In longer-term effects, specific 8-MOP mutations (Briegel et al. 1991) may occur which relax to some degree the stringency of the NF-κB binding site so that more genes may have specific genes upregulated. In this model more class I MHC molecules and changes in cytokine secretion patterns would be the major molecular events induced by photopheresis. (Gasparro 1994; reprinted with permission from the author)

been shown to damage cell membranes either by direct adduct formation with proteins or lipids or through the generation of reactive oxygen species. The activation transcription factors has also been correlated with the UV absorption spectrum of DNA. Furthermore, it was shown that the photoadducts do not need to be "processed" or repaired since transcription factor induction is observed in repair-deficient cells (Stein et al. 1989). In these latter cells lower UV doses are required to induce these transcription factors. Panel C portrays the reprogrammed activity of the cell after 8-MOP/UVA treatment. As a result of transcription factor induction (and new accessibility to binding sites due to concomitant repair process and chromatin remodeling), these cells could have a greater number of class I molecules on their surface and an altered cytokine profile. For simplicity this diagram has been drawn using a single cell to illustrate the impact of photoactivated psoralen on cellular processes. It is possible (and likely) that these effects occur in different cells to different extents. The important message is that activational events can occur which alter the cell's (or cells') ability to regulate a disease process.

DNA damage-induced upregulation of NF-κB coupled with easier access to the binding sites as a result of chromatin remodeling and ongoing repair at specific sites may enhance the recognition and/or binding of these transcription factors. Many studies have shown that the time frame for the response to this type of damage may range from seconds to minutes. Clearly, 8-MOP/UVA-induced events such as those just described could be initiated as the result of a single photopheresis treatment (and perhaps in some cells after just one cycle through the device).

The Potential Role of p53 in Photopheresis

Preliminary studies indicate that a significant fraction of cutaneous T cell lymphoma (CTCL) patients contains mutated p53 (Chooback et al. 1995). Other studies have shown that p53 is induced during photopheresis, which is similar to observations for other DNA-damaging agents (Bennet and Hollstein 1992). Once p53 performs it cellular functions, it would be marked for degradation, which may provide another source of new peptides (and potentially new antigens) for display to the patient's immune system, ultimately resulting in immune-stimulating effects. In some cases p53 mutations have only been detected in the late stages of tumor development. However, nonmutated p53 may be nonfunctional (Ueda et al. 1995). It would be interesting to know the p53 status of CTCL patients (before, during, and after a course of therapy). Of course, there are other parameters that could also contribute to the efficacy of photopheresis – methylation patterns, topoisomerase activity, and the effect of 8-MOP photoadducts on mitochondrial DNA. These are beyond the scope of this presentation.

Houbiers et al. (1993) created a library of oligopeptides (nonamers, decamers, and undecamers) by "walking" along the p53 amino acid sequence. Out of a possible 2112 peptides, 63 were selected because they possessed the correct motif for binding to class I MHC molecules; 41 of the peptides were from wild-type p53 and 22 from mutant p53. A high percentage of the selected peptides showed binding to class I MHC; 44% wild-type and 41% mutant. A human cell line with empty and loadable class I MHC molecules was employed. Once bound to the cells, the oligopeptides were tested for their ability to elicit a subsequent cytotoxic T lymphocyte (CTL) response. CTL clones were obtained which were capable of specifically lysing target cells loaded with wild-type or tumor-specific mutant p53 peptides. In normal cells p53-derived peptides may not be immunogenic because of its very low level of expression. Thus, since the immune system has not become tolerant to p53 peptides, their overexpression as a result of 8-MOP/UVA treatment could lead to spontaneous immune responses which might be exploited therapeutically.

What's Missing – What We Need to Know

Over the last 5 years the progress in characterization of the molecular events induced in cellular biomoieties after 8-MOP/UVA treatment has been remarkable. Although the clinical responses of patients receiving photopheresis have been followed up for many years, the same cannot be said for molecular markers. One could envision a pilot project in which three groups of patients (responders, nonresponders, and untreated) are followed up for a 1- to 2-year period. This would yield a map of molecular markers (e.g., MHC, cytokines, β_2-microglobulin, glutathione, p53, NF-κB – see Gasparro 1994) which could provide clues about important effects induced by photopheresis. A significant difference might be noted between responders and nonresponders. A pattern may evolve that permits predicting which of the new patients will be responders or nonresponders.

In vitro studies should be designed to mimic the experience of physical stress cells during photopheresis. Cells could be pulsed (Sumpio et al. 1994) and/or centrifuged prior to 8-MOP/UVA treatment to determine if there is a synergism induced by the combination of the physical forces (Folkman and Moscona 1978) and subsequent photochemical events.

The efficacy of chemotherapy may also be related to the ability of patients to repair the induced DNA damage. Repair efficiency is known to be compromised by age and disease (Wilhide and Larcom 1993). Since photopheresis inflicts a significant burden of DNA damage, the ability of the patients' cells to respond to this damage may be integral to their response to photopheresis.

Finally, there is no reason why the focus of future studies should not be restricted to human cells – both the normal cells that may play an important role in therapy-induced immune response and malignant lymphoma cells. Whether the lack of the latter is due to purely technical difficulties or a comment on will power can only be evaluated at some future date.

Acknowledgements. This work has been supported by grants from the NIH, Illumenex, and a gift from Therakos, Inc.

References

Baeuerle PA (1991) The inducible transcription activator NF-κB: regulation by distinct protein subunits. Biochim Biophys Acta 1072: 63–80

Bennet W, Hollstein M (1992) Tumor suppressor gene. Princ Prac Oncol 6: 1–12

Bernstein EF, Gasparro FP, Brown DB, Takeuchi T, Uitto J (1996) 8-Methoxypsoralen and ultraviolet radiation A activates human elastin promoter – direct evidence for gene induction in vitro and in vivo. Photochem Photobiol (in press)

Bevilacqua PM, Edelson RL, Gasparro FP (1991) High performance liquid chromatography analysis of 8-methoxypsoralen monoadducts and crosslinks in lymphocytes and keratinocytes. J Invest Dermatol 97: 151–155

Boyer V, Moustacchi E, Sage E (1988) Sequence specificity in photoreaction of various psoralen derivatives with DNA: role in biological activity. Biochemistry 27: 3011–3018

Briegel K, Hentsch B, Pfeuffer I, Deerfling E (1991) One base pair change abolishes the T cell-restricted activity of a kB-like proto-enhancer element from the interleukin 2 promoter. Nucleic Acids Res 19: 5929–5936

Chen E, Karr RW, Frost JP et al (1986) Gamma interferon and 5-azacytidine cause transcriptional elevation of class I major histocompatibility complex gene expression in K562 leukemia cells in the absence of differentiation. Mol Cell Biol 6: 1698–1705

Cheng S, van Houten B, Gamper HB, Sancar A, Hearst JE (1988) Use of psoralen-modified oligonucleotides to trap three-stranded recA-DNA complexes and repair of these cross-linked complexes by ABC excinuclease. J Biol Chem 263: 15110–15117

Chooback L, Felix CA, Salhany KE, Wolfe JT, Salvatore R, Rook AH, Lessin SR (1995) Enhanced expression of p53 in CTCL cells. J Invest Dermatol 104: 674A

Dall'acqua F, Vedaldi D, Bordin F, Rodighiero G (1979) New studies on the interaction between 8-methoxypsoralen and DNA in vitro. J Invest Dermatol 73(2): 191–197

Dimitrov S, Wolffe AP (1995) Chromatin and nuclear assembly: experimental approaches towards the reconstitution of transcriptionally active and silent states. Biochem Biophys Acta 1260: 1–13

Durrin LK, Mann RK, Kayne PS, Grunstein M (1992) Yeast histone H4 N-terminal sequence is required for promoter activation in vivo. Cell 65: 1023–1031

Edelson RL (1975) Cutaneous T-cell lymphoma – perspective. Ann Intern Med 83: 548–552

Edelson R, Berger C, Gasparro F et al (1987) Treatment of cutaneous T-cell lymphoma by extracorporeal photochemotherapy. N Engl J Med 316: 297–303

Felsenfeld G (1992) Chromatin as an essential part of the transcriptional mechanism. Nature 355: 219–224

Folkman J, Moscona A (1978) Role of cell shape in growth control. Nature 273: 345–349

Gasparro FP (1994) Extracoporeal photochemotherapy: clinical aspects and the molecular basis for efficacy. RG Landes Press (Medical Intelligence Unit), Georgetown, TX

Gasparro FP, Weingold D, Goldminz D, Edelson R (1991) Quantification of 8-MOP photoadducts in lymphocytes In: Riklis E (ed) Photobiology – the science and its applications. Plenum, New York, pp 951–962

Gasparro FP, Gattolin P, Olack G, Deckelbaum LI, Sumpio BE (1993a) Visible excitation of 8-MOP: HPLC quantitation of monoadducts and crosslinks. Photochem Photobiol 57: 1007–1010

Gasparro FP, Malane MS, Maxwell VM, Tigelaar RE (1993b) 8-Methoxypsoralen and long wavelength ultraviolet radiation enhances the immunogenicity of tumorigenic P815 mastocytoma cells. Photochem Photobiol 58: 682–688

Gasparro FP, Schmitt IM, Felli A, Edelson RL (1994) 8-Methoxypsoralen/UVA augments class I MHC expression. J Invest Dermatol 102: 604A

Gasparro FP, Dall'Amico R, Goldminz D et al (1989) Molecular aspects of photopheresis. Yale J Biol Med 62: 579–593

Gasparro FP, Bevilacqua PM, Goldminz D et al (1990) Repair of 8-MOP photoadducts in human lymphocytes. In: Sutherland BM, Woodhead AD (eds) DNA damage and repair in human tissues. Plenum, New York, pp 174–187

Gilchrest BA (1979) Methoxsalen photochemotherapy for mycosis fungoides. Cancer Treat Rep 63: 663–667

Gorelik E, Begovic M, Duty L, Herbermann RB (1991) Effect of ultraviolet radiation on MCA102 tumor cell immunogenicity and sensitivity to tumor necrosis factor. Cancer Res 51: 1521–1528

Grether-Beck S, Klammer M, Grewe M, Gyufko K, Olaizola-Horn S, Budnik A, Krutmann J (1994) Differential activation of transcription factors by ultraviolet B versus ultraviolet A1 radiation in human keratinocytes. J Invest Dermatol 102: 577A

Grunstein M (1992) Histones as regulators of genes. Sci Am (Oct): 68–75

Gunther EJ, Yeaskey TM, Gasparro FP, Glazer PM (1995) Mutagenesis by 8-methoxypsoralen and 5-methylangelicin in mouse fibroblasts: mutations at cross-linkable sites induced by monoadducts as well as cross-links. Cancer Res 55: 1283–1288

Han M, Grunstein M (1988) Nucleosome loss activates yeast downstream promoters in vivo. Cell 55: 1137–1145

Hauser SH, Calorini L, Wazer DE, Gattoni-Celli S (1993) Radiation-enhanced expression of major histocompatibility complex class I antigen H-2D^b in B16 melanoma cells. Cancer Res 53: 1952–1955

Heald P, Perez M, Christensen I et al (1989) Photopheresis therapy of cutaneous T cell lymphoma: the Yale-New Haven hospital experience. Yale J Biol Med 62: 629–638

Heald PW, Rook A, Perez M et al (1992) Treatment of erythrodermic cutaneous T-cell lymphoma with extracorporeal photochemotherapy. J Am Acad Dermatol 27: 427–433

Hensling U, Schmidt W, Scholer HR, Gruss P, Hatzopoulos (1990) A transcription factor interacting with the class I gene enhancer is inactive in tumorigenic cell lines which suppress major histocompatibility complex class I genes. Mol Cell Biol 10: 4100–4109

Holbrook NJ, Fornace AJ (1991) Response to adversity: molecular control of gene activation following genotoxic stress. New Biol 9: 825–833

Houbiers JGA, Nijman HW, van der Burg SH et al (1993) In vitro induction of human cytotoxic T lymphocyte responses against peptides of mutant and wild-type p53. Eur J Immunol 23: 2072–2077

Inadomi T, Ross PM (1989) Effects of nuclear isolation on psoralen affinity for chromatin. Biochem Biophys Res Commun 163: 1384–1389

Kayne PS, Kim U-J, Han M, Mullen JR, Yoshizaki F, Grunstein M (1988) Extremely conserved histone H4 N terminus is dispensable for growth but essential for repressing the silent mating loci in yeast. Cell 55: 27–39

Klemm JD, Rould MA, Aurora R, Herr W, Pabo CO (1994) Crystal structure of the OCT-1 POU domain bound to an octamer site: DNA recognition with tethered DNA-binding modules. Cell 77: 21–32

Lambert ME, Ronai Z, Weinstein IB, Garrels JI (1989) Enhancement of major histocompatibility class I protein synthesis by DNA damage in cultured human fibroblasts and keratinocytes. Mol Cell Biol 9: 847–850

Leiden JM, Thompson CB (1994) Transcriptional regulation of T-cell genes during T-cell development. Curr Opin Immunol 6: 231–237

Ljunggren H-G, Stam NJ, Ohlen C et al (1990) Empty MHC class I molecules come out in the cold. Nature 346: 476–480

Mai S, Stein B, van den Berg S et al (1989) Mechanisms of ultraviolet light response in mammalian cells. J Cell Sci 94: 609–615

Marks DI, Fox RM (1991) Mechanism of photochemotherapy-induced apoptotic cell death in lymphoid cells. Biochem Cell Biol 69: 754–760

Maschek U, Pulm W, Hammerling GJ (1989) Altered regulation of MHC class I genes in different tumor cell lines is reflected by distinct sets of DNase I hypersensitive sites. EMBO J 8(8): 2297–2304

McCaffrey J, Hamilton JW (1994) Comparison of effects of direct-acting DNA methylating and ethylating agents on inducible gene expression in vivo. Environ Mol Mutagen 23: 164–170

Moor ACE, Schmitt IM, Patrignelli R, Beijersbergen van Henegouwen GM, Chimenti

S, Edelson R, Gasparro FP (1995) Treatment with 8-methoxypsoralen and UVA enhances MHC class I synthesis in RMA cells; preliminary results. J Photochem Photobiol B29: 193–198

Musajo L, Rodighiero G, Dall'Acqua (1965) Evidences of a photoreaction of the photosensitizing furocoumarins with DNA and pyrimidine nucleosides and nucleotides. Experentia 21: 24–25

Nava G, Ocadiz R, Ortega V, Alfaro G (1992) Damage in B2m genes and DNA methylation of H-2 genes are involved in loss of expression of class I MHC products on the membrane of LR.4, a cell line derivative of the T-cell lymphoma L5178Y. Eur J Immunogen 19: 141–158

Nouri AME, Hussain RF, Oliver RTD (1995) The frequency of major histocompatibility complex antigen abnormalities in urological tumors and their correction by gene transfection or cytokine stimulation. Cancer Gene Ther 1: 119–123

Olack GA, Gattolin P, Gasparro FP (1993) Improved high performance liquid chromatographic analysis of 8-methoxypsoralen monoadducts and crosslinks in polynucleotide, DNA and cellular systems: analysis of split dose protocols. Photochem Photobiol 57: 941–949

Oroskar AA, Gasparro FP, Peak MJ (1993) Relaxation of supercoiled DNA by aminomethyltrimethylpsoralen and UV photons: action spectrum. Photochem Photobiol 57: 648–654

Petersheim UM, Küster W, Gebauer H-J et al (1991) Cytogenetic effects during extracorporeal photopheresis treatment of two patients with cutaneous T-cell lymphoma. Arch Dermatol Res 283: 81–85

Raff MC (1992) Social controls on cell survival and cell death. Nature 356: 397–400

Ronai ZA, Lambert ME, Weinstein IB (1990) Inducible cellular responses to ultraviolet light irradiation and other mediators of DNA damage in mammalian cells. Cell Biol Toxicol 6(1): 105–126

Rook AH, Prystowsky MB, Cassin M et al (1991) Combined therapy of the Sezary syndrome with extracorporeal photochemotherapy and low dose interferon alpha: clinical, molecular and immunologic observations. Arch Dermatol 127: 1535–1549

Ross PM, Yu H-S (1988) Interstrand crosslinks due to 4,5′,8-trimethylpsoralen and near ultraviolet light in specific sequences of animal DNA: effect of constitutive chromatin structure and induced transcription. J Mol Biol 201: 339–351

Sage E, Bredberg A (1991) Damage distribution and mutation spectrum; the case of 8-methoxypsoralen and UVA in mammalian cells. Mutat Res 263: 217–222

Schmitt IM, Gasparro FP (1995) Psoralens and proteins – the forgotten field. J Photochem Photobiol B 27: 101–107

Schmitt IM, Carfos I, Chimenti S, Edelson R, Imaeda S (1995a) Coculture of supernatant from RMA cells treated with 8-MOP/UVA induces an increase in MHC class I expression on untreated cells. J Invest Dermatol 104: 601A

Schmitt IM, Moor ACE, Patrignelli R, Beijersbergen van Henegouwen GJM, Chimenti S, Edelson R, Gasparro FP (1995) Enhanced expression of class I MHC molecules on non-tumorigenic cells obtained from xenogenization of murine mastocytoma cells with 8-methoxypsoralen and long wavelength ultraviolet radiation. Tissue Antigens 46: 45–49

Smith PJ, Paterson MC (1982) Lethality and induction and repair of DNA damage in far, mid or near UV-irradiated human fibroblasts: comparison of effects in normal, xeroderms pigmentosum and Bloom's syndrome cells. Photochem Photobiol 36: 333–343

Spielmann HP, Dwyer TJ, Sastry SS, Hearts JE, Wemmer DE (1995) DNA structural reorganization upon conversion of a psoralen furan-side monoadduct to an interstrand cross-link: implications for DNA repair. Proc Natl Acad Sci USA 92: 2345–2349

Stein B, Rahmsdorf HJ, Steffen A, Litfin M, Herrlich P (1989) UV-induced DNA damage is an intermediate step in UV-induced expression of human immunodeficiency virus type I, collagenase, c-fos and metallothionein. Mol Cell Biol 9: 5169–5181

Sumpio DE, Li G, Deckelbaum LI, Gasparro FP (1994) Inhibition of smooth muscle proliferation by visible light-activated psoralen. Circ Res 75: 208–213

Sumpio BE, Du W, Xu W-J (1994) Exposure of endothelial cells to cyclic strain induces c-fos, fosB and c-jun but not jun-B or jun-D and increases the transcription factor AP-1. Endothelium 2: 149–156

Ueda H, Ullrich SJ, Gangemi JD, Kappel CA, Ngo L, Feitelson MA, Jay G (1995) Functional inactivation but not structure mutation of p53 causes liver cancer. Nature (Gen) 9: 41–47

Vallat VP, Gilleaudeau P, Battat L, Wolfe J, Nabeya R, Heftler N, Hodak E, Gottlieb AB, Krueger JG (1994) PUVA bath therapy strongly suppresses immunological and epidermal activation in psoriasis: a possible cellular basis for remittive therapy. J Exp Med 180: 293–296

van Houten B, Gamper H, Holbrook SR, Hearst JE, Sancar A (1986) Action mechanism of ABC excision nuclease on a DNA substrate containing a psoralen crosslink at a defined position. Proc Natl Acad Sci USA 83: 8077–8081

Vowels BR, Cassin M, Boufal MH et al (1992) Extracorporeal photochemotherapy induces the production of tumor necrosis factor-α by monocytes: implications for the treatment of cutaneous T cell lymphoma and systemic sclerosis. J Invest Dermatol 98: 686–692

Vowels BR, Yoo EK, Gasparro FP. Kinetic analysis of apoptosis induction in human cell lines by 8-MOP and UVA (in press)

Wilhide CC, Larcom LL (1993) An assay for monitoring response to therapy in cancer patients. Ann Clin Lab Sci 23: 207–215

Wolberger C (1993) Transcription factor structure and DNA binding. Curr Opin Struct Biol 3: 3–10

Workman JL, Kingston RE (1992) Nucleosome core displacement in vitro via a metastable transcription factor-nucleosome complex. Science 258: 1780–1784

Yoo EK, Rook AH, Elenitsas R, Gasparro FP, Vowels BR (1995) Apoptosis induction by photochemotherapy: relevance to anti-tumor therapy. J Clin Invest (submitted)

Yun MH, Choi SJ, Shim SC (1992) A novel photoadduct of 4,5′,8-trimethylpsoralen and adenosine. Photochem Photobiol 55: 457–460

Zeh HJ, Leder GH, Lotze MT, Salter RD, Tector M, Stuber G, Modrow S, Storkus WJ (1994) Flow cytometric determination of peptide-class I complex formation. Identification of p53 peptides that bind to HLA-A2. Hum Immunol 39: 79–86

Zmudzka BZ, Strickland AG, Miller SA et al (1993) Activation of the human immunodeficiency virus promoter by UVA radiation in combination with psoralens or angelicins. Photochem Photobiol 58: 226–232

II. Analysis of Cellular Alterations and Growth Dysregulation in Cancer Cells

Cellular Stress Response: Stress Proteins – Physiology and Implications for Cancer

R. Benndorf and H. Bielka

Max-Delbrück-Center for Molecular Medicine, 13122 Berlin, Germany

The Heat Shock Response

The heat shock phenomenon was first observed in *Drosophila* when Ritossa (1962) studied chromosome puffing patterns. In 1974, Tissieres et al. discovered the heat shock proteins (HSPs) by electrophoretically analyzing newly synthesized proteins in heat-shocked *Drosophila* larvae. Heat shock treatment usually results in a strong induction of a set of proteins which have been synthesized before at a low level. Concomitantly, the synthesis of most other proteins is reduced significantly. Induction of HSPs has been found in practically all studied organisms, suggesting the universal importance of this phenomenon. HSP synthesis is part of a general adaptive response towards stresses which also includes changes in cell morphology and in the structure of chromatin and the cytoskeleton. Also, other noxious stress conditions such as arsenite, ethanol, heavy metals, amino acid analogs, oxidative stress, and certain anticancer drugs, as well as physiological stress conditions such as infection, inflammation, and ischemia, may result in the synthesis of HSPs. In addition, several of the HSPs are normally expressed and regulated during physiological processes like differentiation and cell cycle. Today it is generally accepted that HSPs have a protective function for cells and that they are a major cause for a phenomenon called "acquired thermotolerance". The basic observation is that cells or organisms, if exposed to a mild preheating treatment, survive subsequent treatment with an otherwise lethal temperature. Moreover, preheating induces tolerance to other forms of stress and vice versa. Apparently, HSPs induced by moderate stress protect cells or organisms from even more severe stress. Strong evidence for the thermoprotective role of at least HSP25 (also referred to as HSP27, HSP28, 24K-estrogen regulated protein), HSP70, and HSP104 comes from transfection experiments resulting in a constitutive overexpression of HSPs (Landry et al. 1989; Sanchez and Lindquist 1990; Li et al. 1991) and from experiments designed specifically to inactivate single HSPs by antisense RNA, inhibition of HSP gene expression, and microinjection of anti-HSP antibodies (McGarry and Lindquist 1986; Riabowol et al. 1988; Johnston and Kucey 1988). However, there are also several reports showing, that development of thermotolerance and expression of HSPs did not correlate, thus indicating that further critical factors may be involved.

With the exception of the low molecular weight HSPs, the sequences of the other HSPs were highly conserved throughout evolution. Usually, HSPs are distinguished by their molecular mass and grouped in families (HSP110-, HSP90-, HSP70-, HSP60-, HSP20-, and HSP8.5 family). So far, two major functions have been assigned to HSPs: chaperoning (best studied for HSP70, HSP60, but also for HSP90, HSP25), and protein degradation (HSP8.5, ubiquitin). The chaperoning activity of HSPs and of the related constitutively expressed proteins concerns their ability to support correct folding of nascent peptides and to protect the correct structure of other proteins. Chaperoning by HSPs is also involved in translocation of proteins across membranes and in assembly of protein complexes. Under stress conditions, their ability to refold partially denatured proteins becomes important. The second major HSP function, protein degradation, is mediated by ubiquitin.Ubiquitin is conjugated to irreversibly denatured, highly toxic proteins which are subsequently degraded by proteasomes. Some HSPs have obviously more specific chaperone functions. For example, proteins of the HSP90 family bind to steroid receptors and to protein kinases encoded by oncogenic retroviruses. HSP90 is necessary for regulation of steroid receptor activity and for correct insertion of oncogenic protein kinases into the plasma membrane. A specific function of HSP25 is its interaction with actin, which appears to be involved in the regulation of microfilament dynamics (see following). More data on the heat shock response and HSPs are given in the reviews of Morimoto (1991), Burel et al. (1992), Hendrick and Hartl (1993), and Hartl et al. (1994).

The fast and transient induction of the synthesis of HSPs after stress treatment of cells is mainly controlled by a specific transcription factor, HSF1. HSF1 is constitutively expressed, and in unstressed cells it occurs in an inactive, monomeric form. Stress treatment results in trimerization, phosphorylation, and accumulation of HSF1 in the nucleus. This active form binds specifically to heat shock elements (HSE) in the promoter region of *hsp* genes and stimulates their transcription. HSF1 is negatively regulated, i.e., the formation of the active trimer is inhibited in unstressed cells. It is believed that the inactive monomeric form is stabilized by binding to HSP70 (Morimoto et al. 1994). If in cells the level of denatured proteins increases as a result of stress treatment, HSP70 binds them to prevent aggregation and to support their refolding. Thereby HSF is released and, after activation, it binds to the HSE, resulting in an activation of HSP transcription. Dissociation of bound proteins from HSP70 is an ATP-dependent process. Therefore, ATP depletion seems to be critical for the heat shock response. A decreased intracellular ATP level would retain denatured proteins bound to HSP70 and thus reduces the pool of free HSP70 (Beckmann et al. 1992). This leads to dissociation of the HSF-HSP70 complex, leaving HSF free to induce the synthesis of additional HSPs. Recent data suggest that further transcription factors are involved in HSP expression: HSF2 controls the development-related expression of HSPs, while HSF3 appears to be a cell-type specific factor which is also activated by heat but with delayed kinetics.

Heat Shock Proteins in Tumor Diseases

Expression of heat shock proteins has been found in various tumors. Examples are HSP70 expression in brain tumors (Kato et al. 1993) or the elevated expression of HSP90-alpha in breast cancer. Patients with low expression had a significantly more favorable outcome in terms of both overall and disease-free survival (Jameel et al. 1992). A similar conclusion was drawn concerning the prognostic implications of HSP70 in lymph node-negative breast cancer. Patients whose tumors exhibited low expression of HSP70 had significantly longer disease-free survival periods. For patients who received adjuvant therapy, HSP70 was the only independent predictor of disease recurrence (Ciocca et al. 1993a).

In malignant transformation, HSPs seem to be related to several oncproteins. For example, c-*myc* stimulates the synthesis of HSP70 (Taira et al. 1992) and both proteins accumulate in the nucleus. Here, c-*myc* may be kept in an inactive state by HSP70 (Henriksson et al. 1992). HSP70 also binds p53, preferably the mutated form, which prevents its activation and may lead to transformation (Lane et al. 1993).

Recently, exciting data were published with respect to surface expression of HSPs. HSP60 was found on mycobacteria-infected and lymphoma cells, HSP70 on HIV-infected cells, and HSP70 and HSP90 on tumor cells. Despite comparable cytoplasmic HSP induction by stress treatment, the cells of several human tumors are distinguished from normal cells by the surface expression of HSP70 (Multhoff et al. 1995 and references therein). This finding has potential clinical implications. HSP70 appears to be a stress-inducible target for a tumor-specific immune response.

Apoptosis and Heat Shock Proteins

Cell death is a fundamental phenomenon of organisms, occurring as a physiologic process during organogenesis in embryos, in cell turnover in adults, and as a pathologic process in response to injuries. Several lines of investigation have led to the concept that there are two fundamental types of cell death, namely apoptosis and necrosis. Apoptosis, which can be distinguished from necrosis, is an active process characterized by cell shrinkage, DNA degradation, and chromosome condensation and is often followed by fragmentation of the cell into apoptotic bodies. Apoptotic cells and bodies are efficiently phagocytosed in vivo without causing inflammation. In terms of an ideal tumor therapy, controlled apoptosis of tumor cells would be the therapy of choice.

As mentioned, several lines of experimentation strongly suggest that HSPs contribute to the acquisition of stress tolerance, i.e., they prevent the death of cells under stress conditions including therapy-relevant conditions like application of anticancer drugs or hyperthermia. However, almost no data are available whether the necrotic, the apoptotic, or both ways of cell death are affected. Although heat treatment was shown to be one of the inducers of apoptosis as well as of necrosis (Barry et al. 1990), heat pretreatment can protect thymocytes from glucocorticoid-induced cell death (Miglioratti et al. 1992), suggesting that induced HSPs may prevent apoptosis. Recently, more direct evidence came from experiments using the drug quercetin and related flavonoids. These substances are commonly contained in higher plants, and their biological and biochemical effects have been characterized (Hosokawa et al. 1992). Flavonoids have antitumor activity (Sakaguchi et al. 1992) and, most interestingly, specifically inhibit the induction of heat shock proteins by interacting with the heat shock factor (Hosokawa et al. 1992). Consequently, flavonoids were shown to inhibit the acquisition of thermotolerance in a human colon carcinoma cell line (Koishi et al. 1992) and to increase the antitumor effect of hyperthermia in mice (Sakaguchi et al. 1992). In K562 human chronic myeloid leukemic cells it was also shown that apoptosis is induced by quercetin concomitantly with an inhibition of HSP70 synthesis (Wei et al. 1994). Additionally, the same authors showed that treatment with HSP70 antisense oligomers increases the fraction of apoptotic cells and enhances the apoptosis-inducing activity of quercetin.

These data suggest that heat shock proteins may prevent apoptotic cell death under certain stress conditions and it remains a challenging task for future studies to develop a strategy for cancer therapy.

Cytotoxic Hyperthermia and Heat Shock Proteins

Hyperthermia is defined as the raising of cancer tissue to a cytotoxic temperature with the aim of eradicating malignant cells by external means to improve cancer control. The temperature required is between 42° and 43°C, the same range within which proteins begin to denature. The cytotoxic effect of hyperthermia is probably caused by complex damage to several vital cell functions rather than by a single mechanism. It should be mentioned that hyperthermia is no longer recommended as a sole therapeutic modality. But there is growing evidence of a beneficial effect when hyperthermia is combined with irradiation or anticancer drugs such as cisplatin, nitrosoureas, anthracylines, antimetabolites, interferon, tumor necrosis factor, and others (Vernon 1992).

In the clinical setting one of the major impediments to hyperthermic cancer therapy is the development of thermotolerance. It can result in an increase in the survival curve by as much as a factor of 15 which may take several days to return to normal. Thermotolerance can develop during prolonged heating below a critical value or between hyperthermic treatments. Based on the data obtained in cell cultures, it is believed that HSPs also contribute substantially to the acquired thermotolerance in vivo. Thus, efforts should be undertaken to avoid induction of HSPs in tumors during therapy. One way is to add intervals of 5–6 days between treatments (Vernon 1992) to allow the HSP level to return to normal. Another possibility derived from in vitro studies is pharmacological intervention using inhibitors of HSP synthesis (such as quercetin) which can inhibit acquisition of thermotolerance as was shown for a human colon carcinoma cell line (Koishi et al. 1992).

The Small Mammalian Heat Shock Protein HSP25

Structure of the Gene

The murine *hsp25* gene contains three exons which code for 125, 22, and 62 amino acids (209 amino acids in total; calculated molecular weight 23014) and two introns of different sizes (Fig. 1) (Gaestel et al. 1993). By sequence data, HSP25 is closely related to αB-crystallins (Gaestel et al. 1989). The protein segment coded by the second exon is characterized by a high degree of hydrophobicity which may cause HSP25 to aggregate and to form supramolecular structures (see following). The promoter region contains several transcription factor binding elements including two Spl-binding GC-rich sequences, two TATA boxes, one heat shock element (HSE), and one half-palindromic estrogen receptor binding element (ERE). The last two are involved in the activation of the *hsp25* gene by heat shock and estrogens, respectively.

The Protein HSP25

Spectroscopic evaluation of HSP25 reveals primarily β-sheet conformation, with less than 5% α-helix. According to secondary structure predictions, amphiphilic α-helices with a high hydrophobic moment may occur predominantly at the N-terminus which may serve for interactions among proteins (reviewed in DeJong et al. 1993). HSP25 does not exist as a homogeneous protein species inside cells. One reason is its ability to form supramolecular structures (regular

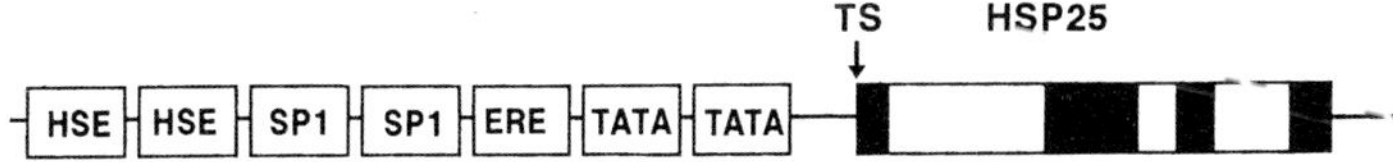

Fig. 1. Molecular organization of the murine *hsp25* structural gene and promoter region according to Gaestel et al. (1993). *HSE*, heat shock element; *SP1*, SP1-binding element; *ERE*, half-palindromic estrogen responsive element; *TATA*, TATA box; *TS*, transcription start point; *HSP25*, structural gene coding for HSP25 (introns and nontranslated regions *black*)

complexes, particles), usually between 200 and 800 kDa, which may increase upon heat shock up to 2 MDa or even more (Arrigo and Welch 1987; DeJong et al. 1992). Isolated particles can be visualized by electron microscopy as more or less regularly shaped, round particles (diameter 10–18 nm) with globular (Arrigo and Welch 1987) or ringlike structures probably composed of 8 monomers (Benndorf et al. 1994). Mixed particles of homologous αB-crystallin and HSP25 were detected in adenovirus-transfected cells (Zantema et al. 1992) and in the human cardiac muscle (Kato et al. 1992a). The complexes may dissociate upon stress (Zantema et al. 1992) or phosphorylation (Kato et al. 1994), a process which might be involved in cellular defense mechanisms for protection against stress. Also, Lavoie et al. (1995) observed a reduction of the multimeric size of HSP25 after phosphorylation by stress-inducing agents or mitogens. Usually HSP25 is located in the cytosol, but after heat shock it redistributes toward the perinuclear region or into the nucleus (Arrigo et al. 1988). Serum-induced phosphorylation of HSP25 was shown to correlate with changes in its intracellular localization and level of oligomerization (Mehlen and Arrigo 1994).

Phosphorylation and Acylation

In cells, murine HSP25 occurs in three isoforms: one non-phosphorylated (HSP25/1) and two phosphorylated forms (HSP25/2, HSP25/3). One prominent feature of HSP25 is its rapid phosphorylation as a cellular response to several mitogens and stress factors. The mitogens include tyrosine kinase receptor-mediated growth factors (e.g., platelet-derived growth factor), GTP-binding protein-mediated agonists (bradykinin, thrombin), cytokines (interleukin-1, tumor necrosis factor), and tumor promoters. In addition to heat treatment further stress factors shown to result in phosphorylation of HSP25 include arsenite, ethyleneglycoltetraacetic acid (EGTA), calcium ionophores, and oxidative stress (Benndorf et al. 1994 and references therein). In Fig. 2, isoform distribution of HSP25 in EAT cells is shown in response to a single heat shock (b), a heat shock followed by a recovery period (c), and to an arsenite treatment (d), as compared with the untreated control (a). Clearly, treatments by a single heat shock and by arsenite increase the portion of phosphorylated HSP25, while during the recovery period HSP25 is shifted largely to the nonphosphorylated isoform (Oesterreich et al. 1990). The major phosphorylation sites of murine HSP25 have been identified as Ser15 and Ser86 within the consensus motif LXRXXS (Gaestel et al. 1991). Phosphorylation of HSP25 was shown to be catalyzed by a new group of protein kinases (HSP25 kinase, MAPKAP kinase-2) that are apparently specific for small heat shock proteins (Benndorf et al. 1992; Engel et al. 1994; Huot et al. 1995). The protein sequence of the HSP25-kinase deduced from mouse cDNA reveals a SH3-binding domain N-terminal to the catalytic region, a MAP-kinase phosphorylation site, and a bipartite nuclear targeting sequence located C-terminal to the catalytic region. The

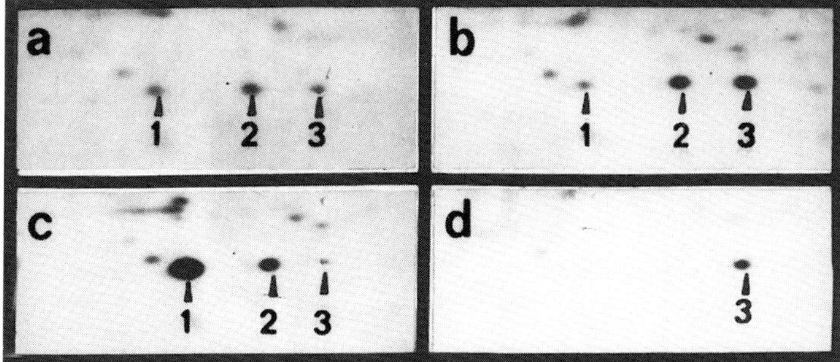

Fig. 2a–d. HSP25 isoform distribution in Ehrlich ascites tumor (EAT) cells after stress treatment according to Oesterreich et al. (1990). Cell proteins were labelled with [^{3}H]-leucine and processed for two-dimensional electrophoresis. **a** Control cells (37 °C). **b** Cells treated with a one-step heat shock (1 h at 41.5 °C). **c** Cells treated with a two-step heat shock with an intermittent recovery period (1 h at 41.5 °C, 2 h at 37 °C, 1 h at 43.5 °C). **d** Cells treated for 2 h with 400 μM sodium arsenite. *1*, nonphosphorylated HSP25/1; *2* and *3*, phosphorylated isoforms HSP25/2 and HSP25/3, respectively

HSP25-kinase is phosphorylated and activated by MAP-kinase which implies its involvement in the signal transduction cascade starting with the proto-oncogen ras (Engel et al. 1994). The fact that both stress and mitogenic stimulation lead to phosphorylation of the same serine residues and that this phosphorylation is catalyzed by the same protein kinase suggests that a common signal transduction mechanism via HSP25 is required for growth and stress response. Recent results suggest that phosphorylation of HSP25 is involved in the regulation of the structure of microfilaments (see following).

Besides phosphorylation, further posttranslational modifications occur. For HSP25, acylation by common fatty acids has been shown (Oesterreich et al. 1991a). Covalently bound palmitic acid, stearic acid, oleic acid, and linolic acid were identified by gas chromatographic analysis. In vivo labeling experiments suggest that the phosphorylated isoforms are acylated preferentially. Acylation might be one reason for size heterogeneity since HSP25 aggregation is known to involve triton-sensitive hydrophobic bonds.

Dimerization of HSP25 Under Oxidative Stress

Oxidative stresses such as H_2O_2, UV radiation, sodium arsenite, and cadmium also induce the synthesis of HSPs and it is hypothesized that this is related to the ability of oxidants to modify cellular thiols, including glutathione, directly. Glutathione itself has been shown to play a role in thermotolerance and in induction of HSPs (Steels et al. 1992). On the other hand, high-level expression of HSPs provides protection during ischemic and reoxygenation episodes (Mestril and Dillman 1995), indicating the additional ability of HSPs to stabilize proteins in cells exposed to oxidative stress. A possible mechanism by which HSP25 can act as an oxidative protectant is dimerization. HSP25 contains one cysteine residue at position 140 enabling the isolated protein to form dimers in the presence of 1 m*M* oxidized glutathion or H_2O_2. Earlier it was shown that dimerization of HSP25 leads to a loss of its activity in the inhibition of actin polymerization (Miron et al. 1988). Treatment of cells containing a high basic level of HSP25, such as breast cancer-derived MaTu cells, with diamide (oxidizes specifically intracellular glutathione), arsenite (binds to and probably oxidizes free sulfhydryls), and H_2O_2 result in a partial dimer formation of HSP25 as compared with corresponding controls (Fig. 3). As judged from the growth characteristics of the treated cells, HSP25 dimerization is a physiological response (not shown). The formation of HSP25 dimers may help to maintain glutathion and other sulfhydryls in a reduced state during an oxidative challenge and thus appears to function as an "oxidative" buffer at least in cells with abundant HSP25.

Function of HSP25

At the cellular level, thermoprotective function of HSP25 is well established. In cDNA transfection studies it was shown that overexpression of this protein is a

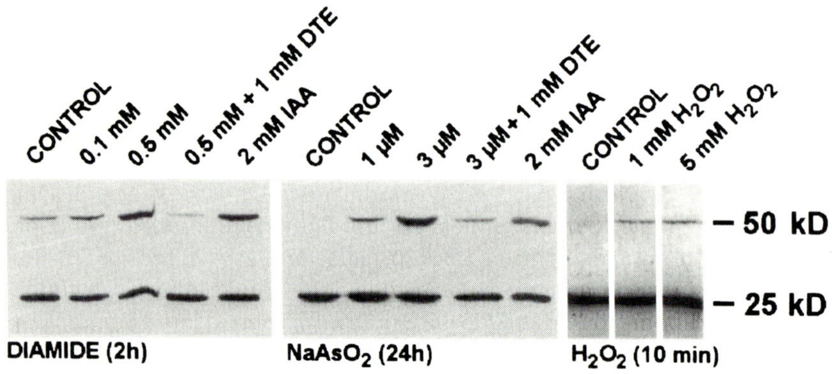

Fig. 3. HSP25 dimerization in MaTu cells exposed to oxidative stress. Cells were treated as indicated and proteins were separated under nonreducing conditions by sodium dodecyl sulfate-polyacrylamide gel electrophoresis (SDS-PAGE) and blotted to nitrocellulose. HSP25 was detected by monospecific rabbit antiHSP25 antibodies/anti-rabbit antibody-alkaline phosphatase conjugate. *25 kD*, position of monomeric HSP25; *50 kD*, position of HSP25 dimers. Note that in control cells (no treatment) the dimer content is subject to a certain variation. The dimerization of HSP25 is diminished by simultaneous incubation of the cells with 1 mM dithioerythritol (*DTE*). If indicated, 2 mM iodoacetamide (substitutes free sulfhydryls) was added to the protein samples of cells treated with 0.5 mM diamide or 3 μM arsenite to exclude dimerization caused by sample processing

sufficient condition for conferring thermoresistance (Knauf et al. 1992; Lavoie et al. 1993). More recently it was shown that only the wild-type protein, but not a phosphorylation site-deficient mutant, confers thermoresistance, emphasizing the importance of phosphorylation for the function of this protein (Lavoie et al. 1995). In this study, evidence was also presented that stabilization of microfilaments is a major target for the protective function of wild-type HSP25, while in cells overexpressing the phosphorylation site-deficient protein microfilaments were thermosensitized. In other studies, it was shown that HSP25 behaves in vitro as an actin barbed-end capping protein which inhibits actin polymerization. This activity is abolished by phosphorylation, dimerization, and organization of HSP25 in supramolecular complexes (Miron et al. 1988, 1991; Benndorf et al. 1994). In summary, these results suggest that HSP25 can function as a regulator of actin organization. The nature of the protective function of HSP25 in stressed cells in unknown, but some data suggest that it may be an extension of the normal phosphorylation-activated function at the level of actin filaments. The available data are summarized in the model shown in Fig. 4.

Besides that, HSP25 appears to have a general chaperoning activity in vitro which is independent of its degree of phosphorylation (Knauf et al. 1994).

Tumor-Associated Occurrence of HSP25

Breast Tumors. Although HSP25 is a widely distributed protein (Klemenz et al. 1993), the basic level in most human tissues including normal breast tissue

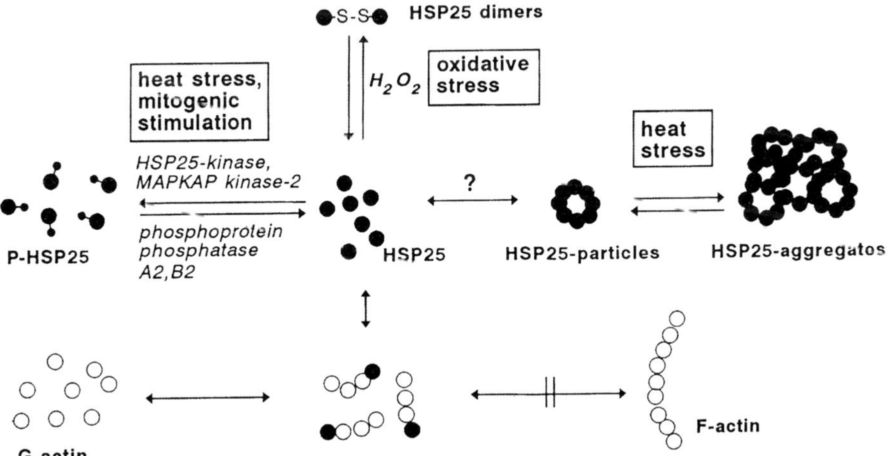

Fig. 4. Model of inactivation of the actin polymerization inhibiting activity of HSP25 by heat stress, mitogenic stimulation, and oxidative stress

[exception: estrogen receptor (ER)-positive tissues like endometrium] is low as compared with the high levels found in many breast cancers as well as in established breast cancer cell lines such as MCF-7, T47D (Dunn et al. 1993) or Ehrlich ascites tumor (EAT) cells (Benndorf et al. 1988a,b). In EAT cells, HSP25 is expressed in vivo depending on the growth phase of the tumor, with a low level in exponentially growing cells and increased amounts in stationary phase cells. Interest in this protein has also arisen from its association to the prognostic markers ER and progesterone receptor (PR) in a variety of estradiol-sensitive cell lines and primary breast tumors, and substantial efforts have been made to use HSP25 as a prognostic marker in breast cancer. HSP25 has been implicated in the estrogen action as an estrogen-regulated protein (Adams and McGuire 1985) and as a protein that will react with activated but not native ER (Dunn et al. 1993).

Regulation of HSP25 expression by estrogens was shown at the protein and mRNA level, resulting in an approximately two fold increase in estrogen-stimulated cells (Moretti-Rojas et al. 1988). In a colocalization study of ER, PR, and HSP25 using human breast cancer tissues, it was found that in 70% of the ER-positive cases the percentage of tumor cells expressing ER was similar to the percentage expressing HSP25. In the remaining 30%, there were tumor cells expressing ER but little or no HSP25. Other research groups described a similar correlation between HSP25 and ER. However, there are also studies which did not confirm this correlation between ER and HSP25 (reviewed in Ciocca et al. 1993b).

Breast cancer patients coexpressing ER and HSP25 were reported to have a better clinical response to hormone therapy than patients expressing ER alone. In other studies it was found that HSP25 overexpression in breast cancer seems to be associated with more aggressive tumors (Ciocca et al. 1993b). Thor et al. (1991) found a significant correlation between HSP25 overexpression, ER content, nodal metastases, advanced T stage, lymphatic or vascular invasion, and also with a shorter disease-free survival time. In a multivariate analysis, however, HSP25 overexpression was not a statistically independent parameter predictive of patient outcome. In another study the prognostic values of ER and HSP25 positivity were compared. ER positivity predicted a good outcome for both disease-free survival (DFS) and survival from first relapse (SR), while HSP25 positivity predicted a prolonged SR but short DFS. Analysis of the different HSP25 and ER-phenotypes revealed significant differences in DFS in the node-negative group only. ER^+HSP25^+ tumors recur more rapidly than ER^+HSP25^- ones, suggesting a positive link between HSP25 and proliferation (Love and King 1994). Why this correlation is obviously confined to the group of node-negative patients remains obscure. Reexamining the data, Fuqua et al. (1994) concluded that HSP25 is a prognosticator only in the subset of ER^+ tumors and indicates a shorter DSF. However, it is not a strong and independent predictor and thus is not recommended for use in medical practice.

Uterine Tumors. In endometrial and cervical hyperplasia and neoplasia, HSP25 is correlated with the degree of tumor differentiation. For example, in cervical cancer, HSP25 is predominantly expressed in well-differentiated and moderately differentiated squamous cell carcinomas (reviewed in Ciocca et al. 1993b).

Malignant Fibrous Histiocytoma. The prognostic significance of HSP25 for this tumor has been investigated in one study (Tetu et al. 1992). High-level expression of HSP25 was found to correlate with a more favorable prognosis.

Brain Tumors. In a few studies expression of HSP25 and of the related αB-crystallin in brain tumors was investigated. HSP25 was detected in 5 of 21 (5/21) meningiomas, 5/11 glioblastomas, 2/5 pituary adenomas, 1/15 astrocytomas, 1/7 medulloblastomas, but no reaction was seen in the tested oligodendrogliomas, schwannomas, and gangliogliomas, suggesting HSP25 expression in certain intracranial tumors (Kato et al. 1992b). One out of three of the glioblastomas coexpressed HSP25 and αB-crystallin (Kato et al. 1993). In neuroblastoma, high-level expression of HSP25 is a feature of differentiated tumors, suggesting that it may play a part in the biology of neuroblastomas with a favorable outcome (Ungar et al. 1994).

Leukemias. Usually, most neoplastic B cell lines express HSP25 constitutively; however, a few were identified which are HSP25-negative (Spector et al. 1992). An involvement of HSP25 in signal transduction during granulocyte differentiation was suggested by Spector et al. (1994). After induction of differentiation of human leukemic HL-60 cells by retinoic acid, the HSP25 level increased transiently concomitantly with the onset of G1 cell cycle arrest. This increase was paralleled by a transient increase of HSP25 phosphorylation. In infant acute lymphoblastic leukemia, a unique, diminished degree of phosphorylation of HSP25 was found in a pre-B cell stage of differentiation of leukemic cells (Strahler et al. 1991).

Drug Resistance and HSP25

Recent data suggest the involvement of small stress proteins in drug resistance. Studying the response of human breast cancer cells to chemotherapeutic drugs, Ciocca et al. (1992) found that both HSP70 and HSP25 were associated with doxorubicin resistance. Evidence that HSP25 is one of the determinants for doxorubicin resistance came from transfection experiments of MCF-7 cells with human HSP25 cDNA in the sense and antisense orientation. An increased HSP25-level was associated with doxorubicin resistance, whereas a reduced HSP25 level was associated with an increased doxorubicin sensitivity (Oesterreich et al. 1993). A similar result was obtained with rodent cells transfected with human HSP25 cDNA resulting in elevated resistance to doxorubicin, colchicine, and vinblastine, but not to 5-fluorouracil (Huot et al. 1991). Conversely, several cytostatic drugs in cytostatically effective concentrations have been shown to induce HSP25 (but not HSP70) in EAT cells. Drugs inducing HSP25 seem to interfere either with DNA replication in S-phase cells (cisplatin, cytosine arabinoside, 3′-fluorodeoxythymidine, doxorubicin, and daunomycin) or with the microtubule system in M-phase cells (colchicine, vincristine) (Oesterreich et al. 1991b; Bielka et al. 1994). Other drugs including 5-fluorouracil, aminopterin, and amethopterin, which interfere with nucleotide metabolism in G1-phase cells, as well as X-irradiation, were found not to induce HSP25. It thus appears that induction of small HSPs by cytostatic drugs is part of the mechanism rendering cells resistant to drugs.

Acknowledgments. This work was supported in part by grants from the Dr. Mildred Scheel Stiftung, Bonn (grant W43/91/Be), the Landesverband Berlin der Deutschen Knebsgesellschaft, and from the Deutsche Forschungsgemeinschaft, Bonn (grant YE5/SFB273). The antiHSP25 antibody was a generous gift from Dr. J. Stahl, Berlin.

References

Adams DJ, McGuire WL (1985) Quantitative enzyme-linked immunosorbent assay for the estrogen-regulated Mr 24,000 protein in human breast tumors: correlation with estrogen and progesterone receptors. Cancer Res 45: 2445–2449

Arrigo A-P, Welch WJ (1987) Characterization and purification of the mammalian 28,000 dalton heat shock protein. J Biol Chem 262: 15359–15369

Arrigo A-P, Suhan JP, Welch WJ (1988) Dynamic changes in the structure and intracellular locale of the mammalian low-molecular-weight heat shock protein. Mol Cell Biol 8: 5059–5071

Barry MA, Behnke CA, Eastman A (1990) Activation of programmed cell death (apoptosis) by cisplatin, other anticancer drugs, toxins and hyperthermia. Biochem Pharmacol 40: 2353–2362

Beckmann RP, Lovett M, Welch WJ (1992) Examining the function and regulation of hsp70 in cells subjected to metabolic stress. J Cell Biol 6: 1137–1150

Benndorf R, Nürnberg P, Bielka H (1988a) Growth phase-dependent proteins of the Ehrlich ascites tumor analyzed by one- and two-dimensional electrophoresis. Exp Cell Res 174: 130–138

Benndorf R, Kraft R, Otto A, Stahl J, Böhm H, Bielka H (1988b) Purification of the growth-related protein p25 of the Ehrlich ascites tumor and analysis of its isoforms. Biochem Int 17: 225–234

Benndorf R, Hayeß K, Stahl J, Bielka H (1992) Cell-free phosphorylation of the murine small heat shock protein hsp25 by an endogenous kinase from Ehrlich ascites tumor cells. Biochim Biophys Acta 1136: 203–207

Benndorf R, Hayeß K, Ryazantsev S, Wieske M, Behlke J, Lutsch G (1994) Phosphorylation and supramolecular organization of murine small heat shock protein HSP25 abolish its actin polymerization inhibiting activity. J Biol Chem 269: 20780–20784

Bielka H, Hoinkis G, Oesterreich S, Stahl J, Benndorf R (1994) Induction of the small stress protein hsp25 in Ehrlich ascites carcinoma cells by anticancer drugs. FEBS Lett 343: 165–167

Burel C, Mezger V, Pinto M, Rallu M, Trigon S, Morange M (1992) Mammalian heat shock protein families. Expression and function. Experientia 48: 629–634

Ciocca DR, Fuqua SAW, Lock-Lim S, Toft DO, Welch WJ, McGuire WL (1992) Response of human breast cancer cells to heat shock and chemotherapeutic agents. Cancer Res 52: 3648–3654

Ciocca DR, Clark GM, Tandon AK, Fuqua SAW, Welch WL, McGuire WL (1993a) Heat shock protein HSP70 in patients with axillary lymph node-negative breast cancer: prognostic implications. J Natl Cancer Inst 85: 570–574

Ciocca DR, Oesterreich S, Chamness C, McGuire WL, Fuqua SAW (1993b) Biological and clinical implications of heat shock protein 27000 (HSP27): a review. J Natl Cancer Inst 85: 1558–1570

DeJong WW, Leunissen JAM, Voorter CEM (1993) Evolution of the α-crystallin/small heat shock protein family. Mol Biol Evol 10: 103–126

Dunn DK, Whelan RDH, Hill B, King RJB (1993) Relationship of HSP27 and estrogen receptor in hormone sensitive and insensitive cell lines. J Steroid Biochem Mol Biol 46: 469–479

Engel K, Plath K, Gaestel M (1994) The MAP kinase-activated protein kinase 2 contains a proline-rich SH3-binding domain. FEBS Lett 336: 143–147

Fuqua SAW, Oesterreich S, Hilsenbeck SG, von Hoff DD, Echardt J, Osborne CK (1994) Heat shock proteins and drug resistance. Breast Cancer Res Treatm 32: 67–71

Gaestel M, Gross B, Benndorf R, Strauss M, Schunck W-H, Kraft R, Otto A, Böhm H, Stahl J, Drabsch H, Bielka H (1989) Molecular cloning, sequencing and expression in Escherichia coli of teh 25-kDa growth-related protein of Ehrlich ascites tumor and its homology to mammalian stress proteins. Eur J Biochem 179: 209–213

Gaestel M, Schröder W, Benndorf R, Lippmann C, Buchner K, Hucho F, Erdmann VA, Bielka H (1991) Identification of the phosphorylation sites of the small murine heat shock protein hsp25. J Biol Chem 266: 14721–14725

Gaestel M, Gotthardt R, Müller T (1993) Structure and organization of a murine gene encoding small heat shock protein HSP25. Gene 128: 279–283

Hartl F-U, Hlodan R, Langer T (1994) Molecular chaperones in protein folding. TIBS 19: 21–25

Hendrick JP, Hartl F-U (1993) Molecular chaperone functions of heat shock proteins. Annu Rev Biochem 62: 349–384

Henriksson M, Classon M, Axelson H, Klein G, Thyberg J (1992) Nuclear colocalization of c-myc protein and HSP70 in cells transfected with human wild-type and mutant c-myc genes. Exp Cell Res 203: 383–394

Huot J, Roy G, Lambert H, Cretien P, Landry J (1991) Increased survival after treatment with anticancer agents of Chinese hamster cells expressing the human Mr 27,000 heat shock protein. Cancer Res 51: 5245–5252

Huot J, Lambert H, Lavoie JN, Guimond A, Houle F, Landry J (1995) Characterization of 45-kDa 54-kDa HSP27 kinase, a stress sensitive kinase which may activate the phosphorylation-dependent protective function of mammalian 27-kDa heat shock protein HSP27. Eur J Biochem 227: 416–427

Hosokawa N, Hirayoshi K, Kudo H, Takechi H, Aoike A, Kawal K, Nagata K (1992) Inhibition of the activation of heat shock factor in vivo and in vitro by flavonoids. Mol Cell Biol 12: 3490–3498

Jameel A, Skilton A, Campbell TA, Chander SK, Coombes RC, Luqman YA (1992) Clinical and biological significance of HSP89 alpha in human breast cancer. Int J Cancer 50: 409–415

Johnston RN, Kucey BL (1988) Competitive inhibition of HSP70 gene expression causes thermosensitivity. Science 242: 1551–1554

Kato K, Shinohara H, Goto S, Inaguma Y, Morishita R, Asano T (1992a) Copurification of small heat shock protein with αB-crystallin from human skeletal muscle. J Biol Chem 267: 7718–7725

Kato M, Herz F, Kato S, Hirano A (1992b) Expression of stress-response (heat shock) protein HSP27 in human brain tumors: an immunohistochemical study. Acta Neuropathol (Berl) 83: 420–422

Kato S, Hirano A, Kato M, Herz F (1993) Comparative study on the expression of stress-response protein (srp) 72, srp 27, αB-crystallin and ubiquitin in brain tumors. An immunohistochemical study. Neuropathol Appl Neurobiol 19: 436–442

Kato K, Hasegawa K, Goto S, Inaguma Y (1994) Dissociation as a result of phosphorylation of an aggregated form of the small stress protein, HSP27. J Biol Chem 269: 11274–11278

Klemenz R, Andres A-C, Fröhli E, Schäfer R, Ayoma A (1993) Expression of the murine small heat shock protein HSP25 and αB-crystallin in the absence of stress. J Cell Biol 120: 639–645

Knauf U, Bielka H, Gaestel M (1992) Over-expression of the small heat-shock protein, hsp25, inhibits growth of Ehrlich ascites tumor cells. FEBS Lett 309: 297–302

Knauf U, Jakob U, Engel K, Buchner J, Gaestel M (1994) Stress- and mitogen- induced phosphorylation of the small heat shock protein HSP25 by MAPKAP kinase-2 is not essential for chaperone properties and cellular thermoresistance. EMBO J 13: 54–60

Koishi M, Hosokawa N, Sato M, Nakai A, Hirayoshi K, Hiraoka M, Abe M, Nagata K (1992) Quercetin, an inhibitor of heat shock protein synthesis, inhibits the acquisition of thermotolerance in a human colon carcinoma cell line. J Cancer Res 83: 1216–1222

Landry J, Chretien P, Lambert H, Hickey E, Weber LA (1989) Heat shock resistance conferred by expression of the human HSP-27 gene in rodent cells. J Cell Biol 109: 7–15

Lane DP, Midgley C, Hupp T (1993) Tumor suppressor genes and molecular chaperones. Philos Trans R Soc Lond 339: 369–373

Lavoie JN, Gingras-Breton G, Tanguay RM, Landry J (1993) Induction of Chinese hamster hsp27 gene expression in mouse cells confers resistance to heat shock. J Biol Chem 268: 3420–3429

Lavoie JN, Lambert H, Hickey E, Weber LA, Landry J (1995) Modulation of cellular thermoresistance and actin filament stability accompanies phosphorylation-induced changes in the oligimeric structure of heat shock protein 27. Mol Cell Biol 15: 505–516

Li GC, Li L, Liu Y, Mak JY, Chen L, Lee WMF (1991) Thermal response of rat fibroblasts stably transfected with the human 70-kDa heat shock protein-encoding gene. Proc Natl Acad Sci USA 88: 1681–1685

Love S, King RJB (1994) A 27 kDa heat shock protein that has anomalous prognostic powers in early and advanced breast cancer. Br J Cancer 69: 743–751

McGarry TJ, Lindquist S (1986) Inhibition of heat shock protein synthesis by heat-inducible antisense RNA. Proc Natl Acad Sci USA 83: 399–403

Mehlen P, Arrigo A-P (1994) The serum-induced phosphorylation of mammalian HSP27 correlates with changes in its intracellular localization and levels of oligomerization. Eur J Biochem 221: 327–334

Mestril R, Dillman WH (1995) Heat shock proteins and protection against myocardial ischemia. J Mol Cell Cardiol 27: 45–52

Miglioratti G, Nicoletti I, Crocicchio F, Pagliacci C, D'Adamio F, Riccardi C (1992) Heat shock induces apoptosis in mouse thymocytes and protects them from glucocorticoid-induced cell death. Cell Immunol 143: 348–356

Miron T, Wilchek M, Geiger B (1988) Characterization of an inhibitor of actin polymerization in vinculin-rich fraction of turkey gizzard smooth muscle. Eur J Biochem 178: 543–553

Miron T, Vancompernolle K, Vanderkerckhove J, Wilchek M, Geiger B (1991) A 25 kDa inhibitor of actin polymerization is a low molecular weight stress protein. J Cell Biol 114: 255–261

Moretti-Rojas I, Fuqua SAW, Montgomery RA, McGuire WL (1988) A cDNA for the estradiol-regulated 24k protein: control of mRNA levels in MCF-7 cells. Breast Cancer Res Treat 11: 155–163

Morimoto RI (1991) Heat shock: the role of transient inducible responses in cell damage, transformation and differentiation. Cancer Cells 3: 295–301

Morimoto RI, Tissieres A, Georgopoulos C (1994) The biology of heat shock proteins and molecular chaperones. Cold Spring Harbor Laboratory Press Cold Spring Harbor

Multhoff G, Botzler C, Wiesnet M, Müller E, Meier T, Willmanns W, Issels R (1995) A stress-inducible 72-kDa heat shock protein (HSP72) is expressed on the surface of human tumor cells, but not on normal cells. Int J Cancer 61: 1–8

Oesterreich S, Benndorf R, Bielka H (1990) The expression of the growth-related 25kDa protein of Ehrlich ascites tumor cells is increased by hyperthermic treatment (heat shock). Biomed Biochim Acta 49: 219–226

Oesterreich S, Benndorf R, Reichmann G, Bielka H (1991a) Phosphorylation and acylation of the growth-related murine small stress protein p25. NATO Asi Ser H56: 489–493

Oesterreich S, Schunck H, Benndorf R, Bielka H (1991b) Cisplatin induces the small stress protein hsp25 and thermotolerance in Ehrlich ascites tumor cells. Biochem Biophys Res Commun 180: 243–248

Oesterreich S, Weng C-N, Qiu M, Hilsenbeck SG, Osborne CK, Fuqua SAW (1993) The small heat shock protein HSP27 is correlated with growth and drug resistance in human breast cancer cell lines. Cancer Res 53: 4443–4448

Riabowol KT, Mizzen LA, Welch WJ (1988) Heat shock is lethal to fibroblasts microinjected with antibodies against hsp 70. Science 242: 433–436

Ritossa FM (1962) A new puffing pattern induced by heat shock and DNP in Drosophila. Experientia 18: 571–573

Sakaguchi Y, Maehara Y, Baba H, Kusomoto T, Sugimachi K, Newman RA (1992) Flavone acetic acid increases the antitumor effect of hyperthermia in mice. Cancer Res 52: 3306–3309

Sanchez Y, Lindquist SL (1990) HSP 104 required for induced thermotolerance. Science 248: 1112–1115

Spector NL, Samson W, Rayn C, Gribben J, Urba W, Welch WJ, Nadler LM (1992) Growth arrest of human B lymphocytes is accompanied by induction of the low molecular weight mammalian heat shock protein (HSP28). J Immunol 148: 1668–1673

Spector NL, Mehlen P, Ryan C, Hardy L, Samson W, Levine H, Nadler LM, Arrigo A-P (1994) Regulation of the 28 kDa heat shock protein by retinoic acid during differentiation of human leukemic HL-60 cells. FEBS Lett 337: 184–188

Steels EL, Watson K, Parsons PG (1992) Relationships between thermotolerance, oxidative stress responses and induction of stress proteins in human tumor cell lines. Biochem Pharmacol 44: 2123–2129

Strahler JR, Kuick R, Hanash SM (1991) Diminished phosphorylation of heat shock protein (HSP27) in infant acute lymphoblastic leukemia. Biochem Biophys Res Commun 175: 134–142

Taira T, Neggishi Y, Kihara F, Iguchi-Ariga SMM, Ariga H (1992) c-myc protein complex binds to two sites in human hsp70 promotor region. Biochim Biophys Acta 1130: 166–174

Tetu B, Lacasse B, Bouchard HL, Lagace R, Huot J, Landry (1992) Prognostic influence of HSP27 expression in malignant fibrous histiocytoma: a clinicopathological and immunohistochemical study. Cancer Res 52: 2325–2328

Thor A, Benz C, Moore D, Goldman E, Edgerton S, Landry J, Schwartz L, Mayall B, Hickey E, Weber LA (1991) Stress response protein (srp27) determination in primary human breast carcinomas: clinical, histologic, and prognostic correlations. J Natl Cancer Inst 83: 170–183

Tissieres A, Mitchell HK, Tracy UM (1974) Protein synthesis in salivary glands of Drosophila melanogaster: relation to chromosome puffs. J Mol Biol 84: 389–398

Ungar DR, Hailat N, Strahler JR, Kuick RD, Brodeur GM, Seeger RC, Reynolds P, Hanash SM (1994) HSP27 expression in neuroblastoma: correlation with disease. J Natl Cancer Inst 86: 780–785

Vernon C (1992) Hyperthermia in cancer growth regulation. Biotherapy 4: 307–315

Wei Y, Zhao X, Kariya Y, Fukata H, Teshigawara K, Uchida A (1994) Induction of apoptosis by quercetin: involvement of heat shock protein. Cancer Res 54: 4952–4957

Zantema A, Verlaan-de Fries M, Maasdam D, Bol S, van der Eb A (1992) Heat shock protein 27 and αB-crystallin can form a complex, which dissociates by heat shock. J Biol Chem 267: 12936–12941

Two-Dimensional Polyacrylamide Gel Electrophoresis of Cancer-Associated Proteins

P.J. Wirth, L.-di Luo, T. Hoang, and T. Benjamin

Biopolymer Chemistry Section, Laboratory of Experimental Carcinogenesis, National Cancer Institute, Bethesda, MD 20893, USA

Introduction

It is generally accepted that cancer development is a multistage process involving a variety of cell types (Farber and Cameron 1980). Over the last 20 years considerable effort has been made to define the genetic events involved in the etiology of cancer development. Indeed, molecular genetics has been highly successful in the demonstration that development of certain forms of human cancers, in particular, colorectal, lung, and breast, may arise following a series of four to six distinct genetic alterations in specific target tissues (Fearon and Vogelstein 1990). These mutations may involve either the activation of one or more cellular protooncogene(s) and/or inactivation of one or more tumor suppressor gene(s) and are thought to initiate a cascade of biochemical events that culminate in the dysregulation of normal control mechanisms governing cellular growth and differentiation (Weinberg 1989; Hunter 1991). Regardless of the nature of the oncogenic agent, the observed phenotypic effects on the host cells are remarkably similar. These include characteristic alterations in cellular morphology, adhesiveness and motility, and cell-to-cell communication, as well as dysregulation of cellular growth and differentiation, including loss of contact growth inhibition in vitro, acquisition of anchorage-independent growth in soft agar, and tumorigenicity in susceptible animals.

Rat liver has provided an excellent model to study a variety of biological processes including the regulation of normal cellular growth and differentiation as well as certain disease states such as cancer development (for reviews see Pitot 1979; Sell et al. 1987). While it has generally been thought that hepatocytes are the primary cellular targets for chemical carcinogens and hence represent the cellular precursors for hepatocellular carcinoma development, recent evidence has suggested that chemically induced hepatocarcinogenesis may involve several cell types (Evarts et al. 1987).

Numerous investigators, including ourselves, have established long-term cultures of rat liver-derived epithelial (RLE) cells which may represent a progeny of a hepatic stem cell population capable of differentiating toward the hepatocyte lineage (Evarts et al. 1987, 1989). RLE cells can be transformed in vitro with both chemical carcinogens (McMahon et al. 1986) and specific oncogenes (Garfield et al. 1988), as well as spontaneously as a result of long-term, continuous passage or after chronic maintenance in a confluent state (Huggett et al. 1991). When injected into nude mice these transformed cells produce a wide spectrum of tumor types which are quite similar to those found in the liver following the in vivo administration of various chemical carcinogens (McMahon et al. 1986; Tsao and Grisham 1987). These include hepatocellular carcinomas, sarcomas, "mixed epithelial-mesenchymal" tumors, hepatoblastomas, and undifferentiated tumors. Because of their capacity for neoplastic transformation, it has been postulated that this facultative stem cell compartment may be one of the in vivo cellular targets for hepatocarcinogenesis (Evarts et al. 1987; Tsao and Grisham 1987). Hence, RLE cells have become an appropriate in vitro model to study genotypic and phenotypic alterations during hepatocarcinogenesis.

Working on the hypothesis that the acquisition of the neoplastic phenotype would result in both qualitative and quantitative changes in cellular functions quite different from those observed under normal and/or preneoplastic conditions, and that these changes should be reflected on the protein level, we have undertaken a detailed study of gene expression at the protein level in RLE cells during chemical, viral, and spontaneously induced transformation using high-resolution two-dimensional polyacrylamide gel electrophoresis (2D-PAGE) (Wirth et al. 1992, 1993; Wirth 1994).

Materials and Methods

Cells

The diploid RLE cell line was established from a 10-day-old female Fischer F344 rat as previously described (McMahon et al. 1986). Details describing the derivation and characterization of the various normal and transformed RLE cell lines with respect to growth in monolayer and soft agar cultures, histological classifications, and tumorigenicity have been reported in detail elsewhere (McMahon et al. 1986; Garfield et al. 1988; Huggett et al. 1991).

2D-PAGE

Isoelectric focusing (IEF) 2D-PAGE was performed essentially as described by Hochstrasser et al. (1988). Briefly, IEF separation was performed at room temperature at a constant power of 20 mW/tube per 14 tubes, 13 500 V-h total in 180 mm × 1.0 mm 4% w/v polyacrylamide gels containing 2% carrier ampholytes (1.6% pH 4–8 and 0.4% pH 4–8 and 0.4% pH 3.5–10). First-dimension tube gels were extruded from the basic end directly onto the surface of a second-dimension, 1.5-mm-thick, 7%–15% sodium dodecyl sulfate (SDS) polyacrylamide gradient slab gel. Electrophoresis was carried out at 10 °C using a Bio-Rad Protean IIxi multicell electrophoresis unit (Bio-Rad Laboratories, Melville, NY)

Electroblotting, Microsequencing, and Amino Acid Sequence Analysis

Protein sequencing was performed after electrotransfer of proteins (500 μg) to ProBlott membranes (Applied Biosystems, Foster City, CA, USA) using 10 m*M* 3-[cyclohexylamino]-1-propanesulfonic acid (CAPS) buffer, pH 11, containing 10% methanol at 70 V for 2 h at 4 °C. Protein spots of interest were excised from the dried Ponceau S stained membranes and N-terminal amino acid sequences determined using an Applied Biosystems Model 475A protein sequencer modified with bottle and regulator updates and equipped with an "online" Model 120A phenylthiohydantoin (PTH)-amino acid analyzer. Amino acid sequence comparisons were performed using the FASTA computer program for the screening of protein or nuclei acid databases (Pearson and Lipman 1988). The PIR (Protein Identification Resource) and SWISSPROT (Swiss Protein Sequence Data Bank) sequence data bases were searched.

Results and Discussion

Whole Cell Lysate Polypeptides from Normal, Aflatoxin B_1 (AFB_1)- and Spontaneously Transformed RLE Cells

Figure 1 illustrates the IEF 2D-PAGE separation of approximately 2000 [^{35}S]-methionine-labeled polypeptides form normal RLE cells (A), a representative AFB-transformed RLE cell line, AFB-C2 (B), and ST-C3T, a spontaneously transformed RLE cell line (C). Numerous qualitative and quantitative differences in the expression of individual polypeptides were readily observed among the three cell types. Some of the more prominent alterations have been illustrated on the respective panels of Fig. 1 with the spot identification numbers and the enclosed boxes. For example, the cytosolic polypeptides 791 and 793 and the membrane-associated polypeptides 1359 and 1361 were markedly decreased both in spontaneous and oncogene (v-Ha-*ras*, v-*raf*, or v-*raf*/v-*myc*)-induced transformants and to a lesser extent in AFB-induced transformants, while 1751 was decreased to almost undetectable levels in each of the various transformants. The nuclear polypeptides 1273, 1652, 1860, and 1873 as well as polypeptides 1274 and 1682 were decreased during spontaneous and oncogene-induced transformation but unaffected in AFB transformed cells. Polypeptides 822, 945, 1042, 1055, 1103, 1217, 1694, 1711, and 1729 were markedly increased in the course of AFB-induced transformation but unchanged in either onco-

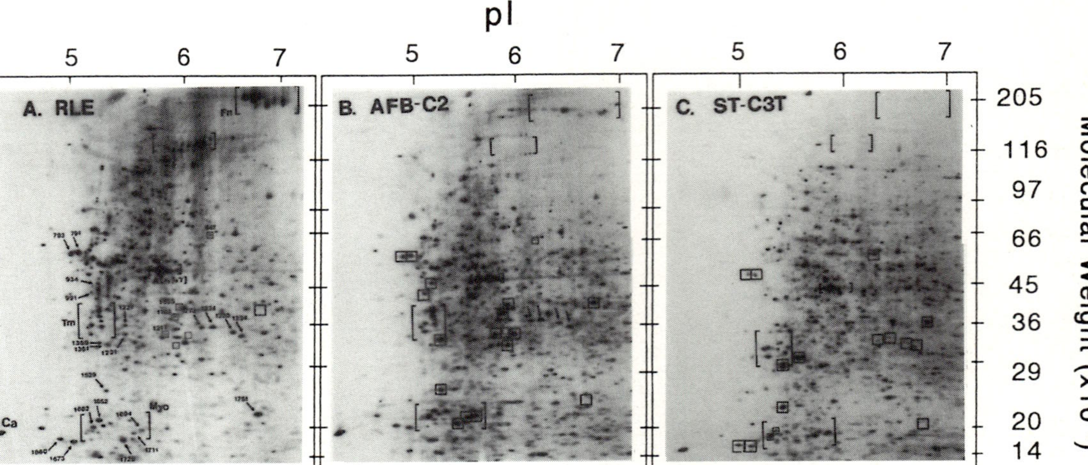

Fig. 1. Two-dimensional polyacrylamide gel electrophoresis (2D-PAGE) separation of [^{35}S] methionine-labeled polypeptides from normal rat liver-derived epithelial (RLE) cells (**A**), a representative AFB-transformed RLE cell line (AFB-C2) (**B**), and a spontaneous transformant (ST-C3T) (**C**). *Fn*, fibronectin; *A* (α, β, γ), actin isoforms; *Tm*, tropomyosins; *Ca*, *calmodulin*, and *Myo*, myosin light chain isoforms. *Numbered polypeptides* indicate those polypeptides whose syntheses are substantially modulated during either aflatoxin B_1 (AFB) or spontaneously induced transformation of RLE cells. *Open boxes* and *brackets* have been positioned to aid in polypeptide spot location. (Adapted from Wirth et al. 1992)

gene or spontaneously transformed RLE cells. The specific subcellular locations of the individual polypeptides described above (e.g., 791 and 1273) have previously been reported and catalogued in the RLE protein database (Wirth et al. 1991). The extracellular matrix protein fibronectin (190–205 kDa/pI 6.5–7.5) (data not shown) and various cytoskeletal components, including the tropomyosin (Tm) family of related polypeptides (30–36 kDa/pI 4.6–5.0) and the actin isoforms (43 kDa/pI 5.2–5.5) (data not shown), were also altered in transformed RLE cells.

Tropomyosin-Related Polypeptides

Figure 2 represents enlarged regions of 2D-PAGE gels illustrating Tm-related polypeptides from normal, and a series of AFB-, spontaneously, and oncogene-transformed RLE cell lines. Comparison of Tm expression in four AFB transformed clones (A-D), four spontaneously transformed lines (E-H), four oncogene-transformed cell lines (I-L), and at succeeding passages of RLEØ13 cells (M-P) revealed that Tm4 and Tm5 were unaltered during transformation of RLE cells. Tm2 and Tm3 were unaltered in AFB transformed RLE cells (Fig. 2A-D), decreased approximately 50% in v-Ha-*ras*-transformed cells (Fig. 2I, L), and markedly decreased during spontaneous transformation (Fig. 2M-P) and in RLE cells transformed with either v-*raf* (Fig. 2J) or v-*raf*/v-*myc* (Fig. 2K). In contrast, Tm1 was markedly increased during AFB-induced transformation (Fig. 2A-D) but showed variable expression during either spontaneous (Fig. 2E-H) or oncogene-induced transformation (Fig. 2I-L). Tm6 was markedly decreased during oncogene and AFB-induced transformation but unchanged of decreased during spontaneously induced transformation. Long-term cultures of RLE cells maintained under selective growth pressures result in spontaneous transformation (Huggett et al. 1991). Comparison of Tm expression in RLEØ13 cells at different passages ranging from passage 26 (Fig. 2M) to passage 44 (Fig. 2P) revealed a progressive loss of expression of Tm2 and Tm3.

At present it is not known how these differences in Tm expression relate to the carcinogenic process (Leavitt et al. 1986). Loss of expression of Tm isoforms has previously been reported in human, murine, and avian fibroblasts transformed by viral oncogenes (Cooper et al. 1985), chemical carcinogens (Leavitt et al. 1986), or following treatment with transforming growth factor α (Cooper et al. 1987). Leavitt et al. (1986) reported that the syntheses of Tm isoforms, Tm1, Tm2, and Tm6, were greatly reduced (80%–90%) in chemically transformed tumorigenic human HuT-14 fibroblasts relative to normal diploid fibroblasts. In contrast, in related "immortalized" HuT fibroblasts, Tm1 and Tm6 were only slightly downregulated while Tm3 was increased 3.5-fold (Leavitt et al. 1986).

Consistent loss of expression of specific Tm isoforms has also been observed in cells cultured from human breast carcinoma (Bhattacharya et al. 1990).

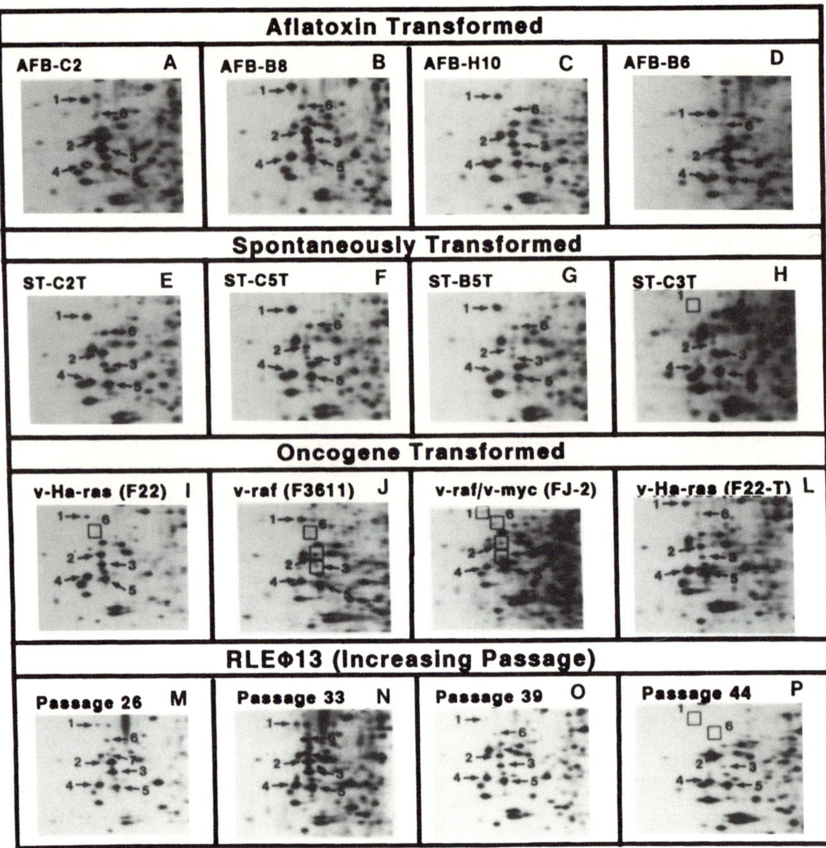

Fig. 2. Expression of tropomyosin-related polypeptides in normal and transformed RLE cells. AFB-transformed RLE cells: AFB-C2, AFB-B8, AFB-H10, and AFB-B6; spontaneously transformed cells; ST-C2T, ST-C5T, ST-B5T, and ST-C3T; and oncogene-transformed: v-Ha-*ras* (F22), v-*raf* (F3611–T2), v-*raf*/v-*myc* (FJ-2), and v-Ha-*ras* (tumor-derived; F22-T); normal RLE cells: passage 26, 33, 39, and 44. The Tm isoforms were numbered according to Matsumura and colleagues (Matsumura and Yamashiro-Matsumura 1985). (Adapted from Wirth 1994)

Recent studies from Cooper's laboratory have demonstrated that the restoration of expression of a 39 kDa Tm isoform, Tm1, previously suppressed as a result of transformation of NIH3T3 mouse fibroblasts by the v-Ki-*ras* oncogene resulted in partial reversion of the transformed phenotype as characterized by the loss of anchorage-independent growth capacity and increased tumor growth latency in these cells (Prasad et al. 1993).

Nuclear Polypeptides

One of the major subcellular organelles that are critically involved in cellular proliferation and differential gene expression is the nucleus. Due to the critical role nuclear proteins play in normal DNA replication and cellular proliferation and their possible involvement in neoplastic transformation, we have undertaken a detailed analysis of nuclear polypeptides from normal and transformed RLE cells. Figure 3 illustrates 2D-PAGE separation of 1550 [^{35}S]-methionine-labeled polypeptides from sucrose gradient purified RLE liver nuclei preparations (Blobel and Potter 1966). Selected transformation-associated RLE nuclear polypeptides whose expression is markedly altered (either increased or decreased) in the course of chemically (AFB-B6) or spontaneously induced transformation (ST-C3T) of RLE cells are highlighted on Fig. 3. For example, polypeptides 1178 (5.2/29 kDa) and 1273 (5.15/22 kDa) are markedly increased in both AFB- and spontaneously transformed cells, whereas polypeptides 367 (5.3/110 kDa), 763 (5.35/42 kDa), and 1342 (6.1/20 kDa) are unaltered during spontaneous transformation (ST-C3T), yet increased dramatically during AFB-induced neoplastic transformation (AFL-B6). Polypeptides 241 (6.15/140 kDa), 270 (5.50/138 kDa), and the isoforms 402 (5.85/105 kDa) and 403 (5.87/105 kDa) are specifically modulated during spontaneous transformation (ST-C3T). Numerous other qualitative and quantitative polypeptide differences are also clearly detected among parental, AFB-, and spontaneously transformed RLE cells and have been recorded in the RLE nuclear protein database (Wirth et al. 1993b).

Numerous RLE nuclear-associated polypeptides have been identified using N-terminal microsequencing and Western immunoblot analysis and are illustrated on Fig. 3. These include calreticulin, glucose-regulated 78-kDa protein, nuclear pore complex protein, ATP synthetase, statin, aldehyde dehydrogenase, vimentin and vimentin degradation products, actin, Tm isoforms, heat shock protein 60, elongation factor eEF-1, phosphatidylinositol-4,5-biphosphate phosphodiesterase, and protein disulfide isomerase. With the exception of Tm, however, none of the transformation-associated polypeptides corresponds to any of these known polypeptides.

Many reports have appeared providing a detailed analysis of nuclear-associated polypeptides from both normal and transformed cell lines and whole tissue samples in attempts to characterize proliferation- and transformation-associated polypeptides. A number of proliferation-associated nuclear proteins have been described (Celis and Bravo 1984; Black et al. 1987; Feuerstein and Mond 1987; Malek et al. 1990) as well as certain tumor-specific or tumor-associated proteins (Takami et al. 1979; Wu et al. 1979; Ruoslahti et al. 1980; Hanash et al. 1986; Menzel and Unteregger 1989). The most notable include Celis's excellent series of experiments characterizing the cell cycle-specific proliferating-cell nuclear and nucleolar antigen (PCNA; pI 5.0/36 kDa) in normal and transformed cell lines (Celis and Bravo 1984); Feuerstein and Mond's characterization of proliferative-associated "numatrin" (pI 5.0/40

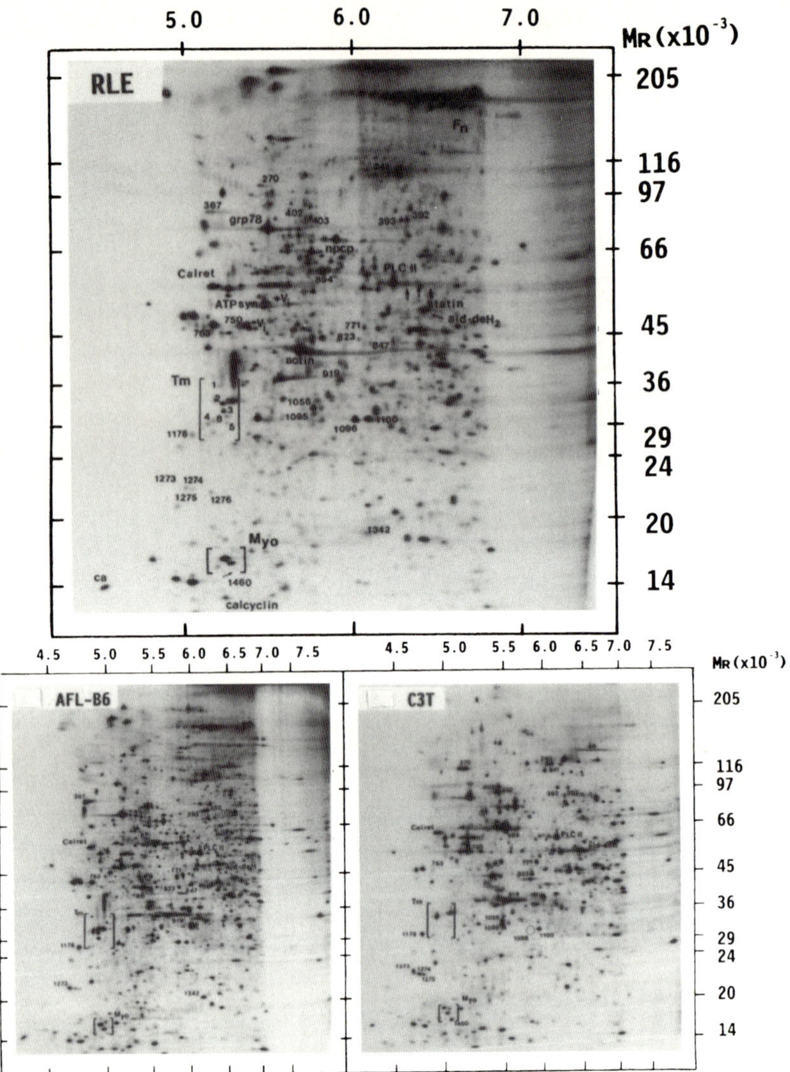

Fig. 3. 2D-PAGE isoelectric focusing (IEF) autoradiogram of [^{35}S] methionine-labeled nuclear polypeptides from normal, AFB-, and spontaneously transformed RLE cells. *Fn*, fibronectin; *Calret*, calreticulin; *Vi*, vimentin degradation products; *grp78*, 78-kDa glucose-regulated protein; *npcp*, nuclear pore complex protein; *ald-deH₂*, aldehyde dehydrogenase; *PLC II*, phospholipase C; *Tm*, tropomyosins; *Ca, calmodulin,* and *Myo*, myosin light chain isoforms. *Numbered polypeptides* indicate selected polypeptides whose syntheses are substantially modulated during either spontaneous or aflatoxin B_1-induced transformation. (Adapted from Wirth et al. 1993)

kDa) (Feuerstein and Mond 1987), which was subsequently identified as Busch's nucleolar B23; and Malek and coworkers' purification of pp32 and pp35 nuclear-associated phosphoproteins, both of which are substrates for caesin kinase II, an enzyme integrally involved in cellular growth and differentiation (Malek et al. 1990).

While it appears that none of the more abundantly expressed, transformation-associated RLE polypeptides (e.g., 367, 771, 823, 1178, or 1274) correspond to either PCNA, B23, or pp32/35, significant qualitative and quantitative alterations do occur in polypeptides localized in the M_r range of 20–100 kDa. These polypeptides represent approximately 20% of the total number of nuclear cytosolic proteins, but they are expressed in relatively minor concentrations (0.01%–0.001% total integrated density of detected protein).

[^{32}P] Orthophosphate-Labeled Polypeptides

One of the major regulatory mechanisms operative in the eucaryotic cell is the reversible phosphorylation/dephosphorylation of cellular polypeptides; as such it is an integral component of such biological regulatory mechanisms as receptor modulation and signal transduction (for reviews see Cohen and Cohen 1989; Hunter 1989; Ullrich and Schlessinger 1990). Protein kinase activity has been shown to be associated with several transforming proteins (Hunter 1989), and the involvement of tyrosine protein kinases in viral oncogenesis and growth factor-mediated signal transduction and growth regulation is well documented (Cantley et al. 1991). Therefore, the analysis of phosphoprotein expression during cellular transformation provides valuable information regarding any alterations in potential regulatory pathways that may be operative during cellular transformation. Figure 4 illustrates [^{32}P] orthophosphate-labeled polypeptide patterns obtained from parental RLE 13 cells (Fig. 4A), a representative AFB-transformed cell line (AFB-B6) (Fig. 4B), and two spontaneously transformed RLE cell lines, ST-B5T (Fig. 4C) and ST-C3T (Fig. 4D). Two sets of polypeptides, (95 [cytosolic/nuclear] and 96) and (87 [cytosolic/nuclear] and 113) were markedly increased during AFB and spontaneous transformation, respectively, whereas the constitutively expressed polypeptide 338 (6.00/16 kDa) was decreased to almost undetectable levels in both AFB- and spontaneously induced transformation. Although significant differences were observed between the parental RLE 13 cells and each of the spontaneously transformed cell lines, phosphoprotein expression in AFB- induced transformants appeared to be altered to a lesser extent. For example, in normal RLE 13 and each of the AFB transformants, three nuclear-associated polypeptides, polypeptides 860, 861, and 881 [pI 5.9–6.1/44 kDa], were expressed as major cellular phosphoproteins, yet following spontaneous transformation (ST-B5T and ST-C3T) their expression was reduced to almost undetected levels, as shown with open brackets in Fig. 4C,D. Conversely, the phosphorylation of polypeptides 275 (5.0/34 kDa) and 298 (4.2–5.0/19 kDa) was greatly

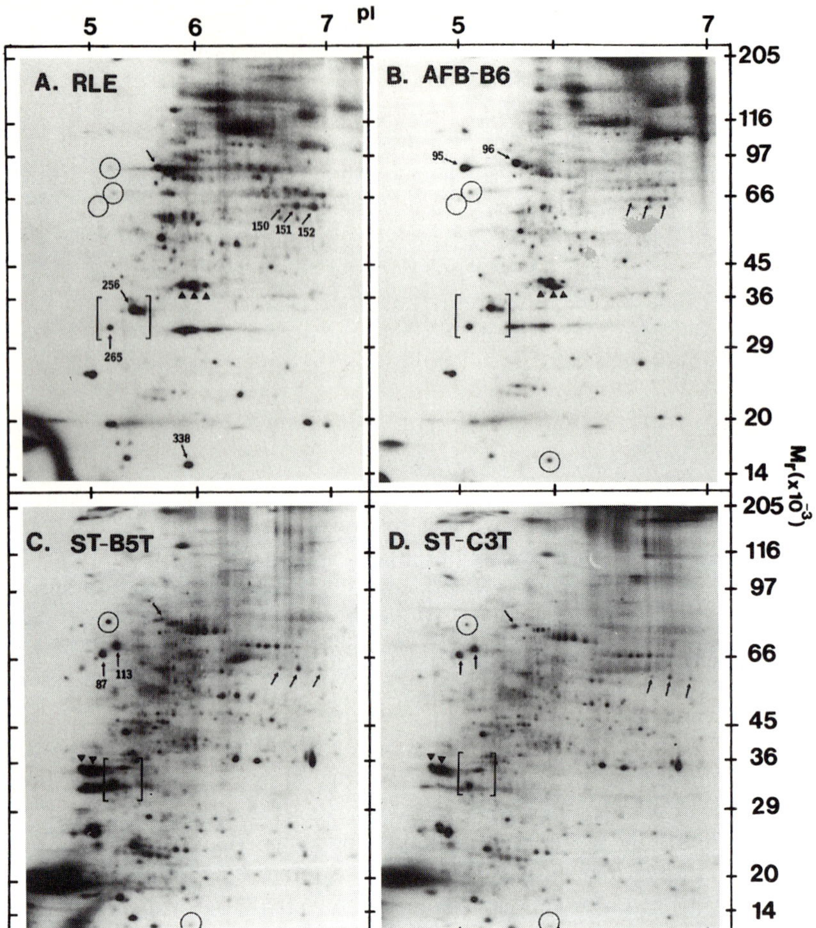

Fig. 4. 2D-PAGE separation of [^{32}P] orthophosphate-labeled polypeptides from normal RLE (**A**), a representative AFB-transformed RLE, AFB-B6 (**B**), and two spontaneously transformed RLE cell lines ST-B5T (**C**) and ST-C3T (**D**). *Numbered arrows* and *arrowheads* illustrate phosphoproteins undergoing significant modulation during transformation. *Open circles* and *brackets* have been positioned on the respective panels to aid in polypeptide spot orientation. Polypeptides 150, 151, 152 indicate the position of the phosphorylated isoforms of lamin-C. (Reprinted with permission from Wirth et al. 1992)

increased during spontaneous transformation. For orientation purposes the phosphorylated isoforms (polypeptides 150, 151, and 152) of lamin-C have been illustrated on Fig. 4A.

Busch and colleagues have identified significant differences in the expression of cytosolic phosphoproteins of normal rat liver, regenerating liver, and Novikoff hepatoma ascites cells (Wu et al. 1979; Black et al. 1987). Seven phosphoproteins found in Novikoff hepatoma were not expressed in normal or regenerating liver; six proteins were found exclusively in regenerating liver, and three spots were common to regenerating liver but not found in normal liver (Wu et al. 1979). In subsequent studies polyclonal and monoclonal antibodies were generated to these and other nuclear-associated polypeptides and were shown to distinguish malignant tissue from normal resting and cycling tissues (Black et al. 1987). Unfortunately, these studies were performed exclusively using 1D electrophoresis, making direct comparisons with our studies impossible.

N-Terminal Amino Acid Microsequencing of Polypeptides

Microsequencing of polypeptides isolated directly from 2D gels has proved invaluable in the characterization of polypeptides (Hochstrasser et al. 1992; Rasmussen et al. 1992). Therefore, we have recently undertaken a systematic approach to microsequencing rodent and human polypeptides in an attempt to integrate protein and DNA information of polypeptides believed to be critically involved in cellular growth and differentiation. Because of our ongoing research interest in growth factor-mediated signal transduction and nuclear transcriptional factors, we have focused our initial efforts on the N-terminal microsequencing of cytosolic nuclear polypeptides. Figure 5 illustrates a Ponceau S-stained membrane of RLE cytosolic nuclear polypeptides. Each step in the microsequencing procedure (e.g., 2D-PAGE gel running procedures, transblotting and staining of Immobiline membranes, and sequencing techniques) was optimized to maximize sequencing sensitivity. Polypeptides that were expressed in significant quantities (e.g., PLC-II, polypeptide 605) as well as polypeptides which appeared to be expressed in minor amounts (e.g., translationally controlled tumor protein, polypeptide 1376) were sequenced in an attempt to determine the sensitivity of our sequencing capabilities. The amount of protein sequenced varied greatly from polypeptide to polypeptide, ranging from 1 pmol (polypeptide 1376) to 14 pmol (PLC-II, polypeptide 605), and yielded 12–20 amino acid residues. Utilizing micropreparative immobilized pH gradients (IPG) 2D-PAGE, we have obtained sequence information from nearly 100 individual human HepG2 proteins from a single Ponceau S-stained membrane (Wirth et al., manuscript submitted). These results are quite exciting since they indicate that with the current high degree of microsequencing sensitivity and efficiency it is possible to identify a large percentage of polypeptides routinely directly from 2D-protein maps.

Concluding Remarks and Perspectives

In this essay I have tried to summarize some of our studies concerning the use of 2D-PAGE in the analysis of specific alterations in protein expression during

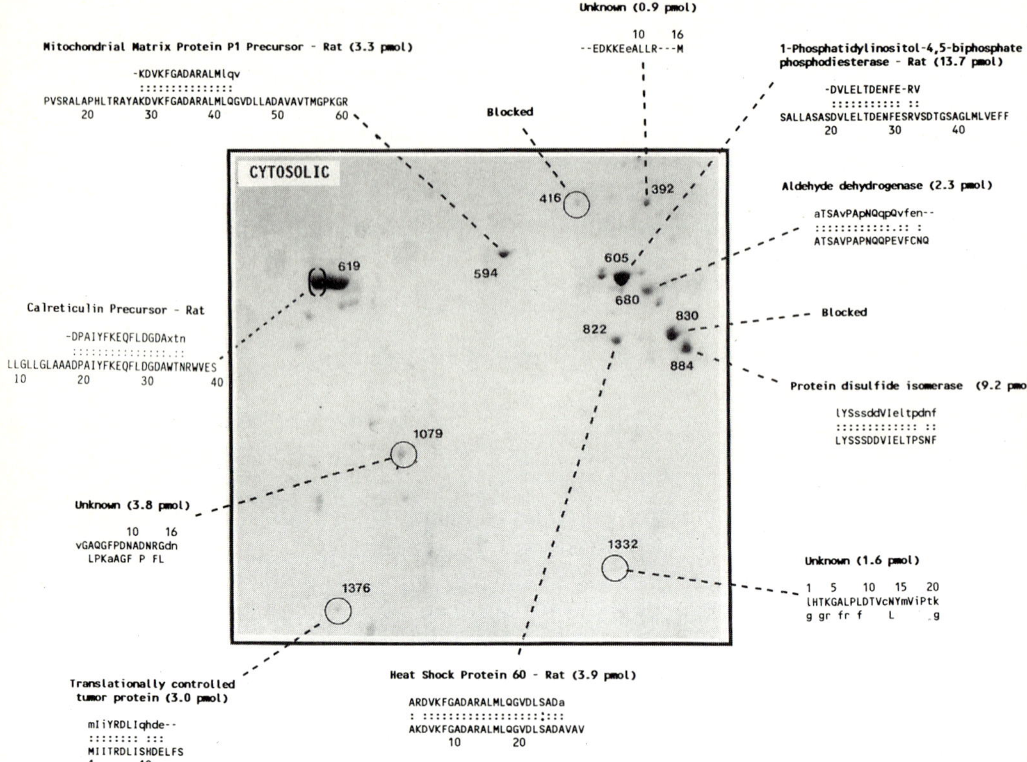

Fig. 5. N-terminal microsequencing of nuclear cytosolic RLE polypeptides. Polypeptides were selected at random for N-terminal microsequencing. Amino acid residues are given in one-letter notation. (*x*) means that the assignment of a phenylthiohydantoin (PTH)-amino acid was not possible. Amino acids shown in *lowercase* represent the most probable assignment. *Upper* amino acid sequences represent sequences obtained from the excised polypeptide spot and *lower sequences* those of known proteins obtained from the respective protein sequence databases. *Numbers below lower sequences* indicate position of identified residues. (Reprinted with permission from Wirth et al. 1993)

chemical, viral, and spontaneously induced hepatocarcinogenesis using an in vitro rat liver epithelial cell model. Since its introduction in 1975 (O'Farrell 1975), 2D-PAGE has become the method of choice for the analysis of complex mixtures of proteins and has found wide applications in a plethora of biological studies. These include the analysis of sequential alterations in protein expression as well as posttranslational modifications such as phosphorylation and changes occurring during cell cycling, differentiation, and transformation.

Several investigators have used 2D-PAGE analysis of normal and malignant tissues to search for changes associated with cancer development. Qualitative and quantitative changes on 2D protein patterns have been performed in breast cancer (Stastny et al. 1984; Wirth et al. 1987), brain tumors (Narayan et al.

1986), fibrosarcomas (Grimstad et al. 1988), colon mucosa and adenocarcinoma (Tracy et al. 1982; Nalty et al. 1988), kidney carcinomas (Ogata et al. 1987), adeno- and squamous cell carcinomas of the lung (Endler et al. 1986; Okuzawa et al. 1994), and leukemic cells (Hanash 1988). While these studies have identified a number of tumor- and transformation-associated protein variants and provided useful markers for carcinogenesis, serious difficulties have been encountered in assigning structural and hence functional identity to these proteins.

Recent advances in 2D-PAGE-associated analytical technologies have now made it possible to obtain N-terminal and internal amino acid microsequence information for polypeptides directly from 2D-PAGE gels (Matsudaira 1987). Partial amino acid sequences obtained for potentially important polypeptides provide the starting point for a wide range of biological studies. Comparison of partial amino acid sequences with existing protein and nucleic acid sequence databases affords a rapid and convenient method of protein identification in the absence of specific antibody preparations. Sequence information can be utilized for the large-scale synthesis of peptides for polyclonal and monoclonal antibody production as well as the design and synthesis of oligonucleotide probes and primers. These reagents can then be used to identify, clone and sequence tumor associated gene(s) for mechanistic studies of hepatocarcinogenesis on the molecular level and its basis in cell biology.

While our work has concentrated on the analysis of polypeptide alterations during experimentally induced rat hepatocarcinogenesis, studies have indicated that a large proportion of rodent and human proteins show a high degree of homology, both at the amino acid and at the nucleotide sequence level (Doolittle et al. 1986). Therefore, it is expected that information obtained concerning the identification and characterization of specific transformation and/or growth regulatory proteins in the RLE in vitro cell system will have direct applications in the screening of a human cDNA library for homologous genes. It is anticipated that animal-based studies such as these will have direct applications to delineating the molecular events during the process of human hepatocarcinogenesis.

References

Bhattacharya B, Prasad GL, Valverius EM, Salomon DS, Cooper HL (1990) Tropomyosins of human mammary epithelial cell lines: consistent defects of expression in mammary carcinoma cell lines. Cancer Res 50: 2105–2112

Black A, Freeman JW, Zhou G, Busch H (1987) Novel cell cycle-related nuclear proteins found in rat and human cells with monoclonal antibodies. Cancer Res 47: 3266–3272

Blobel G, Potter V (1966) Nuclei from rat liver: isolation method that combines purity with yield. Proc Natl Acad Sci USA 154: 1662–1665

Cantley LC, Auger KR, Carpenter C, Duckworth B, Graziani A, Kapeller R, Soltoff S (1991) Oncogenes and signal transduction. Cell 64: 281–302

Celis JE, Bravo R (1984) Synthesis of the nuclear protein cyclin in growing, senescent and morphologically transformed human skin fibroblasts. FEBS Lett 165: 21–25

Cohen P, Cohen PTW (1989) Protein phosphatases come of age. J Biol Chem 264: 21435–21438

Cooper HL, Feuerstein N, Noda M, Bassin RH (1985) Suppression of tropomyosin synthesis, a common biochemical feature of oncogenesis by structurally diverse retroviral oncogenes. Mol Cell Biol 5: 972–983

Cooper HL, Bhattacharya B, Bassin RH, Salomon DS (1987) Suppression of synthesis and utilization of tropomyosin in mouse and rat fibroblasts by transforming growth factor-alpha: a pathway in oncogene action. Cancer Res 47: 4493–4500

Doolittle RF, Feng DF, Johnson MS, McClure MA (1986) Relationships of human protein sequences to those of other organisms. Cold Spring Harbor Symp Quant Biol 51: 447–455

Endler AT, Young DS, Wold LE, Lieber MM, Currie RM (1986) Two-dimensional electrophoresis of proteins in tumours of the lung. J Clin Chem Clin Biochem 24: 981–992

Evarts RP, Nagy P, Marsden E, Thorgeirsson SS (1987) A precursor-product relationship exists between oval cells and hepatocytes in rat liver. Carcinogenesis 8: 1737–1740

Evarts RP, Nagy P, Makatsukasa H, Marsden E, Thorgeirsson SS (1989) In vivo differentiation of rat liver oval cells into hepatocytes. Cancer Res 49: 1541–1547

Farber E, Cameron R (1980) The sequential analysis of cancer development. Adv Cancer Res 31: 125–226

Fearon ER, Vogelstein B (1990) A genetic model for colorectal tumorigenesis. Cell 61: 759–767

Feuerstein N, Mond JJ (1987) Identification of a prominent nuclear protein associated with proliferation of normal and malignant B cells. J Immunol 139: 1818–1822

Garfield S, Huber BE, Nagy P, Cordingley MG, Thorgeirsson SS (1988) Neoplastic transformation and lineage switching of rat liver epithelial cells by retroviral associated oncogenes. Mol Carcinog 1: 189–195

Grimstad IA, Thorsrud AK, Jellum E (1988) Marker polypeptides distinguishing between cancer cell clones with high and low potential for spontaneous metastasis in murine fibrosarcoma cells. Cancer Res 48: 572–577

Hanash S (1988) Contribution of protein electrophoretic analysis to cancer research. Adv Elect 2: 343–384

Hanash SM, Baier LJ, McCurry L, Schwartz SA (1986) Lineage-related polypeptide markers in acute lymphoblastic leukemia detected by two-dimensional gel electrophoresis. Proc Natl Acad Sci USA 83: 807–811

Hochstrasser DF, Harrington MG, Hochstrasser A-K, Miller MJ, Merril CR (1988) Methods for increasing the resolution of two-dimensional protein electrophoresis. Anal Biochem 173: 424–435

Hochstrasser DF, Frutiger S, Paquet N, Bairoch A, Ravier F, Pasquali C, Sanchez J-C, Tissot J-D, Bjellqvist B, Vargas R, Appel RD, Hughes GJ (1992) Human liver protein map: a reference database established by microsequencing and gel comparison. Electrophoresis 13: 992–1001

Huggett AC, Ellis PA, Ford CP, Hampton LL, Rimoldi D, Thorgeirsson SS (1991) Development of resistance to the growth inhibitory effects the transforming growth factor beta-1 during the spontaneous transformation of rat liver epithelial cells. Cancer Res 51: 5929–5936

Hunter T (1989) Protein-tyrosine phosphatases: the other side of the coin. Cell 58: 1013–1016

Hunter T (1991) Cooperation between oncogenes. Cell 64: 249–270

Leavitt J, Latter G, Lutomski L, Goldstein D, Burbeck S (1986) Tropomyosin isoform switching in tumorigenic human fibroblasts. Mol Cell Biol 6: 2721–2726

Malek SN, Katumuluwa AI, Pasternack GR (1990) Identification and preliminary characterization of two related proliferation-associated nuclear phosphoproteins. J Biol Chem 265: 13400–13409

Matsudaira PJ (1987) Sequence from picomole quantities of proteins electroblotted onto polyvinylidene difluoride membranes. J Biol Chem 262: 10035–10036

Matsumura F, Yamashiro-Matsumura S (1985) Purification and characterization of multiple isoforms of tropomyosin from rat cultured cells. J Biol Chem 260: 13851–13859

McMahon JB, Richards WL, del Campo AA, Song M-K, Thorgeirsson SS (1986) Differential effects of transforming growth factor β on the proliferation of normal and malignant rat liver epithelial cells in culture. Cancer Res 46: 4665–4671

Menzel A, Unteregger G (1989) Two-dimensional electrophoretic analysis of nuclear proteins from human tumors. Electrophoresis 10: 554–562

Nalty TJ, Taylor CW, Yeoman LC (1988) Variations in cytosolic protein expression between human colon tumors that differ with regard to differentiation class. Clin Chem 34: 71–75

Narayan RK, Heydorn WE, Creed GJ, Jacobowitz DM (1986) Protein patterns in various malignant human brains tumors by two-dimensional gel electrophoresis. Cancer Res 46: 4685–4694

O'Farrell PH (1975) High resolution two-dimensional gel electrophoresis of proteins. J Biol Chem 250: 4007–4021

Ogata S, Ueda R, Lloyd KO (1987) Comparison of [3H] glucosamine-labeled glycoproteins from human renal cancer and normal epithelial cell cultures by two-dimensional polyacrylamide gel electrophoresis. Proc Natl Acad Sci USA 78: 770–774

Okuzawa K, Franzen B, Lindholm J, Linder S, Hirano T, Bergman T, Ebihara Y, Kato H, Auer G (1994) Characterization of gene expression in clinical lung cancer by two-dimensional polyacrylamide gel electrophoresis. Electrophoresis 15: 382–390

Pearson WR, Lipman DJ (1988) Improved tools for biological sequence comparison. Proc Natl Acad Sci USA 85: 2444–2448

Pitot HC (1979) Biological and enzymic events in chemical carcinogenesis. Annu Rev Med 30: 25–39

Prasad GL, Fuldner RA, Cooper HL (1993) Expression of transduced tropomyosin cDNA suppresses neoplastic growth of cell transformed by the ras oncogene. Proc Natl Acad Sci USA 90: 7039–7043

Rasmussen HH, van Damme J, Puype M, Gesser B, Celis JE, Vandekerckhove J (1992) Microsequence of 145 proteins recorded in the two-dimensional gel protein database of normal human epidermal keratinocytes. Electrophoresis 13: 960–969

Ruoslahti E, Oh E, Jalanko H (1980) Differences in the nuclear proteins of normal and malignant liver cells. Oncodev Biol Med 1: 17–26

Sell S, Hunt JM, Knoll BJ, Dunsford HA (1987) Cellular events during hepatocarcinogenesis in rats and the questions of premalignancy. Adv Cancer Res 48: 37–111

Stastny J, Prasad R, Fosslien E (1984) Tissue proteins in breast cancer, as studied by the use of two-dimensional electrophoresis. Clin Chem 30: 1914–1918

Takami H, Busch FN, Morris HP, Busch H (1979) Comparison of salt-extractable nuclear proteins of regenerating liver, fetal liver, and Morris hepatomas 9618 and 3924 A. Cancer Res 39: 2096–2105

Tracy RP, Wold LE, Currie RM, Young DS (1982) Patterns for normal colon mucosa and colon adenocarcinoma compared by two-dimensional gel electrophoresis. Clin Chem 28: 915–919

Tsao M-S, Grisham JM (1987) Hepatocarcinomas, cholangiocarcinomas, and hepatoblastomas produced by chemically transformed rat liver epithelial cells: a light- and electron-microscopic analysis. Am J Pathol 127: 168–181

Ullrich A, Schlessinger J (1990) Signal transduction by receptors with tyrosine kinase activity. Cell 61: 203–212

Weinberg RA (1989) Oncogenes, antioncogenes, and the molecular basis of multistep carcinogenesis. Cancer Res 49: 3713–3721

Wirth PJ (1994) Two-dimensional polyacrylamide gel electrophoresis in experimental hepatocarcinogenesis studies. Electrophoresis 15: 358–371

Wirth PJ, Egilsson V, Gudnason V, Ingvarsson S, Thorgeirsson SS (1987) Specific polypeptide differences in normal versus malignant human breast tissues by two-dimensional electrophoresis. Breast Cancer Res Treat 10: 177–189

Wirth PJ, Luo L-di, Fujimoto Y, Bisgaard H-C, Olson AD (1991) The rat liver epithelial (RLE) cell protein database. Electrophoresis 12: 931–954

Wirth PJ, Luo L-di, Fujimoto Y, Bisgaard HC (1992) Two-dimensional electrophoretic analysis of transformation-sensitive polypeptides during chemically, spontaneously, and oncogene-induced transformation of rat liver epithelial cells. Electrophoresis 13: 305–320

Wirth PJ, Luo L-di, Benjamin T, Hoang TN, Olson AD, Parmelee DC (1993) The rat liver epithelial (RLE) cell nuclear protein database. Electrophoresis 14: 1199–1215

Wu B, Spohn WH, Busch H (1979) Two-dimensional gel electrophoresis of cytosolic phosphoproteins of Novikoff hepatoma and regenerating liver. Cancer Res 39: 116–122

Mechanisms Leading to the Expression of Recessive Alleles: The Use of Polymorphic Microsatellites and Whole-Chromosome Painting Probes to Analyze Mouse Tumors, Mutants, and Micronuclei

W.J. Caspary[1], H. Stopper[2], J.C. Hozier[3], M.C. Liechty[3], and L.M. Davis[3]

[1]Laboratory of Environmental Carcinogenesis and Mutagenesis, National Institutes of Health, Research Triangle Park, NC 27709, USA
[2]Department of Toxicology, University of Würzburg, 97078 Würzburg, Germany
[3]Applied Genetics Laboratories, 1335 Gateway Drive, Suite 2001, Melbourne, FL 32901, USA

Introduction

Regulatory agencies have the responsibility for assessing the potential risks that chemicals pose to humans. For risk assessment, these agencies evaluate data from in vitro genotoxicity assays (e.g., mutation induction using cells in culture) and from in vivo assays (e.g., micronucleus induction in bone marrow or carcinogenicity testing in rodents). The goal is to develop sensitive models that predict carcinogenic potential in susceptible human populations. Until recently, it was impossible to evaluate whether the genetic events induced by test compounds in the model systems were the same as the genetic events contributing to human cancers. However, new techniques make it possible to evaluate these events in both human and model systems and should aid in evaluating the appropriateness of any particular assay in predicting the disease in humans.

Cancer–a Genetic Disease?

"The unlimited tendency to rapid proliferation in malignant tumor cells [could result] from a permanent predominance of the chromosomes that promote division...Another possibility to explain cancer is the preference of definite chromosomes which inhibit division...Cells of tumors with unlimited growth would arise if those "inhibiting chromosomes" were eliminated...Because each kind of chromosome is represented twice in the normal cell, the depression of only one of these two might pass unnoticed..." (Boveri 1914).

Carcinogenesis is genetically complex, involving multiple lesions in either or both of two families of genes, the oncogenes and/or the tumor suppressor genes. Mutations in oncogenes are expressed dominantly while tumor

Recent Results in Cancer Research, Vol. 143

suppressor gene mutations are expressed recessively; consequently, inactivation of both tumor suppressor alleles is required for the tumorigenic phenotype.

The activation of protooncogenes to oncogenes may disrupt normal cellular functions and lead to neoplastic growth (Bishop 1987). The transforming ability of oncogenes has been associated with overexpression of the protooncogene product or with disruptions of the gene itself that result in a modification of the activity of the oncogene product. These disruptions include point mutations, translocations, or partial deletions.

Tumor suppressor genes are also normal cellular genes. They appear to provide negative signals for cell proliferation, and the activity of both alleles must be lost or significantly impaired for cells to become neoplastic (Barrett and Wiseman 1987). One chromosomal mechanism involved in the loss of tumor suppressor gene function is deletion of either a part or all of a chromosome carrying the normal allele. Whole chromosome loss followed by duplication of the chromosome carrying a mutant allele results in homozygosity of the mutant tumor suppressor locus. Alternatively, if there is no duplication of the remaining chromosome, the mutant tumor suppressor allele will be hemizygous. Another chromosomal mechanism is mitotic recombination after the S phase of the cell cycle between nonsister chromatids of a homologous chromosome pair. The chromatids with the two normal alleles can segregate to one daughter cell and the pair with the mutant alleles to the other daughter cell. If the normal growth control function of the tumor suppressor gene products is lost in the second daughter cell, it may have a growth advantage over the normal cells and this could be a step towards tumor formation.

The first study on the loss of a human tumor suppressor gene was for the retinoblastoma locus at 13q14 (Knudson 1985). The suspicion that there might be a gene at this locus involved in the etiology of cancer came from many cytogenetic studies focusing on this region. Examination of chromosomes from other human tumors such as Wilm's tumor (chromosome 11), acoustic neuroma (chromosome 22), and carcinoma of the lung (chromosome 3) has also revealed cytogenetically visible deletions. Taken together, genetic modifications in the evolving cancer cell include point mutations, gene deletions, gene amplifications, gene rearrangements, recombination, numerical chromosome changes, and modifications in DNA methylation patterns (for reviews see, for example, Hollstein et al. 1991; Weinberg 1991; and Stanbridge 1992).

In vitro and in vivo models have been used to identify chemicals that can induce these lesions. In this paper, we will discuss two more recent techniques that provide additional information on the chromosomal events taking place in the in vitro and in vivo assays. These techniques involve analyses of loss of heterozygosity by restriction fragment length polymorphism (RFLP) or polymerase chain reaction (PCR) analysis and chromosomal aberrations by whole chromosome painting. We present examples applying these techniques in searching for tumor suppressor genes in rodents, in identifying mutagenic lesions in cells in culture, and in identifying chromosomes in micronuclei in vitro. We also show how the two techniques, used together, can assess the role of recombination in mechanisms leading to mutation and demonstrate that mutations in heterozygous cell lines mimic the types of lesions leading to neoplasia.

Loss of Heterozygosity

Cavenee and coworkers applied a technique called RFLP analysis to look for heterozygous DNA segments that become homozygous or hemizygous in various tumors (Cavenee et al. 1983, 1988). This technique is based on variations in the lengths of DNA restriction fragments between homologous chromosomes. The different sizes of DNA can be detected with Southern blots using recombinant DNA probes that are homologous to unique regions in the genome. In tumor tissue that has become homozygous or hemizygous for the mutant allele when previously heterozygous, one of the restriction fragments will be lost on Southern blotting – hence the term "loss of heterozygosity" (LOH). Cavenee and coworkers showed LOH of specific chromosome regions in many kinds of tumors, presumably the result of interstitial deletion, chromosome loss, and duplication or somatic recombination. Nonrandom LOH in a series of tumors suggests that a tumor suppressor gene may be involved in the etiology of that type of tumor.

Although the RFLP technique has many advantages over cytogenetic approaches in searching for tumor suppressor genes, it requires substantial amounts of DNA, is tedious, and requires the preparation of a probe at the site of the polymorphism. More recently, PCR-based techniques for detecting LOH have become popular. Short repetitive stretches of DNA composed of nucleotide repeat sequences, such as $(CA)_n$, punctuate the mammalian genome (Nakamura et al. 1987; Tautz 1989; Weber et al. 1989). They are useful in genetic research because the lengths of these microsatellite repeats in the two chromosomes often differ.

These simple sequence repeats lend themselves well to analysis by PCR if there are identifiable unique primer sets flanking the repeat (Fig. 1). If the microsatellite at a given locus is polymorphic and the PCR products are analyzed electrophoretically, two bands will be seen on the gel (Figs. 2, 3). Generally, these PCR products are 100–200 base pairs in length.

If, in a tumor, one repeat allele is missing because of a deletion or recombination event, then one of the two bands is lost (Fig. 3). Multiple losses of heterozygosity spanning an entire chromosome imply either the loss of the whole chromosome or a somatic recombination event spanning most or all of the chromosome. Smaller and smaller regions of LOH centered at one or two loci in a series of tumors would suggest the location of a putative tumor suppressor gene. Techniques for positional cloning would then be used to begin the search for the gene itself. These techniques have been the subjects of

Homologous
chromosomes
PCR primers
PCR product
Unique sequence
Simple sequence repeat

Fig. 1.

MECHANISM
OF LOSS
GENOTYPE
Point mutation
No LOH
Deletion
Gene
Conversion
Mitotic
Recombination
Chromosome loss
& duplication
Chromosome
loss
Homologous
chromosomes

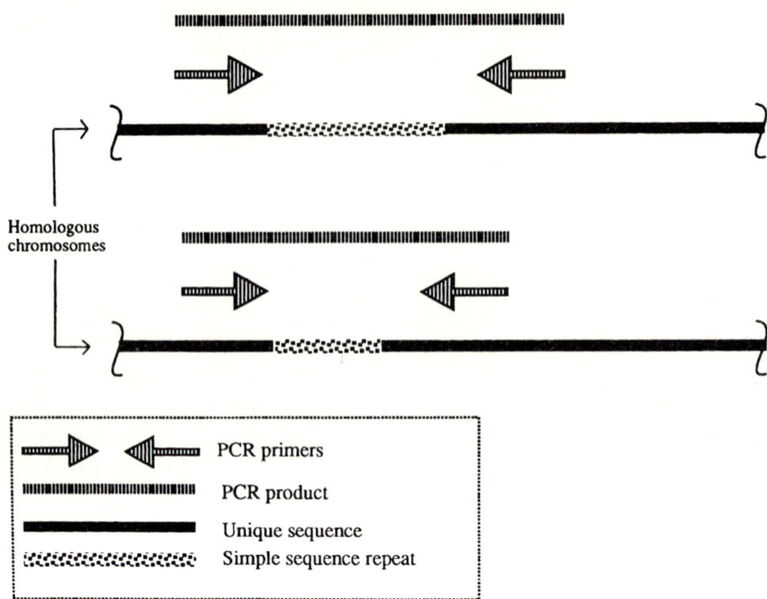

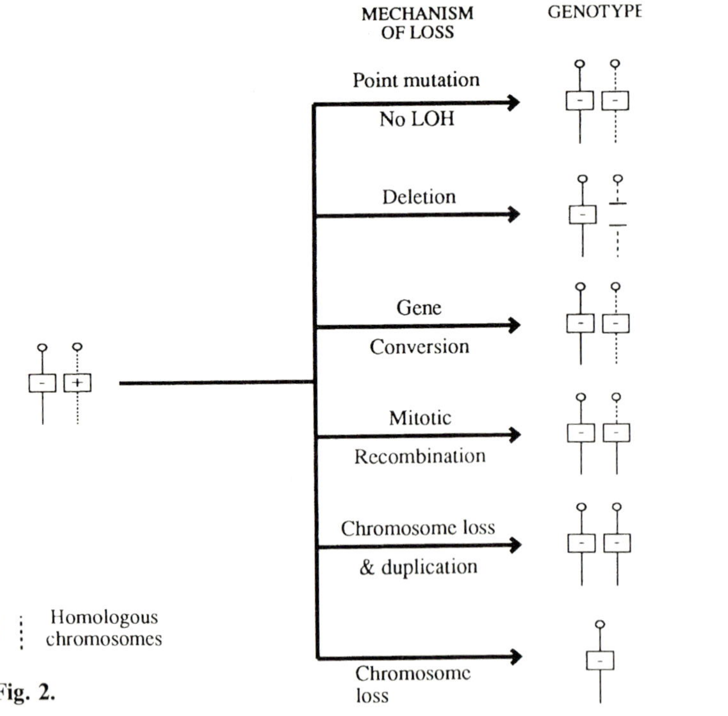

Fig. 2.

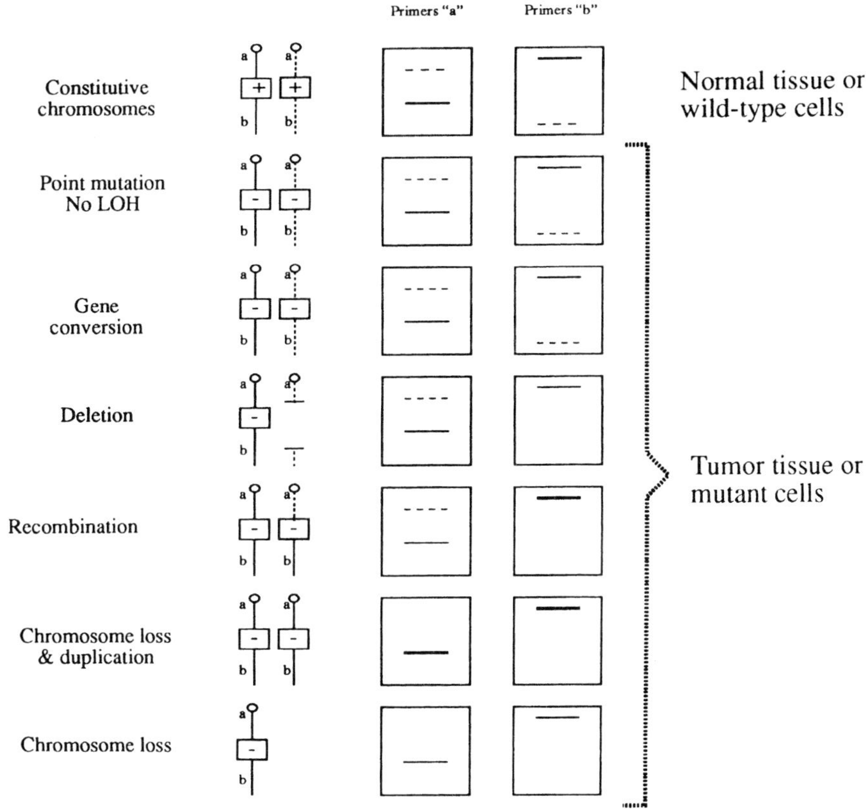

Bands from probing the homologous chromosomes.

Fig. 3. DNA gel of PCR products. This schematic diagram illustrates the number and intensity of the bands revealed upon electrophoresis. Although loss of one chromosome followed by duplication will result in one band of twice the expected intensity, normally such a doubling of intensity cannot be easily detected. Point mutations within and deletions outside the sequences bounded by the primers are not detectable using this technique

Fig. 1. Polymerase chain reaction (PCR) amplification of heteromorphic microsatellite repeats. Repeats that have been previously mapped to a particular locus in the genome are amplified using unique sequence primer pairs that hybridize to both chromosomes at sites flanking the microsatellite repeat sequence. Since the sizes of the two microsatellites are different, two bands will be visible upon electrophoresis. If one of the sites is missing, there will be only one band

Fig. 2. Chromosomal mechanisms leading to loss of heterozygosity. This schematic diagram illustrates the types of chromosomal lesions that can result in loss of heterozygosity (LOH). These lesions include chromosome loss with or without duplication, recombination, gene conversion, and deletions that encompass the microsatellite region. Point mutations or deletions outside the region bounded by the primers will not be detected as losses

numerous review (Collins 1995) and research articles (Ahn et al. 1995) and are beyond the scope of this chapter.

LOH in Mouse Tumors to Identify Tumor Suppressor Genes

There is considerable variation between inbred strains of mice in the lengths of these microsatellite repeats, making them an abundant source of genetically useful polymorphism in hybrid animals. More than 5000 of these simple sequence repeats have been described for the mouse (Dietrich et al. 1992a,b; Hearne et al. 1991; Love et al. 1990; Miller 1992; Montagutelli et al. 1991).

The B6C3F1 mouse, which is used in many countries to gauge the carcinogenic hazard posed by chemicals to humans (Tennant et al. 1987), is a cross between female C57BL/6J and male C3H/HeJ inbred strains of mice (Fig. 4). An assessment of the accuracy of this rodent model to mimic human neoplasia requires an evaluation of the similarities and differences between the genetics of liver tumors in this mouse and in the human. Because the B6C3F1 mouse is heterozygous at many loci, tumors in these mice present a rich opportunity to examine the role of tumor suppressor gene inactivation in

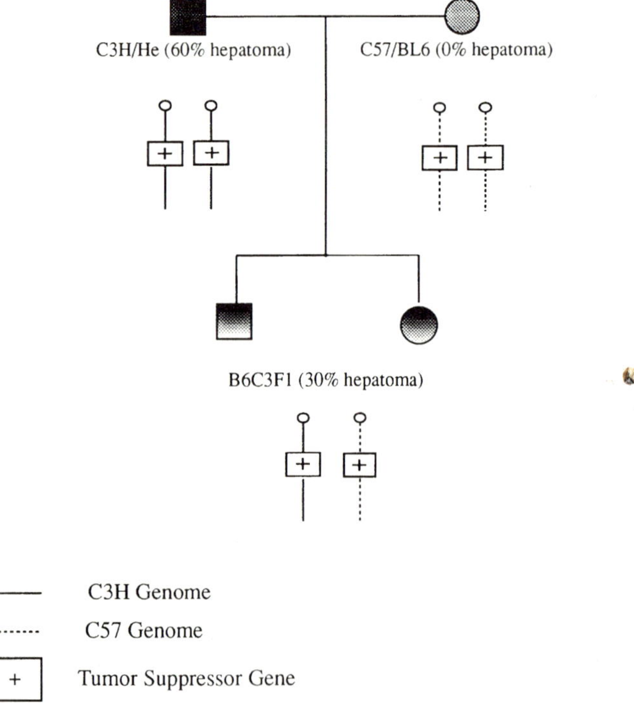

Fig. 4. B6C3F1 mouse. The B6C3F1 mouse is an F1 cross between the C3H/He male and the C57/BL6 female

chemically induced and spontaneous tumors. In addition, the parental origin of lost alleles in these tumors can be easily identified.

To investigate LOH in these liver tumors, DNA from 144 tumors was PCR-amplified at 78 loci randomly distributed throughout the genome (Davis et al. 1994). In this early "global" scan of the tumors, we found significant losses on chromosomes 2, 5, 8 and 18. The global scan also revealed several unexpected features of these liver tumors, including a very low incidence of whole chromosome loss as a significant event. The losses we identified spanned very small segments of specific chromosomes, rather than whole chromosomes. In addition, there was not a high incidence of insignificant "background" loss of chromosomal material. We later focused on those regions of the genome that were implicated by the preliminary scan, and on regions of the genome where the mouse homologs of human tumor suppressor genes had been mapped or would be expected to map. The data from mouse chromosome 18 illustrate these points.

Initially, the tumors were analyzed at two polymorphic loci on chromosome 18 (Fig. 5), and five tumors that lost both loci were identified (Davis et al. 1994). At the time, the available genetic mapping data placed both markers in the approximate middle of the chromosome, so small, centrally located deletions could not be distinguished from losses of the whole chromosome. We decided to investigate the LOH in more detail to locate the region of LOH more accurately. In addition, mouse chromosome 18 harbors three tumor suppressor genes that are known to be involved in human colon cancers: Apc, Mcc, and Dcc. Although there had been no indication that any of these three genes would be involved in human or mouse liver tumors, analysis with a higher density of markers might provide the first indication for involvement of one of these three genes.

We therefore analyzed the set of tumors at 11 additional loci distributed throughout the chromosome but with a concentration in the region around the Apc and Mcc gene. Loci close to Apc or Dcc did not undergo LOH, eliminating the possibility of loss of either of those two genes in these tumors. The pattern of LOH in this higher density analysis clearly defined a small region of LOH of four loci centered on the genetic interval that includes Mcc. However, the precise linear relationship of these five loci within the interval is unknown. Nineteen tumors underwent LOH of at least one of four central loci that all map to a region within 1 cM of Mcc. Because of the close proximity of the Mcc gene and the region of LOH, the possibility that Mcc might be involved in the etiology of these tumors was considered. However, there are other observations suggesting that these data may not represent a simple case of Mcc gene involvement.

First, a recent comprehensive report (Curtis et al. 1994) described a study of 80 human colon carcinomas in which LOH at both Apc and Mcc was detected in 21 cases. These genes map very close to each other on human chromosome 5 at band 5q21, in a region that is homologous to the region of mouse chromosome 18 where we are seeing LOH. All 21 tumors underwent LOH at both Apc and Mcc but there was no evidence for mutation in the Mcc gene in any of the tumors. The authors suggest that LOH of Mcc in these tumors may be more a consequence of its proximity to Apc than its involvement in tumorigenesis. In addition, there have been no reports of mutations in the Mcc gene in any tumors other than six tumors in the original publications of the gene (Kinzler et al. 1991; Nishisho et al. 1991), thus casting doubt on the role of Mcc as a tumor suppressor gene.

Second, there are two recent reports of LOH in human hepatocellular carcinoma (HCC) in which noncirrhotic HCC (but not cirrhotic HCC) undergoes LOH at a locus on the long arm of chromosome 5 mapping to a locus much more distal than the Apc-Mcc locus, at 5q31 (Ding et al. 1991). This analysis included 6 out of 6 noncirrhotic HCC that are informative at both Apc and Mcc that do not undergo LOH at either Apc or Mcc but do undergo LOH at the 5q31 locus (Ding et al. 1993). This information suggests there is another tumor suppressor gene on human chromosome 5q31, and this region of human 5q is homologous to the region where the mouse liver tumors are undergoing LOH. Because Mcc is beginning to appear not to be a tumor suppressor gene, and because the more recently described putative tumor suppressor gene at 5q31 is involved in human hepatocellular carcinomas, it is possible that the mouse homolog of the human 5q31 gene may be involved in these mouse liver tumors. Thus, by expanding our LOH analysis from 2 loci to 13 loci, we were able to increase our panel of tumors with LOH from 5 to 19, we were able to locate the region of significant LOH to a 1-cM interval, and we were able to eliminate the possibility that either Apc or Dcc were involved in these tumors.

Chromosome Painting Probes

Before the availability of LOH as a means to investigate chromosomal aberrations, the only available technique was cytogenetic examination. This is limited to identification of events such as translocations or large interstitial or terminal deletions. Cytogenetic examination also frequently requires tumor cells to be grown in culture, which can be difficult. It also requires expertise in chromosome identification.

Loss of heterozygosity analysis also has limitations. For example, whether the analysis is by PCR amplification of microsatellites or by Southern blotting, chromosomal material translocated to another chromosome will appear normal upon LOH analysis if the translocation breakpoint does not fall directly within the segment under examination. If these translocated sequences were small, they might not be detected by standard cytogenetic banding techniques either. Similarly, LOH analysis will not detect point mutations and cannot distinguish between deletions and recombination events.

Chromosome painting probes used in conjunction with LOH analysis could overcome some of these difficulties. Chromosome painting probes are DNA sequences that uniquely hybridize to a particular region of the genome (e.g., a chromosome or segment of a chromosome). These sequences are labeled with biotin or digoxigenin, hybridized to metaphase chromosome spreads and/or interphase nuclei and detected immunocytochemically. These probes produce specifically painted fluorescent chromosomes against a background of nonhomologous unpainted chromosomes counterstained for visibility.

Painting probes for the human chromosomes have been prepared by isolating chromosomal material from monochromosomal somatic cell hybrids (Ledbetter et al. 1990) or from human cells (Cremer et al. 1988; Lichter et al. 1988a,b). Although appropriate for human chromosomes, this technique is not readily applicable to production of mouse probes because monochromosomal hybrids for the mouse are generally not available and normal mouse chromosomes cannot be sorted because of the similar sizes of many of the chromosomes.

Tucker and coworkers prepared probes for mouse chromosomes by flow-sorting Robertsonian translocations followed by degenerate oligonucleotide-primed PCR amplification (Breneman et al. 1993). These probes paint two different chromosomes simultaneously. Although there have been two reports in which flow-sorting has been fortuitously used to prepare mouse chromosome probes (Miyashita et al. 1994; Weier et al. 1994), this approach cannot be expected to be a routine method. Another potential problem with flow-sorted material is that it can contain DNA from regions of the genome other than the one of interest (Gray et al. 1987; Telenius et al. 1993). This can complicate the interpretation of results. In addition, this technique limits the probes to those that paint whole or translocated chromosomes and it is not possible to produce subchromosomal painting probes.

We have used chromosome microdissection as a means to prepare whole-chromosome painting probes, chromosome band-specific painting probes, centromere painting probes, and even multichromosome painting probes (Liechty et al. 1995b). Chromosomes or subchromosomal segments can be microdissected directly from metaphase spreads prepared by using standard cytogenetic techniques. We use a micromanipulator controlled by a stepper motor with coarse and fine controls, mounted on an inverted microscope with a rotating stage, to position a heat-drawn glass needle relative to the chromosome of interest to remove the chromosome from the slide. The dissected chromosomes are PCR-amplified using a degenerate oligonucleotide primer. The primer has a six-base degeneracy in the central region, with specific sequences at the 3′ and 5′ termini (Telenius et al. 1993; Zhang et al. 1993). The PCR is in two stages: The first stage consists of eight cycles at reduced annealing and extension temperatures to encourage annealing between the primer sequence and the chromosomal DNA at many sites, including many mismatches. These first eight cycles use Sequenase for the extension reaction. The second stage consists of 25 additional cycles under standard PCR cycling conditions using Amplitaq polymerase. This approach has been used to prepare paints for human chromosomes (Guan et al. 1993, 1994; Meltzer et al.

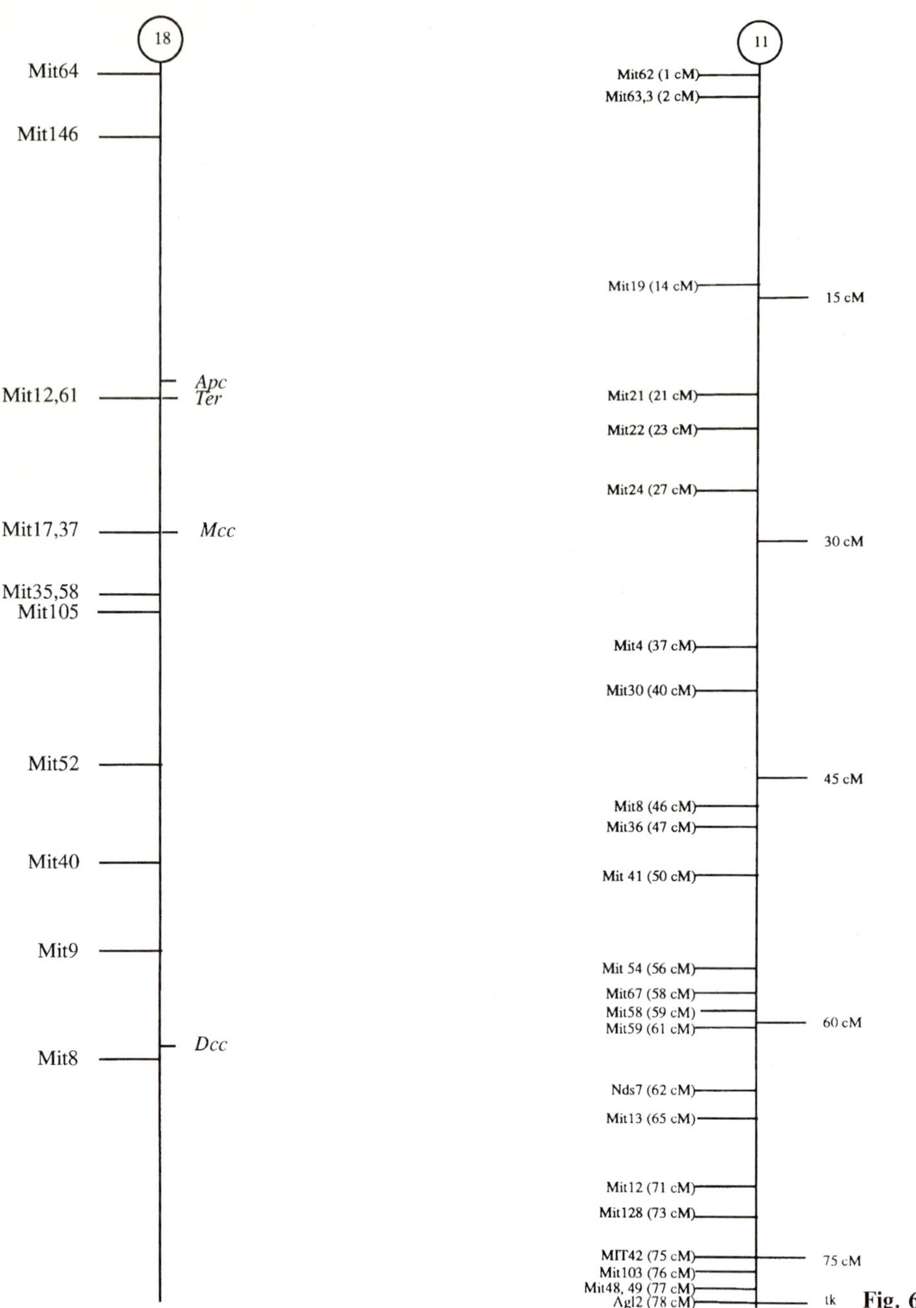

Fig. 5. Mouse chromosome 18. The diagram shows the locations of the polymorphic microsatellites that we used in our examination of chromosome 18

Fig. 6. Mouse chromosome 11. The diagram shows locations of the 28 chromosome 11 polymorphic loci in mouse lymphoma cells. The polymorphic locus Ag12 is located in the region between exons 6 and 7 within the tk gene

1992; Zhang et al. 1993). We have used it to prepare a whole-chromosome painting probe for mouse chromosome 11 by dissecting ten copies of that chromosome from metaphase spreads prepared from an outbred mouse (Liechty et al. 1995b). This painting probe and others are available from Clontech Laboratories, Palo Alto, CA, USA (Clontech 1995). The painting probes were hybridized to the chromosomes and revealed by fluorescence using standard fluorescence in situ hybridization techniques (Hozier et al. 1994).

Application of LOH and Chromosome Paints to Identify Mutagenic Lesions

Genetic, epidemiological, molecular, and cytogenetic data suggest that the expression of multiple, independent recessive genes by aberrant mitotic lesions plays a major role in carcinogenesis. These lesions include intragenic mutations as well as chromosomal lesions, such as nondisjunction, mitotic recombination, and deletion. An appropriate in vitro model for studying carcinogenesis should be responsive to all of these lesions. Many studies on mutagenesis have targeted hemizygous loci (one active allele/no homologous allele) where the missing region on the nonactive chromosome is usually extensive. Such loci may not be useful for studying chromosomal mechanisms because large lesions that incorporate essential genes which are already missing on the inactive homologous chromosome may be lethal to the cell. Cells that are heterozygous at the selectable gene (one active and one inactive allele) may survive because of the presence of the essential allele on the homologous chromosome. The L5178Y mouse cell line, clone 3.7.2C (Clive et al. 1972), is heterozygous at the tk locus (Liechty et al. 1993). Both chemical and physical agents can induce trifluorothymidine (TFT) resistance in this cell line (Caspary et al. 1988a,b; Clive et al. 1979) by producing the homozygote with both tk alleles made inactive.

L5178Y mouse mutants display a wide range of genetic lesions (Blazak et al. 1986a, 1989; Clive et al. 1990, 1991; Hozier et al. 1985, 1991; Liechty et al. 1993). All the lesions so far identified have also been implicated in tumorigenesis (Applegate et al. 1990; Hozier et al. 1992). Our objective in applying LOH and FISH analysis to mutants derived from L5178Y mouse cells is to determine whether types of lesions leading to mutation in this cell line mimic those leading to tumorigenesis.

Although L5178Y mouse cells were derived from an inbred mouse strain and would therefore be expected to be homozygous at all microsatellite loci, the cell line has been in cell culture for many generations and microsatellite sequences are highly mutable (Aaltonen et al. 1993; Tautz 1989; Thibodeau et al. 1993). We have identified informative microsatellites that span the entire chromosome 11 and are heteromorphic in the L5178Y mouse cell line (Liechty et al. 1994). These polymorphic microsatellites include a complex CA repeat within one of the introns of the tk gene (Liechty et al. 1995a).

We analyzed 122 spontaneous TFT-resistant colonies derived from L5178Y mouse cells at 28 heteromorphic microsatellites to assess the types of genomic alterations in these mutants (Fig. 6). These heteromorphic loci span chromosome 11 from 1 centiMorgan (cM) distal to the centromere to 78 cM distal to the centromere at the tk gene. We have no microsatellite heteromorphism for the centromeric region or the region distal to the tk gene. Thus, our analysis does not include these two regions. When analyzed at the heteromorphic locus within the tk gene using the primer set Ag12 (Liechty et al. 1995a), 36 of the mutants had two bands indicating that both tk alleles were present. These 36 mutant colonies harbor either intragenic mutations or deletions distal to the tk gene.

Of the remaining 86 mutant colonies, 85 lost heterozygosity at the polymorphic microsatellite within the tk gene and revealed LOH at at least one other locus. Of the 122 mutants, 23 lost all polymorphic loci, probably originated by loss of the entire tk^+ chromosome or a large part of it. Sixty-three colonies underwent LOH of subchromosomal regions including the tk gene, with breakpoints apparently spanning the entire chromosome. In every case of LOH, the lost microsatellite sequence alleles resided on the tk^+ chromosome, which would be expected if this loss were etiologically related to the mutant phenotype.

The results reveal the utility of using LOH to analyze polymorphic microsatellite repeats to learn the extent of the lesions in mutant cells. The main advantages of this approach compared to cytogenetic techniques are that the skills necessary for its performance and interpretation are common and the necessary reagents are readily available, while the resolution possible is at least as good as for cytogenetic techniques. LOH analysis is not a perfect substitute for cytogenetic analysis because there is poor correlation between the genetic and physical maps in mouse and because LOH analysis alone cannot distinguish between a deletion and a recombination, whereas cytogenetic analysis can.

We can gain even more information concerning the nature of the lesions by coupling LOH analysis with cytogenetic techniques, and since chromosome paints are available, such analyses are accessible to many laboratories lacking chromosome recognition skills. To illustrate this, we painted chromosome 11 from some of these same mutants. This analysis depends on the previous observation that the two centromeres from chromosomes 11 are heteromorphic with the tk^+ centromere being the larger of the two (Blazak et al. 1986a; Hozier et al. 1982). We examined ten to 20 metaphase spreads or banded preparations to assess the relative centromeric sizes (data not shown). The following four mutants are examples from the 122 spontaneous mutants we isolated.

Mutant 42b (Fig. 7A) lost microsatellites from the tk^+ chromosome at all loci examined, suggesting the loss of all or most of the chromosome. Chromosome painting revealed two whole chromosomes 11. Both chromosome painting data and banded chromosome data revealed two tk^-

centromeres. This mutant, therefore, lost the tk$^+$ chromosome and duplicated the tk$^-$ chromosome. The two chromosomes are of unequal length, suggesting that one of the chromosomes lost or gained some chromatin material.

Mutant 41b (Fig. 7B) also lost microsatellite alleles from the tk$^+$ chromosome at all loci examined. This again suggested loss of the whole chromosome or a large part of it. However, when hybridized with the chromosome 11 painting probe, we also saw two apparently normal chromosomes 11. Here the sizes of the two centromeres from mutant 41b are different. When we consider the LOH, paint, and centromere size data together, it appears that an extensive recombination occurred between the chromosomes that replaced most of the tk$^+$ chromosome sequences with tk$^-$ chromosome sequences, preserving the centromeres.

Mutant 142a (Fig. 7C) lost microsatellite alleles between the tk$^+$ allele and D11Nds7, inclusive, suggesting a terminal deletion. When painted, the two chromosomes 11 possess differing centromere sizes. Our interpretation is that sequences from the tk$^-$ chromosome replaced the lost 16 cM of sequence on the tk$^+$ chromosome, probably by recombination. However, unlike mutant 41b where recombination did not alter the size of the chromosome, the tk$^+$ chromosome is longer than the tk$^-$ chromosome, suggesting that the recombination that occurred was an unequal crossover event.

The tk$^+$ chromosome from mutant 3b (Fig. 7D) lost microsatellite alleles between the tk$^+$ allele and D11Mit21, suggesting a large deletion. Painting shows that the tk$^+$ chromosome has some non-11 material translocated to it, but the 11 portion is of apparently normal length, again suggesting a recombination rather than a deletion. However, it is not possible to determine if the mutation in the tk gene arose as a result of the translocation or the recombination. In this particular mutant, the tk$^-$ chromosome has been duplicated, but this is probably not relevant to mutant formation.

The mutants shown here are just four of the spontaneous mutants that were isolated using the in situ procedure. Our data show that this cell system detects mutations due to mitotic recombination, nondisjunction and reduplication, and translocations and that because of the unequal sizes of the two centromeres, we are able to distinguish conclusively between recombination and nondisjunction. The data support the suggestions by others (Gille et al. 1994; Hozier et al. 1992; Li et al. 1992; Little 1989; Smith et al. 1993; Xia et al. 1994; Zhu et al. 1993) that recombination plays a major role in mutation in mammalian cells and that heterozygous loci are able to detect chromosomal lesions that are known to be involved in tumorigenesis.

Application of Chromosome Paints to Micronucleus Analysis

Our interests lie in mechanisms leading to LOH and the expression of recessive genes. One possible mechanism for whole or partial chromosome loss involves micronucleus induction. Micronuclei consist of chromatin material en-

A Mutant 42b
11-
11-
B Mutant 41b
62
tk
11-
11+
C Mutant 142a
Nds7
tk
11-
11+
D Mutant 3b
21
tk
11-
11-
11+

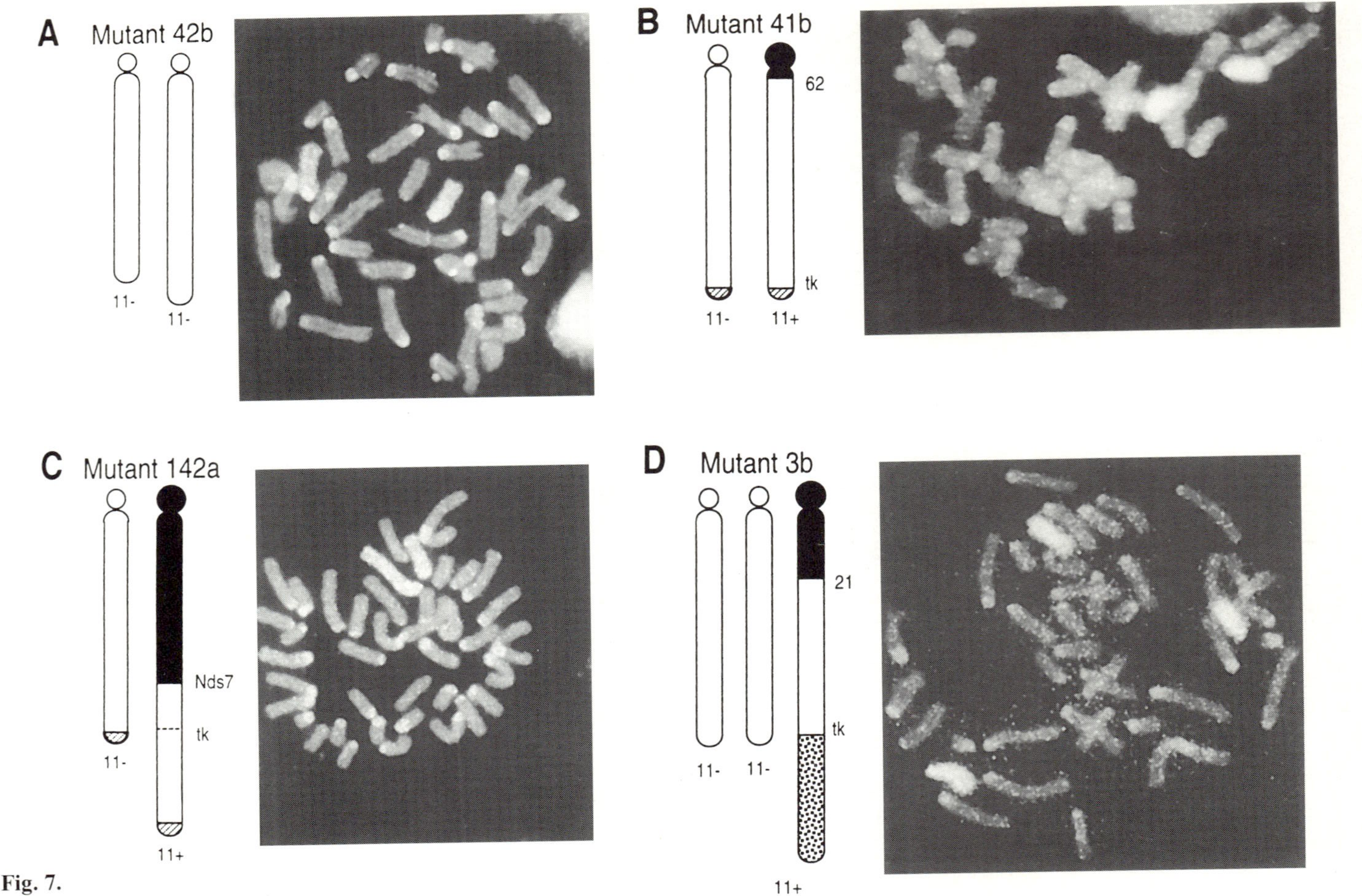

Fig. 7.

capsulated within a membrane and are found in the cytoplasm of cells. Some micronuclei contain whole chromosomes and others contain chromosome fragments. The two types of micronuclei can usually be distinguished from one another by antikinetochore-antibody staining. Unless there is a damaged kinetochore, whole chromosomes stain positively with antikinetochore antibody. Most chromosomal fragments, except those containing the centromere, do not stain with antikinetochore antibody.

Micronucleus formation is a widely used toxicological endpoint in vivo (mouse bone marrow assay; Gudi et al. 1992) and in vitro (short-term tests in cultured cells; Combes et al. 1995; Fritzenschaf et al. 1993; Matsuoka et al. 1993), as well as in the biomonitoring of human populations (Fenech 1993). Little is known about the fate of the chromosome or chromosomal fragment in a micronucleus. Micronucleus formation may in certain cases lead to cell death. It is relevant to ask whether the use of this assay in toxicity testing is appropriate because the biological consequences of those cells that survive micronucleus induction are not known. One possibility is that the micronucleus is eventually lost after a few cell divisions. We are investigating the possibility that micronucleus induction is an early step towards chromosome loss or fragmentation (Stopper et al. 1994).

When mutation is measured at the tk locus, a number of investigators have shown that, with the resolution available with the light microscope, the L5178Y mouse lymphoma cell line is capable of detecting the same kinds of lesions that are known to be involved in tumorigenesis (Applegate et al. 1990), including cytogenetically detectable chromosome aberrations (Blazak et al. 1986a,b, 1989; Hozier et al. 1981, 1985, 1989). In this chapter we present further evidence verifying this conclusion by subjecting mutants from this heterozygous cell line to molecular analysis. We used a protocol to provide the greatest chance of

◄

Fig. 7A–D. Chromosome paints of four mutants. Four spontaneous mutants from L5178Y mouse lymphoma cells were hybridized with the chromosome 11 paint. The ideograms on the *left* of each picture represent the results from the LOH data and our interpretation of the results of both the LOH and chromosome paint data. The text to the *right* of the chromosome identifies the limits of loss of heterozygosity (LOH). We can distinguish the centromeres from the two chromosomes 11 from each other because of a size heteromorphism, with the tk$^+$ centromere being the larger of the two. Our assessment of the sizes of the centromeres comes from examination of multiple metaphases of these mutants, of which the ones shown here are a representative sample. *White areas*, loci of tk- chromosome 11 origin; *black areas*, loci of tk$^+$ chromosome 11 origin; *diagonally shaded areas*, chromosome 11, not known whether tk$^-$ or tk$^+$; *stippled areas*, non-chromosome 11 material. **A** Mutant 42b shows chromosome loss and duplication and either a loss or gain of sequences in one of the two chromosomes. **B** Mutant 41b represents mutants that are trifluorothymidine (TFT)-resistant because of a large recombination event. **C** Mutant 142a also shows a large recombination event in which the initiation of the recombination did not occur at homologous loci on the two chromosomes. **D** Mutant 3B is trisomic with duplication of the tk$^-$ chromosome and a translocation of non-tk$^+$ chromosomal material onto the distal end of the tk$^+$chromosome

detecting mutants containing whole chromosome losses (Rudd et al. 1990; Spencer and Caspary 1994; Spencer et al. 1994). We have also established that L5178Y mouse cells are suitable for measuring chemically induced micronucleus formation (Stopper et al. 1994). Thus, the L5178Y cell line provides the opportunity to assay both mutation and micronucleus induction in one cell system and to investigate whether micronuclei can lead to LOH, which could result in the expression of recessive genes such as tumor suppressor genes.

In an initial analysis, we compared the fraction of micronuclei and mutations induced when L5178Y cells were treated with one of four aneugens: colcemid, diethylstilbestrol, griseofulvin, and vinblastine (Stopper et al. 1994). All four compounds induced micronuclei, more than 85% of which stained positive for the presence of kinetochores. Although the kinetochore assay detects only the centromeric region and cannot distinguish between centromeric fragments of chromosomes and whole chromosomes, our assumption is that most of these micronuclei contained whole chromosomes. However, these same compounds were unable to induce TFT resistance under three different treatment regimens. We concluded that these compounds, under conditions where they induce primarily kinetochore-positive micronuclei, were not able to induce viable mutations. This suggested that the induction of micronuclei containing whole chromosomes was not an early event leading to phenotypically expressed mutations in these cells.

One explanation may be that micronuclei do not contain chromosome 11, which harbors the selectable gene, at a frequency that would be detectable in a mutation assay. We assumed that the chromosome carrying the functional tk allele, which in the mouse is located in chromosome 11, would be lost via micronucleus formation and loss. In our experiments, we used aneugens at doses that induced approximately 40 or more micronuclei per 2000 cells. There are 40 chromosomes in the mouse. If we assume that whole chromosomes are being sequestered in a micronucleus and then lost with equal probability, then the number of cells that form micronuclei containing the chromosome 11 carrying the functional tk allele should be one per 2000 cells. If each of these cells were to survive and form a $tk^{-/-}$ mutant by loss of the micronucleus, we could expect an induced mutation fraction of 500 mutations per million cells. The spontaneous mutation fractions in our experiments were generally between 100 and 300 mutations per million cells. Thus, if the micronucleated cells survived and divided, the additional induced mutation fraction of 500 mutations per million cells should be detectable. Therefore, we might conclude that cells containing that chromosome in a micronucleus are not viable and thus cannot form a countable colony in the mutation assay. If this were the case L5178Y mouse cells could not measure lesions that involve loss of the whole chromosome 11 with the functional tk allele. An alternative explanation is that the chromosome with the functional tk allele is preferentially inhibited from forming micronuclei.

Little is known about the fate or identity of a chromosome or chromosomal fragment in a micronucleus. Since karyotyping of micronuclei is not possible due to the uncondensed state of the chromatin, in situ hybridization provides the first technique with the potential to determine the identity of chromosomes or chromosome fragments found in a micronucleus. Fluorescent in situ hybridization with whole-chromosome painting probes does not depend on metaphase chromosome structure and may therefore be a successful technique for this purpose. Chromosome-specific centromeric DNA probes are only suitable for this type of analysis if exclusively whole chromosomes are included in micronuclei. The first question that we addressed is whether painting probes can detect chromosomes or chromosomal fragments in micronuclei. In Fig. 8, we demonstrate that it is possible by showing a human chromosome 16 paint of micronuclei from cholchicine-treated human lymphocytes. Therefore, chromosome paints should allow us to assess whether the number of micronuclei containing chromosome 11 is sufficient to produce the mutant numbers required to be observed in the mutation assay. In our studies we are also interested in developing a subchromosomal paint specific for the region around

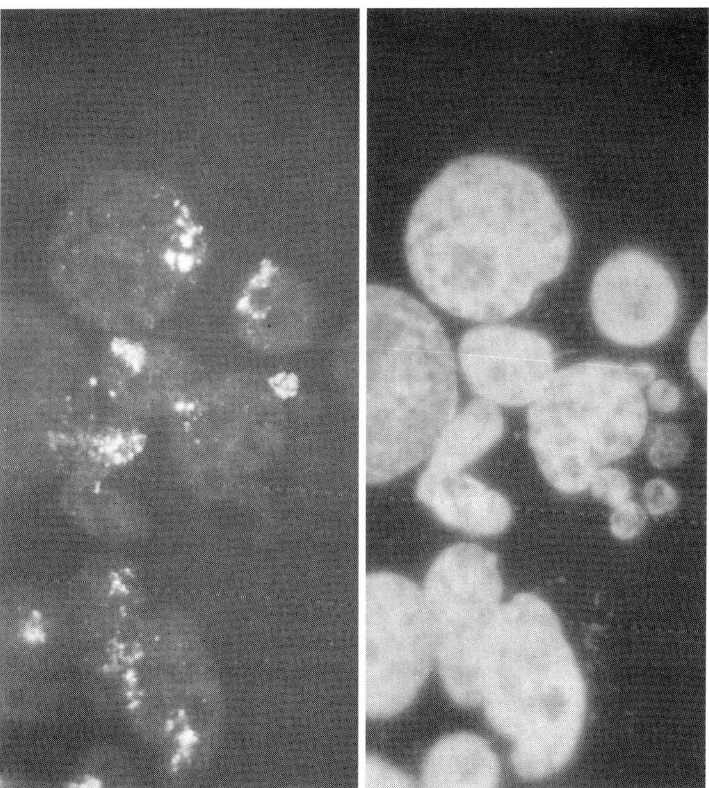

Fig. 8. Painting of chromosome 16 in micronuclei and interphase nuclei of human lymphocytes. *Left*, painting signals and propidium iodide total DNA counterstain; *right*, total DNA staining with bisbenzimid

the tk gene so that we can assess mutation induced by loss of the tk gene and the presence of the tk gene within micronuclei.

Clastogenic agents induce formation of micronuclei containing chromosomal fragments. The genome has fragile sites, although it is not known whether micronuclei harbor chromosomal fragments resulting from breakage at fragile sites. We analyzed micronuclei in the lymphocytes of a carrier of the rare fragile site fra(16)(q22) for the presence of fragments of chromosome 16 using chromosome painting (Fig. 8; Stopper et al. 1995) to test the hypothesis that the induction of the fragile site may lead to breakage of the chromosome at this site and formation of a micronucleus. However, in the cells of the one carrier examined, we observed no increase over the controls (untreated and aneugen-treated cells) in the percentage of signal-positive micronuclei (ranging between 7 and 10%). Thus, we concluded that the distal part of the fragile chromosome 16 was not included in the micronuclei of this patient.

These examples show the role that chromosome painting can play in an understanding of the mechanism of micronucleus formation and the potential role of micronuclei in mutation and neoplastic cell transformation. As such it would provide an underpinning for a role for micronucleus assays in genotoxicity testing and its possible role in the expression of recessive genes.

Acknowledgment. We thank Dr. Julian Preston of the Chemical Industry Institute of Toxicology (CIIT) and Dr. Ronald Cannon of the National Institute of Environmental Health Sciences (NIEHS) for their comments on this manuscript. We also thank Ms. Inge Eckert, Mr. Reinhard Gerhard, Ms. Diane Spencer, Mr. Herbert Crosby, Ms. A. Murthy, Mr. Bryan K. Hall, and Ms. Jane M. Scalzi for their contributions. This study was supported by the NATO (CRG programme).

References

Aaltonen LA, Peltomäki P, Leach FS, Sistonen P, Pylkkänen L, Mecklin J-P, Järvinen H, Powell S, Jen J, Hamilton SR, Petersen GM, Kinzler KW, Vogelstein B, de la Chapelle A (1993) Clues to the pathogenesis of familial colorectal cancer. Science 260: 812–816

Ahn J, Lüdecke H-J, Lindow S, Horton WA, Lee B, Wagner MJ, Horsthemke B, Wells DE (1995) Cloning of the putative tumour suppressor gene for hereditary multiple exostoses (EXT 1), Nature Genet 11: 137–143

Applegate ML, Moore MM, Broder CB, Burrell A, Juhn G, Kasweck KL, Lin PF, Wadhams A, Hozier JC (1990) Molecular dissection of mutations at the heterozygous thymidine kinase locus in mouse lymphoma cells. Proc Natl Acad Sci USA 87: 51–55

Barrett J, Wiseman R (1987) Cellular and molecular mechanisms of multistep carcinogenesis: relevance to carcinogen risk assessment. Environ Health Perspect 76: 65–70

Bishop J (1987) The molecular genetics of cancer. Science 235: 305–311

Blazak W, Stewart B, Galperin I, Allen K, Rudd C, Mitchell A, Caspary W (1986a) Chromosome analysis of trifluorothymidine-resistant L5178Y mouse lymphoma cell colonies. Environ Mutagen 8: 229–240

Blazak W, Stewart B, Galperin I, Allen K, Rudd C, Mitchell A, Caspary W (1986b) Stable dicentric chromosomes induced by chemical mutagens in L5178Y mouse lymphoma cells. Mutat Res 173: 263–266

Blazak WF, Los FJ, Rudd CJ, Caspary WJ (1989) Chromosome analysis of small and large L5178Y mouse lymphoma cell colonies. Comparison of trifluorothymidine-resistant and unselected cell colonies from mutagen-treated and control cultures. Mutat Res 224: 197–208

Boveri T (1914) Zur Frage der Entstehung maligner Tumoren. Fischer, Jena

Breneman JW, Ramsey MJ, Lee DA, Eveleth GG, Minkler JL, Tucker JD (1993) The development of chromosome-specific composite DNA probes for the mouse and their application to chromosome painting. Chromosoma 102: 591–598

Caspary W, Lee YJ, Poulton S, Myhr B, Mitchell A (1988a) Evaluation of the mouse L5178Y lymphoma system as an indicator of the mutagenic activity of chemicals: quality control criteria and response categories. Environ Mol Mutagen 12 [Suppl. 13]: 19–36

Caspary WJ, Myhr B, Mitchell A (1988b) Evaluation of the mouse L5178Y lymphoma system as an indicator of the mutagenic activity of chemicals: V. interlaboratory reproducibility and assessment. Environ Mol Mutagen 12: 195–229

Cavenee W, Dryja T, Phillips R (1983) Expression of recessive alleles by chromosomal mechanisms in retinoblastoma. Nature 205: 779–784

Cavenee W, Koufos A, Hansen M (1988) Recessive mutant genes predisposing to human cancer. Mutat Res 168: 3–14

Clive D, Flamm WG, Machesko MR, Bernheim NJ (1972) Mutational assay system using the thymidine kinase locus in mouse lymphoma cells. Mutat Res 16: 77–87

Clive D, Johnson K, Spector J, Batson A, Brown MM (1979) Validation and characterization of the L5178Y/tk mouse lymphoma mutagen assay system. Mutat Res 59: 61–108

Clive D, Glover P, Applegate M, Hozier J (1990) Molecular aspects of chemical mutagenesis in L5178Y/tk$^{+/-}$ mouse lymphoma cells. Mutagenesis 5: 191–187

Clive D, Glover P, Krehl R, Poorman-Allen P (1991) Mutagenicity of 2-amino-N^6-hydroxyadenine (AHA) at three loci in L5178Y/tk$^{+/-}$ mouse lymphoma cells: molecular and preliminary cytogenetic characterizations of AHA-induced tk$^{-/-}$ mutants. Mutat Res 253: 73–82

Clontech (1995) Clontechniques X: 14–15

Collins F (1995) Positional cloning moves from perditional to traditional. Nature Genet 9: 347–350

Combes RD, Stopper H, Caspary WJ (1995) The use of L5178Y mouse lymphoma cells to assess mutagenic, clastogenic and aneugenic activity of chemicals. Mutagenesis (in press)

Cremer T, Lichter P, Borden J, Ward DC, Manuelidis L (1988) Detection of chromosome aberrations in metaphase and interphase tumor cells by in situ hybridization using chromosome-specific library probes. Hum Gene 80: 235–246

Curtis LJ, Bubb VJ, Gledhill S, Morris RG, Bird CC, Wyllie AH (1994) Loss of heterozygosity of MCC is not associated with mutation of the retained allele in sproadic colorectal cancer. Hum Mol Genet 3: 443–446

Davis LM, Caspary WJ, Sakallah SA, Maronpot R, Wiseman R, Barrett JC, Elliott R, Hozier JC (1994) Loss of heterozygosity in spontaneous and chemically induced liver tumors from the B6C3F1 mouse. Carcinogenesis 15: 1637–1645

Dietrich W, Katz H, Lincoln SE, Shin H-S, Friedman J, Dracopoli NC, Lander ES (1992a) A genetic map of the mouse suitable for typing intraspecific crosses. Genetics 131: 423–447

Dietrich W, Miller J, Katz H, Joyce D, Stean R, Lincoln S, Daly M, Reeve MP, Goodman N, Dracopoli N, Lander ES (1992b) SSLP microsatellite map. In:

O'Brien SJ (ed) Genetic maps, nonhuman vertebrates, vol 4, 6th edn. Cold Spring Harbor Laboratory Press, Cold Spring Harbor, pp 110–142

Ding SF, Habib NA, Dooley J, Wood C, Bowles L, Delhanty DA (1991) Loss of constitutional heterozygosity on chromosome 5q in hepatocellular carcinoma without cirrhosis. Br J Cancer 64(6): 1083–1087

Ding SF, Delhanty JDA, Dooley JS, Bowles L, Wood CB, Habib NA (1993) The putative tumor suppressor gene on chromosome 5q for hepatocellular carcinoma is distinct from the MCC and APC genes. Cancer Detect Prevention 17: 405–409

Fenech M (1993) The cytokinesis-block micronucleus technique: a detailed description of the method and its application to genotoxicity studies in human populations. Mutat Res 285: 35–44

Fritzenschaf H, Kohlpoth M, Rusche B, Schiffmann D (1993) Testing of known carcinogens and noncarcinogens in the Syrian hamster embryo (SHE) micronucleus test in vitro: correlation with in vivo micronucleus formation and cell transformation. Mutat Res 319: 47–53

Gille JJ, van Berkel CG, Joenje H (1994) Mutagenicity of metabolic oxygen radicals in mammalian cell cultures. Carcinogenesis 15: 2695–2699

Gray JW, Dean PN, Fuscoe JC, Peters DC, Trask BJ, van den Ength GJ (1987) High speed chromosome sorting. Science 238: 323–329

Guan X-Y, Trent JM, Meltzer PS (1993) Generation of band-specific painting probes from a single microdissected chromosome. Hum Mol Genet 2: 1117–1121

Guan X-Y, Meltzer PS, Trent J (1994) Rapid generation of whole chromosome painting probes (WCPs) by chromosome microdissection. Genomics 22: 101–107

Gudi R, Xu Y, Thilager A (1992) Assessment of the in vivo aneuploidy/micronucleus assay in mouse bone marrow cells with 16 chemicals. Environ Mol Mutagen 20: 106–116

Hearne CM, McAleer MA, Love JM, Aitman TJ, Cornall RJ, Ghosh S, Knight AM, Prins JB, Todd JA (1991) Additional microsatellite markers for mouse genome mapping. Mammalian Genome 1: 273–282

Hollstein M, Sidransky D, Vogelstein B, Harris CC (1991) P53 mutations in human cancers. Science 253: 49–53

Hozier J, Sawyer J, Moore M, Howard B, Clive D (1981) Cytogenetic analysis of the L5178Y/tk+/– to tk–/– mouse lymphoma mutagenesis assay system. Mutat Res 84: 169–181

Hozier J, Sawyer J, Clive D, Moore M (1982) Cytogenetic distinction between the TK^{+} and TK^{-} chromosomes in the L5178Y $TK^{+/-}$ 3.7.2C mouse-lymphoma cell line. Mutat Res 105: 451–456

Hozier J, Sawyer J, Clive D, Moore MM (1985) Chromosome 11 aberrations in small colony L5178Y $TK^{-/-}$ mutants early in their clonal history. Mutat Res 147: 237–242

Hozier J, Sawyer JR, Moore MM (1989) High-resolution cytogenetic analysis of L5178Y $TK^{+/-}$ 3.7.2c cells: variation in chromosome 11 breakpoints among small-colony $TK^{-/-}$ mutants. Mutat Res 214: 195–199

Hozier J, Scalzi J, Sawyer J, Carley N, Applegate M, Clive D, Moore M (1991) Localization of the mouse thymidine kinase gene to the distal portion of chromosome 11. Genomics 10: 827–832

Hozier J, Applegate M, Moore MM (1992) In vitro mammalian mutagenesis as a model for genetic lesions in human cancer. Mutat Res 270: 201–209

Hozier J, Graham R, Westfall T, Siebert P, Davis L (1994) Preparative in situ hybridization: selection of chromosome region-specific libraries on mitotic chromosomes. Genomics 19: 441–447

Kinzler KW, Nilbert MC, Su L-K, Vogelstein B, Bryan TM, Levy DB, Smith KJ, Preisinger AC, Hedge P, McKechnie D, Finniear R, Markham A, Groffen J, Boguski MS, Altschul SF, Horii A, Ando H, Miyoshi Y, Miki Y, Nishisho I, Nakamura Y (1991) Identification of FAP locus genes from chromosome 5q21. Science 253: 661–664

Knudson A (1985) Hereditary cancer, oncogenes and antioncogenes. Cancer Res 45: 1437–1443

Ledbetter SA, Nelson DL, Warren ST, Ledbetter D (1990) Rapid isolation of DNA probes within specific chromosome regions by interspersed repetitive sequence polymerase chain reaction. Genomics 6: 475–481

Li CY, Yandell DW, Little JB (1992) Molecular mechanisms of spontaneous and induced loss of heterozygosity in human cells in vitro. Somat Cell Mol Genet 18: 77–87

Lichter P, Cremer T, Borden J, Manuelidis L, Ward DC (1988a) Delineation of individual chromosomes in metaphase and interphase cells by in situ suppression hybridization using recombinant DNA libraries. Hum Genet 80: 224–234

Lichter P, Cremer T, Tang CC, Watkins PC, Manuelidis L, Ward DC (1988b) Rapid detection of human chromosome 21 aberrations by in situ hybridization. Proc Natl Acad Sci USA 85: 9664–9668

Liechty MC, Rauchfuss HS, Lugo MH, Hozier JC (1993) Sequence analysis of tk_a^{-} –1 and $tk_b^{+\text{-}1 \text{ alleles in L5178Ytk}^{+/-}}$ mouse-lymphoma cells and spontaneous $tk^{-/-}$ mutants. Mutat Res 286: 299–307

Liechty MC, Hassanpour Z, Hozier JC, Clive D (1994) Use of microsatellite DNA polymorphisms on mouse chromosome 11 for in vitro analysis of thymidine kinase gene mutations. Mutagenesis 9: 423–427

Liechty MC, Crosby H, Murthy A, Davis LM, Caspary WJ, Hozier JC (1995a) Identification of a polymorphic microsatellite within the tk gene in L5178Y mouse lymphoma cells. Nucleic Acids Res (in press)

Liechty MC, Hall BK, Scalzi JM, Davis LM, Caspary WJ, Hozier JC (1995b) Mouse chromosome-specific painting probes generated from microdissected chromosomes. Mammal Genome (in press)

Little JB (1989) In vitro models of carcinogenesis: expression of recessive genes by chromosomal mutations. Environ Health Perspect 81: 63–66

Love JM, Knight AM, McAleer MS, Todd JA (1990) Towards construction of a high resolution map of the mouse genome using PCR-analysed microsatellites. Nucleic Acids Res 18: 4123–4130

Matsuoka A, Yamasaki N, Suzuki T, Hayashi N, Sofuni T (1993) Evaluation of the micronucleus test using a Chinese hamster cell line as an alternative to the conventional in vitro chromosomal aberration test. Mutat Res 272: 223–236

Meltzer PS, Guan X-Y, Burgess A, Trent JM (1992) Rapid generation of region specific probes by chromosome microdissection and their application. Nat Genet 1: 24–28

Miller J (1992) Genetic map of the mouse. Whitehead Institute/MIT Center for Genome Research, Cambridge, MA

Miyashita K, Voojis MA, Tucker JD, Lee DA, Gray JW, Pallavicini MG (1994) A mouse chromosome library generated from sorted chromosomes using linker-adapter polymerase chain reaction. Cytogenet Cell Genet 66: 54–57

Montagutelli X, Serikawa T, Guenet J (1991) PCR analysed microsatellites: data concerning laboratory and wild-derived mouse inbred strains. Mammal Genome 11: 225–259

Nakamura Y, Leppert M, O'Connell P, Wolff R, Holm T, Culver M, Martin C, Fujimoto E, Hoff M, Kumlin E, White R (1987) Variable number of tandem repeat (VNTR) markers for human gene mapping. Science 235: 1616–1622

Nishisho I, Nakamura Y, Miyoshi Y, Miki Y, Ando H, Horii A, Koyama K, Utsunomiya J, Baba S, Hedge P, Markham A, Krush AJ, Petersen G, Hamilton SR, Nilbert MC, Levy DB, Bryan TM, Preisinger AC, Smith KJ, Su L-K, Kinzler KW, Vogelstein B (1991) Mutations of chromosome 5q21 genes in FAP and colorectal cancer patients. Science 253: 665–669

Rudd C, Daston D, Caspary WJ (1990) Spontaneous mutation rates in mammalian cells: effect of differential growth rates and phenotypic lag. Genetics 126: 435–442

Smith LE, Grosovsky AJ (1993) Genetic instability on chromosome 16 in a human B lymphoblastoid cell line. Somat Cell Mol Genet 19: 515–527

Spencer DL, Caspary WJ (1994) In situ and suspension protocols for mutation in L5178Y mouse cells: dose response and colony size distribution, Mutat Res 322: 291–300

Spencer DL, Hines KC, Caspary WJ (1994) An in situ protocol for measuring the expression of chemically induced mutations in mammalian cells. Mutat Res. 312: 85–98

Stanbridge EJ (1992) Functional evidence for human tumor suppressor genes: chromosome and molecular genetic studies. Cancer Surv 12: 5–24

Stopper H, Körber C, Schiffmann D, Caspary WJ (1993a) Cell cycle dependent micronucleus formation and mitotic disturbances in mammalian cells treated with 5-azacytidine. Mutat Res 300: 165–177

Stopper H, Körber C, Spencer DL, Kirchner S, Caspary WJ, Schiffmann D (1993b) An investigation of micronucleus and mutation induction by oxazepam in mammalian cells. Mutagenesis 8: 449–455

Stopper H, Eckert I, Schiffmann D, Spencer D, Caspary WJ (1994) Is micronucleus induction by aneugens an early event in mutagenesis? Mutagenesis 9: 411–416

Stopper H, Diener U, Schwefel I, Bittner D (1995) Does the presence of a fragile site lead to micronucleus formation? J Cancer Clin Onc 121(2): M26

Tautz D (1989) Hypervariability of simple sequences as a general source for polymorphic DNA markers. Nucleic Acids Res 17: 6463–6471

Telenius H, de Vos D, Blennow E, Willat LR, Ponder BA, Carter NP (1993) Chromatid contamination can impair the purity of flow-sorted metaphase chromosomes. Cytometry 14: 97–101

Tennant R, Margolin B, Shelby M, Zeiger E, Haseman J, Spalding J, Caspary W, Resnick M, Stasiewicz S, Anderson B, Minor R (1987) Prediction of chemical carcinogenicity in rodents from in vitro genetic toxicity assays. Science 236: 933–941

Thibodeau SN, Bren G, Schald D (1993) Microsatellite instability in cancer of the proximal colon. Science 260: 815–819

Weber JL, May PE (1989) Abundant class of human DNA polymorphisms which can be typed using the polymerase chain reaction. Am J Hum Genet 44: 388–396

Weier HUG, Polikoff D, Fawcett JJ, Greulich KM, Lee KH, Cram S, Chapman VM, Gray JW (1994) Generation of five high-complexity painting probe libraries from flow-sorted mouse chromosomes. Genomics 21: 641–644

Weinberg RA (1991) Tumor suppressor genes. Science 254: 1138–1146

Xia F, Amundson SA, Nickoloff JA, Liber HL (1994) Different capacities for recombination in closely related human lymphoblastoid cell lines with different mutational responses to X-irradiation. Mol Cell Biol 14: 5850–5857

Zhang J, Meltzer P, Jenkins R, Guan X-Y, Trent J (1993) Application of chromosome microdissection probes for elucidation of BCR-ABL fusion and variant Philadelphia chromosome translocation in chronic myelogenous leukemia. Blood 81: 3365–3371

Zhu Y, Stambrook PJ, Tischfield JA (1993) Loss of heterozygosity: the most frequent cause of recessive phenotype expression at the heterozygous human adenine phosphoribosyltransferase locus. Mol Carcinogen 8: 138–144

Formation of Micronuclei and Inhibition of Topoisomerase II in the Comet Assay in Mammalian Cells with Altered DNA Methylation

H. Stopper[1], I. Eckert[1], P. Wagener[1], and W.A. Schulz[2]

[1]Department of Toxicology, University of Würzburg, Versbacher Str. 9, 97078 Würzburg, Germany
[2]Department of Physiological Chemistry, Heinrich-Heine University, 40001 Düsseldorf, Germany

Introduction

In mammalian DNA, 3%–5% of cytosine residues are present as 5-methylcytosine (Holiday and Grigg 1993). This methylation is involved in several epigenetic processes, including genomic imprinting and gene expression (Tilghman 1993). DNA hypomethylation is one of the possible causes and one of the consequences of mammalian neoplasia and also occurs in cultured cells after treatment with certain carcinogenic drugs (Spruck et al. 1993). Changes in DNA methylation can affect DNA conformation (Bird 1992).

Our hypothesis (Stopper et al. 1993; Kirchner et al. 1995) about the relationship between the DNA methylation pattern and genomic instability suggests that the function of certain DNA-binding proteins is disturbed when the methylation pattern is changed and DNA conformation changes occur. For example, a disturbed function of the kinetochore complex results in displaced metaphase chromosomes, which can be included in micronuclei (Kirchner et al. 1993). Inhibition of the activity of topoisomerase II is known to disturb chromatid separation during mitosis (Downes et al. 1991). This leads to the formation of chromatid bridges, which may rupture (Gaulden 1987). The resulting chromatin fragments may be included in micronuclei (Kirchner et al. 1995; Stopper et al. 1993).

In an earlier investigation we showed that the hypomethylating agent 5-azacytidine induced micronucleus formation and cell transformation in Syrian hamster embryo (SHE) fibroblasts but was unable to induce unscheduled DNA synthesis (Stopper et al. 1992). 5-Azacytidine also induced micronuclei in L5178Y cells (Stopper et al. 1993), the cell line used by us and others to study the mutagenicity of this compound (Amacher and Turner 1987; McGregor et al. 1989; Spencer et al. 1994). We were interested whether an increase in micronucleus frequency could also be observed in a cell system in which changes in the pattern of DNA methylation occur endogenously and are not induced by a chemical. The mouse teratocarcinoma F9 cell system is suitable for such an investigation. F9 cells treated with retinoic acid differentiate into extraembryonic endoderm (Alonso et al. 1991). The differentiation process is accompanied by a decrease in total DNA methylation (Razin et al. 1986). Specifically, methylation analysis using a mouse minor satellite probe that hybridizes to mouse chromosomes within the centromeric region revealed that this region was highly methylated in undifferentiated F9 cells (Teubner and Schulz 1994). During differentiation about 40% of all CCGG sites in the minor satellite sequence became demethylated (Teubner and Schulz 1994). The state of the centromeric region is important for the function of the kinetochore complex as well as for the topoisomerase II-dependent separation of chromatids at anaphase.

We determined the occurrence of micronuclei in F9 mouse teratocarcinoma cells during the course of in vitro differentiation. Using kinetochore staining and in situ hybridization (minor satellite DNA probe) we investigated the role of the kinetochore complex in micronucleus formation. We then assayed the efficiency of topoisomerase II activity throughout differentiation by using single cell gel electrophoresis (SCGE, comet assay). In addition, the frequency of micronuclei generated by topoisomerase II inhibitors after the induction of hypomethylation was assayed in mouse L5178Y cells.

Materials and Methods

Cell Culture

F9 Mouse embryonal carcinoma cells were cultured in gelatin-coated tissue culture flasks in DMEM supplemented with 10% heat-inactivated fetal calf serum, 2 m*M* glutamine, and antibiotics. Differentiation (into parietal endoderm-like cells) was induced in F9 cells seeded at low density by addition of 0.5 μM retinoic acid and 50 μM dibutyryl cyclic AMP. Cell cultures were grown in a humidified atmosphere with 5% CO_2 in air at 37 °C.

Mouse L5178Y cells were cultured in suspension in RPMI-1640 supplemented with 10% heat-inactivated horse serum, 0.25 mg/ml L-glutamine, 107 μg/ml sodium pyruvate, and antibiotics. Cell cultures were grown in a humidified atmosphere with 5% CO_2 in air at 37 °C.

Micronucleus Assay During Differentiation

F9 cells were trypsinized at the indicated time points during differentiation and placed on glass slides by cytospin centrifugation. L5178Y cells were treated with the same inducers used to differentiate F9 cells, and slides were prepared at the indicated time points. Cells were fixed with methanol (–20 °C, 1 h). To stain nuclei and micronuclei, slides were washed with distilled water, incubated with bisbenzimide 33258 (5 μg/ml, 5 min), washed three times with distilled water, mounted for microscopy, and the number of nuclei and micronuclei was scored using a magnification of ×1250. Each data point represents the mean of at least three slides from one experiment with 2000 nuclei evaluated per slide. Experiments were repeated with consistent results.

Micronucleus Assay for Genotoxicity Testing of Chemicals

Exponentially growing mouse L5178Y cells were treated for 4 h with a final concentration of 0.25 μg/ml 5-azacytidine or solvent (control). This compound was removed by washing the cells in culture medium and the cells were allowed to recover for 5 h. Then, to both 5-azacytidine pretreated and solvent control cells, amsacrine, berenil, etoposide or solvent were added to a final concentration of 3 ng/ml, 20 μg/ml, 25 ng/ml, and 1%, respectively. After an incubation time of 4 h, these compounds were again removed by washing the cells with culture medium, and the cells were allowed to recover for 15 h. The solvent for the chemicals was dimethylsulfoxide (DMSO) and the solutions were prepared such that the final concentration of DMSO was 1% in the cell cultures. The cells were then placed on glass slides by cytospin centrifugation, fixed, stained, and evaluated as described above for F9 cells. This experiment was repeated with consistent results.

Kinetochore Staining

We stained kinetochores by incubating the fixed cell preparations (after washing 5 min in PBS/0.1% Tween 20) with human anti kinetochore antiserum as provided by Biermann, Bad Nauheim, Germany, for 75 min in a humidified chamber at 37 °C. After washing twice for 5 min in PBS/0.5% Tween 20, pH 7.4 we incubated the cells for 30 min with fluorescein isothiocyanate (FITC)-conjugated goat-antihuman antibody that had been diluted 1:100 in PBS/0.5% Tween 20, pH 7.4. They were then washed twice in PBS/0.1% Tween 20 and counterstained with bisbenzimide 33258.

In Situ Hybridization

Fixation of F9 cells was performed in methanol-acidic acid (3:1; –20 °C) for 30 min and slides were then air-dried. For hybridization, cells were dehydrated by putting the slides through an ethanol series (70%, 80%, 95%, 100%, 2 min each). The cellular DNA on the slides was then denatured in 70% formamide/2×SSC (pH 7.0, 2 min, 70 °C). Subsequently, they were again dehydrated as described above. A mixture of 50% formamide/2×SSC/10% dextrane sulphate, containing 20–50 ng of centromeric probe, was incubated at 70 °C for 10 min and then put on ice for 10 min. For hybridization, slides were incubated overnight at 37 °C with the above mixture containing the centromeric probe. The centromeric probe was mouse minor satellite DNA (Wong and Rattner 1988), labeled with fluorescein-deoxyuridine triphosphate (dUTP). Slides were counterstained with bisbenzimide as described above and mounted for fluorescence microscopy.

Comet Assay

F9 cells were incubated with either 50 ng/ml etoposide, 6 ng/ml amsacrine, 250 μg/ml ethylmethanesulfonate (EMS; positive control), or solvent control (DMSO; final concentration 1%) for 4 h. Cells were then washed and embedded in low melting agarose (0.5%) which was layered onto slides that had been coated with a layer of 0.75% normal agarose. A final layer of 0.5% low melting agarose was added on top. Slides were put in a buffer containing 1% Triton X-100, 10% DMSO, and 89% of 10 m*M* Tris/1% Na-Sarcosinat/2.5 *M* NaCl/100 m*M* Na_2 ethylenediaminetetraacetate (EDTA) (pH 10) for lysis (1 h). Then, slides were pretreated for 15 min in electrophoresis buffer (300 m*M* NaOH/1 m*M* Na_2 EDTA, pH 10) and after that exposed to 25V/300 mA for 20 min. Slides were then neutralized for 3×5 min in 0.4 *M* Tris, pH 7.5 and DNA was stained by adding 50 μl of ethidium bromide (20 μg/ml) onto each slide. Cells were scored using computer-aided image analysis. This was done by selecting two areas in each picture: the whole cellular DNA including the comet region and a region containing the comet region including only the border of the nuclear DNA. Using the software program NIH-image the integrated densities (sum of the gray values of each pixel in the selection) were measured in each selection and the percent of all staining intensity that was located in the comet region (including just the border of the nuclear DNA region) was calculated. This number represents the amount of DNA in the comet region and is referred to as "% comet" in the figure. The average of at least 50 cells and the standard deviation from each slide are given.

Results

The micronucleus frequency during differentiation in F9 cells was determined (Fig. 1). An increase was observed that was most pronounced during the second half of the differentiation period. The chemicals used for the induction of differentiation were tested in L5178Y mouse lymphoma cells but were only weakly active in producing micronuclei (Fig. 1).

To investigate the role of impaired function of the kinetochore complex we stained micronuclei that occurred in F9 cells during differentiation by immunofluorescence (Table 1). The percentage of kinetochore-positive micronuclei was constant over most of the time span and increased at the

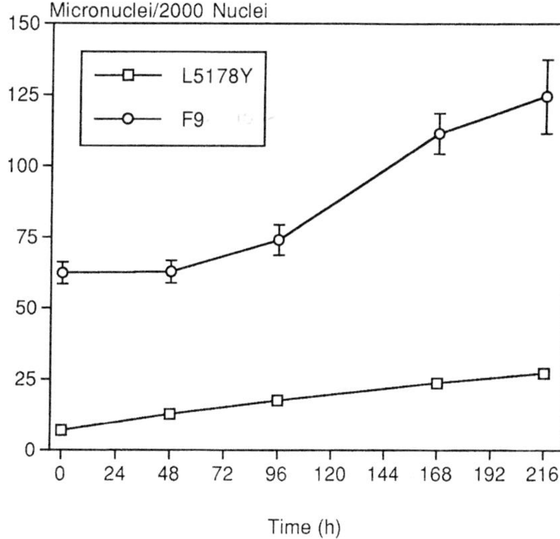

Fig. 1. Formation of micronuclei in F9 cells during differentiation. Also shown is the induction of micronuclei by the compounds used for F9 cell differentiation in L5178Y cells

last time point assayed. In situ hybridization of the micronuclei using mouse minor satellite DNA to reveal the presence of the DNA in the centromeric region yielded similar percentages of signal-positive micronuclei, supporting the data of kinetochore staining (Table 1).

Next, we investigated topoisomerase II activity. We used the method of single cell gel electrophoresis (SCGE; "comet assay"; Fig. 2). Agents such as amsacrine and etoposide stabilize the so-called "cleavable complex" formed between topoisomerase II and DNA. In certain assays like the comet assay this can be measured as an elevated frequency of DNA strand breaks. Thus,

Table 1. Presence of kinetochore signals and centromer DNA signals in micronuclei of F9 cells during differentiation

Time (hours)	No.Mn	%K+	No.Mn	%C+
0	400	18.5	97	11.3
48	300	19.7		
96	100	25.0	97	17.5
168	300	21.0		
216	300	35.3	100	31.0

Given are the numbers of micronuclei evaluated (No. Mn) and the percentages of micronuclei that showed a kinetochore signal (%K+) and a centromer (minor satellite) DNA in situ hybridization signal (%C+).

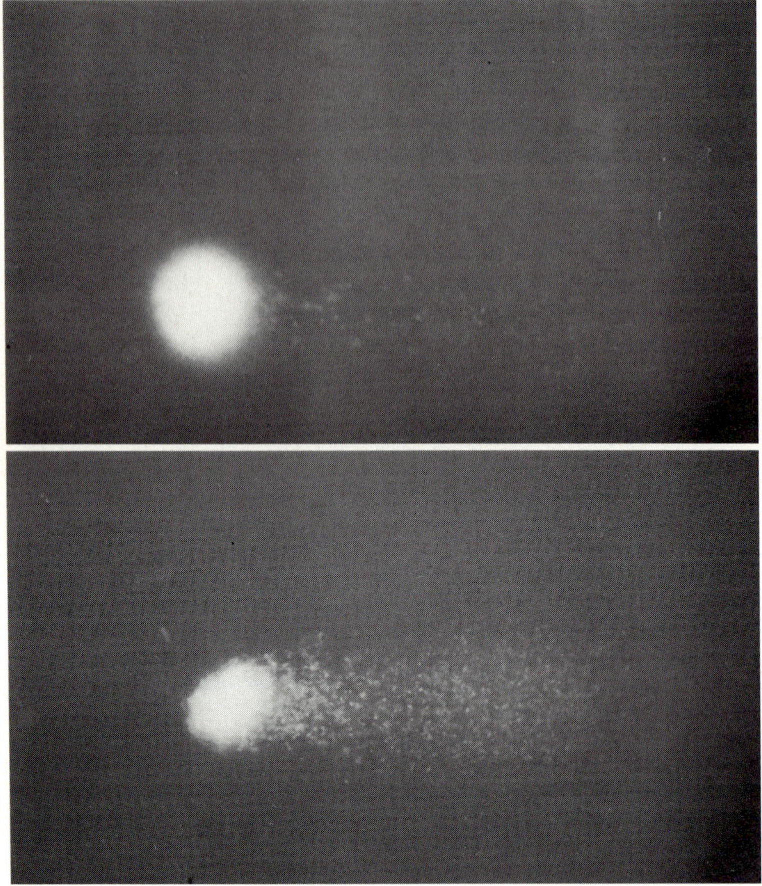

Fig. 2. Formation of comets in the single cell gel electrophoresis assay (comet assay). A control cell (*top*) and a chemically treated cell (*bottom*) are shown

amsacrine and etoposide-mediated DNA break frequencies were used as parameter of topoisomerase II activity and were followed throughout the in vitro differentiation of F9 cells (Fig. 3). Both amsacrine and etoposide induced comets in F9 cells at the beginning of their differentiation but were unable to induce comets at 96 or more h of differentiation, although the positive control substance EMS induced comets throughout the differentiation period.

For further investigation of the possible relationship between topoisomerase II activity and DNA methylation we assayed the induction of micronuclei in mouse L5178Y cells (Table 2). The cells were pretreated with the hypomethylating agent 5-azacytidine and then treated with the topoisomerase II inhibitors amsarcine, berenil, and etoposide. Treatment with the topoisomerase II inhibitors elevated the micronucleus frequencies. Pretreatment with the hypomethylating agent 5-azacytidine also induced micronuclei. The combina-

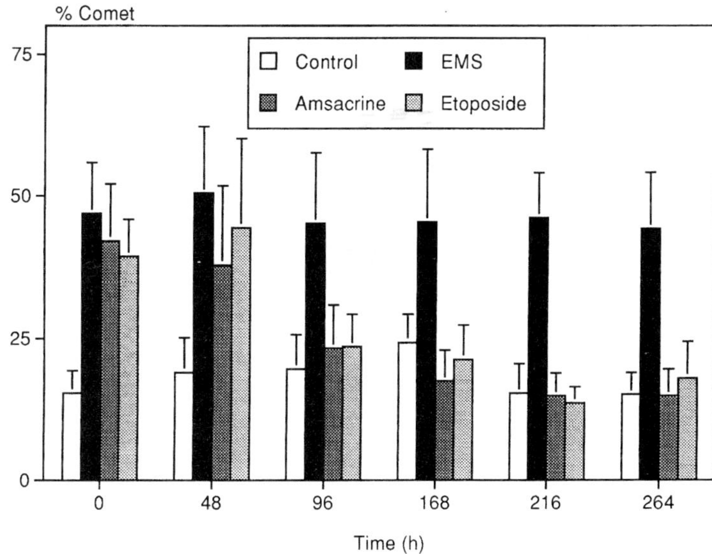

Fig. 3. Induction of comets by amsacrine, etoposide, and ethylmethanesulfonate (EMS) in F9 cells during differentiation. For explanation of evaluation, see "Materials and Methods"

Table 2. Induction of micronuclei in mouse L5178Y cells

Pretreatment	Treatment	Mn/2000[a]	Ind.Mn	%K+[b]
Solvent control	Solvent control	9.3 ± 0.5	0	29.9 ± 1.7
	Amsacrine	100 ± 12	91	17.9 ± 2.0
	Berenil	17.6 ± 2.3	8	21.8 ± 4.0
	Etoposide	158 ± 8.1	149	19.4 ± 2.7
5-Azacytidine	Solvent control	32.2 ± 4.6	23	22.4 ± 1.2
	Amsacrine	194 ± 15	185	20.0 ± 2.4
	Berenil	57 ± 7.0	48	18.1 ± 2.2
	Etoposide	303 ± 16.5	294	17.3 ± 1.7

[a]Mn/2000 is the number of micronuclei counted when 2000 nuclei were evaluated from each slide. The averages and standard deviations from five slides are given. Ind.Mn gives the (rounded) number of micronuclei after subtraction of the frequency in the solvent control. For explanation of treatment procedures, see "Materials and Methods."
[b]Percentage of micronuclei showing kinetochore signals in L5178Y cells. For each treatment, about 100 micronuclei on each of three slides were evaluated and the average percentages of signal-positive micronuclei (%K+) and standard deviations were calculated.

tion of both treatments induced micronucleus frequencies which were more than the sum of both single treatments (synergism). For example, 5-azacytidin induced 23 and amsacrine induced (without pretreatment) 91 micronuclei. These numbers would yield a sum of 114 micronuclei. However, the combined treatment yielded 185 micronuclei, which is 1.6 times the expected number. The factors for berenil and etoposide are 1.6 and 1.7, respectively. Kinetochore staining (Table 2) yielded percentages of around 20 for all treatments as well as for the control. Unless kinetochore binding was impaired or kinetochores damaged, this suggests that in all cases predominantly chromosome fragments and not whole chromosomes were included in the micronuclei.

Discussion

The purpose of this study was to investigate a possible relationship between changes in endogenous cytosine methylation of DNA and disturbance of mitosis resulting in genotoxic effects. We used two mammalian cell lines. F9 mouse embryonal carcinoma cells can be induced to differentiate in vitro (Alonso et al. 1991). This process was investigated on a molecular level (Teubner and Schulz 1994) and it was shown that the methylation pattern changed dramatically. Mouse L5178Y cells are widely used in genotoxicity studies and have been found to be suitable for studying chemically induced micronuclei (Stopper et al. 1994). To assess genotoxicity, we measured the formation of micronuclei and the formation of DNA strand breaks in the comet assay. Both can develop as a result of chromosomal breakage. However, the comet assay directly quantifies the occurrence of single and double strand DNA breaks, whereas the formation of micronuclei is an indirect measure of chromosomal breakage.

The frequency of micronuclei increased during differentiation in F9 cells. This could only in part be due to the genotoxicity of the chemicals used for the differentiation induction, since they were only weakly active when tested in L5178Y cells. The formation of additional micronuclei supports our hypothesis that the changes in methylation pattern and especially the hypomethylation at the minor satellite region in the centromer impair the function of DNA-binding proteins that are necessary for mitosis.

Kinetochore staining in F9 cells revealed percentages of signal positive micronuclei around 20% during most of the differentiation period. If whole chromosomes were displaced from the chromatin and included in micronuclei, a percentage of around 80 would have been expected (Stopper et al. 1994). Even if only part of the induced micronuclei were due to the enclosure of whole chromosomes, a change in the percentage of kinetochore-positive micronuclei during the differentiation period would have been expected. This was only seen at the latest time point where the frequency increased to 35%. However, the binding of the kinetochore may have been not only impaired but totally disturbed, and thus whole chromosomes without a kinetochore protein would have been included in the micronuclei. Kinetochore staining would then not have adequately reflected the presence of whole chromosomes in micronuclei. The results obtained with in situ hybridization with mouse minor satellite DNA probe which binds to the DNA in the centromeric region (Wong and Rattner 1988) supported our kinetochore data. We concluded that the function of the kinetochore complex at the centromeric DNA was only affected at the end of differentiation. Since the hypomethylation in the minor satellite region is also most pronounced at the time (Teubner and Schulz 1994), the formation of micronuclei may be related to kinetochore function under conditions where hypomethylation is very pronounced. However, most of the micronuclei must have been formed through a different mechanism.

The possible involvement of topoisomerase II in the observed micronucleus formation was investigated using the comet assay in F9 cells. The reduced comet induction at later time points may be interpreted as impaired topoisomerase II function under conditions of significantly altered methylation pattern (Teubner and Schulz 1994). However, it cannot be excluded that altered expression of topoisomerase II also contributed to the observed changes.

The topoisomerase II inhibitors amsacrine and etoposide as well as the hypomethylating agent 5-azacytidine induced micronuclei in L5178Y cells. If 5-azacytidine was applied first and the topoisomerase II inhibitors after that, a synergistic effect occurred. Therefore, DNA hypomethylation seemed to act as topoisomerase II inhibitor in this assay.

The sensitivity of DNA-binding proteins to changes in cytosine methylation has been described for several proteins. Methylated CpG-rich regions of DNA are more resistant to micrococcal nuclease digestion than bulk DNA (Razin and Cedar 1977; Keshet et al. 1986). MspI, which cuts CCGG sequences in naked DNA whether or not the internal C is methylated, is unable to cleave methylated CpGs in nuclei. Recently, DNA binding proteins which specifically bind to methylated DNA (MeCPs) have been identified (Lewis and Bird 1991). Cytosine methylation patterns are altered during cell differentation as well as during carcinogenesis and the importance of these processes requires further clarification of the underlying mechanisms. For example, it has been suggested that hypermethylation can silence tumor suppressor genes (Greger et al. 1994), that hypermethylation serves to "mark" regions of chromosomes for deletion with loss of tumor suppressor genes (Makos et al. 1993) and that hypomethylation facilitates aberrant gene expression involved in tumor promotion (Counts and Goodman 1994).

To understand the nature of these relationships completely, studies on the molecular level will be necessary. However, the data presented here support our hypothesis that changes in DNA methylation that occur after that the treatment with carcinogenic substances as well as during cell differentiation have genotoxic effects by altering the activity of certain DNA-binding proteins such as the kinetochore complex and topoisomerase II.

Acknowledgments. We thank Mr. Reinhard Gerhard for excellent technical assistance. This work was supported by the Deutsche Forschungsgemeinschaft (SFB 172) and the NATO (CRG programme).

References

Alonso A, Breuer B, Steuer B, Fischer J (1991) The F9-EC cell line as a model for the analysis of differentiation. Int J Dev Biol 35(4): 389–397

Amacher D, Turner G (1987) The mutagenicity of 5-azacytidine and other inhibitors of replication DNA synthesis in the L5178Y mouse lymphoma cell. Mutat Res 176: 123–131

Bird A (1992) The essentials of DNA-methylation. Cell 70: 5–8

Counts JL, Goodman JI (1994) Hypomethylation of DNA: an epigenetic mechanism involved in tumor promotion. Mol Carcinog 11: 185–188

Downes CS, Mullinger AM, Johnson RT (1991) Inhibitors of topoisomerase II prevent chromatid separation in mammalian cells but do not prevent exit from mitosis. Proc Natl Acad Sci USA 88: 8895–8899

Gaulden ME (1987) Hypothesis: some mutagens directly alter specific chromosomal proteins (DNA topoisomerase II and peripheral proteins) to produce chromosome stickiness, which causes chromosome aberrations. Mutagenesis 2: 357–365

Greger V, Debus N, Lohmann D, Hopping W, Passarge E, Horsthemke B (1994) Frequency and parental origin of hypermethylated RB1 alleles in retinoblastoma. Hum Genet 94: 491–496

Holiday R, Grigg GW (1993) DNA-methylation and mutation. Mutat Res 285: 61–67

Keshet I, Lieman-Hurwitz J, Cedar H (1986) DNA-methylation affects the formation of active chromatin. Cell 44: 535–545

Kirchner S, Stopper H, Papp T, Eckert I, Yoo HJ, Vig BK, Schiffmann D (1993) Cytogenetic changes in primary, immortalized and malignant mammalian cells. Toxicol Lett 67: 283–295

Kirchner S, Schiffmann D, Stopper H (1995) The influence of DNA-methylation on topoisomerase II activity and genomic instability. Toxicol In Vitro (in press)

Lewis J, Bird A (1991) DNA-methylation and chromatin structure. FEBS Lett 285: 155–159

Makos M, Nelkin BD, Reiter RE, Gnarra JR, Brooks J, Isaacs W, Linehan M, Baylin SB (1993) Regional DNA-hypermethylation at D17S5 precedes 17p structural changes in the progression of renal tumors. Cancer Res 53: 2719–2722

McGregor DB, Brown AG, Cattanach P, Shepherd W, Riach C, Daston DS, Caspary WJ (1989) TFT and 6TG resistance of mouse lymphoma cells to analogs of azacytidine. Carcinogenesis 10: 2003–2008

Razin A, Cedar H (1977) Distribution of 5-methylcytosine in chromatin. Proc Natl Acad Sci USA 74: 2725–2728

Razin A, Szyf M, Kafri T, Roll M, Giloh H, Scarpa S, Carotti D, Cantoni GL (1986) Replacement of 5-methylcytosine by cytosine: a possible mechanism for transient DNA-demethylation during differentiation. Proc Natl Acad Sci USA 83: 2827–2831

Spencer DL, Hines KC, Caspary WJ (1994) An in situ protocol for measuring the expression of chemically induced mutations in mammalian cells. Mutat Res 312: 85–98

Spruck CH III, Rideout WM III, Jones PA (1993) DNA-methylation and cancer. In: Jost JP, Saluz HP (eds) DNA-methylation: molecular biology and biological significance. Birkhäuser Basel, pp 487–509

Stopper H, Pechan R, Schiffmann D (1992) 5-Azacytidine induces micronuclei in and morphological transformation of Syrian hamster embryo fibroblasts in the absence of unscheduled DNA synthesis. Mutat Res 283: 21–28

Stopper H, Körber C, Schiffmann D, Caspary WJ (1993) Cell cycle dependent micronucleus formation and mitotic disturbances in mammalian cells treated with 5-azacytidine. Mutat Res 300: 165–177

Stopper H, Eckert I, Schiffmann D, Spencer DL, Caspary WJ (1994) Is micronucleus induction by aneugens an early event leading to mutagenesis? Mutagenesis 9(5): 411–416

Teubner B, Schulz W (1994) Exemption of satellite DNA from demethylation in immortalized derivatives of F9 mouse embryonal carcinoma cells. Exp Cell Res 210: 192–200

Tilghman S (1993) DNA-methylation: a phoenix rises. Proc Natl Acad Sci USA 90: 8761–8762

Wong AKC, Rattner JB (1988) Sequence organization and cytological localization of the minor satellite of mouse. Nucleic Acid Res 16(24): 11645–11661

Poly(ADP-Ribosyl)ation and Nuclear Matrix/Intermediate Filament Proteins in Renal Carcinogenesis

S. Vamvakas, H. Richter, and D. Bittner

Department of Toxicology, University of Würzburg, Versbacher Str. 9, 97078 Würzburg, Germany

Introduction

Extragenomic changes play a crucial role in the regulation of gene expression and consequently in cell proliferation and differentiation. Hence, changes in cellular components other than the genome may influence – promote or inhibit – the process of malignant transformation. Among these extragenomic cellular components, the histones and the proteins of the nuclear matrix, consisting mainly of the nuclear pore complex and the nuclear lamins, are directly involved in the regulation of gene expression. Posttranslational modification of these proteins may have a direct impact on the three-dimensional organization of the genome and hence, on the availability of specific DNA sequences for repair, replication, or transcription.

One of the most efficient posttranslational modifications of nuclear proteins is by poly(ADP-ribosyl)ation. The branched poly(ADP-ribose)conjugates contain ribose-ribose linkages alternating with pyrophosphate bonds, an adenine base being attached to every second ribose. The changes in chromatin structure brought about by poly(ADP-ribosyl)ation of histones and numerous proteins of the nuclear matrix may be best described as a reduction of the degree of chromatin condensation at certain parts of the genome. The degree of chromatin condensation is of paramount importance for all major nuclear events, since gene transcription, DNA repair, and replication predominantly occur in decondensed chromatin fractions. Poly(ADP-ribose)conjugates may act by opening up the higher-order chromatin structure or by removing core histone octamers from DNA, because they weaken DNA-histone interactions by addition of negative charges (Poirier et al. 1982; Boulikas 1992a). Poly(ADP-ribose)polymerase, the key enzyme catalyzing this modification, initially gained recognition as a DNA repair enzyme (Durkacz et al. 1980). Among the different types of DNA damage, DNA double-strand breaks are the most potent inducers of poly(ADP-ribosyl)ation (Boulikas 1992b, 1993b). Increased poly(ADP-ribosyl)ation is usually found in rapidly proliferating and

Recent Results in Cancer Research, Vol. 143

comparatively poorly differentiated cells (Althaus et al. 1982), indicating that this process may play a role in tumor formation. Indeed, it has been reported that poly(ADP-ribosyl)ation may be involved in the hepatocarcinogenicity of *N*-nitrosodiethylamine and benzo[*a*]pyrene (Denda et al. 1988) as well as in the tumor-promoting effects of 12-*0*-tetradecanoylphorbol-13-acetate in mouse fibroblasts (Singh 1990a,b) and of phenobarbital in rat liver (Tsujiuchi et al. 1990).

In addition to tumor-associated posttranslational protein modification, tumor-specific changes in the composition of the nuclear matrix and intermediate filament proteins have recently been demonstrated by two-dimensional electrophoretic analysis (for review see Puck and Krystosek 1992).

The nuclear matrix, sometimes termed also the karyo- or nucleoskeleton, is the detergent-insoluble residue of the nucleus, consisting mainly of the nuclear pore complexes and the nuclear lamina. The major proteins of the lamina are called lamins, and three forms are found in mammalian cells, termed lamin A, B, and C. Changes in the nuclear matrix flow into changes in the three-dimensional organization of the DNA (Puck et al. 1990; Nakayasu and Berezney 1991; Getzenberg et al. 1992).

The composition of the cytoskeleton is much better understood than that of the nuclear matrix. The mammalian cytoskeleton consists of (a) microtubules, mainly α- and β-tubulin; (b) the microfilaments, among which the β- and γ-isoforms of actin are found in most mammalian cells; and (c) the intermediate filaments. Epithelial cells contain some 20 isoforms of intermediate filament, while cells of mesenchymal origin express only vimentin. Unlike tubulin and actin, intermediate filaments are elongated molecules that penetrate into the nuclear space and exhibit marked homology to the nuclear lamins. In fact, lamin sequences suggest that these two groups of nuclear and cytoskeletal proteins belong to the same family.

Both in vitro and in vivo experiments and studies in human tumor specimens support the idea of involvement of nuclear matrix and cytoskeletal proteins in the regulation of nuclear processes and consequently in the cellular differentiation status. In the course of malignant transformation a major reorganization of the cytoskeletal proteins takes place, e.g., from the fibrous array characteristic of vimentin in normal fibroblasts to a highly condensed state in transformed clones (Chan et al. 1989). Other examples include reorganization of the nuclear matrix – intermediate filament scaffold in cultured cells exposed to tumor promoters, altered cytokeratin expression in aflatoxin-induced liver tumors, or alterations in actin architecture in human thyroid cancers (Fey and Penman 1984; Green et al. 1990; Getzenberg et al. 1991a,b). Vimentin is normally not expressed in epithelial cells; in contrast, this mesenchymal intermediate filament protein has repeatedly been reported to be coexpressed with keratin in tumors of epithelial origin, e.g., in adenomas and carcinomas of the breast and the salivary gland, in thyroid tumors, and in mesotheliomas (Miettinen et al. 1984; Yanada et al. 1988; Wada et al. 1992). Vimentin is also expressed in malignant clear-cell and chromophilic (granular) renal cell tumors, which have a remarkable metastatic capability, while it is not found in the benign renal oncocytomas, indicating that specific changes in the protein composition may be developed as prognostic tools in the future (Pitz et al. 1987).

Recently, analysis of the composition of the nuclear matrix and intermediate filament proteins by two-dimensional gel electrophoresis provided more precise information, not only on quantitative but also on qualitative changes occurring in specific cell types undergoing morphological and malignant transformation and tissues in the course of tumor formation (Getzenberg et al. 1991a; Keese et al. 1994). These studies demonstrated that the composition of the nuclear matrix is tissue- and cell type-specific and undergoes distinct changes in the course of differentiation as well as dedifferentiation/malignant transformation processes (Fey and Penman 1988; Getzenberg and Coffey 1990; Brancolini and Schneider 1991). Nuclear matrices derived from normal human breast tissue and breast carcinoma tissue share common protein components, but they also demonstrate specific differences which appear to occur with the acquisition of the cancer phenotype (Khanuja et al. 1993). Similarly, several nuclear matrix proteins are consistently found only in malignant tissue of the prostate or colon, while they are not expressed in the normal adjacent epithelia (Getzenberg et al. 1991a: Keese et al. 1994). Furthermore, elevated levels of certain nuclear matrix proteins were determined with monoclonal antibodies in the serum of cancer patients, indicating the potential of this parameter to be developed as a clinical marker for diagnosis and monitoring of cancer (Miller et al. 1992).

The following sections describe some new insights into the role of poly(ADP-ribosyl)ation and the composition of nuclear matrix/intermediate filament proteins in renal carcinogenesis.

Induction of Poly(ADP-ribosyl)ation in the Rat Kidney After Application of Renal Carcinogens with Different Mechanisms of Action

Studies on the role of poly(ADP-ribosyl)ation in tumorigenesis had been carried out in tissues other than the kidney so far (for review see Boulikas 1993a). Hence, little information is available on the contribution of poly(ADP-ribosyl)ation to the formation of renal cell tumors. Dichlorovinylcysteine, the key metabolite responsible for the nephrocarcinogenicity of trichloroethene and dichloroacetylene (Dekant et al. 1989; Kanhai et al. 1989), induced DNA double-strand breaks followed by increased poly(ADP-ribosyl)ation of nuclear proteins in cultured renal LLC-PK_1 cells (Vamvakas et al. 1992). This raised the question whether poly(ADP-ribosyl)ation is involved in the process of renal tumorigenesis and which mechanisms are responsible for its induction. In the study described in the following section, several renal carcinogens with different mechanisms of action, e.g., dichlorovinylcysteine, potassium bromate, ferric nitrilotriacetate, dimethylnitrosamine, and trimethylpentane were administered to male Wistar rats and the extent of poly(ADP-ribosyl)ation was determined in isolated nuclei from the renal cortex by the incorporation of ^{32}P-NAD (McLaren et al. 1994). Since DNA double-strand breaks are the most potent inducers of poly(ADP-ribosyl)ation among the different types of DNA damage (Benjamin and Gill 1980; Boulikas 1989), the effects of the administered renal carcinogens on DNA double-strand break formation in renal cortex and the temporal relationship between induction of poly(ADP-ribosyl)ation and DNA double-strand breaks were also studied.

Dichlorovinylcysteine is mutagenic in bacteria (Dekant et al. 1986) and induces DNA repair in the cultured kidney cell line LLC-PK_1 (Vamvakas et al. 1989). In addition, dichlorovinylcysteine also increases intracellular Ca^{2+} concentrations in LLC-PK_1 cells; this results in activation of Ca^{2+}-dependent endonucleases and in an increased formation of DNA double-strand breaks followed by increased poly(ADP-ribosyl)ation of nuclear proteins (Vamvakas et al. 1990, 1992). Intraperitoneal application of dichlorovinylcysteine to male rats resulted in the induction of poly(ADP-ribosyl)ation, which was preceded by increased formation of DNA double-strand breaks (Fig. 1). The increase in the poly(ADP-ribosyl)transferase activity was maintained throughout the experiment (96 h), whereas the rates of DNA double-strand breaks returned to control values at 72 h after dosing. The temporal relationship between the induction of DNA double-strand breaks and poly(ADP-ribosyl)ation indicated that DNA fragmentation induced by dichlorovinylcysteine may cause increased poly(ADP-ribosyl)ation. Poly(ADP-ribosyl)ation maintained in the absence of DNA double-strand breaks could be accounted for by the presence of significant amounts of DNA single-strand breaks because, in a previous study, administration of 100 mg/kg dichlorovinylcysteine to male rabbits resulted in a threefold increase of DNA single-strand breaks compared with controls (Jaffe et al. 1985).

Potassium bromate ($KBrO_3$) is an oxidizing agent previously (in some countries still) used as a food additive. It is nephrocarcinogenic in rats and nephrotoxic in both humans and experimental animals when given orally (Kurokawa et al. 1990). $KBrO_3$ is a complete carcinogen, with both initiating and promoting activities; it has weak mutagenic activity in microbial assays, but a relatively strong potential for inducing chromosomal aberrations both in vivo and in vitro. Ferric nitrilotriacetate is a chelating agent found as a substitute for polyphosphates in some detergents. Although it induces a high incidence of renal adenocarcinomas (Okada and Midorikawa 1982), it is negative in the Ames test (Li et al. 1987). Both $KBrO_3$ and ferric nitrilotriacetate have oxidizing properties implicating active oxygen species in their initiation/promotion activity in vivo. Both compounds form 8-hydroxydeoxyguanosine, which has been shown to cause a loss of fidelity of DNA synthesis at the residue itself and also the pyrimidine next to it (Kuchino et al. 1987). Hence, this may be an important source of mutations causally involved in the formation of renal tumors. Induction of poly(ADP-ribosyl)ation in the renal

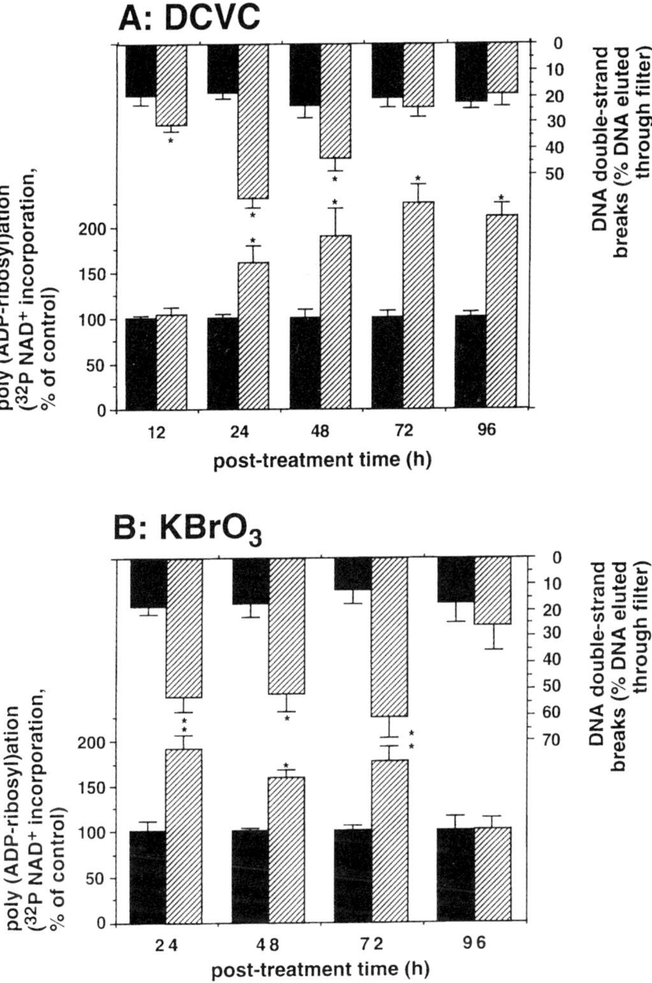

Fig. 1. Poly(ADP-ribosyl)ation and DNA double-strand break formation after the administration of 70 mg/kg dichlorovinylcysteine (*DCVC*, **A**) and of 80 mg/kg potassium bromate (*KBrO$_3$*, **B**) to male Wistar rats in vivo. Vehicle (*solid bars*), DCVC (*hatched bars*, **A**), or KBrO$_3$ (*hatched bars*, **B**) were administered by i.p injection. Animals were killed and cortical nuclei isolated at the posttreatment times indicated. Data are shown as means ± SD of nine samples from three separate animals. The *asterisk* indicates significant difference ($P < 0.01$) compared with controls as determined by Student's *t*-test

cortex after in vivo administration of either drug was paralleled by increased formation of DNA double-strand breaks, implicating DNA fragmentation as the cause of the induction (Fig. 1). To date DNA double-strand breaks had only been reported with ferric nitrilotriacetate in vitro (Toyokuni and Sagripanti 1993). DNA double-strand breaks upon exposure to H_2O_2 and other factors that primarily induce sinlge-strand breaks by a free-radical mechanism may arise from overlapping or closely spaced single-strand breaks. These may result from multiple radical attacks or from incision opposite a preexisting single-strand break (Siddiqi and Bothe 1987; Ward 1990). An additional interesting mechanism for the formation of a double-strand break by a single radical involves radical transfer to the opposite DNA strand: the end of the (first) broken strand on which the radical resides swings over and abstracts a hydrogen from a deoxyribose on the opposite strand followed by reaction of this second product to form the second strand break. The causal link between DNA single- and double-strand breaks induced by reactive oxygen species is supported by the finding that free radical-induced DNA double-strand breaks are usually observed at high levels of single-strand breaks. Approximately 30%–40% of the DNA molecules must have at least one single-strand break before DNA double-strand breaks can be detected (Toyokuni and Sagripanti 1993). These mechanisms are likely to be involved in the double-strand break induction observed in the renal cortex after application of $KBrO_3$ and ferric nitrilotriacetate.

Dimethylnitrosamine is a methylating agent that undergoes cytochrome P450 2E1-catalyzed demethylation reaction to give a reactive methyl diazonium intermediate, which is the primary toxic metabolite in the liver (Yang et al. 1985). Both toxic cell death and liver neoplasms require dimethylnitrosamine metabolism, and tumor formation is quantitatively associated with alkylation of DNA and the persistence of alkylation at O^6 guanosine (Pegg 1988). Kidney tumors can be induced with a single high dose of dimethylnitrosamine (Swann et al. 1980). However, in the present study, exposure of rats to a dose of dimethylnitrosamine known to be nephrocarcinogenic did not result in significant induction of poly(ADP-ribosyl)ation or formation of DNA double-strand breaks (data not shown). Dimethylnitrosamine causes DNA fragmentation in the liver by alkylation and as a result of activating Ca^{2+}-dependent endonucleases but previous studies have shown little DNA fragmentation in extrahepatic tissues (Parodi et al. 1978; Petzold and Swenberg 1978; Ray et al. 1992). The possibility of DNA single-strand break formation due to repair of methylation products cannot be ruled out. However, the extent of their formation must be minimal because this type of DNA fragmentation can also induce poly(ADP-ribosyl)ation, and this was not observed. Alternatively, these DNA adducts may be removed from the DNA by repair mechanisms not involving incision.

Trimethylpentane, a major constituent of unleaded gasoline, is converted to 2,4,4-trimethyl-2-pentanol by cytochrome P450-catalyzed oxidation. Its nephrocarcinogenicity results from the reversible binding of this metabolite to the male rat specific protein α_{2u}-globulin rendering the protein, which is actually synthesized in high amounts in the male rat under androgen control, indigestible by renal lysosomal proteases. The increased concentration of α_{2u}-globulin in the lysosomes results in lysosomal rupture and cell lysis due to the release of lysosomal degradative enzymes. This leads to massive compensatory cell proliferation in the proximal tubules, and the increased cell turnover may contribute to the formation of renal cell tumors by enhancing the likelihood of spontaneous mutational events or by promoting clonal expansion of otherwise initiated cells (Borghoff et al. 1990). Exposure of rats to trimethylpentane in vivo did not result in the formation of DNA double-strand breaks or in the induction of poly(ADP-ribosyl)ation (data not shown), which is in line with the proposed nongenotoxic mechanism of action.

In conclusion, the renal carcinogens dichlorovinylcysteine, $KBrO_3$, and ferric nitrilotriacetate induced elevated levels of poly(ADP-ribosyl)ation in the renal cortex. The crucial role of this posttranslational modification of nuclear proteins in DNA repair and replication and also in gene expression indicates that the increased levels of poly(ADP-ribosyl)ation observed after treatment with dichlorovinylcysteine, $KBrO_3$, and ferric nitrilotriacetate may play an important role in the malignant transformation of renal cells and in the formation of renal cell tumors by these compounds.

Alterations in the Composition of the Nuclear Matrix and Intermediate Filament Proteins in Dedifferentiated Clones of LLC-PK_1 Cells Induced on Long-Term Exposure to Dichlorovinylcysteine

Dichlorovinylcysteine at concentrations greater than 100 μM exerts potent acute toxicity in the cultured renal cell line LLC-PK_1. In contrast, exposure to low, not cytotoxic doses of dichlorovinylcysteine, i.e., ≤ 5 μm, for a period of 4 to 8 weeks induces morphological and biochemical dedifferentiation of LLC-PK_1 cells that remains stable after removal of the drug. In addition to the loss of the physiological cuboidal morphology, the impaired formation of domes and the diminished uptake of glucose indicate disruption of the membrane transport systems and/or of the formation of tight junctions in the dichlorovinylcysteine-derived clones (Fig. 2A–C). Furthermore, the decreased pH-dependent ammonia production indicates impairment of the intramitochondrial phosphate-dependent glutaminase pathway, the predominant pathway of ammonia production in LLC-PK_1 cells and also in the kidney in vivo (Sahai et al. 1989). Since polarization of the plasma membrane, glucose uptake, and ammonia production are the main markers of the physiological integrity of LLC-PK_1 cells and their in vivo counterpart, the proximal tubule cells of the kidney, exposure of LLC-PK_1 cells to dichlorovinylcysteine induces dedifferentiation. This conclusion is strongly supported by the fact that dedifferentiation of LLC-PK_1 cells induced by the prototype dedifferentiating agent 12-*0*-tetradecanoylphorbol-13-acetate and hypoxia-induced dedifferentiation also includes loss of membrane polarity and impairment of glucose transport and ammonia production (Sahai et al. 1992).

Furthermore, higher poly(ADP-ribose)transferase activities were determined in the dedifferentiated dichlorovinylcysteine-induced LLC-PK_1 clones

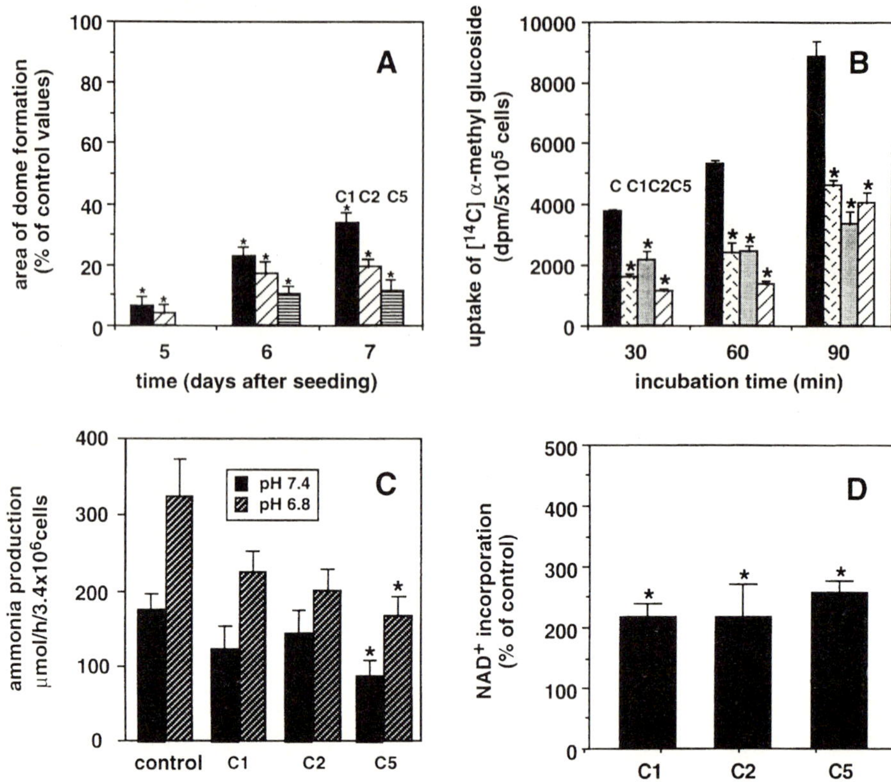

Fig. 2A–D. Change in morphological and biochemical parameters in dedifferentiated LLC-PK_1 clones upon long-term exposure to dichlorovinylcysteine. **A** Impairment of dome formation in dichlorovinylcysteine-induced clones compared with normal LLC-PK_1 cells. The areas occupied by domes in confluent monolayers of the clones derived from exposure to 1 μM (C1, C2) and 5 μM dichlorovinylcysteine (C5) were compared to the dome area in normal LLC-PK_1 monolayers (control areas were set at 100%). Data are from the days 5 (first day of confluency), 6, and 7 after seeding. In contrast to C1 and C2, the C5 clone did not exhibit dome formation on day 5. **B** Time course of the α-methyl glucoside uptake in untreated control LLC-PK_1 cells (C), the 1 μM dichlorovinylcysteine exposure-derived clones C1 and C2, and the 5 μM dichlorovinylcysteine exposure-derived clone C5. **C** Ammonia production in untreated LLC-PK_1 cells (control), in the 1 μM dichlorovinylcysteine exposure-derived clones C1 and C2, and in the 5 μM dichlorovinylcysteine exposure-derived clone C5 at two different pH levels (pH 7.4 and pH 6.8). **D** Poly(ADP-ribosyl)transferase activity in normal LLC-PK1 cells (control), in the 1 μM dichlorovinylcysteine exposure-derived clones C1 and C2, and in the 5 μM dichlorovinylcysteine exposure-derived clone C5. The poly(ADP-ribosyl)transferase activity of the control was set at 100%. Data in **A–D** represent means ± SD from nine determinations of three separate experiments. The *asterisk* indicates significant difference ($p < 0.01$) compared to controls as determined by Student's *t*-test

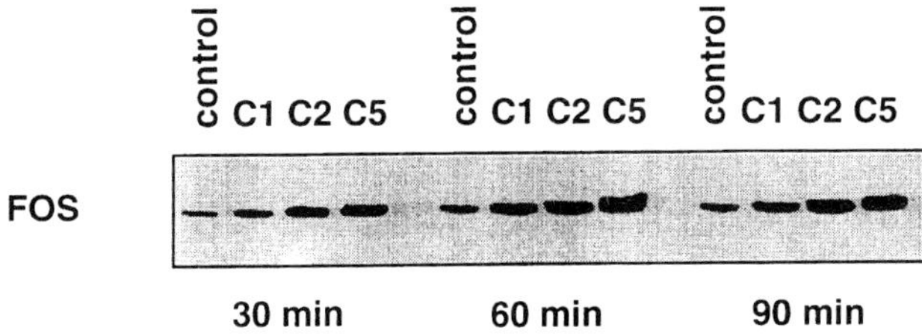

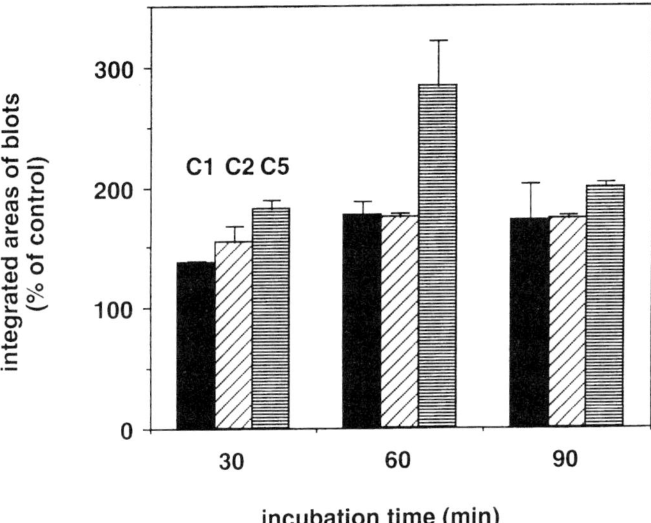

Fig. 3. Effects of long-term dichlorovinylcysteine treatment on c-*fos* expression in LLC-PK_1 cells. **Top** Immunoblot analysis of c-*fos* expression in untreated control cells (control); clones derived from treatment with 1 μM dichlorovinylcysteine (C1 and C2) and 5 μM dichlorovinylcysteine (C5) after 30, 60, and 90 min incubation in Dulbecco's modified Eagle medium (DMEM) supplemented with 10% fetal calf serum (FCS) following 24 h serum deprivation (DMEM/0.2% FCS). Protein was loaded from whole cell lysates at 25 μg/well. The immunoblot shown is from one typical experiment out of three. **Bottom** Content of FOS protein in the three clones (C1, C2, and C5) expressed as percent of the protein in untreated control LLC-PK_1 cells. *Incubation time*, time after supplementation with 10% FCS following 24 h serum deprivation (0.2% FCS). The FOS bands were quantified densitometrically. Data represent means ± SD from three separate experiments

compared with the untreated controls (Fig. 2D). As described above, high concentrations of poly(ADP-ribosyl)conjugates weaken DNA-histone interactions by adding negative charges to the histones, thus unraveling DNA-binding sites for proteins and facilitating gene expression. This may be reflected in the higher levels of FOS protein determined in the dichlorovinylcysteine-induced clones (Fig. 3), although the present experiments cannot provide proof of the causal link between the increased poly(ADP-ribosyl)ation and the induction of c-*fos* expression.

Analysis of the intermediate filament and nuclear matrix protein composition by two-dimensional gel electrophoresis revealed both qualitative and quantitative changes between the wild-type LLC-PK_1 cells and the dichlorovinylcysteine-induced LLC-PK_1 clones (Fig. 4). Compared with the untreated cells, the nuclear matrix of the clones contained at least five new proteins, while four other proteins present in the untreated control cells could not be detected in the nuclear matrix isolated from the clones. In addition, at least four proteins were present with clearly higher concentrations in the nuclear matrix of the dichlorovinylcysteine-clones. Hence, the changes in the dedifferentiated LLC-PK_1 clones induced with the key metabolite of the nephrotoxic and nephrocarcinogenic solvents trichloroethylene and dichloroacetylene may be involved in the malignant transformation of renal tubule epithelia and the

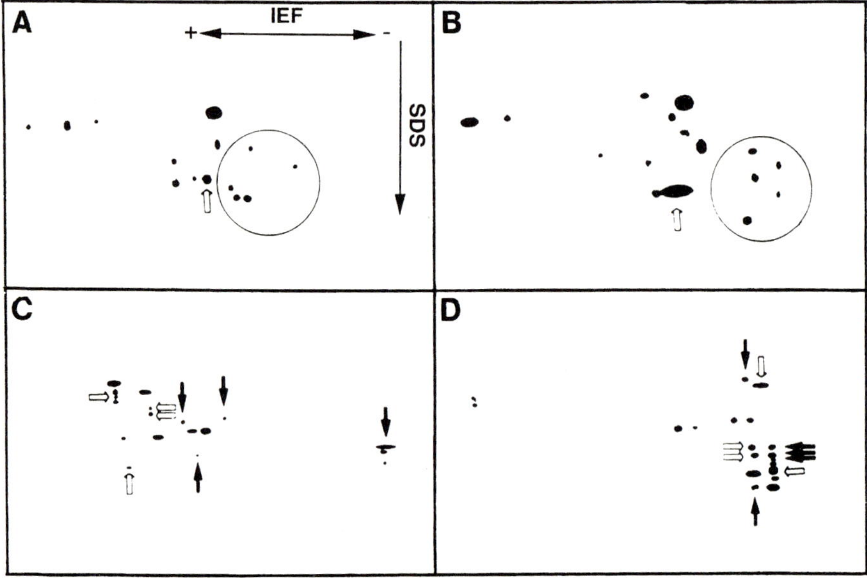

Fig. 4A–D. Comparison of the protein composition of the intermediate filament fractions (*upper panels)* and of the nuclear matrix fractions (*lower panels)* in untreated control LLC-PK_1 cells **(A,C)** and a clone induced with 5 μM dichlorovinylcysteine **(B,D)**. The intermediate filament and the nuclear matrix proteins were examined by equilibrium two-dimensional gel electrophoresis. The *circled areas* in the upper panels indicate clear qualitative differences in the intermediate filament protein composition between the control cells and the dichlorovinylcysteine-derived clone. The *shaded arrows* (↑)represent proteins which are unique for the untreated control LLC-PK_1 cells or for the dedifferentiated clone. The *open arrows* (⇑) indicate protein spots found both in control cells and in the dedifferentiated clone but at different concentration levels. Data are from one typical experiment out three

formation of renal cell tumors observed in the rat and also in workers chronically exposed to trichloroethylene (NTP 1988, 1990; Puck and Krystosek 1992; Vamvakas and Köster 1993; Henschler et al. 1995).

We are currently investigating the nuclear matrix and intermediate filament protein composition in specimens from human renal cell tumors in comparison with the tissue of origin, the adjacent normal renal parenchyma, aiming to answer the following questions: (a) Are specific changes in the protein composition characteristic of the malignant tissue? (b) Are these changes related to the tumor stage (size, metastases), and do they have a predictive value for the patients' prognosis? Furthermore, experiments are currently in progress aiming to identify the altered proteins with specific antibodies and by sequencing of the proteins contained in the gel spots.

References

Althaus FR, Lawrence SD, Sattler GL, Pitot HC (1982) ADP-Ribosyltransferase activity in cultured hepatocytes. J Biol Chem 257: 5528–5535

Benjamin R, Gill DM (1980) Poly(ADP-ribose) synthesis in vitro programmed by damaged DNA. A comparison of DNA molecules containing different types of strand breaks. J Biol Chem 255: 10502–10508

Borghoff SJ, Short BG, Swenberg JA (1990) Biochemical mechanisms and pathobiology of alpha 2u-globulin nephropathy. Annu Rev Pharmacol Toxicol 30: 349–367

Boulikas T (1989) DNA strand breaks alter histone ADP-ribosylation. Proc Natl Acad Sci USA 86: 3499–3503

Boulikas T (1992a) Poly(ADP-ribose)synthesis in blocked and damaged cells and its relation to carcinogenesis. Anticancer Res 12: 885–898

Boulikas T (1992b) Poly(ADP-ribosyl)ation, repair, chromatin and cancer. Curr Perspect Mol Cell Oncol 1: 1–9

Boulikas T (1993a) Poly(ADP-ribosyl)ation of variant histones and possible implications in carcinogenesis. Int J Oncol 2: 105–110

Boulikas T (1993b) Poly(ADP-ribosyl)ation, DNA strand breaks, chromatin and cancer. Toxicol Lett 67: 129–150

Brancolini C, Schneider C (1991) Change in the expression of a nuclear matrix-associated protein is correlated with cellular transformation. Proc Natl Acad Sci USA 88: 6936–6940

Chan D, Goate A, Puck TT (1989) Involvement of vimentin in the reverse transformation reaction. Proc Natl Acad Sci USA 86: 2747–2751

Dekant W, Vamvakas S, Berthold K, Schmidt S, Wild D, Henschler D (1986) Bacterial β-lyase-mediated cleavage and mutagenicity of cysteine conjugates derived from the nephrocarcinogenic alkenes trichloroethylene, tetrachloroethylene and hexachlorobutadiene. Chem Biol Interact 60: 31–45

Dekant W, Vamvakas S, Anders MW (1989) Bioactivation of nephrotoxic haloalkenes by glutathione conjugation: formation of toxic and mutagenic intermediates by cysteine conjugate β-lyase. Drug Metab Rev 20: 43–83

Denda A, Tsutsumi M, Yokose Y (1988) Effect of 3-aminobenzamide on the induction of γ-glutamyltranspeptidase-positive foci by various chemicals in rat liver. Cancer Lett 39: 29–36

Durkacz BW, Omidiji O, Gray DA, Shall S (1980) (ADP-ribose) participates in DNA excision repair. Nature 283: 593–596

Fey EG, Penman S (1984) Tumor promoters induce a specific morphological signature in the nuclear matrix-intermediate filament scaffold on Madin-Darby canine kidney (MDCK) cell colonies. Proc Natl Acad Sci USA 81: 4409–4413

Fey EG, Penman S (1988) Nuclear matrix proteins reflect cell type of origin in cultured human cells. Proc Natl Acad Sci USA 85: 121–125

Getzenberg RH, Coffey DS (1990) Tissue specificity of the hormonal response in sex accessory tissues is associated with nuclear matrix protein patterns. Mol Endocrinol 4: 1336–1342

Getzenberg RH, Pienta KJ, Huang EY, Coffey DS (1991a) Identification of nuclear matrix proteins in the cancer and normal rat prostate. Cancer Res 51: 6514–6520

Getzenberg RH, Pienta KJ, Huang EYW, Murphy BC, Coffey DS (1991b) Modifications of the intermediate filament and nuclear matrix networks by the extracellular matrix. Biochem Biophys Res Commun 179: 340–344

Getzenberg RH, Pienta KJ, Ward WS, Coffey DS (1992) Nuclear structure and the three-dimensional organization of DNA. J Cell Biochem 47: 289–299

Green JA, Carthew P, Heuillet E, Simpson JL, Manson MM (1990) Cytokeratin expression during AFB1-induced carcinogenesis. Carcinogenesis 11: 1175–1182

Henschler D, Vamvakas S, Lammert M, Dekant W, Kraus B, Thomas B, Ulm K (1995) High incidence of renal cell tumors in a cohort of cardboard workers exposed to trichloroethene. Arch Toxicol 69: 291–299

Jaffe DR, Hassall CD, Gandolfi AJ, Brendel K (1985) Production of DNA single strand breaks in renal tissue after exposure to 1,2-dichlorovinylcysteine. Toxicology 35: 25-33

Kanhai W, Dekant W, Henschler D (1989) Metabolism of the nephrotoxin dichloroacetylene by glutathione conjugation. Chem Res Toxicol 2: 51–56

Keese SK, Meneghini MD, Szaro RP, Wu Y-J (1994) Nuclear matrix proteins in human colon cancer. Proc Natl Acad Sci USA 91: 1913–1916

Khanuja PS, Lehr JE, Soule HD, Noto AC, Choudhury S, Chen R, Pienta KJ (1993) Nuclear matrix proteins in normal breast cancer cells. Cancer Res 53: 3394–3398

Krystosek A, Chan DC (1990) Genome regulation in mammalian cells. Somat Cell Mol Genet 16: 257-265

Kuchino Y, Mori F, Kasai H, Inoue H, Iwai S, Miura K, Ohtsuka E, Nishimura S (1987) DNA templates containing 8-hydroxydeoxyguanosine are mistread both at the modified base and at adjacent residues. Nature 327: 77–79

Kurokawa Y, Maekawa A, Takahashi M, Hayashi Y (1990) Toxicity and carcinogenicity of potassium bromate – a new renal carcinogen. Environ Health Perspect 87: 309–335

Li JL, Okada S, Hamazaki S, Ebina Y, Midorikawa O (1987) Subacute nephrotoxicity and induction of renal cell carcinoma in mice treated with ferric nitrilotriacetate. Cancer Res 47: 1867–1869

McLaren J, Boulikas T, Vamvakas S (1994) Induction of poly(ADP-ribosyl)ation in the kidney after in vivo application of renal carcinogens. Toxicology 88: 101–112

Miettinen M, Franssila K, Lehto V-P, Paasivuo R, d Virtanen I (1984) Expression of intermediate filament proteins in thyroid gland and thyroid tumors. Lab Invest 50: 262–270

Miller TE, Beausang LA, Winchell LF, Lidgard GP (1992) Detection of nuclear matrix proteins in serum from cancer patients. Cancer Res 52: 422–427

Nakayasu H, Berezney R (1991) Nuclear matrix: identification of the major nuclear matrix proteins. Proc Natl Acad Sci USA 88: 10312–10316

NTP (1988) National toxicology program. Toxicology and carcinogenesis studies of trichloroethylene in four strains of rats (ACI, August, Marshall, Osborne-Mendel) (gavage studies). US Department of Health and Human Services TR no 273

NTP (1990) Carcinogenesis studies of trichloroethylene (without epichlorohydrin) in F344/N rats and B6C3F1 mice (gavage studies). US Department of Health and Human Services TR no 243

Okada S, Midorikawa O (1982) Induction of the rat renal adenocarcinoma by Fe-nitrilotriacetate. Jpn Arch Intern Med 36: 41–47

Parodi S, Taningher M, Santi L, Cavanua M, Sciaba L, Maura A, Brambilla G (1978) A practical procedure for testing DNA damage in vivo proposed for a pre-screening of chemical carcinogens. Mutat Res 54: 39–44

Pegg AE (1988) Alkylation and subsequent repair of DNA after exposure to dimethylnitrosamine and related carcinogens. Rev Biochem Toxicol 5: 83–95

Petzold GL, Swenberg JA (1978) Detection of DNA damage induced in vivo following exposure of rats to carcinogens. Cancer Res 38: 1589–1597

Pitz S, Moll R, Störkel S, Thoenes W (1987) Expression of intermediate filament protein in subtypes of renal cell carcinomas and in renal oncocytomas. Distinction of two classes of renal cell tumors. Lab Invest 56: 642–653

Poirier GG, de Murcia G, Jongstra-Bilen J, Niedergang C, Mandel P (1982) Poly(ADP-ribosyl)ation of polynucleosomes causes relaxation of chromatin structure. Proc Natl Acad Sci USA 79: 3423–3432

Puck TT, Krystosek A (1992) Role of the cytoskeleton in genome regulation and cancer. Int Rev Cytol 132: 75–108

Ray SD, Sorge CL, Kamendulis LM, Corcoran GB (1992) Ca^{++}-activated DNA fragmentation and dimethylnitrosamin-induced hepatic necrosis: effects of Ca^{++}-endonuclease and poly(ADP-ribose)polymerase inhibitors in mice. J Pharmacol Exp Ther 263: 387–394

Sahai A, Cole LA, Tannen RL (1989) Pathways and regulation of ammoniagenesis by the LLC-PK_1 cells in culture. J Lab Clin Med 114: 285–293

Sahai A, Xu G, Sandler RS, Tannen RL (1992) Hypoxia-mediated impaired differentiation by LLC-PK_1 cells: evidence based on the protein kinase C profile. Kidney Int 42: 1145–1152

Siddiqi MA, Bothe E (1987) Single- and double-strand break formation in DNA irradiated in aqueous solution: dependence on dose and OH radical scavenger concentration. Radiat Res 112: 449-463

Singh N (1990a) A comparative study on the effect of tumor promoters on poly-ADP-ribosylation in A431 cells. Int J Cancer 46: 648–651

Singh N (1990b) Effect of tumor promoters on poly-ADP-ribosylation in human epidermoid carcinoma HeP2 cells. Int J Exp Pathol 71:809–902

Swann PF, Kaufman DG, Magee PN, Mace R (1980) Induction of kidney tumours by a single dose of dimethylnitrosamine: dose response and influence of diet and benzo[a]pyrene pretreatment. Br J Cancer 41: 285–294

Toyokuni S, Sagripanti J-L (1993) DNA single- and double-strand breaks produced by ferric nitrilotriacetate in relation to renal tubular carcinogenesis. Carcinogenesis 14: 223–227

Tsujiuchi T, Tsutsumi M, Denda A, Kondoh S, Nakae D, Maruyama H, Konishi Y (1990) Possible involvement of poly ADP-ribosylation in phenobarbital promotion of rat hepatocarcinogenesis. Carcinogenesis 11: 1783–1787

Vamvakas S, Köster U (1993) The nephrotoxin dichlorovinylcysteine induces expression of the protooncogenes c-*fos* and c-*myc* in LLC-PK_1 cells – a comparative investigation with growth factors and 12-*O*-tetradecanoylphorbolacetate. Cell Biol Toxicol 9: 1–13

Vamvakas S, Dekant W, Henschler D (1989) Assessment of unscheduled DNA synthesis in a cultured line of renal epithelial cells exposed to cysteine *S*-conjugates of haloalkenes and haloalkanes. Mutat Res 222: 329–335

Vamvakas S, Sharma VK, Shen S-S, Anders MW (1990) Perturbations of intracellular calcium distribution in kidney cells by nephrotoxic haloalkenyl cysteine *S*-conjugates. Mol Pharmacol 38: 455–461

Vamvakas S, Bittner D, Dekant W, Anders MW (1992) Events that precede and that follow *S*-(1,2-dichlorovinyl)-*l*-cysteine-induced release of mitochondrial Ca^{2+} and their association with cytotoxicity to renal cells. Biochem Pharmacol 44: 1131–1138

Wada T, Yasutomi M, Hashmura K, Kunikata M, Tanaka T, Mori M (1992) Vimentin expression in benign and malignant lesions in the human mammary gland. Anticancer Res 12: 1973–1982

Ward JF (1990) The yield of DNA double-strand breaks produced intracellularly by ionizing radiation: a review. Int J Radiat Biol 57: 1141–1150

Yanada K, Shinohara H, Takai Y, Mori M (1988) Monoclonal antibody-detected vimentin distribution in pleomorphic adenomas of salivary glands. J Oral Pathol 17: 348–353

Yang CS, Tu YY, Koop D, Coon MJ (1985) Metabolism of nitrosamines by purified rabbit liver cytochrome P-450 isoenzymes. Cancer Res 45: 1140–1146

Genotoxic and Chronic Toxic Effects in the Carcinogenicity of Aromatic Amines

A. Bitsch, J. Fecher, M. Jost, P.-C. Klöhn, and H.-G. Neumann

Department of Toxicology, University of Würzburg, Versbacher Str. 9, 97078 Würzburg, Germany

Introduction

Many polycyclic aromatic amines are mutagenic, and their genotoxic properties are held responsible for their biological effects. The genotoxic effects are explained by the formation of metabolites that react with macromolecules by forming adducts (Kriek 1969; Franz et al. 1986). DNA adducts may cause mutations which are responsible for tumorigenic effects. Results from comparative studies, however, indicate that tissue-specific and species-specific tumor formation caused by arylamines cannot be explained readily by the extent of DNA modifications. Long-term feeding of 2-acetylaminofluorene (AAF) typically produces liver tumors; 2-acetylaminophenanthrene (AAP), mammary tumors; and *trans*-4-acetylaminostilbene (AAS), Zymbal's gland tumors in rats (Neumann et al. 1970). All three arylamines are genotoxic. They generate comparable DNA adduct levels in rat liver, and in liver more extensively than in any other tissue (Neumann 1983; Ruthsatz and Neumann 1988; Gupta et al. 1989). But only AAF is a complete carcinogen in rat liver. AAS and AAP are able to produce liver tumors in rats only, if initiation is followed by some promotion treatment (Hammel 1989). Therefore, DNA binding may reflect the formation of some critical lesions related to tumor initiation but is not sufficient to explain carcinogenic effects. This raises two questions: (1) Do differences in genotoxic initiating effects contribute to tissue specificity? and (2) What are the additional promoting properties of AAF that distinguish it from the incomplete liver carcinogens?

Our aim is to characterize mutagenic initiating and promoting properties of the above arylamines. Different types of experiments will be described.

1. In an initiation-promotion model according to Peraino et al. (1981), we studied the initiating potency of the arylamines in vivo. Rat liver tumors were initiated with the three amines, and phenobarbital was used for promotion. GST-P, a fetal protein that is highly expressed in neoplastic and preneoplastic foci, was investigated by immunohistochemistry.

Recent Results in Cancer Research, Vol. 143

2. In the mammalian cell culture AS52, we investigated whether amine-specific differences exist in the primary DNA lesions. AS52 cells are hypoxanthine-guanine phosphoribosyltransferase (HPRT)-deficient CHO cells that are transfected with the bacterial xanthine-guanine phosphoribosyltransferase gene (gpt) (Mulligan and Berg 1981). Mutations in the gpt gene that induce 6-thioguanine resistance were quantified.
3. In human hepatoma (HepG2) cells the expression of stress proteins, so-called heat shock proteins (HSPs), was analyzed. Heat shock proteins are believed to play a cytoprotective role within the cell. A series of these proteins (HSP90, HSP70, HSP20/30, and ubiquitin) is induced by environmental stress like temperature shock and exposure to chemicals (Welch 1992). Our question was whether stress induced by exposure to carcinogenic arylamines could be demonstrated by changes in the expression of HSPs.
4. Isolated rat liver mitochondria were used for biochemical studies with the AAF metabolite 2-NOF. The involvement of liver mitochondria was indicated by recent investigations of tumor-promoting properties of AAF. Following up the observation that oxygen consumption of rat liver increases upon AAF feeding, a highly specific mechanism of producing oxidative stress in mitochondria was proposed (Neumann et al. 1992).
5. AAF was chronically administered to adult animals for up to 16 weeks. Mitochondria were isolated from treated livers in order to confirm results from in vitro experiments on isolated mitochondria. Furthermore, livers were investigated by histochemistry to study correlations between mitochondrial injuries and cirrhosis-like transformation of the liver.

Methods

Chemicals

2-Acetylaminofluorene (AAF) was obtained from Merck (Darmstadt, Germany), and phenobarbital (PB) from Serva (Heidelberg, Germany). 2-Acetylaminophenanthrene (AAP) and trans-4-acetylaminostilbene (AAS) were synthesized and characterized according to Calder and Williams (1974) and Metzler and Neumann (1971). Nitrosofluorene was synthesized from 2-nitrofluorene (Lotlikar et al. 1965), and the synthesis of nitrosophenanthrene followed the method of Gupta et al. (1989) with some modifications.

Animals and Treatment

Newborn Wistar rats were used for an initiation-promotion experiment. Rats were randomly divided into five treatment groups. The three aromatic amines were dissolved in tinned milk and orally administered at days 5, 7, 9, and 11 postnatally: AAF and AAP (1.5 mmol/kg body weight), AAS (0.15 mmol/kg).

Control groups were treated with the solvent only. The rats were maintained on normal diet with Altromin 1324 (Altrogge, Lage, Germany) and water ad libitum under standard conditions. Promotion with phenobarbital (500 ppm in the drinking water) was started at day 35. Rats were killed after 26, 52, and 104 weeks. Tumors, if present, were prepared from the surrounding tissue.

For long-term application of AAF, male Wistar rats (180–200 g) were maintained under standard conditions with free access to diet, either standard Altromin 1324 or diet supplemented with 0.02% AAF. Rats were killed after 2, 4, 6, and 16 weeks of feeding.

Histochemistry

Formalin-fixed, paraffin-embedded 4- to 6-μm liver sections were stained with hematoxylin/eosin (HE). The tumor marker glutathione-S-transferase (GST-P) was investigated on 4- to 6-μm cryosections by immunohistochemistry according to the method of Sato et al. (1984).

Isolated Liver Mitochondria

Intact liver mitochondria were isolated by differential centrifugation as described (Weinbach 1961). All procedures were performed at 4 °C. The final mitochondrial pellet was dissolved in isolation buffer at protein concentrations of 20 mg/ml.

The rate of respiration was measured polarographically with a clark oxygen electrode DW1 (Bachofer, Reutlingen, Germany). Respiration was supported by glutamate/malate. Respiration control ratios (RCR) were determined as the ratio of state-3/state-4 respiration. Mitochondria (2.5 mg/ml) in respiration buffer (pH 7.4, containing 0.3 *M* sucrose, 5 m*M* (*N*-2-morpholino)propane sulfonic acid (MOPS), 2 m*M* ethyleneglycoltetraacetic acid (EGTA), 5 m*M* KH_2PO_4, 5 m*M* $MgSO_4$, and 0.1% bovine serum albumin (BSA) (fatty acid-free)) were incubated at 25 °C with 5 m*M* succinate and 5 μM Rotenon. After 5 min, nitroso derivatives were added and O_2 consumption under non-phosphorylating conditions was measured (state-4). After 1 min adenosine diphosphate (ADP) (150 μM) was added and O_2 consumption under phosphorylating conditions (state-3) was recorded.

Contents of cytochromes $a+a_3$, b, and $c+c_1$ in rat liver mitochondria were quantified by dual-wavelength spectrophotometry. The extinction coefficient used for the determination of cytochrome $a+a_3$ was $\Delta\varepsilon$ (605–630 nm) = 24 $mM^{-1} \times cm^{-1}$, and those for cytochrome b and cytochrome $c+c_1$ were $\Delta\varepsilon$ (560–575 nm) = 23.4 $mM^{-1} \times cm^{-1}$ and $\Delta\varepsilon$ (542–550 nm) = 18.7 $mM^{-1} \times cm^{-1}$, respectively (von Jagow and Klingenberg 1972).

Cell Cultures

AS52 cell lines (gpt+) and conditions for their growth have been described previously by Stankowski et al. (1986). Stock cultures were maintained in monolayer in flasks in MPA medium ($F_{12}FCM_5$ containing 250 μg/ml xanthine, 25 μg/ml adenine, 50 μM thymidine, 3 μM aminopterin, and 10 μg/ml mycophenolic acid) with 10% fetal calf serum (FCS) at 37 °C and 100% humidity in 5% CO_2 in air. HepG2 cells were cultured under standard conditions (37 °C, 100% humidity, 5% CO_2 in air) in DMEM (Dulbecco's modified Eagle's medium with 1 g/l glucose) medium with 10% FCS. Incubation with 50 μM AAF solubilized in dimethylsulfoxide (DMSO) was carried out for 4 h at 37 °C, and proteins were isolated.

Cytotoxicity and Mutation Frequency

Cytotoxicity and mutations to thioguanine resistance were determined in AS52 cells as described previously by Stankowski et al. (1986). Briefly, duplicate cultures of approximately 10^6 cells per flask were treated with arylamines for 2.5 h at 37 °C in Ham's F_{12} in the presence and absence of an exogenous activation system (S9-mix). Treatment with ethylmethanesulfonate served as a control for the test system. The metabolic activation system consisted of AAF-induced rat liver homogenate (S9-mix), supplemented with nicotinamide adenine dinucleotide phosphate, reduced (NADPH) and citrate. Cytotoxicity was measured as cell survival on day 1 and day 8 after treatment. Then, 10^6 cells were again subcultured and allowed to express the thioguanine-resistant phenotype. Colonies were stained with Giemsa (Merck, Darmstadt, Germany) on day 8, and mutant frequencies calculated as mutants/10^6 clonable cells, corrected for cloning efficiency.

Protein Analysis

Proteins from HepG2 cells were resolved in a lysis buffer (O' Farrell 1975). Equal amounts of protein from each sample were separated in the first dimension on a gel system for IEF (isoelectric focusing). Sodium dodecyl sulfate (SDS)-polyacrylamide gel electrophoresis was performed for the second dimension (Laemmli 1970). Proteins were blotted onto nitrocellulose membrane and immunostained with an antibody raised against HSP 72/73 (Biochemical, Santa Cruz, CA, USA). Gels were fixed in 45% methanol, 9% acetic acid, and silver stained for proteins. Molecular weights were estimated using a protein standard (carboanhydrase 29 kD, ovalbumin 45 kD, glutamic dehydrogenase 55 kD, albumin 66 kD, and phosphorylase b 97 kD).

Results

Genotoxic Properties of Aromatic Amines In Vivo

In the initiation-promotion experiment early changes of the tumor marker GST-P were demonstrated in rat livers (Fig. 1). Although no macroscopic changes were seen in rat livers 26 weeks after initiation, a large number of GST-P-positive foci was already detected. AAF and AAP were given at a dose tenfold higher than that of AAS; nevertheless, in all initiated livers comparable numbers of GST-P-positive foci occurred. The number of foci per cm^2 is generally greater in male than in female animals. The first tumors developed 52 weeks after initiation. Tumor incidences do not differ significantly in the different groups of treatment (data not shown).

Genotoxic Properties of Aromatic Amines In Vitro

AS52 cells were used as an in vitro test system to compare and distinguish the cytotoxic and mutagenic effects of the three aromatic amines. Enzyme patterns in these cells are not yet well defined. Therefore, experiments were done with and without exogenous activation systems. Mutation rates without exogenous activation are within the control level, indicating a low metabolic capacity of AS52 cells. Additional activation with S9-mix revealed AAF and AAP equally but with less mutagenicity and cytotoxicity than AAS (Fig. 2). Furthermore, cytotoxicity and mutagenicity of several metabolites of AAF were investigated. 2-NOF was more cytotoxic than N-OH-AAF (Fig. 3).

Chronic Toxic Properties of AAF In Vitro

O_2 consumption is increased in perfused livers from AAF-treated rats. Therefore mitochondria were considered to be involved in tumor-promoting effects of AAF (Neumann et al. 1992).

We found that 2-NOF, a metabolite of AAF, withdraws electrons from the inner site of the b/c_1 complex of the mitochondrial respiration chain, which has an impact on control mechanisms of oxidative phosphorylation (Fig. 4). 2-NOF is reduced to the corresponding nitroxyl radical, which readily autoxidizes to form cytotoxic O_2^-. As a result of redox cycling, 2-NOF uncouples oxidative phosphorylation in a dose-dependent manner (Klöhn and Neumann, submitted). In isolated mitochondria, redox cycling of 2-NOF and 2-NOP, which are metabolites of AAF and AAP, induce uncoupling of oxidative phospho-rylation, at concentrations as low as 1 nmol/mg mitochondrial protein. 2-NOF is approximately twice as effective as the phenanthrene derivative 2-NOP (Fig. 5).

The expression of stress proteins was studied in a simple in vitro system. Human (HepG2) hepatoma cells in culture were incubated with AAF. Heat

A

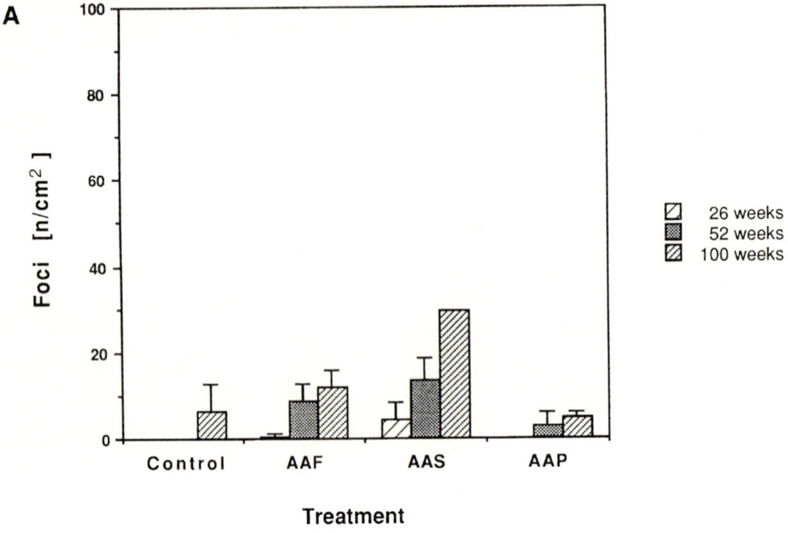

B

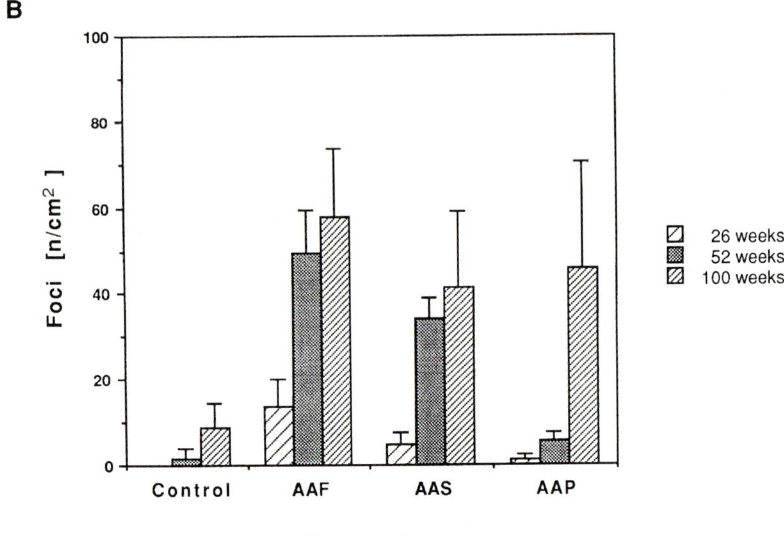

Fig. 1. Number of glutathione-S-transferase (GST-P)-positive foci in livers of female (**A**) and male (**B**) rats from an initiation-promotion experiment. Rats were treated with 2-acetylaminofluorene (AAF), 2-acetylaminophenanthrene (AAP) (1.5 mmol/kg, and *trans*-4-acetylaminostilbene (AAS) (0.15 mmol/kg) as initiators and phenobarbital as a tumor promoter. Livers were taken after indicated times

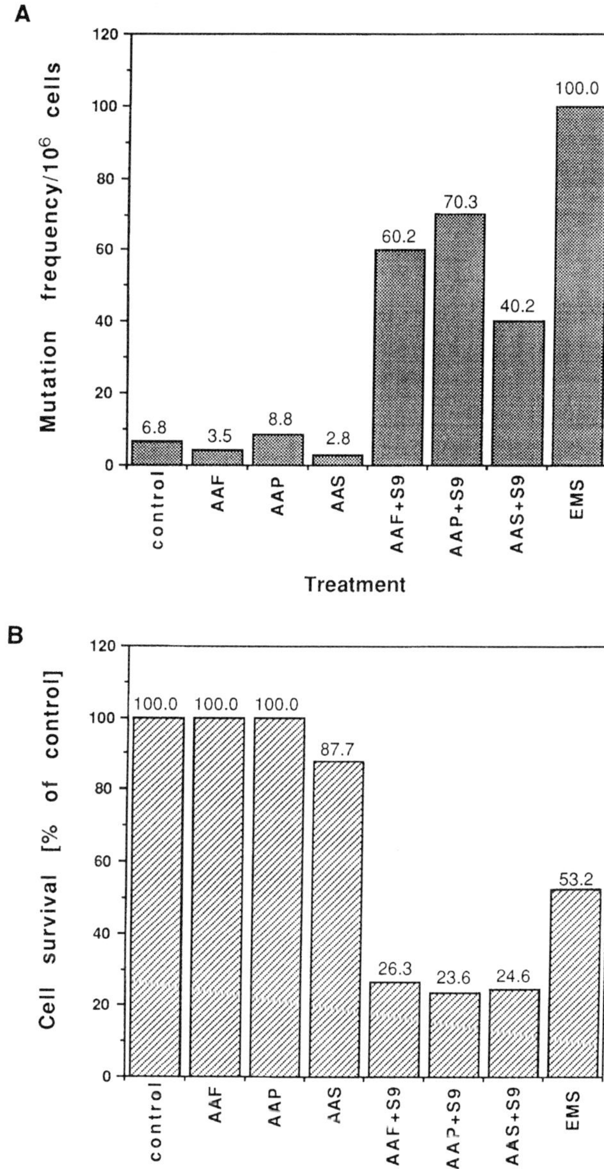

Fig. 2. Mutagenic (**A**) and cytotoxic (**B**) effects of aromatic amines in AS52 cells. AS52 were treated with 30 μM AAF, 30 μM AAP, and 3 μM AAS for 2.5 h with and without exogenous activation (S9-mix). Cell survival was determined on day 1, mutation frequencies on day 8 after treatment. *EMS*, ethylmethanesulfonate (250 μM)

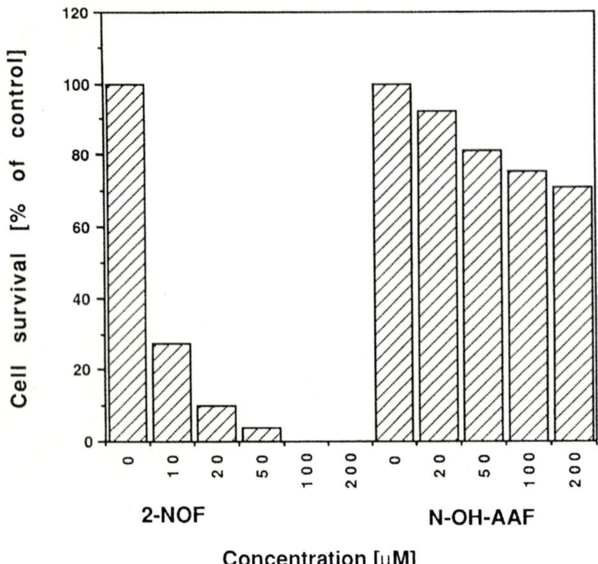

Fig. 3. Cytotoxic effects of AAF metabolites in AS52 cells. AS52 cells were treated with indicated concentrations of 2-NOF and N-OH-AAF for 2.5 h without exogenous activation. Cell survival was determined on day 3 after treatment

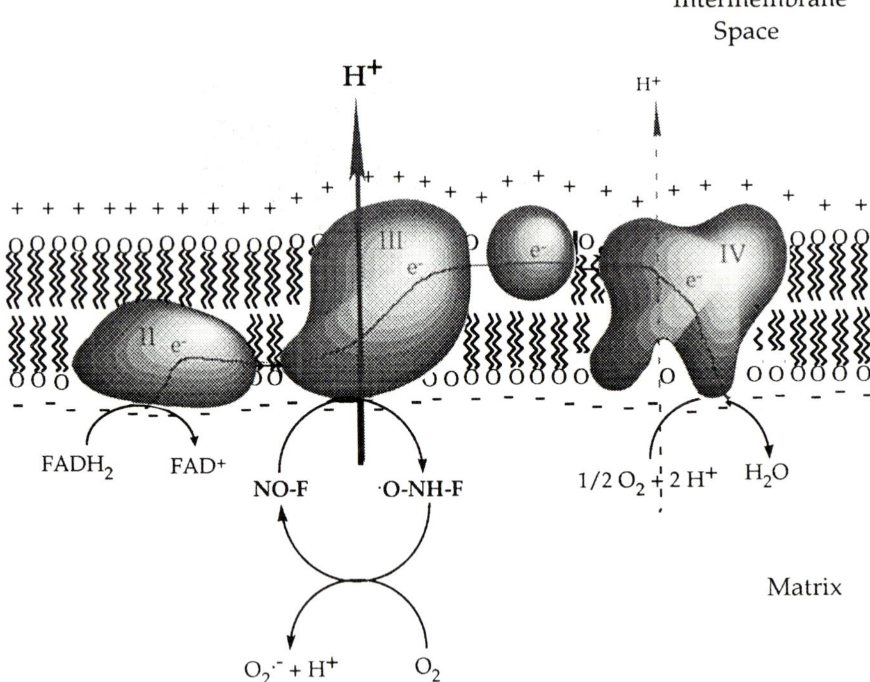

Fig. 4. Schematic presentation of redox cycling of 2-NOF in mitochondria. 2-NOF uncouples oxidative phosphorylation by impairing transmembrane electrochemical proton gradient

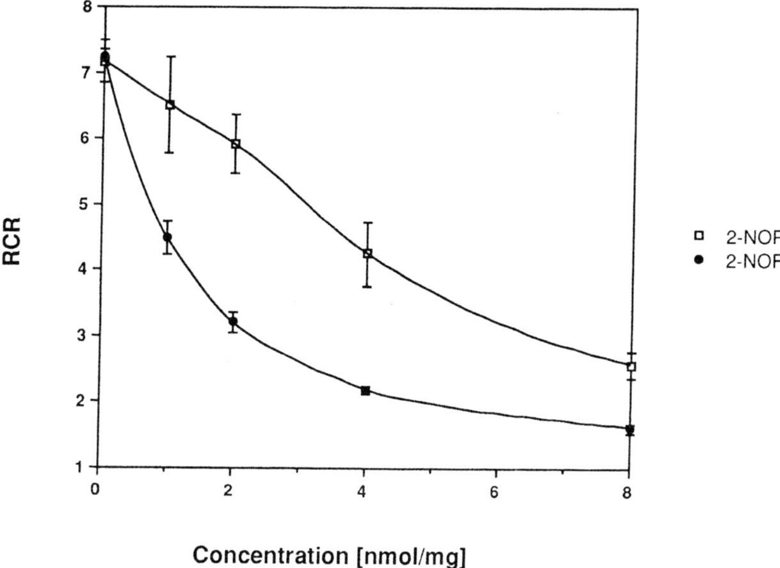

Fig. 5. Comparison of 2-NOF and 2-NOP effects on uncoupling oxidative phosphorylation in isolated mitochondria. The rate of respiration was measured in isolated mitochondria polarographically with an oxygen electrode. Respiration was supported by glutamate/malate. Respiration control ratio (RCR) values were determined as the ratio state-3/state-4 respiration

treatment of the cells served as a positive control. Isolated proteins were separated on 2D gel electrophoresis and immunoblotted for HSP72/73. In preliminary experiments we demonstrated alterations in the expression of heat shock proteins with this approach. Cells incubated with AAF express – in addition to the proteins induced by solvents or heat – other isoforms of the hsp70 family (Fig. 6).

Chronic Toxic Properties of AAF In Vivo

An increase of cytochromes was demonstrated in liver mitochondria after long-term feeding of rats with 0.02% AAF. The content as well as the activity of mitochondrial cytochrome-c-oxidase increased significantly after 8 weeks of 2-AAF feeding. In controls cytochrome-c-oxidase shows a zonal distribution of activity. The activity is higher in oxygen-rich zones. After 4–6 weeks of feeding, the total activity increased, while the zonal distribution leveled off (data not shown). The content of cytochrome a/a_3 and of cytochrome c/c_1 is elevated, but not that of b-cytochromes (cytochrome b_{566} and cytochrome b_{562}) (Fig. 7).

At the same time (6 weeks), the number of eosinophilic hepatocytes increases in the periportal region and foci appear in the liver lobule. Oval cells

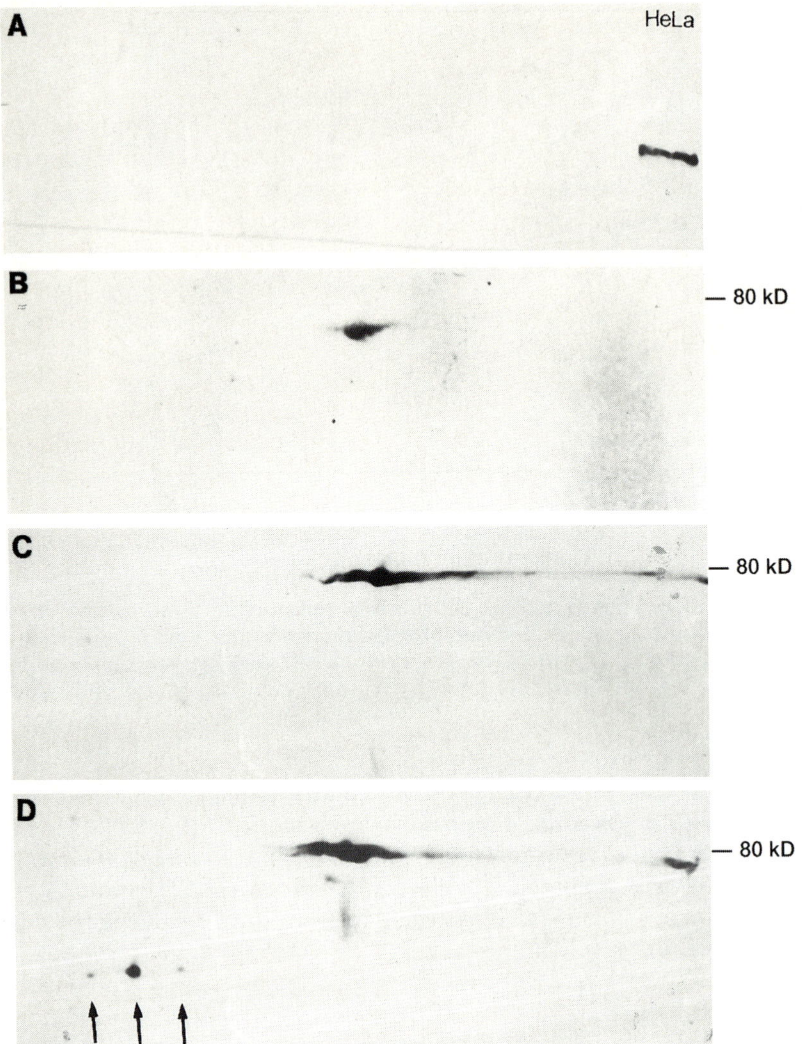

Fig. 6A–D. Expression of HSP72/73 in AAF-treated human hepatoma (HepG2) cells. HepG2 cells were treated with 50 μM AAF for 4 h at 37 °C or 43 °C, respectively. Proteins were separated by 2-D gel electrophoresis, blotted and immunostained for HSP70s. **A** Control (with HeLa cells as positive control). **B** Heat treatment. **C** Solvent. **D** AAF treatment

appear after 4–6 weeks in the area of bile ducts of the periportal field and start to penetrate the parenchyma along the sinusoids (Fig. 8). After 16 weeks of AAF feeding they form septa around the parenchyma.

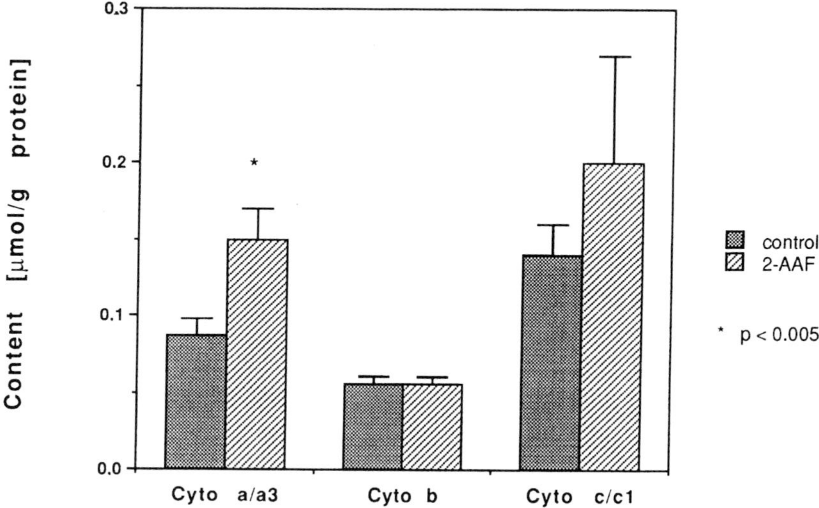

Fig. 7. Effects of AAF on the content of cytochromes in rat liver mitochondria. Male Wistar rats were fed with 0.02% AAF in diet, liver mitochondria were isolated, and the content of cytochrome was quantified by dual-wavelength spectrophotometry

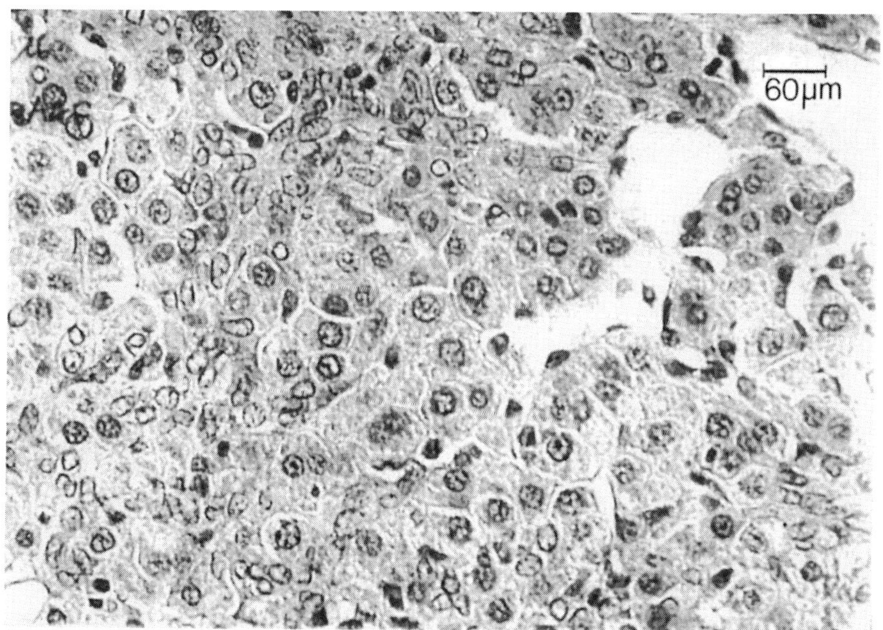

Fig. 8. Oval cell proliferation in the periportal area of rat liver after 6 weeks of long-term feeding. Male Wistar rats were fed with 0.02% AAF in diet; formalin-fixed liver sections were stained with H&E

Discussion

Cellular alterations that take place during chemically induced liver carcinogenesis include the expression of several fetal proteins in enzyme-altered foci. One of these fetal proteins is GST-P, whose expression correlates well with the formation of preneoplastic and neoplastic foci. The formation of GST-P-positive foci in the initiation-promotion experiment clearly indicates the tumor-initiating properties of all three amines, which confirms previous observations (Bitsch et al. 1993). In general, the number of foci per cm^2 is greater in male than in female animals. Sex-specific effects of two aromatic amines in combination have already been reported previously (Hammerl et al. 1994). Considering the lower dose of AAS, the initiating potency decreased AAS > AAF = AAP in both sexes. AAF, which is the only complete carcinogen in rat liver, was not the most potent initiator.

Although the mutagenic and cytotoxic effects of AAF have been thoroughly investigated (McGregor 1988), no in vitro assay has been used so far to compare directly the genotoxic properties of the three amines. Following metabolic activation all three compounds were mutagenic and cytotoxic. In agreement with the results from the initiation-promotion experiment, AAS was the most mutagenic and cytotoxic amine. The comparative studies in these two systems demonstrate AAF and AAP to be equally but less efficient than AAS. This suggests that only a combination of genotoxic and specific toxic properties can explain why AAF is a complete carcinogen in rat liver.

Mitochondria were therefore considered a possible target for AAF toxicity (Neumann et al. 1992). 2-NOF, a metabolite of AAF, which may be formed in vivo in microsomes by deacylation of N-OH-AAF and subsequent oxidation, induced cyanide-resistant O_2 consumption in isolated mitochondria (Neumann et al. 1994). A role for free radical processes in 2-NOF metabolism was first proposed by Floyd et al. (1976), who demonstrated a reaction with lipid membranes. Our experiments with isolated mitochondria suggest that tumor-promoting effects of AAF are related to oxidative stress induced by mitochondrial redox cycling of 2-NOF and uncoupling of oxidative phosphorylation (Neumann et al. 1992; Klöhn et al. 1995). Recently, the proposed superoxide anion formation was able to be confirmed (Massalha et al. 1994).

The mechanism of uncoupling by the nitroso derivatives 2-NOF and 2-NOP is associated with an impairment of the transmembrane electrochemical proton gradient. In comparative studies of 2-NOF and 2-NOP we now show that 2-NOF uncouples oxidative phosphorylation twice as much as 2-NOP, which may explain the higher toxicity of AAF. Redox cycling of 2-NOF induces decreased energy conversion in addition to the oxidative stress. This is supported by in vivo observations in AAF-treated rat livers, which reveal an increase of cytochrome-c-oxidase activity and cytochrome contents as an adaptive response to this impairment. The results obtained by detailed studies with mitochondria in vitro may well explain the chronic toxic effect observed in vivo. Oval cell proliferation was observed after feeding AAF-containing diet in the periportal zones of rat liver, which are rich in mitochondria. We propose that cytotoxic events in hepatocytes precede the emergence of oval cells.

Liver tissue may thus respond to AAF-induced stress by various adaptive responses that lead to a cirrhosis-like transformation of the liver (Ambs 1992).

A conserved response of cells to environmental stress including heat and chemical exposure is the synthesis of heat shock proteins (HSPs; Lindquist and Craig 1988). The HSPs are a diverse family of proteins consisting of both constitutively expressed and stress-induced members. They are involved in a wide range of cellular processes including folding of nascent proteins, protein targeting, and many protein-protein interactions (Rothman 1990). Heat shock proteins are thought to prevent aberrant proteins from precipitating in the cell (Beckmann et al. 1990). Donati et al. (1990) demonstrated a heat shock response to oxidative injury. We therefore asked whether hepatoma cells exposed to AAF react to oxidative stress by increasing HSP levels.

Preliminary results suggest that there is indeed a specific effect of AAF on the expression of members of the HSP70 family. These effects may represent another adaptive response of cells to oxidative stress induced by redox cycling of 2-NOF, and they encourage further studies.

AAF triggers at least two independent processes, the generation of initiated cells by genotoxic effects and the transformation of the liver lobule by chronic toxicity. Both properties together are proposed to be necessary to make it a complete rat liver carcinogen.

Acknowledgements. These studies were supported by the Deutsche Forschungsgemeinschaft. We gratefully acknowledge the skillful help of Christian Günther for the synthesis of 2-NOP and of W. Caspary for the gift of AS52/XPRT cells. We also would like to thank I. Fenske for her technical assistance in histology.

References

Ambs S (1992) Die Bedeutung von oxidativem Stress in Rattenlebermitochondrien für die Erzeugung chronisch toxischer Effekte durch karzinogene aromatische Amine. Dissertation, Naturwissenschaftliche Fakultät, University of Würzburg

Beckmann RP, Mizzen LA, Welsh WJ (1990) Interaction of hsp70 with newly synthesized proteins: implications for folding and assembly. Science 248: 850–854

Bitsch A, Röschlau H, Deubelbeiss C, Neumann H-G (1993) The structure and function of the H-ras-protooncogene are not altered in rat liver tumors initiated by 2-acetylaminofluorene, 2-acetylaminophenanthrene and trans-4-acetylaminostilbene. Toxicol Lett 67: 173–186

Calder IC, Williams PJ (1974) The synthesis and reactions of some carcinogenic N-(2-phenanthryl)hydroxylamine derivatives. Aust J Chem 27: 1791–1795

Donati YR, Slosman DO, Polla BS (1990) Oxidative injury and the heat shock response. Biochem Pharmacol 40: 2571–2577

Floyd RA, Soong LM, Walker RN, Stuart M (1976) Lipid hydroperoxide activation of N-hydroxy-N-acetylaminofluorene via a free radical route. Cancer Res 36: 2761–2767

Franz R, Schulten HR, Neumann H-G (1986) Identification of nucleic acid adducts from trans-4-acetylaminostilbene. Chem Biol Interact 59: 281–293

Gupta RC, Earley K, Fullerton NF, Beland FA (1989) Formation and removal of DNA adducts in target and nontarget tissues of rats administered multiple doses of 2-acetophenanthrene. Carcinogenesis 10: 2025–2033

Hammerl R (1989) Zur synergistischen Wirkung aromatischer Amine bei der Initiierung von Tumoren in der Rattenleber. Dissertation, Tiermedizinische Fakultät, University of Munich

Hammerl R, Kirchner T, Neumann H-G (1994) Synergistic effects of trans-4-acetylaminostilbene and 2-acetylaminofluorene at the level of tumor initiation. Chem Biol Interact 93: 11–28

Klöhn PC, Massalha H, Neumann H-G (1995) A metabolite of carcinogenic 2-acetylaminofluorene, 2-nitrosofluorene, induces redox cycling in mitochondria. Biochim Biophys Acta 1229: 363–372

Kriek E (1969) On the mechanism of action of carcinogenic aromatic amines. I. Binding of 2-acetylaminofluorene and N-hydroxy-2-acetylaminofluorene to rat liver nucleic acids in vivo. Chem Biol Interact 1: 3–17

Laemmli UK (1970) Cleavage of structural proteins during the assembly of the head of bacteriophage T4. Nature 227: 680–685

Lindquist S, Craig EA (1988) The heat shock proteins. Annu Rev Genet 22: 631-677

Lotlikar PD, Miller EC, Miller JA, Margreth A (1965) The enzymatic reduction of the N-hydroxy derivatives of 2-acetylaminofluorene and related carcinogens by tissue preparations. Cancer Res 25: 1743–1752

Massalha H, Klöhn P-C, Neumann H-G (1994) 2-Nitrosofluorene effects on rat liver mitochondria: superoxide production, lipid peroxidation and a dual effect on respiration. Naunyn Schmiedebergs Arch Pharmacol [Suppl] 349: R128

McGregor D (1988) The activities of 2-acetylaminofluorene, 4-acetylaminofluorene, benzo(a)pyrene and pyrene in in vitro assays for genetic toxicity. In: Ashby J, de Serres FJ, Shelby MD, Margolin BH, Ishidate M Jr, Becking GC (eds) Report of the international programme on chemical safety's collaborative study on in vivo assays, vol. 2. Cambridge University Press, Cambridge, pp 345–350

Metzler M, Neumann H-G (1971) Zur Bedeutung chemisch-biologischer Wechselwirkungen für die toxische und krebserzeugende Wirkung aromatischer Amine. III Synthese und Analytik einiger Stoffwechselprodukte von trans-4-Dimethylaminostilben, cis-4-Dimethylaminostilben und 4-Dimethylaminobibenzyl. Tetrahedron 27: 2225–2246

Mulligan RC, Berg P (1981) Selection for animal cells that express the *Escherichia coli* gene coding for xanthine guanine phosphoribosyl transferase. Proc Natl Acad Sci USA 78: 2072–2076

Neumann H-G (1983) Role of extent and persistence of DNA modifications in chemical carcinogenesis by aromatic amines. In: Rentchnick P, Herfarth C, Senn HJ (eds) Recent results in cancer research, vol 84. Springer, Berlin Heidelberg New York, pp 77–89

Neumann H-G (1986) The role of DNA damage in chemical carcinogenesis of aromatic amines. J Cancer Res Clin Oncol 112: 100–106

Neumann H-G, Metzler M, Brachmann I, Thomas C (1970) Zur Bedeutung chemisch-biologischer Wechselwirkungen für die toxische und krebserzeugende Wirkung aromatischer Amine. I. Krebserzeugende Wirksamkeit einiger 4-Aminostilben- und 4-Aminobibenzyl-Verbindungen. Z Krebsforsch 74: 200

Neumann H-G, Ambs S, Hilleshein H (1992) The biochemical basis of hepatotoxicity. In: Dekant W, Neumann H-G (eds) Tissue specific toxicity, biochemical mechanisms. Academic Press, London, pp 139–162

Neumann H-G, Ambs S, Bitsch A (1994) The role of nongentoxic mechanisms in arylamine carcinogenesis. Environ Health Perspect 102 [Suppl 6]: 173–176

O' Farrel PH (1975) High resolution two-dimensional electrophoresis of proteins. J Biol Chem 250: 4007–4021

Peraino C, Staffeldt EF, Ludeman VA (1981) Early appearance of histochemically altered hepatocyte foci and liver tumors in female rats treated with carcinogens one day after birth. Carcinogenesis 2: 463–465

Rothman JR (1990) Polypeptide chain binding porteins: catalysts of protein folding and related processes in cells. Cell 59: 591–601

Ruthsatz M, Neumann H-G (1988) Synergistic effects on the initiation of rat liver tumors by trans-4-acetylaminostilbene and 2-acetylaminofluorene, studied at the level of DNA adduct formation. Carcinogenesis 9: 265–269

Sato K, Kithara A, Satoh H (1984) The placental form of glutathione-S-transferase as a marker protein for neoplasia in rat chemical hepatocarcinogenesis. GANN 75: 199–202

Stankowski LF, Tindall KR, Hsie AW (1986) Quantitative and molecular analyses of ethylmethanesulfonate- and ICR191 induced mutations in AS52 cells. Mutat Res 160: 133–147

Von Jagow G, Klingenberg M (1972) Close correlation between antimycin titer and cytochrome b_T content in mitochondria of chloramphenicol-treated *Neurospora crassa*. FEBS Lett 24: 278–282

Weinbach EC (1961) A procedure for isolating stable mitochondria from rat liver and kidney. Anal Biochem 2: 335–343

Welch WJ (1992) Mammalian stress response: cell physiology, structure/function of stress proteins, and implications for medicine and disease. Physiol Rev 72: 1063–1081

Analysis of Genetic Factors and Molecular Mechanisms in the Development of Hereditary and Carcinogen-Induced Tumors of Xiphophorus

A. Schartl, M. Pagany, M. Engler, and M. Schartl

Department of Physiological Chemistry I, Theodor Boveri Institute, Biocenter, University of Würzburg, Am Hubland, 97074 Würzburg, Germany

Introduction

The number and amount of carcinogenic agents in our environment has raised steadily increasing public concern and led to a decline in interest in another aspect of turmorigenesis, namely the involvement of genetic factors in the processes that lead to malignant tumors. It is becoming evident that both the noxious influences in the environment and the genetic makeup of cells or of the whole individual are involved in cancerous processes to a similar extent. Animal models offer unique possibilities to analyze the extreme complexity of the interaction of multiple genetic factors and various molecular mechanisms underlying tumor formation. A well-accepted system for tumor development is the *Xiphophorus* melanoma model.

In the late 1920s it was discovered that certain hybrids of the platyfish (*Xiphophorus maculatus*) and the swordtail (*X. helleri*) spontaneously develop malignant melanoma (Gordon 1927; Kosswig 1928; Häussler 1928). The tumors originate from small, black spot patterns of the platyfish which are composed of a peculiar pigment cell type, the macromelanophore. In hybrids the macromelanophore spots can grow unrestricted. The severity of the resulting melanoma ranges from benign in some individual animals to highly malignant in others. Highly malignant melanomas grow invasively and/or exophytically and are fatal (Fig. 1). The malignancy of these fish melanoma is impressively documented by their ability to grow progressively in thymus-aplastic ("nude") mice (Schartl and Peter 1988).

Based on crossing experiments and cytological observations, a genetic model has been developed to explain tumor formation in *Xiphophorus* (Ahuja and Anders 1976). The macromelanophore locus was formally equated with a sex chromosomal locus whose critical constituent was designated "tumor gene" (*Tu*). *Tu* was defined by its capacity for neoplastic transformation of pigment cells. Melanoma formation was then attributed to the uncontrolled activity of *Tu*. In nontumorous fish, *Tu* activity was proposed to be negatively controlled

Recent Results in Cancer Research, Vol. 143

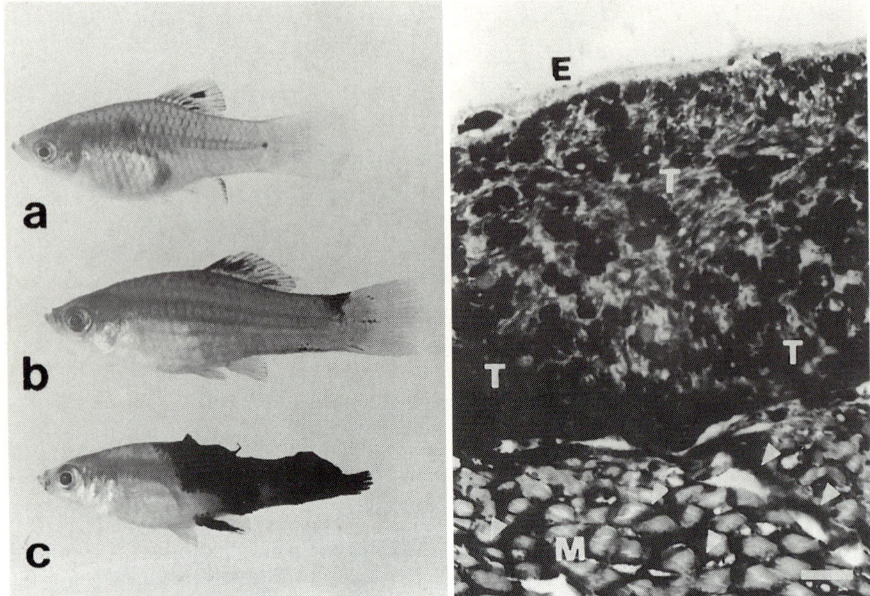

Fig. 1. *Left*, melanoma formation due to unrestricted growth of macromelanophores after crossing of *Xiphophorus maculatus* and *X. helleri*. **a** *X. maculatus* with macromelanophore spot in the dorsal fin. **b** F_1 hybrid with increased number of macromelanophores leading to melanosis in the dorsal fin and the peduncle. **c** Backcross hybrid with malignant melanoma. *Right*, histological section of a fish with malignant melanoma exhibiting three-dimensional exophytic growth and invasion of the underlying muscles by tumor cells. *E*, epidermis, *T*, tumor; *M*, muscle; *arrowheads*, invading tumor cells. *Bar*, 50 μm; H&E

by regulatory genes or tumor suppressor genes (*R* genes). The platyfish, for instance, contains the *Tu* locus on the X-chromosome and the corresponding major *R* on an autosome, while the swordtail is proposed to contain neither of these loci. Thus, crossing and further backcrossing of the platyfish with the swordtail results, in effect, in the progressive replacement of *R*-bearing chromosomes of the platyfish by *R*-free chromosomes of the swordtail. This stepwise elimination of regulatory genes is thought to allow expression of the *Tu* phenotype, leading to benign pigment cell lesions if one functional allele of *R* is still present (e.g., in F_1 animals and a certain fraction of backcross hybrids; Fig. 1b) or malignant melanoma if *R* is absent (Fig. 1c).

The *Tu* Locus Encodes the Novel Growth Factor Receptor Oncogene X*mrk*

Using strategies of positional cloning that were aided by precise knowledge of the chromosomal location of *Tu* and a plethora of chromosomal mutants affecting this region, a candidate gene was isolated that maps to the *Tu* locus

(Schartl 1988; Zechel et al. 1988; Wittbrodt et al. 1989). It encodes a novel growth factor receptor of the superfamily of receptor tyrosine kinases which is intimately related in structure and biochemical properties to the epidermal growth factor receptor (Wittbrodt et al. 1989, 1992). It was designated X*mrk* for *X*iphophorus *m*elanoma *r*eceptor *k*inase. There is another copy of this gene in addition to the *Tu*-encoded X*mrk*. While the X*mrk* copy from the *Tu* locus is present only in fish that have the genetic predisposition to develop melanoma following the appropriate crossings, the second copy is found in all *Xiphophorus* fish regardless of the presence of a *Tu* locus. It represents the corresponding protooncogene whose biological function so far is unknown. The *Tu*-encoded X*mrk* gene is abundantly expressed in malignant melanoma. The premalignant lesions, however, have only small amounts of this transcript. No mRNA of this gene has been detected in any normal organ so far (Wittbrodt et al. 1989).

The molecular structure of the growth factor that is the corresponding ligand to the Xmrk receptor is still unknown. Biochemical experiments have revealed that the fish melanoma cells secrete a protein factor, most likely the Xmrk ligand, that stimulates the Xmrk protein to become a highly active growth signal transducer (Malitschek et al. 1994). Thus the X*mrk* overexpressing *Xiphophorus* melanoma cells are an autocrine and thereby growth-autonomous system.

Like other members of the epidermal growth factor receptor (EGFR) family of receptor tyrosine kinases (RTKs), the Xmrk protein is dependent on a specific signal transduction machinery to transmit its growth-promoting activity to the nucleus (see Winkler et al. 1994). Several Xmrk substrates that bind to the activated receptor have been identified. They include phospholipase Cγ, Grb2, and phosphoinositol-3-kinase, all of which are common downstream effectors of EGFR-like receptors. However, the cytoplasmic kinase Xfyn, which is associated with Xmrk via SH2 domain binding and stimulated upon Xmrk activation, was found as a novel substrate for subclass I RTKs and appears to contribute to the specificity of the Xmrk signal transduction pathway (Wellbrock et al. 1995).

All known properties of X*mrk* are in accordance with what can be expected for a dominant oncogene and its protein product. However, as with other genes isolated by positional cloning as candidate genes, more evidence was required to determine whether X*mrk* is the *Tu* gene. The most stringent question is whether X*mrk* is necessary and sufficient for tumor formation. The first part was readily answered by analyzing the genomic organization of X*mrk* in a mutant that had lost the capacity to develop melanoma. The mutant genotype was found to contain a large insertion in one exon of the kinase domain of X*mrk* (Wittbrodt et al. 1989). This gene disruption abolishes the *Tu* phenotype, thereby proving that X*mrk* is necessary for melanoma formation. To answer the second part of the question, transgenic fish were employed. A X*mrk* minigene was introduced into a closely related fish species, the Japanese medaka (*Oryzias latipes*) which – unlike the live-bearing *Xiphophorus* – is egg-laying and therefore more suited for gene transfer experiments. Tumors appeared at high frequencies after a few days in the injected embryos (Winkler et al. 1994). The remarkably short latency period excludes the possibility that additional events such as mutations that lead to activation of host oncogenes or inactivation of tumor suppressor genes were required for tumor formation in the X*mrk* transgenics. Thus X*mrk* alone appears to be sufficient for tumor formation.

Evolutionary Origin and Control of the Melanoma Oncogene

Examination of the genomic organization of the X*mrk* protooncogene and comparison to the oncogene revealed the following explanation: at some point in the evolutionary history of *Xiphophorus,* the coding region of X*mrk* was duplicated and the new copy was fused for a foreign 5′ regulatory region originating from an anonymous locus, designated *D*. The new compound locus is the *Tu* locus with the oncogenic version of X*mrk*. As a consequence, the protooncogene and oncogene are subject to different transcriptional regulation (Adam et al. 1991, 1993). This has several implications for our understanding of the *Xiphophorus* melanoma system. A pigment cell lineage-specific overexpression of the X*mrk* oncogene in hybrid genotypes is responsible for melanoma formation. The *R* locus-dependent transcriptional control of the oncogene promoter allows high levels of expression only in pigment cells of certain hybrid genotypes, but not in nonhybrids. This explains why the dominant oncogene is ineffective in purebred *Xiphophorus* strains and is a nonhazardous constituent of the genome in natural populations for many generations.

Spontaneous Melanoma in Nonhybrid *Xiphophorus*

The formation of melanoma of a strict hereditary origin in *Xiphophorus* hybrids is a peculiar situation which might be analogous to the familial melanoma of humans. In rare cases malignant melanoma even develops spontaneously in nonhybrid fish taken from their natural habitats. Such melanoma were also found to overexpress the Xmrk receptor tyrosine kinase (Schartl et al. 1995). Thus the deleterious character of the X*mrk* oncogene can become apparent.

The nonhybrid melanoma in *Xiphophorus*, whose etiology is still unclear, but might well be due to environmentally noxious agents (carcinogens, tumor promoters) or internal factors like hormonal imbalance in an aging organism, appear to be caused by the same molecular event as the melanoma of hybrids, namely overexpression of X*mrk* (Schartl et al. 1995). This supports the common expectation in research on hereditary cancers in man, namely that the same gene that is responsible for the inherited form of a tumor might also be instrumental in so-called spontaneous forms of the same tumor. It is, however, important to note that nonhybrid melanomas are consistently found in only a few populations and that they are always associated with certain *Tu* (=X*mrk*) alleles.

Carcinogen-Induced Tumors

Cancer diseases of strict hereditary etiology like the *Xiphophorus* hybrid melanoma represent only a minority of mammalian tumors. By far the largest number of tumors is generally believed to be caused by carcinogens. When individuals from purebred strains of wild *Xiphophorus* were treated with known effective chemical carcinogens, they were found to be relatively resistant. The tumor rate was as low as less than 1%. Hybrid genotypes, however, showed a markedly increased susceptibility. Following the same protocol for treatment, the tumor rate surprisingly increased to more than 10% (Anders et al. 1984; Anders 1990). Such increased hybrid susceptibility for carcinogen induction of neoplasms has also been noted for melanoma in the medaka (Hyodo-Taguchi and Matsudaira 1987). Neither the genetics nor the molecular biology of this phenomenon has been investigated so far, although this appears to be an appealing task.

To find out if the phenomenon of hybrid sensitivity versus wild fish resistance is a common feature of poeciliid fish in general or confined to the genus *Xiphophorus* and if the hybrid susceptibility can be assigned to certain chromosomes or linkage groups we have started a large-scale carcinogenesis treatment experiment. To this end 800 fish (435 wild-type fish of *Xiphophorus* and related species and 240 hybrids between different *Xiphophorus* species) were exposed to the DNA-alkylating agents *N*-ethylnitrosourea (ENU) or *N*-methylnitrosourea (MNU). Some offspring from treated fish received a second treatment when having grown to preadulthood. The optimal treatment protocol was very much dependent on the type of fish (body size, age, general physical constitution, etc.); an average of three treatments at weekly intervals with concentrations ranging from 1 to 5 mM of either MNU or ENU was effective in inducing tumors of different tissue origin. Notably, the latency period for tumor development was quite long (6–9 months). Thus, the number of cancerous lesions so far is too low to permit analyzing correlations of histiotype and tumor incidence to the genetic makeup. Some peculiar effects were observed in some newborn fish that were exposed to carcinogenic treatment as embryos. Besides higher lethality due to preterm delivery, severe malformations occurred. Interestingly, one *G. affinis* neonate had a large hyperpigmented area made up of unusually large, black pigment cells. The cells grew at a higher density than the wild-type melanophores of *G. affinis* and were morphologically similar to the *Xiphophorus* macromelanophores, which are the cells giving rise to malignant melanoma. Histological analysis revealed that besides the dermal location, pigment cells are also present in the underlying muscles (Fig. 2).

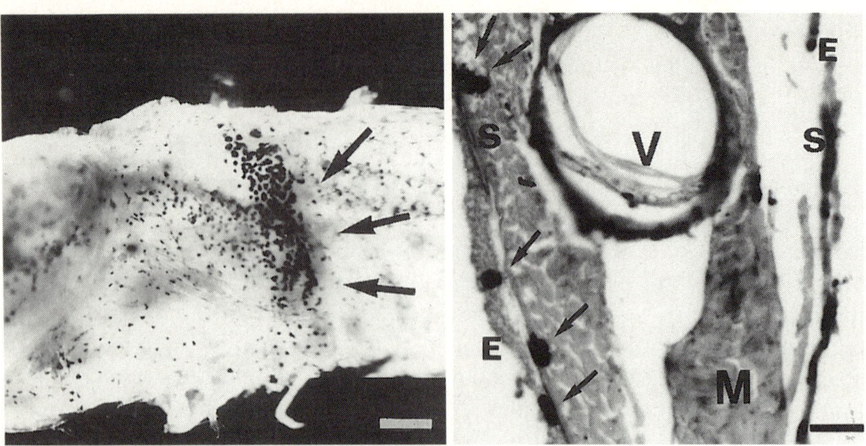

Fig. 2. *Left*, hyperpigmented area (*arrows*) on the bodyside of a neonate of *G. affinis*; *bar* represents 3 mm. *Right*, transversal section showing large pigment cells in the epidermis, dermis, and the trunk muscles (*arrows*). *E*, epidermis; *M*, muscle; *S*, scale; *V*, vertebra. *Bar* 50 μm; H & E

In a pilot study melanoma from *Xiphophorus* that were induced by chemical carcinogens and which are indistinguishable by all histopathological parameters from hereditary melanoma of backcross hybrids showed no expression of X*mrk* (Mäueler et al. 1993). Thus, X*mrk*, the melanoma-inducing gene of hereditary melanoma, seems to be insignificant for the development of carcinogen-triggered melanoma. Tumor genes other than X*mrk* appear to be instrumental in causation of carcinogen-induced melanoma. Obviously, several pathways exist on the molecular level that lead to an identical phenotype, namely a malignant melanoma. The prediction is that the situation will increase in complexity when tumors of other histiotypes are included in the analysis. For such analysis the collection of an extended data set on the molecular biology of carcinogen-induced tumors is required. A variety of homologous probes from *Xiphophorus* protooncogenes is already available (see Table 1). Other important candidate genes that are suspected to play a crucial role in the development of carcinogen-induced tumors (tumor suppressor genes like p53 or DNA repair genes) are currently under scrutiny (Fig. 3).

Genotypic differences in cancer susceptibility may be suspected to be related to differences in such general phenomena as DNA repair or genomic instability. This, for instance, is reflected in the formation of micronuclei which have proven to be a reliable assay system for those parameters commonly used to test genotoxicity (De Flora et al. 1993). The phenomenon of micronuclei formation has thus far not been reported from *Xiphophorus*. A *Xiphophorus* melanoma cell line (PSM: platyfish/swordtail hybrid melanoma cell line) and an embryonal epithelial cell line (A2) were tested for micronuclei

Table 1. Cloned *Xiphophorus* protooncogenes and related genes with oncogenic potential

Gene ("alias")	cDNA	Genomic clones	Protein	Expression in tumors		Ref.
				Hered. mel.	Carcinog. ind.	
X*mrk* ("*Tu*" "X*erb* B^{a*}")	Full-length	Entire coding region + 5′ upstr.	160 kD Receptor tyrosine kinase	Highly overexpressed	Not detectable	Wittbrodt et al. 1989, 1992; Malitschek et al. 1994
X*src*	Full-length	Kinase + SH2-3 coding region	60 kD Cytoplasmic kinase	High expression	High to overexpressed	Raulf and Robertson, unpublished; Mäueler et al. 1988, 1993
X*yes*	Full-length	Kinase domain	61 kD Cytoplasmic kinase	High expression	n.d.	Hannig et al. 1991
X*fyn*	Full-length	n.a.	60 kD Cytoplasmic kinase	High expression	n.d.	Hannig et al. 1991; Wellbrock et al. 1995
X*egfr* ("*erbB*")	n.a.	2 Exons from kinase domain	n.d.	Low expression	Not detectable	Mäueler et al. 1988, 1993; Wittbrodt et al. 1989; Zechel et al. 1988
X*t3/r* ("*erbA*")	n.a.	1 Exon from DNA binding domain	n.d.	Low expression	n.d.	Zechel et al. 1989

n.a., not available; n.d., not determined; Hered. mel., hereditary melanoma; Carcinog. ind., carcinogen-induced; upstr., upstream.

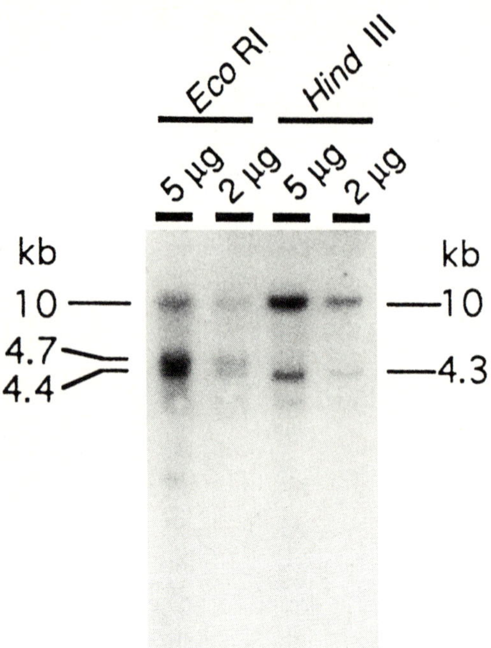

Fig. 3. Southern blot of *X. maculatus* DNA hybridized to mouse p53. Hybridization conditions: 35% formamide, 42 °C. Washing conditions: 55 °C, 1 × sodium saline citrate (SSC)

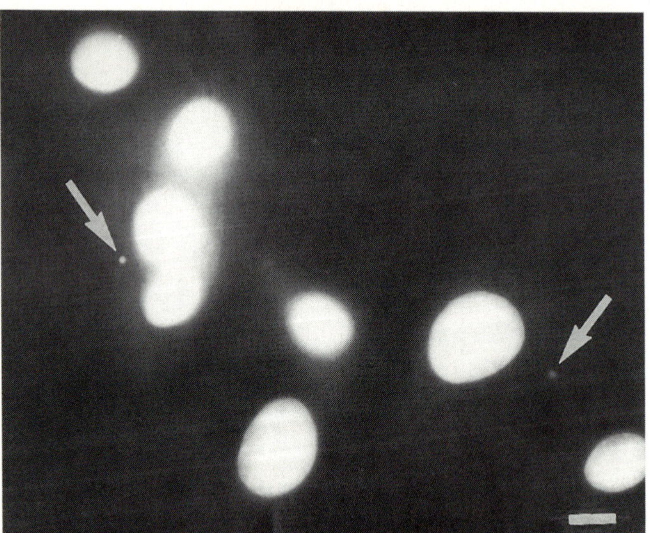

Fig. 4. Platyfish/swordtail hybrid melanoma (PSM) cells with micronuclei (*arrows*). Untreated, Hoechst stain. *Bar*, 5 μm

Table 2. Increased number of micronuclei after treatment with MMS

Concentration	Micronuclei/cell				Micronuclei/2000 cells
	1	2	3	4	Total
Control[a]	12	0	0	0	12
25 μg MMS/ml	117	6	0	0	129
50 μg MMS/ml	192	11	1	0	217
75 μg MMS/ml	216	11	2	1	248

MMS, methylmethanesulfonate.
[a]Treated with solvent [dimethylsulfoxide (DMSO)] alone.

formation using standard assay conditions (Stopper et al. 1994). The rate of spontaneous micronuclei (Fig. 4) was 0.5%–1% in both cell lines. Following treatment with methylmethanesulfonate (MMS) the rate was increased in a typical dose-dependent manner (Table 2) up to 75 μg/ml. Higher concentrations showed severe cytotoxic effects. The rate of micronuclei observed was highest 60 h after treatment (Fig. 5). These parameters are in accordance with data from higher vertebrates (Stopper et al. 1994). Based on this, cells from different genotypes can now be tested for differential sensitivity and rate of micronuclei induction.

Conclusions

The advantage of *Xiphophorus* as a genetic system for basic research on cancer is that it permits the identification and functional analysis of genes that control the onset of tumor formation. Due to the large variety of strains and mutants that affect the tumor phenotype (compartment of occurrence, severity and

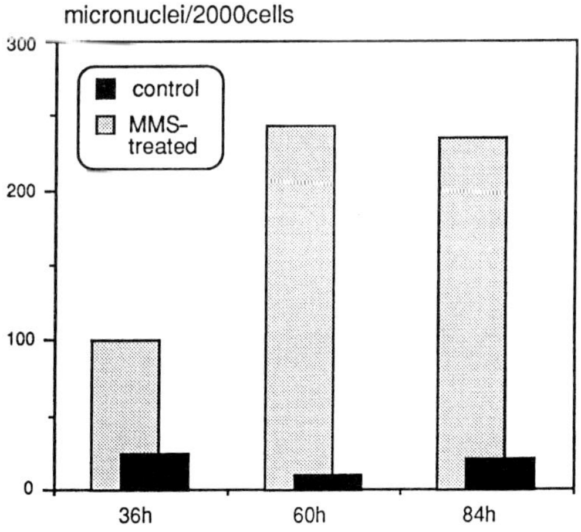

Fig. 5. Time course of micronuclei induction by methylmethanesulfonate (*MMS*): micronuclei counted in MMS-treated (50 μg/ml; 8 h) melanoma cells. Given are the time points after substance withdrawal

prognosis, cell-type specificity), there is a considerable potential for future work on genes that modulate the malignant phenotype, genetic factors that are involved in tumor-related genetic instability, tumor susceptibility genes, tissue-specific and nonspecific tumor suppressors, and DNA repair genes.

Acknowledgements. We acknowledge the expert technical assistance of Robin Wacker in the histopathological analysis and of Hugo Schwind, Georg Schneider, and Petra Weber in breeding the fish. This work was supported by the Deutsche Forschungsgemeinschaft through Sonderforschungsbereich 172 (Teilprojekt C-11) and partly by the European Commission (BIO2CT-930430).

References

Adam D, Mäueler W, Schartl M (1991) Transcriptional activation of the melanoma inducing X*mrk* oncogene in Xiphophorus. Oncogene 6: 73–80

Adam D, Dimitrijevic N, Schartl M (1993) Tumor suppression in Xiphophorus by an accidentally acquired promoter. Science 259: 816–819

Ahuja MR, Anders F (1976) A genetic concept of the origin of cancer, based in part upon studies of neoplasms in fishes. Prog Exp Tumor Res 20: 380–397

Anders F (1990) A biologist's view of human cancer. In: Neth R, Frolova E, Gallo RC, Greaves MF, Afanasiev BV, Elstner E (eds) Modern trends in human leukemia, vol 8. Springer, Berlin Heidelberg New York

Anders F, Schartl M, Barnekow A, Anders A (1984) Xiphophorus as an in vivo model for studies on normal and defective control of oncogenes. Adv Cancer Res 42: 191–275

De Flora S, Vigano L, D'Agostini F, Camoirano A, Bagnasco M, Bennicelli C, Melodia F, Arillo A (1993) Multiple genotoxicity biomarkers in fish exposed in situ to polluted river water. Mutat Res 319(3): 167–177

Gordon M (1927) The genetics of viviparous top-minnow Platypoecilus: the inheritance of two kinds of melanophores. Genetics 12: 253–283

Hannig G, Ottilie S, Schartl M (1991) Conservation of structure and expression of the c-*yes* and *fyn* genes in lower vertebrates. Oncogene 6: 361–369

Häussler G (1928) Über Melanombildungen bei Bastarden von *Xiphophorus maculatus var. rubra.* Klin Wochenschr 7: 1561–1562

Hyodo-Taguchi Y, Matsudaira H (1987) Higher susceptibility to N-methyl-N′-nitro-N-nitrosoguanidine-induced tumorigenesis in an interstrain hybrid of the fish, *Oryzias latipes* (medaka). Jpn J Cancer Res (Gann) 78: 487–493

Kosswig C (1928) Über Kreuzungen zwischen den Teleostiern *Xiphophorus helleri* und *Platypoecilus maculatus.* Z Indukt Abstammungs Vererbungsl 47: 150–158

Mäueler W, Raulf F, Schartl M (1988) Expression of proto-oncogenes in embryonic, adult, and transformed tissue of Xiphophorus (Teleostei: Poeciliidae). Oncogene 2: 421–430

Mäueler W, Schartl A, Schartl M (1993) Different expression patterns of oncogenes and proto-oncogenes in hereditary and carcinogen-induced tumors of Xiphophorus. Int J Cancer 55: 288–296

Malitschek B, Wittbrodt J, Fischer P, Lammers R, Ullrich A, Schartl M (1994) Autocrine stimulation of the X*mrk* receptor tyrosine kinase in Xiphophorus melanoma cells and identification of a source for the physiological ligand. J Biol Chem 269: 10423–10430

Schartl M (1988) A sex chromosomal restriction-fragment-length marker linked to melanoma-determining *Tu* loci in Xiphophorus. Genetics 119: 679–685

Schartl M, Peter RU (1988) Progressive growth of fish tumors after transplantation into thymus-aplastic (*nu*/*nu*) mice. Cancer Res 48: 741–744

Schartl A, Malitschek B, Kazianis S, Borowsky R, Schartl M (1995) Spontaneous melanoma formation in non-hybrid Xiphophorus. Cancer Res 55: 159–165

Stopper H, Kühnel A, Podschun B (1994) Combination of the chemotherapeutic agent 5-fluoro-uracil with an inhibitor of its catabolism results in increased micronucleus induction. Biochem Biophys Res Commun 203: 1124–1130

Wellbrock C, Lammers R, Ullrich A, Schartl M (1995) Association between the melanoma-inducing receptor tyrosine kinase Xmrk and src family tyrosine kinases in Xiphophorus. Oncogene 10: 2135–2143

Winkler C, Wittbrodt J, Lammers R, Ullrich A, Schartl M (1994) Ligand-dependent tumor induction in medakafish embryos by a X*mrk* receptor tyrosine kinase transgene. Oncogene 9: 1517–1525

Wittbrodt J, Adam D, Malitschek B, Mäueler W, Raulf F, Telling A et al (1989) Novel putative receptor tyrosine kinase encoded by the melanoma-inducing *Tu* locus in Xiphophorus. Nature 341: 415–421

Wittbrodt J, Lammers R, Malitschek B, Ullrich A, Schartl M (1992) The X*mrk* receptor tyrosine kinase is activated in Xiphophorus malignant melanoma. EMBO J 11: 4239–4246

Zechel C, Schleenbecker U, Anders A, Anders F (1988) v-*erb*B related sequences in Xiphophorus that map to melanoma determining Mendelian loci and overexpress in a melanoma cell line. Oncogene 3: 605–617

Zechel C, Schleenbecker U, Anders A, Pfütz M, Anders F (1989) Search for genes critical for the early and/or late events in carcinogenesis: studies in Xiphophorus (Pisces, Teleostei). In: Neth R, Frolova E, Gallo RC, Greaves MF, Afanasiev BV, Elstner E (eds) Modern trends in human leukemia, vol 8. Springer, Berlin Heidelberg New York, pp 366–385

The Role of Raf Kinases in Development and Growth of Tumors

U. Naumann, I. Eisenmann-Tappe, and U.R. Rapp

Institute of Medical Radiation and Cell Research, University of Würzburg, Versbacher Str. 5, 97078 Würzburg, Germany

Introduction

Cancer is a disease that is caused predominantly by genetic alterations. A critical group of genes involved in malignant transformations includes the so-called oncogenes. There are four categories of protooncogenes from which oncogenic products can emerge: (1) peptide factors that act as ligands for cell surface receptors, (2) the receptors themselves, (3) intracellular signal transducers, and (4) transcription factors. Mutations of oncogenes leading to cancer frequently cause constitutive activity of the gene products. This results in an unregulated and enhanced transduction of mitogenic signals from the cell membrane to the nucleus.

Raf proteins belong to the third category of protooncogene products. They are serine/threonine kinases that are now known to play a central role in mediating the mitogenic response of cells to numerous growth factors and cytokines. Once a receptor is activated by its extracellular ligand, the signal is transported via cytoplasmic kinase cascades to the nucleus where transcription of specific genes is induced through phosphorylation and activation of transcription factors. Long-term cellular behavior like suppression of apoptosis, proliferation, and differentiation are regulated by those signaling events. Currently three distinct kinase cascades are known in vertebrates, but others may yet be found (Cano and Mahadevan 1995). The best-understood and the only clearly growth-regulatory cascade is the Ras/Raf/MEK/ERK pathway (Fig. 1). Cytokine receptors as well as receptor-protein tyrosine kinases (RPTKs) link to this pathway via activation of the Ras protein, a protooncogene that is found altered in more than 75% of colon cancers and about 30% of all human cancers (Ando et al. 1991; Boland 1993). Ras activation is achieved by translocation to the plasma membrane of the Grb-2/Sos complex that binds to an autophosphorylation site in the RPTK itself, or to a substrate or docking protein phosphorylated by a nonreceptor protein tyrosine kinase. Juxtaposition of Sos and Ras at the plasma membrane results

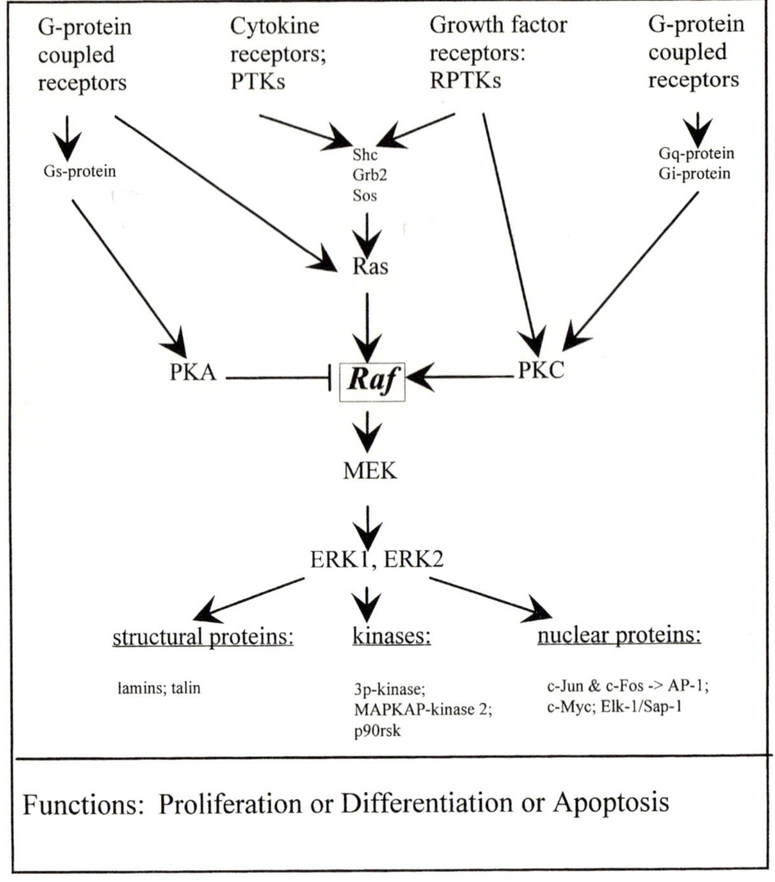

Fig. 1. Simplified model of Raf-dependent signal transduction. Raf is activated upon stimulation of a variety of receptors and, together with MEK and ERK, forms a cytoplasmic kinase cascade. ERKs act on a panel of targets that finally regulate important cellular functions. *Arrows* indicate direct or indirect activation, *blocked lines,* inactivation

in exchange of GDP for GTP on Ras. Only the GTP-bound form of Ras is able to bind to an N-terminal sequence of Raf, termed the Ras-binding-domain (RBD), thus recruiting Raf to the membrane. There, an as yet uncharacterized event activates Raf, which subsequently phosphorylates and activates MEK, which in turn phosphorylates and activates the MAP-kinases ERK1/ERK2. In contrast to Raf and MEK, both of which are able to recognize only one substrate, MAP-kinases can activate a panel of target proteins as indicated in Fig. 1 (reviewed in Daum et al. 1994).

Raf and Cancer

There are several lines of evidence that point to the role of Raf kinases in malignant transformation. Raf first came into view as part of an acute transforming murine virus (Rapp et al. 1983). Furthermore, transforming versions of *raf* genes have been detected in fibroblasts following transfection with DNA from various tumor cells including primary human stomach cancer cells (Shimizu et al. 1985), a human glioblastoma cell line (Fukui et al. 1985), cells derived from renal and breast carcinoma and a lung carcinoid (Stanton and Cooper 1987) as well as chemically induced rat hepatocarcinoma cells (Ishikawa et al. 1985, 1986, 1987). The oncogenic mutations detected were 5′ deletions of *c-raf-1* resulting in N-terminally truncated or fused Raf proteins. However, the mutations could not be detected in the primary tumors and it appears that the oncogenic Raf versions were generated by DNA breakage during transfection (Ishikawa et al. 1986, 1987; Stanton and Cooper 1987).

A function of Raf in tumor development was examined on the level of chromosomal aberrations and cellular expression. There are three functional *raf* genes known in vertebrates, called *A-raf, B-raf* and *c-raf-1*. In mice *raf* genes are differentially expressed in tissues such that *A-raf* is present in urogenital tissues, *B-raf* is most abundant in cerebrum and testes, while c-*raf-1* is ubiquitously found in all tissues (Storm et al. 1990; Wadewitz et al. 1993). Little is known about the functional consequences of tissue-specific Raf expression and extensive research is in progress to elucidate isozyme-specific Raf effects. In humans as in mice the three functional *raf* genes are located on different chromosomes. Human *A-raf* is located on chromosome X region p11.2, *B-raf* on 7q34, and *c-raf-1* on 3p25. The chromosomal region Xp11.2 is known to be altered in a variety of human diseases, e.g., Norrie's disease, Wiskott-Aldrich-syndrome, and Cone dystrophy (Bleeker-Wagemakers et al. 1985; Kwan et al. 1988). However, no functional correlations between these diseases and alterations of the *A-raf* gene locus have been described so far. Alterations in 3p25 were observed in familiar renal carcinomas, certain salivary gland tumors, and ovarian carcinomas (Rapp et al. 1988). In small cell lung cancer (SCLC), loss of heterozygosity was frequently found in chromosome 3p regions involving the *c-raf-1* gene in 80% of analyzed tumor tissues. Along with this phenomenon Raf-1 appears to be constitutively activated (Sithanandam et al. 1989; Graziano et al. 1991).

In order to study *c-raf-1* as a potential target in lung carcinogenesis we have designed a mouse tumor model for rapid induction of lung tumors. Tumors were induced by in utero exposure of F1 mice from NFS x AKR matings to 1-ethyl-1-nitrosourea (ENU) on day 16 of gestation. This strain combination was expected to be particularly susceptible to induction of lung tumors and lymphomas based on earlier work by Diwan and Meier (1974). Tumor promotion was achieved by treating weanling mice with weekly intraperitoneal injections of the antioxidant butylated hydroxytoluene BHT which has been shown to cause lung lesions and hyperplasia in mice (Witschi and Saheb 1974).

In this system nearly 100% of the offspring developed lung adenocarcinomas and 70% additionally developed T-cell lymphomas. When tumors were examined for altered expression or structure of tumor-associated genes it was found that one allele of *c-raf-1* was consistently mutated in all tumors, along with a conspicuous lack of mutations of the Raf-activator Ras. Furthermore, no mutations in the tumor-suppressor gene p53, which is known to be altered in many types of human cancers, could be detected (Müller and Naumann, unpublished data). The prevalent mutation in the *raf* gene was an exchange of serine to phenylalanine in position 533 of the kinase subdomain VIII. Additional mutations also clustered in that region, whereas no other mutations could be detected throughout the rest of the Raf molecule. The consistently mutated region apparently forms the surface of the substrate pocket (Fig. 2). This was suggested by computer modeling based on the available coordinates of protein kinase A. Although the mutated allele of *c-raf-1* was not constitutively active, an increased activity of Raf after stimulation by coexpression with Ras

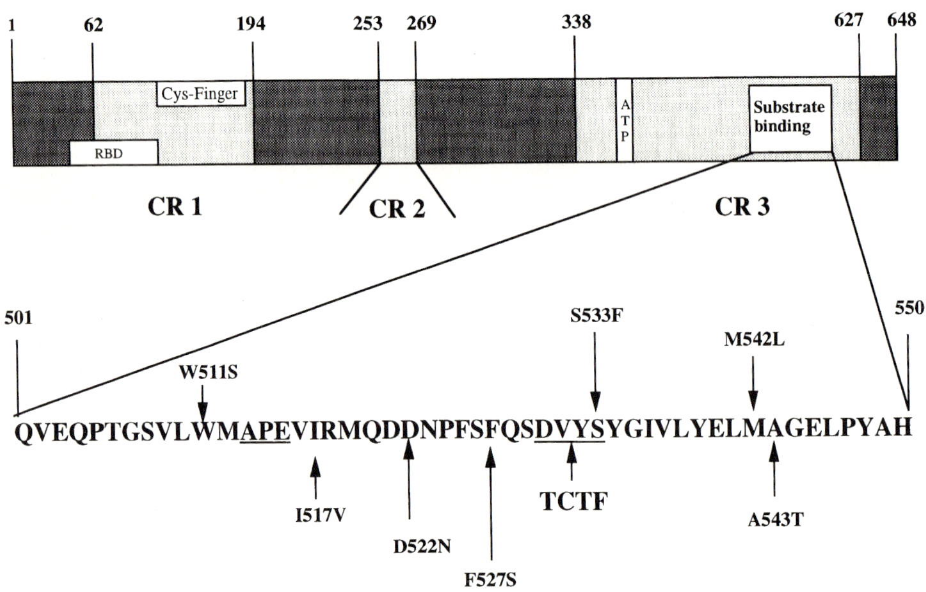

Fig. 2. Clustering of mutations in the murine *c-raf-1* gene after 1-ethyl-1-nitrosourea/butylated hydroxytoluene (ENU/BHT) treatment. Raf family proteins contain three conserved regions named *CR1, CR2,* and *CR3*. The N-terminal part of the Raf kinase contains regulatory elements, e.g., the Ras binding domain and a zinc finger motif in CR1, and regulatory phosphorylation sites in CR2 (for details see Daum et al. 1994; Avruch et al. 1994). The carboxy terminal half of the molecule comprises CR3, the catalytic kinase domain. All of the identified mutations cluster in a small area around the APE-site (conserved sequence located in subdomain VIII), apparently at the surface of the substrate pocket. Amino acid sequence is that of wt-murine *c-raf-1* with *arrows* indicating substitutions

and the nonreceptor tyrosine kinase Lck in insect cells could be demonstrated for the most common mutations (Storm et al., in preparation).

In addition to mutational activation of Raf, its level of expression may be a determinant of cellular transformation as suggested by cooperative transformation experiments with wild-type *ras* and *c-raf-1* in NIH3T3 fibroblasts (Cuadrado et al. 1993). Cooperation was only seen when overexpressing Raf together with oncogenic, i.e., constitutively active, Ras expressed at low levels, or wt-Ras expressed at high levels. This indicates that Raf is limiting for Ras-mediated transformation under conditions where only few activated Ras molecules are present at the inner face of the plasma membrane.

In our mouse model Northern and Western blot analysis revealed elevated levels of *c-raf-1* mRNA as well as Raf protein in all tumors compared to normal tissue. Additionally, one member of the *myc* gene family (either *c-*, *N-*, or *L-myc*) was overexpressed in each case. Also, of the *ras* genes at least one member (*Ki-, Ha-,* or *N-ras)*, and often more than one, was found to be expressed at elevated levels (Storm and Rapp 1993). A synergism between Raf- and Myc-dependent pathways in tumor development has already been described (Rapp et al. 1986). Examination of the role of *raf* genes in human diseases in the future should include the search for point mutations. If clustering of such mutations were observed, similar to the finding in our mouse model, it might be possible to develop inhibitors that can distinguish between normal and oncogenic Raf kinase.

Inhibitors of Raf Kinases

Specific inhibitors are valuable tools for biochemical characterizations of enzymes. There are many gaps in the understanding of the mechanisms of Raf kinase activation and of how activation is regulated. The use of specific Raf inhibitors may elucidate still-unknown regulatory events, and the detection of putative Raf-specific inhibitors might be an important step in the development of anticancer drugs.

The U.S. National Cancer Institute (NCI) natural product database offers growth inhibitory data for approximately 21 000 extracts predominantly derived from plants and fungi that have been tested for anticancer activity in the NCI panel of human tumor cell lines. We tested eight of those extracts (natural products, NPs) for their ability to inhibit the growth of normal and Ras- or Raf-transformed cell lines. The eight extracts were chosen because they had shown growth inhibitory patterns strongly correlating with those that had been obtained in preliminary experiments using antisense *Ki-ras* oligonucleotides. This approach could principally detect inhibitors of either Ras or downstream members of a Ras-dependent signaling cascade. For the growth inhibitory studies we utilized normal NIH3T3 mouse fibroblasts, 3T3 cells transformed with *c-Ha-ras* under the transcriptional control of an SV40 promoter, and 3T3 cells transformed by a mutant *c-raf-1 gene* (lacking the amino terminal 90 amino acids of wt Raf-1) under the transcriptional control of a Rous sarcoma virus promoter. The Ha-ras-transformed 3T3 cells were found to be more sensitive to growth inhibition by NPs than either wild-type or mutant *c-raf-1*-transformed cells (Housey et al., submitted). Since Raf-1 functions directly downstream of Ras in mitogen-activated signal transduction, we performed in vitro kinase assays to test the ability of the NPs to inhibit activated Raf-1-mediated phosphorylation and activation of MEK. For these experiments we utilized the Raf/MEK/ERK coupled assay system which was described by Housey et al. (submitted). For comparison we included well-characterized specific as well as nonspecific protein kinase inhibitors: H7, tamoxifen, and staurosporine. At final concentrations of 10 to 1000 μg/ml, seven of eight NPs exhibited substantial inhibition of Raf-mediated phosphorylation of MEK (Table 1), whereas H7, tamoxifen, and staurosporine had no or only weak inhibitory effects at comparable concentrations.

Future experiments will attempt to characterize precisely the nature of the inhibitory extracts and to learn about the mechanisms involved. First results point to an interference with Ras/Raf binding in the case of two of the NPs (Housey et al., submitted).

Raf-Deficient Mice

The generation of Raf-deficient mice may provide a means of studying the role of Raf kinases in development and cancer. To prevent the expression of a functional protein, an exon near the 5′ end of the target gene is disrupted by insertion of a marker gene. In case of *c-raf-1* as well as *B-raf* exon 2 was chosen to be interrupted by a neomycine gene (L. Wajnowski and U.R. Rapp, unpublished data). Using standard techniques we were able to generate either *c-raf-1*

Table 1. Inhibition of Raf kinase activity by natural products (Housey et al., submitted)

NP	Organism	Inhibition of Raf-mediated MEK phosphorylation	Concentration (μg/ml)
1	Plant	yes	100
2	Plant	yes	1000
3	Plant	yes	10
4	Plant	yes	10
5	Lichen	yes	1000
6	Plant	yes	10
7	Plant	yes	100
8	Fungus	no	1000

NP, natural product.

or *B-raf*-negative stem cell lines and chimeric mice. Examination of these mice showed that the size of the animals is inversely correlated with the grade of chimerism, indicating a functional role of Raf kinases in embryonic development (L. Wagnowski and U.R. Rapp 1995). Further studies have to await the production of homozygous knockout mice. As to the involvement of Raf kinases in carcinogenesis, it would be interesting to know if mice with Raf-1-deficient lung tissue can be bred and what effect the deficiency might have on lung tumor development after treatment with ENU/BHT as described for our lung tumor model.

Acknowledgement. This work was supported by the Sonderforschungsbereich 172 of the Deutsche Forschungsgemeinschaft.

References

Ando M, Maruyama M, Oto M, Takemura K, Endo M, Yuasa Y (1991) Higher frequency of point mutations in the c-K-ras 2 gene in human colorectal adenomas with severe atypia than in carcinomas. Jpn J Cancer Res 82: 245–249

Avruch J, Zhang X, Kyriakis JM (1994) Raf meets Ras: completing the framework of a signal transduction pathway. Trends Biochem Sci 19: 279–283

Bleeker-Wagemakers LM, Friedrich U, Gal A, Wienker TF, Warburg M, Ropers HH (1985) Hum Genet 71: 211–214

Boland CR (1993) The biology of colorectal cancer. Cancer [Suppl] 71: 4180–4186

Cano E, Mahadevan LC (1995) Parallel signal processing among mammalian MAPKs. Trends Biochem 20: 117–122

Cuadrado A, Bruder JT, Heidaran MA, App H, Rapp UR, Aaronson SA (1993) H-ras and raf-1 cooperate in transformation of NIH3T3 fibroblasts. Oncogene 8: 2443–2448

Daum G, Eisenmann-Tappe I, Fries HW, Troppmair J, Rapp UR (1994) Ins and outs of raf kinases. Trends Biochem 19: 474–480

Diwan BA, Meier H (1974) Strain- and age-dependent transplacental carcinogenesis by 1-ethyl-1-nitrosourea in inbred strains of mice. Cancer Res 34: 764–770

Fukui M, Yamamoto T, Kawai S, Maruo K, Toyoshima K (1985) Detection of a raf-related and two other transforming DNA sequences in human tumors maintained in nude mice. Proc Natl Acad Sci USA 81: 5954–5958

Graziano SL, Pfeifer AM, Testa JR, Johnson BE, Hallinan EJ, Pettengill OS, Sorenson GD et al (1991) Involvement of the RAF1 locus, at band 3p25, in the 3p deletion of small-cell lung cancer. Genes Chrom Dev 3: 283–293

Ishikawa F, Takaku F, Ochiai M, Hayashi K, Hirohashi S, Terada M, Takayama S et al. (1985) Activated c-raf gene in a rat hepatocellular carcinoma induced by 2-amino-3-methylimidazole (4,5-F) quinoline. Biochem Biophys Res Commun 132: 186–192

Ishikawa F, Takaku F, Hayashi K, Nagao M, Sugimura T (1986) Activation of rat c-raf during transfection of hepatocellular carcinoma DNA. Proc Natl Acad Sci USA 83: 3209–3212

Ishikawa F, Takaku F, Nagao M, Sugimura T (1987) Rat-c-raf oncogene activation by rearrangement that produces a fused protein. Mol Cell Biol 7: 1226–1232

Kwan SP, Sandkuyl LA, Blaese M, Kunkel LM, Bruns G, Parmley R, Skarhaug S et al (1988) Genetic mapping of the Wishott-Aldrich syndrome with two highly-linked polymorphic DNA markers. Genomics 3: 39–43

Rapp UR, Goldsborough MD, Mark GE, Bonner TI, Groffen J, Reynolds FH Jr, Stephenson JR (1983) Structure and biological activity of v-raf, a unique oncogene transduced by a retrovirus. Proc Natl Acad Sci USA 80: 4218–4222

Rapp UR, Cleveland JL, Storm SM, Beck TW, Huleihel M (1986) Transformation by raf and myc oncogenes. Princess Takamatsu Symp 17: 55–74

Rapp UR, Cleveland JL, Bonner TI, Storm SM (1988) The raf oncogenes. In: Reedy EP, Skalka AM, Curran T (eds) The oncogene handbook. Elsevier Science, Amsterdam, pp 213–253

Shimizu K, Nakasu Y, Sekisuchi M, Hokamura K, Tanaka K, Terada M, Sugimura T (1985) Molecular cloning of an activated human oncogene, homologous to v-raf, from primary stomach cancer. Proc Natl Acad Sci USA 82: 5641–5645

Sithanandam G, Dean M, Brennscheidt U, Beck T, Gazdar A, Minna JD, Brauch H et al (1989) Loss of heterozygosity at the c-raf locus in small cell lung carcinoma. Oncogene 4: 451–455

Stanton V Jr, Cooper GM (1987) Activation of human raf transforming genes by deletion of normal amino-terminal coding sequences. Mol Cell Biol 7: 1171–1179

Storm SM, Rapp UR (1993) Oncogene activation: c-raf-1 gene mutations in experimental and naturally occurring tumors. Toxicol Lett 67: 201–210

Storm SM, Cleveland JL, Rapp UR (1990) Expression of raf family proto-oncogenes in normal mouse tissues. Oncogene 5: 345–351

Wadewitz AG, Winer MA, Wolgemuth DJ (1993) Developmental and cell lineage specificity of raf family gene expression in mouse testis. Oncogene 8: 1055–1062

Witschi H, Saheb W (1974) Stimulation of DNA synthesis in mouse lung following intraperitoneal injection of butylated hydroxytoluene. Proc Soc Exp Biol Med 147: 690–693

Apoptosis Regulation by Raf, Bcl-2, and R-Ras

J. Troppmair and U.R. Rapp

Institute of Medical Radiation and Cell Research, University of Würzburg, Versbacher Str. 5, 97078 Würzburg, Germany

Introduction

The cellular response to environmental stimuli is triggered by signaling cascades which connect receptor activation at the cell membrane with intracellular changes resulting in proliferation, differentiation, survival, or cell death. One of the best-studied signaling pathways is the cytoplasmic cascade which channels signals originating from a variety of different receptors (with both intrinsic and associated protein tyrosine kinase (PTK) activity, and G protein-coupled receptors) through the cytoplasmatic serine threonine kinase Raf-1 (Rapp 1991; Daum et al. 1994; Rapp et al. 1994). Activation of Raf-1 is essential for the induction of growth by most mitogens in mammalian cells as well as in *D. melanogaster* and *C. elegans*. In NIH3T3 fibroblasts, microinjection of activated but not wild-type Raf-1 was sufficient to replace the growth factor for the induction of cell cycle entry (Smith et al. 1990). However, in the strictly interleukin (IL)-3 dependent myeloid cell line 32D, expression of oncogenic Raf-1 was insufficient to induce factor-independent proliferation which was readily achieved by the ectopic expression of protein tyrosine kinase oncogenes (Cleveland et al. 1994). Only in combination with v-*myc*, which synergizes with v-*raf* in the transformation of cells derived from several lineages (Rapp et al. 1994), did v-*raf* sustain proliferation of 32D cells in the absence of growth factors (Troppmair et al. 1992). To delineate the contribution of these two oncogenes to factor-independent growth, 32D cells constitutively expressing v-*myc* or v-*raf* were established and analyzed in the presence or absence of the growth factor IL-3. These studies demonstrated that constitutive expression of *myc* – though beneficial to cell cycle progression in the presence of IL-3 – accelerated cell death after factor removal (Askew et al. 1991). 32D cells expressing v-*raf* showed a shortened G1 phase and lowered IL-3 requirement in the presence of IL-3. In its absence, v-*raf* expression significantly prolonged cell survival (Cleveland et al. 1994).

Recent Results in Cancer Research, Vol. 143

Apoptosis Regulation by Bcl-2 and Raf-1

Several gene products have been identified as either repressors or inducers of apoptosis. Among them bcl-2 represents the prototype of a negative regulator of apoptosis. Bcl-2, first discovered at the site of a t(14;18) translocation in non-Hodgkin's lymphomas, has been shown to suppress apoptosis induced by a variety of stimuli (Reed 1994). Its gene product encodes a 26-kDa intracellular protein predominantly located in the outer mitochondrial membrane, the nuclear envelope, and parts of the endoplasmic reticulum (ER) (Reed 1994). Recently it has been shown that Bcl-2 interacts with R-Ras (see next), a member of the Ras family of small GTP binding proteins which binds to Raf-1 in a fashion previously demonstrated for p21 Ras (Spaargaren et al. 1994). To test for possible involvement of Raf-1 in apoptosis suppression by Bcl-2, a weakly transforming version of Raf-1 called EC12 (Heidecker et al. 1990) was expressed constitutively alone or in combination with bcl-2 in 32D cells. These experiments demonstrated that Raf-1 and Bcl-2 synergized in their ability to suppress apoptosis (Wang et al. 1994). Biochemical analysis of cells coexpressing Raf-1 and Bcl-2 showed that Bcl-2 can be coimmunoprecipitated with Raf-1. Analysis of Raf-1 deletion mutants further demonstrated that the C-terminal half (kinase domain) of Raf-1 is sufficient for this interaction and did not require an active Raf-1 kinase. Further, binding of Bcl-2 to constitutively active Raf-1 does not result in the phosphorylation of Bcl-2, nor did Bcl-2 affect the activation of Raf-1 by Ras and the PTK lck or its ability to phosphorylate its physiological substrate MEK.

The functional consequence of the observed Raf-1/Bcl-2 interaction remains elusive. Based on the differences in the subcellular localisation between Raf-1 and Bcl-2 we speculate that Bcl-2 might function by translocating bound Raf-1 to cellular compartments where it can access components of the apoptosis-regulating machinery.

R-Ras-Induced Apoptosis Occurs via Bcl-2-Suppressible Mechanisms

In addition to the association with Raf-1 just demonstrated, Bcl-2 has been shown recently to associate with p23 R-Ras, a member of the Ras family of small G proteins (Fernandez-Sarabia and Bischoff 1993; Rey et al. 1994). This association requires the full-length Bcl-2 protein but only the 60 C-terminal amino acids of R-Ras (Fernandez-Sarabia and Bischoff 1993). In a fashion similar to p21-Ha-Ras, p23-R-Ras can interact with Raf-1 as well as rasGAP and NF-1 (Rey et al. 1994). Amino acid exchanges in R-Ras at positions which render Ha-ras oncogenic had only moderate effects on the ability to transform NIH3T3 fibroblasts and failed to induce DNA synthesis or membrane ruffling in Swiss 3T3 cells (Saez et al. 1994). In our work we have analyzed the significance of the R-Ras/Bcl-2/Raf-1 interaction in the regulation of cell death (Wang et al. 1995). These experiments demonstrated that the expression of a mutant R-Ras-38V (glycine at position 38 replaced by valine) in 32D cells increased the rate of cell death after IL-3 removal. Analysis of independent clones demonstrated the correlation of rates of apoptosis with levels of R-Ras (38V) protein. This apoptosis-promoting effect of R-Ras was not restricted to IL-3 deprived 32D cells but was also observed for FL5.12 and NIH3T3 cells. We were further able to demonstrate that the effect of R-Ras was sensitive to the inhibition by Bcl-2 as had been shown for a variety of apoptotic stimuli.

In search for a possible mechanism for the protective effect of Bcl-2 on R-Ras-induced apoptosis under conditions of growth factor removal we analyzed the effect of Bcl-2 on the GTP binding and GTPase activity of R-Ras and R-Ras-38V as well as on the ability of R-Ras to bind to other proteins. Addition of purified biologically active Bcl-2 protein to GST wild-type and mutant R-Ras protein had no effect on the intrinsic GTPase activity and did not alter the ratio of GDP/GTP bound to wild-type or mutant R-Ras as well as the total amount of guanidine nucleotides bound.

Further studies with baculovirus-expressed R-Ras (wild type and mutant), Raf-1, and Bcl-2 proteins were carried out in Sf9 cells to study the effect of Bcl-2 on the Ras/Raf-1 interaction. Mutant R-Ras and to a lesser extent wild-type R-Ras were found associated with Raf-1. In the case of p23-Ras V38 this interaction resulted in the activation of Raf-1 as demonstrated by its ability to phosphorylate MEK. Presence of Bcl-2 did not alter Raf-1 kinase activity, suggesting that Bcl-2 does not nullify R-Ras effects by interfering with Raf-1 activation.

Conclusion

We have previously demonstrated that activated Raf-1 can suppress apoptosis induced in 32D cells by growth factor removal. The mechanism by which Raf-1 affects cell death remains enigmatic but recent findings have shown that Raf-1 can physically associate with the antiapoptotic protein Bcl-2 as well as the apoptosis-inducing R-Ras protein. In the case of Bcl-2 this interaction with the kinase domain of Raf-1 does not alter the phosphorylation status of Bcl-2 nor could we find any effect of constitutively expressed Bcl-2 on Raf kinase activity (Reed et al. 1991). Expression of mutant R-Ras protein in 32D cells results in the induction of apoptosis, which is sensitive to inhibition by Bcl-2. Although not analyzed in 32D cells, coexpression of mutant R-Ras with wild type Raf-1 in Sf-9 cells lead to the activation of Raf-1 kinase. Although the possibility has to be considered that R-Ras-induced apoptosis is mediated through Raf-1-independent pathways, these results raise the possibility that activated Raf plays a role in the induction as well as suppression of apoptosis. Raf-interacting proteins like R-Ras or Bcl-2 might function by shuttling Raf-1 to new subcellular locations and thereby alter substrate interactions. The data are compatible with the following model: Raf may function as the effector of Bcl-2. The primary role of Bcl-2 would be as a locator of Raf, which it may bring to

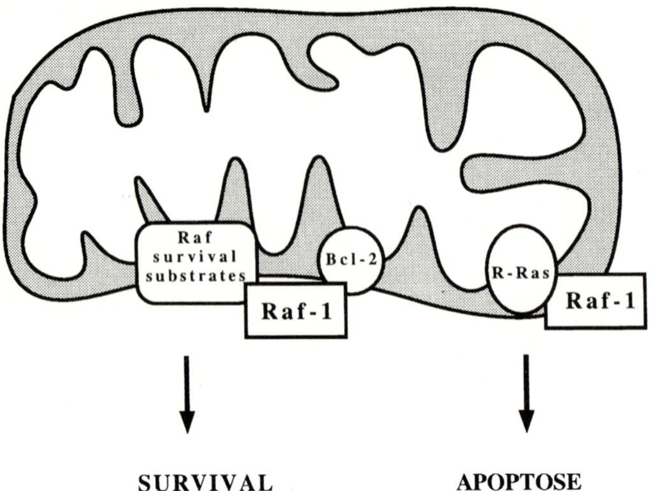

Fig. 1. Model for the potential interactions of Raf-1 with Bcl-2 or R-Ras at the outer mitochondrial membrane

substrates/activators present in the outer mitochondrial and/or nuclear membrane. R-Ras may compete with Bcl-2 for Raf in these locations and block access to substrates involved in the suppression of apoptosis. Bcl-2 has been shown to localize to the outer mitochondrial membrane (Reed 1994). Such a location is also proposed for R-Ras.

A model for the potential interactions of Raf-1 with Bcl-2 or R-Ras at the outer mitochondrial membrane is given in Fig. 1. Interaction with Bcl-2 allows Raf-1 to access substrates required for the transmission of a survival signal. Raf-1 bound to R-Ras is excluded from this interaction, thereby blunting Raf-1 survival activity.

References

Askew DS, Shmun RA, Simmons BC, Cleveland JL (1991) Constitutive c-myc expression in an IL-3 dependent myeloid cell line suppresses cell cycle arrest and accelerates apoptosis. Oncogene 6: 1915–1922

Cleveland JL, Troppmair J, Packham G, Askew DS, Lloyd P, Gonzales-Garcia M, Nunez G, Ihle JN, Rapp UR (1994) v-raf suppresses apoptosis and promotes growth of interleukin-3-dependent myeloid cells. Oncogene 9: 2217–2226

Daum G, Eisenmann Tappe I, Fries HW, Troppmair J, Rapp UR (1994) Ins and outs of raf kinase. TIBS 19: 474–480

Fernandez-Sarabia MJ, Bischoff JR (1993) Bcl-2 associates with the ras-related protein R-Ras p23. Nature 366: 274–275

Heidecker G, Huleihel M, Cleveland JL, Kolch W, Beck TW, Lloyd P, Pawson T, Rapp UR (1990) Mutational activation of c-raf-1 and definition of the minimal transforming sequence. Mol Cell Biol 10: 2503–2512

Rapp UR (1991) Role of Raf-1 serine/threonine protein kinase in growth factor signal transduction. Oncogene 6: 495–500

Rapp UR, Bruder JT, Troppmair J (1994) Role of Raf signal transduction pathway in fos/jun regulation and determination of cell fates. In: Angel P, Herrlich P (eds) The fos jun families of transcription factors. CRC, Boca Raton, pp 221–247

Reed JC (1994) Bcl-2 and the regulation of programmed cell death. J Cell Biol 124: 1–6

Reed JC, Yum S, Cuddy MP, Turner BC, Rapp UR (1991) Differential regulation of the p72-74 RAF-1 kinase in 373 fibroblasts expressing ras or src oncogenes. Cell Growth Differ 2: 235–243

Rey I, Taylor-Harris P, van Erp H, Hall A (1994) R-ras interacts with ras GAP, neurofibromin and c-raf but does not regulate cell growth or differentiation. Oncogene 9: 685–692

Saez RA, Chan ML, Miki T, Aaronson A (1994) Oncogenic activation off human R-ras by point mutations analogous to those of prototype H-ras oncogenes. Oncogene 9: 2977–2982

Smith MR, Heidecker G, Rapp UR, Kung HF (1990) Induction of transformation and DNA synthesis after microinjection of raf proteins. Mol Cell Biol 10: 3828–3833

Spaargaren M, Martin GA, McCormick F, Fernandez-Sarabia MJ, Bischoff JR (1994) The ras related protein R-Ras interacts directly with Raf-1 in a GTP-dependent manner. Biochem J 300: 303–307

Troppmair J, Cleveland JL, Askew DS, Rapp UR (1992) v-Raf/v-Myc synergism in abrogation of IL-3 dependence: v-Raf suppresses apoptosis. In: Capron A, Compans RW, Cooper M et al. (eds) Current topics in microbiology and immunology, vol 182. Springer, Berlin Heidelberg New York, pp 453–460

Wang H-G Miyashita T, Takayama S, Sato T, Torigoe T, Krajewski S, Tanaka S, Hovey L, Troppmair J, Rapp UR, Reed JC (1994) Apoptosis regulation by interaction of Bcl-2 protein and Raf-1 kinase. Oncogene 9: 2751–2756

Wang H-G, Millan JA, Cox AD, Der CD, Rapp UR, Beck T, Zha H, Reed JC (1995) R-Ras promotes apoptosis caused by growth factor deprivation via a bcl-2 suppressible mechanism. J Cell Biol 129: 1103–1114

New Cell Cycle-Regulated Genes in the Yeast Saccharomyces cerevisiae

T. Schuster[1], C. Price[2], W. Rossoll[1], and B. Kovacech[1]

[1]Institute for Medical Radiation and Cell Research, University of Würzburg, Versbacher Straβe 5, 97078 Würzburg, Germany
[2]Krebs Institute, Department of Molecular Biology and Biotechnology, University of Sheffield, P.O. Box 594, Western Bank, Sheffield S10 2UH, UK

Introduction

Primary carcinogenic changes involve mutations in genes which contribute to the ordered events that control the eucaryotic cell cycle. It has been demonstrated that many protooncogenes take part in the regulation of cell growth. Prad1, for instance, has been identified as cyclin D1. Myc is involved in early cell cycle events while p53, one of the growing number of tumor suppressors, blocks the cell cycle in G1 in response to DNA damage. These proteins interfere with certain cell cycle control elements and cause either induction or repression of specific regulatory events. However, when mutated these regulators may be unable to fulfill their proper function which can then lead to inappropriate cell cycle progression. This may result in cell death or in transformation from quiescence to uncontrolled proliferation. Thus, the investigation of the cell cycle will lead to a better understanding of the molecular events which result in malignant cell growth.

Ongoing work has described a general model of how a cell regulates its progression through the cell cycle (Murray 1989; Lewin 1990; Pines and Hunter 1990; Pines 1993a,b). Currently, it is thought that specific serine/threonine kinases in conjunction with cyclins play a central role in the regulation of these events (Pines and Hunter 1990; Reed and Wittenberg 1990). Work on *Saccharomyces cerevisiae* has demonstrated that the gene product of *CDC28*, p34*CDC28*, forms a complex with any one of the G1 cyclins, Cln1, Cln2, and Cln3, in the G1 stage of the cell cycle (Hadwiger et al. 1989; Richardson et al. 1989; Reed 1991). The p34-cyclin complexes constitute active protein kinases that directly promote budding (Cvrckova and Nasmyth 1993). At around the same time when this G1-kinase is formed, p34*CDC28* assembles with one of two B-type cyclins. Clb5 and Clb6, to form kinases which activate replication (Schwob and Nasmyth 1993). Furthermore, it has been shown that later in the cell cycle, in G2 prior to mitosis, p34*CDC28* is able to generate complexes with G2 cyclins, which in budding yeast are Clb1 to Clb4, to form

Recent Results in Cancer Research, Vol. 143

active kinases whose activity then leads to progression into M phase (Reed and Wittenberg 1990; Surana et al. 1991). This mitotic kinase has initially been described as the maturation promoting factor (MPF) first identified in studies on frog oocytes (Masui and Markert 1971; Gerhart et al. 1984; Newport and Kirschner 1984). In all cases disassembly of the complexes and degradation of the cyclin parts are thought to be required to inactivate the kinase function and release the cell into the following cell cycle stages (Draetta et al. 1989).

Work on yeast and vertebrates has shown that this mechanism of regulation of cell growth is conserved throughout evolution. The model involves mainly posttranslational events, such as complex formation, protein modification, and degradation. However, cell cycle-specific transcriptional activation also seems to be required to control the discontinuous processes of the cell cycle. It has been estimated that in budding yeast as many as 250 genes may be regulated in a cell cycle-specific manner (Price et al. 1991). Many of them are activated in early and late G1, others during S-phase, and some are transcribed during G2 and mitosis. Genes that have been found to be activated in early G1 are involved in cell separation, like *CTS1* encoding chitinase (Dohrmann et al. 1992, *EGT1* (Kovacech and Schuster, unpublished), and *EGT2* (Kovacech et al., submitted). Another gene, *SIC1*, which is upregulated during early G1, seems to code for a protein that inactivates the S-phase promoting kinase (Schwob et al. 1994). In late G1, all genes containing SCB- and MCB-*cis*-acting elements in their promoter region are activated. The SCB-element containing genes encode G1-cyclins like Cln1, Cln2, and Hcs26 (Wittenberg et al. 1990; Ogas et al. 1991; Nasmyth and Dirick 1991) and the double-strand endonuclease HO, which is involved in mating type switching (Nasmyth 1985; Breeden and Nasmyth 1987; Andrews and Herskowitz 1989). The genes containing MCB sequences in their promoters, on the other hand, are generally involved in DNA replication, e.g., *POL1, TMP1*, and *CDC9* (McIntosh 1993). The cyclin genes *CLB5* and *CLB6* as well as *SPK1*, which encodes an essential S-phase specific kinase, and *SWI4* encoding one of the SCB binding transcription factors also contain MCB-elements in their promoters (Breeden and Mikesell 1991; Epstein and Cross 1992; Schwob and Nasmyth 1993; Zheng et al. 1993; Foster et al. 1993). While during S-phase all the histone genes are expressed (Osley 1991), in late S-phase and during G2 the B-type cyclin genes *CLB1* to *CLB4* are transcribed, the gene products of which form the mitotic kinase, in conjunction with p34*CDC28* (Nasmyth 1993; Amon et al. 1993). More recently genes have been identified which are expressed exclusively during mitosis, e.g., *DBF2* encoding a protein kinase (Parks and Johnson 1992), and *MST1* and *MST2* which code for related membrane proteins that resemble some known receptors containing seven membrane-spanning domains (Price et al. 1991; Rossoll and Schuster, unpublished). All these data suggest a significant role of cell cycle-dependent transcriptional activation for the regulation of cell growth. A systematic search for cell cycle-regulated genes should identify novel genes whose cell cycle-dependent transcriptional activity is crucial for normal cell growth. We have undertaken such a search using the unicellular eukaryotic organism *Saccharomyces cerevisiae*.

Isolation of Novel Cell Cycle Regulated Genes

To find genes of that kind our strategy was first to search for all cell cycle-regulated genes in *S. cerevisiae* and then later to test each for their function. We decided to proceed using northern blot analysis as the most sensitive method for identifying cell cycle-regulated genes. Our approach relied on the existence of an ordered yeast genomic library provided to us by Maynard Olson which encompasses 80%–90% of the haploid yeast genome subcloned in 855 overlapping phage of type λ (Olson et al. 1986; Riles et al. 1993). In the primary screen, individual *Eco*RI/*Hind*III DNA restriction fragments, which correspond to those which have been ordered into a map of yeast chromosomes by M. Olson and coworkers, were isolated from the recombinant phage. They were used as probes in northern blots against RNA samples out of six different cell cycle stages. Transcripts identified as being cell cycle-regulated in this screen were further analyzed by a secondary screen which consists of northern blots of temporal staged RNAs isolated from synchronously growing cultures. Figure 1 shows some candidate genes out of our collection of genes detected as being cell cycle-regulated. This secondary screen enabled us to establish whether or not these transcripts exhibit genuine periodicity (Price et al. 1991). Thus far, we have examined over 60% of the library using more than 4500 northern hybridizations.

This approach has the advantage that we are able to detect all those genes which cannot be found by standard genetic techniques. It is known that many genes are refractory to mutagenesis, while others can be redundant in sequence or function. Additionally, we were able to map the chromosomal location of every gene of interest immediately, which helps us to distinguish genes which have previously been isolated.

Characterization of the Isolated Genes

Four of the genes we have identified in our screen as being cell cycle-dependently expressed are *EGT2* (*e*arly *G*1 *t*ranscript), *MST1* and *MST2* (*m*itosis-*s*pecific *t*ranscript), and *KIN3* (*Kin*ase 3, Kambouris et al. 1993). In Northern blots using RNAs isolated from cell cultures synchronized by using the thermosensitive allele *cdc15* (arrest at the restrictive temperature in mitosis) we were able to show (Fig. 1) that peak expression levels of *EGT2* appear early in G1 shortly after the peak expression levels of *MST1, MST2*, and *KIN3* (not shown) which are expressed in mitosis. As controls we used the *URA3* gene that is expressed constitutively throughout the cell cycle and the gene encoding

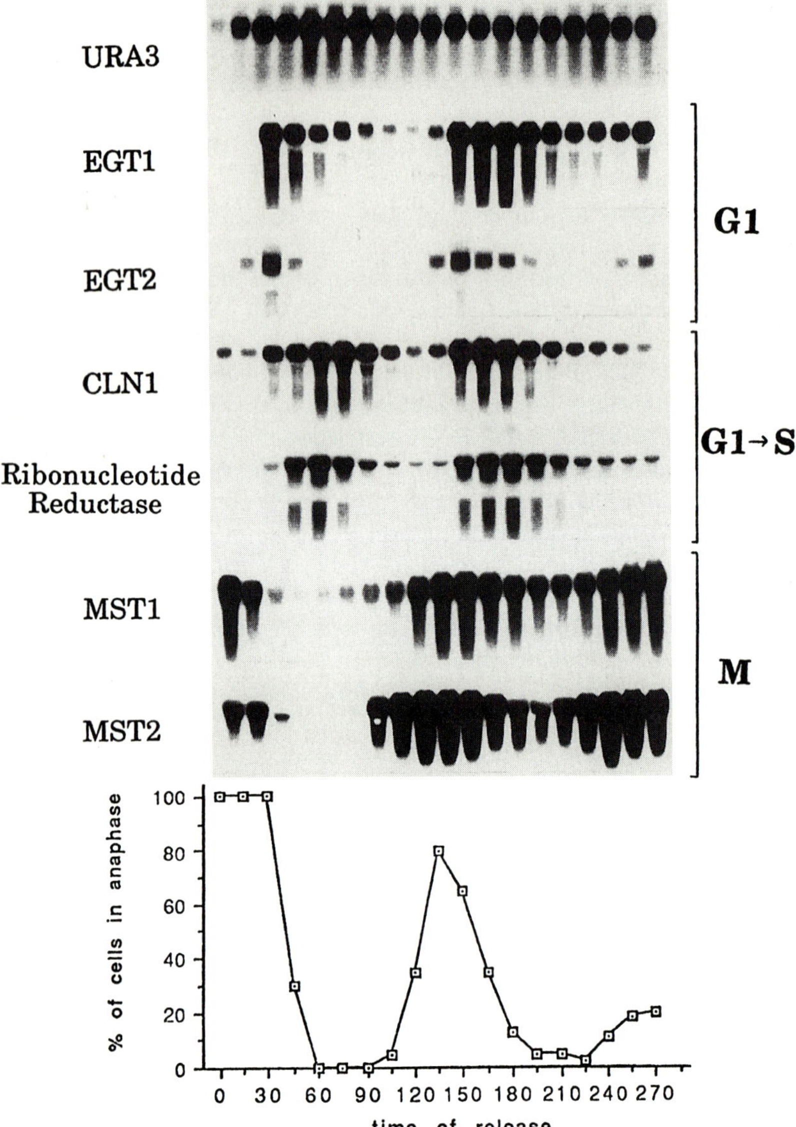

Fig. 1. Cell cycle dependent expression in *cdc15*^{ts}-synchronized yeast cell cultures. Exponentially growing cells were arrested in mitosis by incubation at the restrictive temperature (37 °C) and subsequently released by growth at the permissive temperature (25 °C). Samples were taken every 15 min up to 270 min. The zero time point was taken immediately prior to the release from the temperature arrest. Synchrony was determined by scoring for the presence of anaphase spindles following in situ immunofluorescence with rat antitubulin monoclonal antibodies. 10 μg of total RNA from each time point was electrophoresed on 1% agarose formaldehyde gels and the gene probes used for hybridization are indicated in the figure

the large subunit of ribonucleotide reductase (*RNR1*) which is expressed shortly after cells have passed Start. The graph indicates the percentage of cells being in mitosis identified by antitubulin staining of mitotic spindles.

To elucidate the specific functions of the genes we have isolated, we are applying reverse genetic techniques. This should identify genes whose specific transcriptional fluctuation during the cell cycle is a requirement for the ordered steps of cell growth. An additional important question we ask is which regulatory cell cycle events lead to activation and which ones lead to inactivation of transcription of the genes we isolate in our screen. The answer to this question will give information about the connection of the cell cycle with the transcriptional machinery.

EGT2 Is Involved in Cell Separation

EGT2 encodes a protein of 1041 amino acids in length. It contains a potential 20-amino-acid leader peptide at its N-terminus that could lead the peptide into the secretory pathway. In its C-terminal half it has nine direct repeats of a novel type (marked by boxes). The consensus of these repeats is shown (see Fig. 2).

Microscopic investigation revealed a delay of cell separation if *EGT2* is deleted. Contrary to wild-type cells, *egt2*- cells do not separate in G1 but create small clusters of three to four cells which consist of connected mother and daughter cells, both already budding and replicating their DNA. This leads us to conclude that Egt2 protein is involved in mother-daughter cell disjunction.

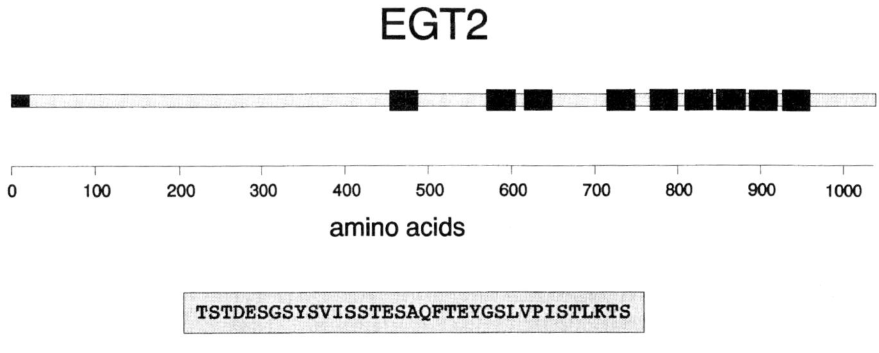

Fig. 2. A graphic representation of the *EGT2* gene. According to our database searches, the Egt2 protein does not show any similarity to other known gene products. It contains nine homologous sequences at its C-terminal part *(dark shadowed boxes)* whose consensus is outlined. Its potential leader sequence at the amino terminus is indicated as a *black box*

EGT2 Is Expressed at the Boundary Between Mitosis and Early G1 but Before Start

The appearance of *EGT2* expression has been studied by hybridizing Northern blots of temporal staged RNA. The RNAs were isolated out of cells synchronized by several different methods (B. Kovacech et al. 1996). These experiments show that *EGT2* is expressed immediately after mitosis but before Start in G1. It is, therefore, the first cell cycle-regulated gene that has been identified as being expressed at such an early cell cycle stage. Our analysis revealed that the transcription factor which induces *EGT2* transcription is Swi5, which is known to be one of the transactivators of the *HO* gene. While Swi5 activates *EGT2* in early G1, it induces *HO* transcription during late G1 and early S-phase in conjunction with Swi4 and Swi6 (B. Kovacech et al. 1996). This is the first time that a transcription factor has been described which is able to activate two different genes at two different cell cycle stages. Since the early G1-stage of the cell cycle is crucial for the developmental fate of a eukaryotic cell, further investigation of the transcriptional regulation of genes expressed during this cell cycle stage will help us understand how a cell regulates its own fate.

The MST Gene Family

In our screen we have identified several unknown periodically expressed genes, most of which exhibit expression at the late G1/S boundary and are presumably involved in progression into S-phase or in DNA replication. Two of them, however, showed strong expression when cells are in mitosis. We called them *MST1* (Price et al. 1991) and *MST2* which stands for *M*itosis-*S*pecific *T*ranscript *1* and *2*.

Sequence analysis revealed that the *MST* genes are highly related and code for membrane proteins possessing seven putative membrane-spanning domains (Fig. 3). Antibodies directed against the aminoterminal part of Mst1 revealed that the proteins are located in the plasma membrane (unpublished).

Much effort has been aimed at elucidating the role these two genes play in the development of a yeast cell. So far, we have not been able to ascribe a function to these genes. The great similarity the hydrophobic domains show to the light-driven proton pump bacteriorhodopsin suggests the possibility that both genes encode membrane proteins performing ion channel functions. However, since Mst1 and Mst2 seem to belong to the same class of membrane proteins as the G protein-coupled receptors, it is also possible that they exhibit receptor function. This is supported by our finding of a gene, *HSP30*, encoding a membrane protein with an identity of only 35% to Mst1 and Mst2. Hsp30 is the first membrane protein that is a heat shock protein (Regnacq and Boucherie 1993; Piper et al. 1994). Since the domains most homologous to the Mst proteins are positioned between the membrane-spanning domains at

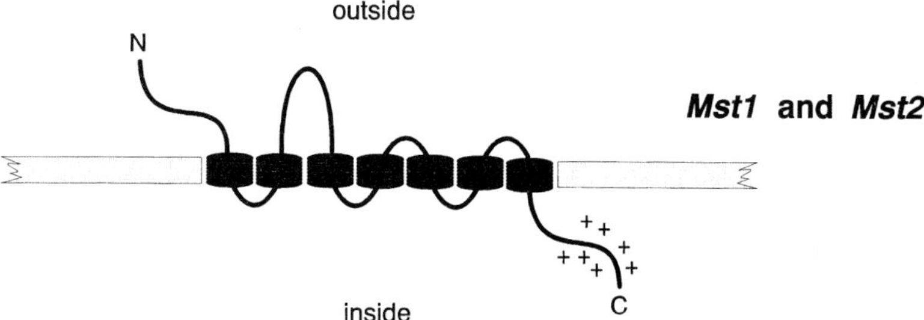

Fig. 3. *MST1* and *MST2* encode highly related cytoplasmic membrane proteins. This graphic representation of the *MST1* and *MST2* gene products describe their location in the plasma membrane. Sequence analysis revealed that their carboxy termini are positively charged

locations we think are placed at the outside of the cell, the domains may bind the same ligand and transmit presumably different signals. If this hypothesis proves to be correct, the *MST* gene family could be involved in a novel signal transduction pathway. The deletion of *MST1, MST2,* and *HSP30,* however, revealed that even the triple deletion is not lethal for the cell. Currently, further functional analysis is examining the growth behavior of strains deleted for all three genes under different growth conditions.

Transcriptional Regulation of the MST Gene Family

MST1 and *MST2* were the first genes detected in *S. cerevisiae* which are exclusively expressed during mitosis. Studying the regulation of their expression will lead to the understanding of how the individual cell cycle -dependent steps governing the entry of a cell into mitosis are involved in activation of these genes and which steps lead to their repression again later in the cell cycle. Our analysis revealed that transcriptional activation of both genes is dependent on the activity of mitotic kinase (p34*CDC28*-Clb2). Their transcriptional inactivation, however, requires active G1-kinase (p34*CDC28*-Cln3). The *HSP30* gene, however, is expressed only during certain stress conditions such as heat shock, starvation, and pheromone arrest. If it turns out that this gene family is indeed involved in sensing environmental stress conditions, the different transcriptional activation patterns of the genes might be crucial for a correct response to distinct environmental cues.

The KIN3 Gene

KIN3 codes for a putative serine/threonine protein kinase with an unknown function (Schweitzer and Philippsen 1992). Its homology to *nimA* – a gene of the filamentous fungus *Aspergillus nidulans* that is required for progression into mitosis (Osmani et al. 1988) – suggests a possible role in controlling mitotic events. Its deletion, however, does not have any effect on cell growth. Overexpression, on the other hand, shows dramatic effects on cytokinesis and nuclear division. Additionally, we have shown that *KIN3* is regulated in a cell cycle-dependent manner and that expression of *KIN3* peaks in mitosis (unpublished).

The fact that the deletion of *KIN3* has no effect on growth may be due to the existence of a homologous gene which complements a *KIN3* functional defect. This makes it very difficult to analyze *KIN3* for the functional role it may have in division control. Therefore, we employed a colony color assay to screen for synthetic lethal mutations in yeast cells with no functional *KIN3* gene in the genetic background. We identified several mutants which depend on ectopic expression of *KIN3*. This will enable us now to study *KIN3* function under genetic conditions where it has become an essential gene. In an initial experiment we transformed one synthetic lethal mutant with a genomic yeast library. We identified five different clones which could complement the mutant phenotype. One plasmid carried the *KIN3* gene. The other clones contained the gene *CCR4* (=*c*arbon *c*atabolite *r*epressor; Malvar et al. 1992) which is required for the expression of genes involved in nonfermentative growth. It is thought, however, that *CCR4* plays a general role in transcription and is not only involved in carbon catabolite repression. Currently, we are examining the phenotype of the synthetic lethal mutants in the absence of *KIN3* expression.

Conclusion

To investigate the role of transcriptional activation in governing the timing and order of events of the cell cycle we are searching the genome of the yeast *S. cerevisiae* for cell cycle-dependently transcribed genes and testing them for a possible function in the regulation of cell growth. For this purpose we have chosen a northern blot approach which is able to screen for periodically expressed genes. Classic genetic screens have turned up a large number of genes which are important for normal cell growth and development. Many genes, however, cannot be identified this way, since they are either refractory of mutagenesis or they consist of multigene families whose products possess redundant functions. For example, histone genes have never been found as temperature-sensitive mutants in yeast, which is a prerequisite for classic genetic screens. On the other hand, the deletion of one or even two of the three G1-cyclin genes (*CLN1* to *CLN3*) in yeast does not lead to cell death. There are also four different B-type cyclins present in *S. cerevisiae*. A deletion of just one of them is not lethal for a yeast cell. These findings argue in favor of an employment of our Northern approach which should identify most if not all cell cycle-regulated transcriptional units. This screen enabled us to identify a large collection of periodically expressed genes, some of which are now under investigation in our laboratory. Since the deletion of these genes is not lethal for a yeast cell, none of them would have been detected in a classic genetic screen. Even the triple deletion of the whole *MST* gene family did not reveal any phenotype. Therefore, reverse genetic techniques have to be employed to identify a specific function for the individual genes. These kinds of experiments identified the function of *EGT2* as well as the nature of its transcriptional regulation (B. Kovacech et al., submitted). Next, we expect to clarify the function of *KIN3* and the *MST* gene family. The transcriptional regulation of these genes is also under current investigation. Our ongoing research should enable us to understand the significance of the relationship between cell cycle-dependent activation of transcription and the function of the genes we have identified so far and which we will detect in the near future.

References

Amon A, Tyers M, Futcher B, Nasmyth K (1993) Mechanisms that help the yeast cell cycle clock tick: G2 cyclins transcriptionally activate and repress G1 cyclins. Cell 74: 993–1007

Andrews BJ, Herskowitz I (1989) The yeast Swi4 protein contains a motif present in developmental regulators and is part of a complex involved in cell-cycle-dependent transcription. Nature 342: 830–833

Breeden L, Mikesell GE (1991) Cell cycle-specific expression of the SWI4 transcription factor is required for the cell cycle regulation of HO transcription. Genes Dev 5: 1183–1190

Breeden L, Nasmyth K (1987) Cell cycle control of the yeast HO gene: cis- and trans-acting regulators. Cell 48: 389–397

Cvrckova F, Nasmyth K (1993) Yeast G1 cyclins CLN1 and CLN2 and a Gap-like protein have a role in bud formation. EMBO J 12: 5277–5286

Dohrman PR, Butler G, Tamai K, Dorland S, Green JR, Thiele DJ, Stillman D (1992) Parallel pathways of gene regulation: homologous regulators SW15 and ACE2 differentially control transcription of HO and chitinase. Genes Dev 6: 93–104

Draetta G, Luca F, Westendorf J, Brizuela L, Ruderman J, Beach D (1989) Cdc2 protein kinase is complexed with both cyclin A and B: evidence for proteolytic inactivation of MPF. Cell 56: 829–838

Epstein CB, Cross FR (1992) CLB5, a novel B cyclin from budding yeast with a role in S-phase. Genes Dev 6: 1695–1706

Foster R, Mikesell GE, Breeden L (1993) Multiple SWI6-dependent cis-acting elements control SWI4 transcription through the cell cycle. Mol Cell Biol 13: 3792–3801

Gerhart J, Wu M, Kirschner M (1984) Cell cycle dynamics of an M-phase-specific cytoplasmic factor in Xenopus laevis oocytes and eggs. J Cell Biol 98: 1247–1255

Hadwiger JA, Wittenberg C, Richardson HE, de Barros Lopez M, Reed SI (1989) A family of cyclin homologs that control the G1 phase in yeast. Proc Natl Acad Sci USA 86: 6255–6259

Kovacech B, Nasmyth K, Schuster T (1996) EGT2 gene transcription is induced predominantly by Swi5 in early Gl. Mol Cell Biol 16: in press

Lewin B (1990) Driving the cell cycle: M phase kinase, its partners, and substrates. Cell 61: 743–752

Malvar T, Biron RW, Kaback DB, Denis CL (1992) The CCR4 protein from Saccharomyces cerevisiae contains a leucine-rich repeat region which is required for its control of ADH2 gene expression. Genetics 132: 951–962

McIntosh EM (1993) MCB elements and the regulation of DNA replication in yeast. Curr Genet 24: 185–192
Masui Y, Markert CL (1971) Cytoplasmic control of nuclear behavior during meiotic maturation of frog oocytes. J Exp Zool 177: 129–145
Murray AW (1989) The cell as a cdc2 cycle. Nature 342: 14–15
Nasmyth K (1985) A repetitive DNA sequence that confers cell-cycle START (CDC28)-dependent transcription of the HO gene in yeast. Cell 42: 225–235
Nasmyth K (1993) Control of the yeast cell cycle by the Cdc28 protein kinase. Curr Opin Cell Biol 5: 166–179
Nasmyth K, Dirick L (1991) The role of SWI4 and SWI16 in the activity of G1 cyclins in yeast. Cell 66: 995–1013
Newport JW, Kirschner MW (1984) Regulation of the cell cycle during early Xenopus development. Cell 37: 731–742
Ogas J, Andrews BJ, Herskowitz I (1991) Transcriptional activation of CLN1, CLN2, and a putative new G1 cyclin (HCS26) by Swi4, a positive regulator of G1-specific transcription. Cell 66: 1015–1026
Olson MV, Dutchik JE, Graham MY, Brodeur GM, Helms C, Frank M, Mc Collin M, Scheinman R, Frank T (1986) Random-clone strategy for genomic restriction mapping in yeast. Proc Natl Acad Sci USA 83: 7826–7830
Osley M (1991) Regulation of histone synthesis in the cell cycle. Annu Rev Biochem 60: 827–861
Osmani SA, Pu RT, Morris NR (1988) Mitotic induction and maintenance by over-expression of a G2-specific gene that encodes a potential protein kinase. Cell 53: 237–244
Parks V, Johnston LH (1992) SPO12 and SIT4 suppress mutations in DBF2, which encodes a cell cycle protein kinase that is periodically expressed. Nucleic Acids Res 20: 5617–5623
Pines J (1993a) Cyclin-dependent kinases. Curr Biol 3: 544–547
Pines J (1993b) Cyclins and cyclin-dependent kinases: take your partners. TIBS 18: 195–197
Pines J, Hunter T (1990) p34cdc2: The S and M kinase. New Biol 2: 389–401
Piper PW, Talreja K, Panaretou B, Moradas-Ferreira P, Byrne K, Praekelt UM, Meacock P, Regnacq M, Boucherie H (1994) Induction of major heat-shock proteins of Saccharomyces cerevisiae, including plasma membrane Hsp30, by ethanol levels above a critical threshold. Microbiology 140: 3031–3038
Price C, Nasmyth K, Schuster T (1991) A general approach to the isolation of cell cycle-regulated genes in the budding yeast, Saccharomyces cerevisiae. J Mol Biol 218: 543–556
Reed SI (1991) G1-specific cyclins: in search of an S-phase promoting factor. TIG 7: 95–99
Reed SI, Wittenberg C (1990) Mitotic role for the Cdc28 protein kinase of Saccharomyces cerevisiae. Proc Natl Acad Sci USA 87: 5697–5701
Regnacq M, Boucherie H (1993) Isolation and sequence of HSP30, a yeast heat-shock gene coding for a hydrophobic membrane protein. Curr Genet 23: 435–442
Richardson HE, Wittenberg C, Cross F, Reed SI (1989) An essential G1 function for cyclin-like proteins in yeast. Cell 59: 1127–1133
Riles L, Dutchik JE, Baktha A, McCauley BK, Thayer EC, Leckie MP, Braden VV, Depke JE, Olson MV (1993) Physical maps of the six smallest chromosomes of Saccharomyces cerevisiae at a resolution of 2.6 kilobase pairs. Genetics 134: 81–150
Schweitzer B, Philippsen P (1992) NPK1, a nonessential protein kinase gene in Saccharomyces cerevisiae with similarity to Aspergillus nidulans nimA. Mol Gen Genet 234: 164–167

Schwob E, Nasmyth K (1993) CLB5 and CLB6, a new pair of B cyclins involved in DNA replication in Saccharomyces cerevisiae. Genes Dev 7: 1160–1175

Schwob E, Böhm T, Mendenhal MD, Nasmyth K (1994) The B-type cyclin kinase inhibitor $p40^{SIC1}$ controls the G1 to S transition in S. cerevisiae. Cell 79: 233–244

Surana U, Robitsch HH, Price C, Schuster T, Fitch I, Futcher AB, Nasmyth K (1991) The role of CDC28 and cyclins during mitosis in the budding yeast S. cerevisiae. Cell 65: 145–161

Wittenberg C, Sugimoto K, Reed SI (1990) G1-specific cyclins of S. cerevisiae: cell cycle periodicity, regulation by mating pheromone, and association with p34CDC28 protein kinase. Cell 62: 225–237

Zheng P, Fay DS, Burton J, Xiao H, Pinkham JL, Stern DF (1993) SPK1 is an essential S-phase specific gene of Saccharomyces cerevisiae that encodes a nuclear serin/threonine/tyrosine kinase. Mol Cell Biol 13: 5829–5842

The Role of Workhorse Protein Kinases in Coordinating DNA Metabolism and Cell Growth

E. Christenson, A.J. DeMaggio, and M.F. Hoekstra

ICOS Corporation, 22021-20th Ave S.E., Bothell, WA 98021, USA

Introduction

Cells are continually experiencing various forms of DNA damage. External factors such as environmental agents and radiation or internal factors such as oxidative damage or replication errors can all lead to potentially mutagenic or lethal DNA lesions. UV irradiation and DNA strand interruptions, for example, stimulate transcription and genetic recombination, lead to the activation of DNA repair proteins, cause cell cycle arrest, and initiate nuclear signal transduction cascades (Hartwell 1992; Hartwell and Weinart 1989; Hibi et al. 1993).

A single DNA double-strand break is a dominant lesion that is toxic if left unrepaired. In the baker's yeast *Saccharomyces cerevisiae*, strains that contain the HO endonuclease and mutations in recombination-repair genes such as *RAD52* are nonviable (Malone and Esposito 1980). HO is a site-specific double-strand endonuclease that makes a double-strand break at the mating-type locus that initiates mating-type interconversion. Rad52p is a DNA repair protein that interacts with Rad51p, a recA-like protein in yeast. Rad52p is required for the repair of DNA double-strand breaks introduced by ionizing radiation and by alkylating agents like methyl methanesulfonate (MMS); it is also essential for yeast to proceed through meiosis I. The nonviability of *HO rad52* strains is thought to be due to the inability of *rad52* mutants to tolerate and repair the double-strand break introduced by the HO protein.

In mammalian cells, a similar paradigm is observed for the tolerance and repair of DNA double-strand breaks. Wahl and coworkers (DiLenardo et al. 1994) have shown that DNA damage triggers a prolonged G1 arrest. This arrest is dependent on p53 and it has been suggested that p53 helps maintain genetic stability in normal human diploid fibroblasts by mediating a permanent cell cycle arrest when low amounts of unrepaired DNA damage are present in G1 (DiLenardo et al. 1994).

Recent Results in Cancer Research, Vol. 143

The complex physiology of cellular responses to DNA damage, and in particular DNA strand breaks, begs the question of whether all the factors responsible for the tolerance and repair of DNA strand interruptions have been identified. In other words, have all the components for double-strand break repair been identified and is the repair pathway saturated? The most likely answer is that further components will be identified and, because the repair response to DNA strand breaks is predominantly postreplicative and occurs through recombinational mechanisms, genetic means to identify additional components can rely on a variety of approaches. For example, since a single unrepaired double-strand break is toxic, genetic screens based on conditional cellular viability could be employed to identify mutants in double-strand break repair. Further, since the repair is recombinational, mutants with double-strand break-induced recombination defects could also be employed to identify additional components. Both of these strategies have been fruitfully applied and have resulted in the identification of a large number of potential DNA repair mutants. The remainder of this article will be a discussion of the identification and characterization of a conserved protein kinase gene family that was first identified through an associated mutant DNA repair defect in baker's yeast.

S. cerevisiae Isoforms of Casein Kinase I

The *S. cerevisiae HRR25* gene was identified in a mutant hunt devised to identify yeast strains that were sensitive to persistent DNA strand interruptions (Hoekstra et al. 1991). A wild-type yeast strain containing galactose-regulated *HO* endonuclease gene was mutagenized, and survivors were screened for isolates that were unable to grow on galactose-containing medium. A large collection of mutants was identified, and among these was a single isolate (*hrr25-1*) that appeared to encode a potential regulator of DNA strand break repair. *Hrr25-1* mutants were sensitive to persistent HO expression and to MMS. This mutant was resistant to UV treatment yet was unable to sporulate, a defect that was attributed to an inability to repair the high level of DNA strand breaks that occur during meiosis I genetic recombination. Finally, the *hrr25-1* mutant strain was proficient at intrachromosomal mitotic recombination, suggesting that the cells contained the basic recombination apparatus. These data further suggested that Hrr25p played a role, directly or indirectly, in the response to DNA strand breaks.

A deletion allele of *hrr25* revealed additional phenotypic defects that were not found with *hrr25-1*. *Hrr25*Δ strains showed nuclear segregation defects that resulted in a small population of anucleate cells. *Hrr25*Δ strains had a severe growth defect with a doubling time eight- to tenfold slower than in the wild type. Furthermore, these strains were aberrantly shaped, and cell cycle analysis revealed that much of a logarithmic population has a G2/M content of DNA. These pleiotrophic phenotypes suggested that Hrr25p played an important role in coordinating the proper execution of DNA metabolism with cell growth and division.

Hrr25p encodes a protein kinase with structural similarity to the serine/theronine protein kinase superfamily (Fig. 1). The enzyme is active when expressed in *Escherichia coli* (DeMaggio et al. 1992), indicating that an associated regulatory subunit is not required for its ability to phosphorylate proteins. Further, the *E. coli*-produced protein showed dual-specificity, i.e., the enzyme phosphorylated serine, threonine, and tyrosine residues in protein substrates (Hoekstra et al. 1994). The primary structure of Hrr25p is most closely related to the mammalian casein kinase I (CKI) protein kinase family (approximately 65% identical to mammalian CKIα, Fig. 1; Rowles et al. 1991; DeMaggio et al. 1992; Hoekstra 1995), and in vitro experiments confirmed that casein was a preferred substrate for Hrr25p. Furthermore, an isoquinoline-based inhibitor of mammalian CKI that shows little effect on other protein kinases (CKI-7) inhibited Hrr25p activity. The in vitro inhibition of Hrr25p by CKI-7, coupled with its high degree of primary sequence identity, indicates that

Hrr25p	MDL-RVGRKF	RIGRKIGSGS	FGD-------	----------	IYHGTNLISG	32
Yck1p	D.STI..LHY	K..K...E..	..V-------	----------	LFE...M...	92
Yck2p	D.STI..LHY	K..K...E..	..V-------	----------	LFE...M...	99
Cki3p	SSQHI..IHY	AV.P...E..	..VIFEGENI	LHSCQAQTGS	KRDSSIIMAN	54
Hhp1	ALDL.I.N.Y	....	...-------	----------	..L...VV..	34
Hhp2	VVDIKI.N.Y	....	..Q-------	----------	..L.L.TV..	35
Cki1	GQNNV..VHY	KV..R..E..	..V-------	----------	.FE....LNN	35
Cki2	SQTSV..VHY	.V.....E..	..V-------	----------	.FD.M..LNN	35
Rag8	D.STI..LHY	K..K...E..	..V-------	----------	LFE.V.M..N	100
C03C10.1	VKDFI.AT.Y	KLI.......	...-------	----------	..VSI.VT..	39
ATU12857	.EP-...N..	.L........	..E-------	----------	..L...IHTN	32
CKIα1	KAEFI..G.Y	KLV.......	...-------	----------	..LAI.ITN.	40
CKIβ	KTDVL..GRY	KLV.E..F..	..H-------	----------	V.LAID.T.H	40
CKIδ	.E.-...NRY	.L........	...-------	----------	..L..DIAA.	32
CKIγ	SGVLM..PN.	.V.K...C.N	..E-------	----------	LRL.K..YTN	74
CKIε	.E.-...N.Y	.L........	...-------	----------	..L.A.IA..	73

Hrr25p	EEVAIKLESI	RSRHPQLDYE	SRVYRYLSGG	VGIPFIRWFG	REGEYNAMVI	82
Yck1p	VP....F.PR	..EA...RD.	YKT....N.T	PN..YAYY..	Q..LH.I...	142
Yck2p	LP....F.PR	..EA...KD.	Y.T....A.T	P...QEYY..	Q..LH.I...	149
Cki3p	.P....F.PR	H.DA...RD.	F.A....N.C	....HAYY..	Q..MH.ILI.	104
Hhp1	.........T	.AK....E..	Y.........	.....V....	V.CD.....M	84
Hhp2	.Q..V...PL	.A..H..E..	F...N..K.N	I...T.....	VTNS.....M	85
Cki1	QQ....F.PR	..DA...RD.	Y.T.KL.A.C	T...NVYY..	Q..LH.VL..	85
Cki2	QLI...F.PK	K.EA...RD.	Y.T.KL.V.N	A...NVYY..	Q..LH.IL..	85
Rag8	VP F.PR	..DA...KD.	Y.T......S	E...QAYY..	Q..LH.I...	150
C03C10.1	.........N	.A.....L..	.K.....Q..	....II..Y.	T.R V..M	89
ATU12857	..L.....NV	..K.Q..L..	.KL....Q..	T.V.NVK...	V..D..V..M	82
CKIα1	....V....Q	.A.....L..	.KL....Q..	....H...Y.	Q.KD..V..M	90
CKIβ	.Q..V....E	N..Q.R.LH.	KEL.NF.Q..	....Q...Y.	Q.TD..V..M	90
CKIδ	CV	..K....HI.	.KI..MMQ..	....T...C.	A..D..V..M	82
CKIγ	.Y......PM	...A...HL.	Y.F..Q.GS.	D...QVYY..	PC.K.....L	124
CKIε	CV	..K....HI.	.KF..MMQ..	....S.K.C.	A..D..V..M	123

Hrr25p	DLLGPSLEDL	FNYCHRRFSF	KTVIMLALQM	FCRIQYIHGR	SFIHRDIKPD	132
Yck1p	....	.DW.G.K..V	...VQV.V..	.TL..DL.AH	DL.Y......	192
Yck2p	....	.DW.G....V	...VQV.V..	.TL..DL.AH	DL.Y......	199
Cki3p	....	.EW.G.K..V	..TC.V.K..	.D.VRA..DH	DL.Y......	154
Hhp1	....	..F.N.K..L	....L..D.L	.S...F..SK	..L.......	134
Hhp2	....	.C..G.K.TL	....L..D.L	.S....V.SK	..L.......	135
Cki1	....	LDL.G.K..V	...A.A.K..	LA.V.S..EK	.LVY......	135
Cki2	....	.EW.G.R..V	...A.T.K..	LS.V.T..EK	NLVY......	135
Rag8	....	.DW.G....I	...VHV.I..	.TL..EL.DH	DL.Y......	200
C03C10.1	....	..F.S...TM	.......D..	.G....V.VK	N.........	139
ATU12857	....	..F.S.KL.L	.S.....D..	.N.V.FF.SK	..L...L.QT	132
CKIα1	....	..F.S...TM	.......D..	.S....V.TK	N.........	140
CKIβ	....	..F.S....M	.......D..	.S....V.S.	NL........	140
CKIδ	E.........	..F.S.K..L	....L..D..	.S......SK	N.....V...	132
CKIγ	E.........	.DL.D.T..L	.....I.I.L	.S.M..V.SK	NL.Y..V..E	174
CKIε	E.........	..F.S.K..L	....L..D..	.S......SK	N.....V...	173

Fig. 1

```
Hrr25p      NFLMG-VGR-  ----------  -----R-GST  VHVIDFGLSK  KYRDFNTHRH  164
Yck1p       ...I.RP.Q-  ----------  -----PDA.N  I.L....M..  Q...PK.K..  226
Yck2p       ...I.RP.Q-  ----------  -----PDA.K  ..L....M..  Q...PK.K..  233
Cki3p       ...ISQYQ.I  SPEGKVIKSC  ASSSNNDP.L  IYMV...M..  Q...PR.K..  204
Hhp1        .....-I.K-  ----------  -----.-..Q  .NI.......  ....HK..L.  166
Hhp2        ....KKHSN-  ----------  ---------V  .TM.......  .....K..V.  165
Cki1        ...IGRP---  ----------  ---NSKNANM  IY.V...MV.  F...PV.KQ.  169
Cki2        ...IGRP---  ----------  ---SS.NANM  .YMV...MA.  Y...PK.KQY  169
Rag8        ...I.RPNQ-  ----------  -----PDA.M  ..L....M..  L...PK.K..  234
C03C10.1    .....-I..-  ----------  ------HC.K  LFL.......  ....SR.RT.  171
ATU12857    .....-L..-  ----------  ------RA.Q  .YI.......  ....MT....  164
CKIα1       .....-I..-  ----------  ------HC.K  LFL.......  ....NR.R..  172
CKIβ        .....-T.P-  ----------  ------QWKK  LFLV......  ....NR.G..  172
CKIδ        .....-L.K-  ----------  ------K..L  .YI.......  ....AR....  164
CKIγ        ...I.RP.N-  ----------  -----KTQQV  I.I.......  E.I.PE.KK.  208
CKIε        .....-L.K-  ----------  ------K..L  .YI.......  ....AR....  205

Hrr25p      IPYRENKSLT  GTARYASVNT  HLGIEQSRRD  DLESLGYVLI  YFCKGSLPWQ  214
Yck1p       .....K...S  .....M.I..  ...R......  .M.A..H.FF  ..L..H....  276
Yck2p       .....K...S  .....M.I..  ...R......  .M.AM.H.FF  ..L..Q....  283
Cki3p       .....R...S  .....M.I..  .F.R......  ......H.FF  ..L.......  254
Hhp1        .......N..  .......I..  ..........  .........V  ..........  216
Hhp2        ....D..N..  .......I..  .I........  .........L  ..........  215
Cki1        .....K.N.S  .....M.I..  ...R......  ...A..H.FM  ..LR......  219
Cki2        ...S.R...S  .....M.I..  ...R......  ......H.FM  ..LR......  219
Rag8        .....K...S  .....M.I..  ...R......  .M.A..H.FF  ..L..Q....  284
C03C10.1    .....D.N..  .......I.A  ..........  .M.......M  ..N..T....  221
ATU12857    .......N..  .......M..  ..........  ..K....I.M  ..L.......  214
CKIα1       .....D.N..  .......I.A  ..........  .M.......M  ..N.T.....  222
CKIβ        ..H.SG..FI  ..PFC..ISA  ..........  .M..I....M  ..N.......  222
CKIδ        .......N..  .......I..  ..........  .........M  ..NL......  214
CKIγ        .....H....  .....M.I..  ...K......  ...A..HMFM  ..L.......  258
CKIε        .......N..  .......I..  ..........  .........M  ..NL.L....  255

Hrr25p      GLKATTKKQK  YDRIMEKKLN  VSVETLC---  ---SGLPLEF  QEYMAYCKNL  258
Yck1p       ....PNN...  ....G...RS  .N.YD.A---  ---Q...VQ.  GR..EIV.S.  320
Yck2p       ....PNN...  ....G...RL  .N.YD.A---  ---Q...IQ.  GR..EIV...  327
Cki3p       ....PNN.L.  ....GMT.QK  LNPDD.L---  -LNNAI.YQ.  AT..K.A.S.  300
Hhp1        ..........  ........IS  .PT.V..---  ---R.F.Q..  SI..N.T.S.  260
Hhp2        ..Q.D..E..  .Q..RDT.IG  .PL.V..---  ---K...E..  IT..C.T.Q.  259
Cki1        ....A.N...  .E..G...QS  TPLRE..---  ---A.F.E..  YK..H.AR..  263
Cki2        ....ANN.H.  .EK.S...QS  T.ISE..---  ---A.F.N..  SK..T.VRS.  263
Rag8        ....ANN.L.  ....G...RS  .N.YD.S---  ---Q...VQ.  GR..EIV...  328
C03C10.1    ....A.....  ....S...MT  .S..H..---  ---K.F.A..  PM..S.T.G.  265
ATU12857    ....G...K.  ....S...VS  .SI.A..PIE  ALCR.Y.S..  AS.FH...S.  264
CKIα1       ....A.....  ....S...MS  .P..V..---  ---K.F.A..  AM..N...G.  266
CKIβ        ....A.L...  C...S.M.MT  .P.DV..---  ---K.F.I..  AM..K..LR.  266
CKIδ        ....A..R..  ....S...MS  .PI.V..---  ---K.Y.S..  AT..NF..S.  258
CKIγ        ....D.L.ER  .Q..GDT.RA  .PI.V..---  ---ENF.E.M  AT..R.V.R.  302
CKIε        ....A..R..  ....S...MS  .PI.V..---  ---K.Y.S..  ST..NF..S.  299

Hrr25p      KFDEKPDYLF  LARLFKDLSI  KLEYHNDHLF  DWTMLRYTKA              298
Yck1p       S.E.C...EG  Y.K.LLSVLD  D..ETA.GQY  ..MK.NDGRG              360
Yck2p       S.E.T...EG  Y.M.LLSVLD  D..ETA.GQY  ..MK.NGGRG              367
Cki3p       ....D...D.  .IS.MD.ALR  LNDLKD.GHY  ..MD.NGG.G              340
Hhp1        R..D....A.  ..K..R..FC  RQS.EF..M.  ..--------              292
Hhp2        S.T...N.A.  ..K..R..L.  RK..QY..V.  ..MI.K.Q.-              298
Cki1        A..AT...DY  .QG..SKVLE  R.NTTE.EN.  ..NL.NNG.G              303
Cki2        E...E...A.  .QE..D.VLR  ANGDT..GVY  ..ML.NDG.G              303
Rag8        G.E.T...EG  Y.K.LLSVLD  E..QKL.GEY  ..MK.NGGRG              368
C03C10.1    R...S...M.  ..Q..RI.FR  T.NHQY..T.  .....K----              300
ATU12857    R..D....A.  .K.I.R..F.  RE.FQF..V.  ...I.K----              300
CKIα1       R.E.A...M.  ..Q..RI.FR  T.NHQY..T.  .....K----              302
CKIβ        S.E.A...R.  ..Q..RL.FR  ..S.QH..A.  ..IV.-----              301
CKIδ        R..D....S.  ..Q..RN.FH  RQ.FSY..V.  ..N..KFGAS              298
CKIγ        D.F.....D.  ..K..T..FD  RK..MF..EY  ..IGKQLPTP              352
CKIε        R..D....S.  ..Q..RN.FH  RQ.FSY..V.  ..N..KFGA.              339
```

Fig. 1. Sequence alignment of casein kinase I (CKI) isoforms from a variety of organisms. An alignment of the protein kinase domains of CKI proteins from different organisms is shown. Hrr25p, Yck1p, Yck2p, and Cki3p are from *S. cerevisiae*. Hhp1, Hhp2, Cki1, and Cki2 are from *S. pombe*. Rag8 is from *K. lactis*. C03C10.1 is from *C. elegans*. ATU12857 is from *Arabidopsis*. CKIα, *β*, *γ*, *δ*, and ε are mammalian forms of CKI. The protein kinase domains are compared to Hrr25p, with *dots* indicating amino acid identity and *dashes* revealing insertions

Hrr25p is a yeast isoform of CKI. The identification of a yeast CKI protein kinase mutant with sensitivity to DNA damaging agents like MMS is the first physiological indication that CKI might participate in a specific regulatory capacity in vivo.

Roles for Hrr25p-Like Protein Kinases in *S. pombe*

An important concept to emerge from investigation in basic cell biology has been the linkage of yeast genetics to studies in other organisms. This concept has been extended to *HRR25*. Structural and functional homologues called *hhp1*$^{+}$ and *hhp2*$^{+}$ have been identified in the fission yeast *Schizosaccharomyces pombe*. These isoforms of CKI play a redundant role in responding to ionizing radiation, and *hhp1*$^{+}$ is essential for the tolerance of MMS-created DNA strand breaks (Dhillon and Hoekstra 1994).

The strongest evidence supporting the notion that *hhp1*$^{+}$ and *hhp2*$^{+}$ are isoforms of *HRR25* and CKI comes from direct complementation experiments. Both *S. pombe* protein kinases show high structural identity to Hrr25p and to mammalian CKI, and expression of *hhp1*$^{+}$, for example, in *S. cerevisiae hrr25* mutants, suppresses the MMS sensitivity and growth defects. Further evidence that *hhp* protein kinases are analogous to Hrr25p comes from in vitro measurements of their phosphotransferase activity. Hhp1 and hhp2 are active in *E. coli* and both show dual specificity activity (Hoekstra et al. 1994).

Mutational analysis of *hhp* genes has been informative of their regulatory capacity. Mutations in these *S. pombe* genes show some similarities to *hrr25* mutants. However, the *S. pombe* mutants reveal subtle differences from *S. cerevisiae* that give additional insight into their function. *Hhp1* mutants are most reminiscent of *hrr25*. Cells lacking *hhp1* are sensitive to MMS and these cells have a modest mitotic delay. *Hhp2* mutants are indistinguishable from wild type in their cell cycle progression and are as resistant as wild type to a variety of DNA-damaging treatments. The lack of a discernable phenotype for *hhp2* mutants does not indicate that this gene product is without a role in DNA repair or cell cycle progression. *Hhp1 hhp2* double mutant strains have additional defects not seen in either single mutant: double mutant cells are sensitive to ionizing radiation, have a severe growth rate defect, and the double mutant reveals a nuclear segregation defect and a severe mitotic delay. These data indicate a redundant role for *hhp1* and *hhp2* in the regulation of responses to certain forms of DNA strand interruptions (Dhillon and Hoekstra 1994).

A direct role for *hhp1* and *hhp2* in responding to DNA strand interruptions was revealed by physical analysis of strand break repair. Pulse field gel electrophoresis of *S. pombe* chromosomes showed that *hhp1* mutants were unable to correctly rejoin MMS-created DNA strand lesions whereas *hhp1 hhp2* mutants were unable to repair X-ray-created strand breaks. These data confirmed the sensitivity of these mutants to the DNA-damaging agents and suggest that the toxicity of these agents was due directly to the DNA strand interruptions.

In *S. pombe,* a variety of DNA repair checkpoints and replication feedback controls have been described (reviewed by Sheldrick and Carr 1993 and Carr and Hoekstra 1995). These controls determine whether specific aspects of growth control have been fulfilled in order for cell division to occur correctly. Starting in the G1 phase of the cell cycle, some of the aspects which appear to be regulated by feedback or checkpoint controls include determining if the previous mitosis has occurred correctly, if cell size is correct, and if sufficient nutrients are present to exit to G1. During S phase, feedback controls and DNA structure-specific checkpoints examine DNA replication and coordinate proper DNA synthesis with cell cycle progression. In G2/M, DNA repair checkpoints monitor whether unrepaired DNA lesions are present, whether chromosomes have condensed and aligned with mitotic spindles, and whether segregation is proceeding correctly. Clearly, mutations in *hhp1*$^{+}$ and *hhp2*$^{+}$ confer differential and overlapping sensitivity to DNA-damaging agents. They also affect cell division-related events including cell size, the timing of nuclear segregation, and cell shape. Nevertheless, *hhp1* and *hhp2* do not have a checkpoint function *per se. Hhp1* and *hhp2* mutants arrest normally in response to DNA-damaging treatments (Fig. 2). To separate the growth defects from the effects of DNA metabolism, genetic interactions between *hhp1* and *hhp2* mutations with *cdc*, checkpoint, and DNA repair mutants were investigated.

The *hhp* related mitotic delay (Fig. 2 and Dhillon and Hoekstra 1994) could be due to defects in the cell size pathway. In part, the *wee1*$^{+}$ protein kinase controls this pathway by negatively regulating p34^{cdc2}. *wee1* mutants enter mitosis permaturely (Russell and Nurse 1987; Gould and Nurse 1989; Featherstone and Russell 1991). The interaction between *hhp* mutants with the temperature-conditional *wee1-50* allele was examined. The *hhp1* and *hhp1 hhp2* mitotic delay was independent of Wee1 activity. *Wee1-50 hhp1* double mutants and *wee1-50 hhp1 hhp2* triple mutants were elongated at 36° C. This indicates that the cell cycle delay associated with loss of Hhp activity is independent of the direct inactivation of p34^{cdc2} by p80^{wee1} and the cell size control pathway.

The *hhp1* delay may be due to incomplete DNA replication activating an S phase-mitosis checkpoint or spontaneous damage activating the radiation checkpoint. If correct, the mitotic delay should be lost in the absence of these controls. We examined the interactions of *hhp* mutations with *chk1/rad27* [a radiation checkpoint mutant (A1-Khodairy et al. 1994)], *rad17* [a radiation checkpoint and replication checkpoint mutation (A1-Khodairy and Carr 1992; Carr and Hoekstra 1995)], and *cdc2-3w* [an allele of p34^{cdc2} that bypasses the p80^{cdc25} phosphatase requirement and which is deficient for the replication checkpoint (Enoch and Nurse 1990)].

The *hhp1* and *hhp1 hhp2* mitotic delay is independent of the *chk1/rad17*-mediated radiation checkpoint and the *cdc2-3w/rad17*-mediated replication checkpoint as *chk1 hhp1*, *rad17 hhp1,* and *cdc2-3w hhp1* double mutants, as well

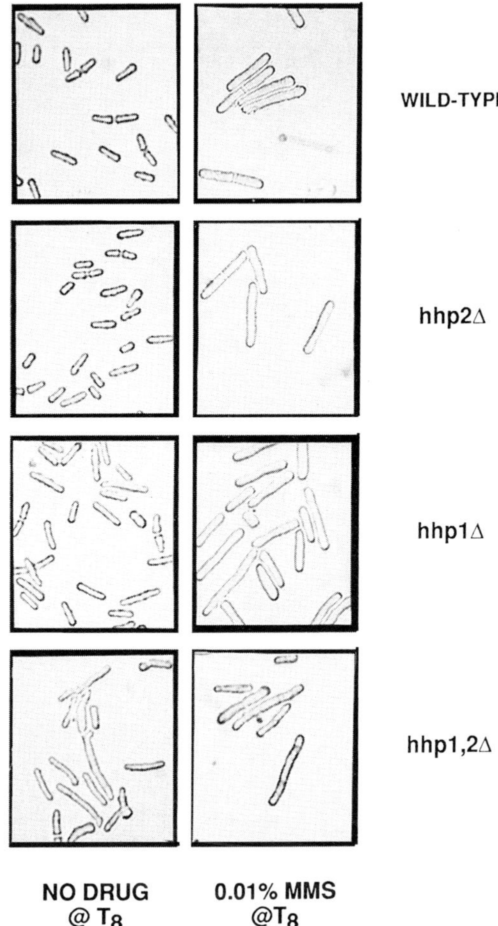

Fig. 2. Hhp mutants arrest in response to DNA-damaging Treatments. Midlog-phase wild-type and *hhp* mutant strains of *S. pombe* were treated with methyl methanesulfonate (MMS) for 8 h. Cells were fixed and examined by phase-contrast microscopy for the ability to elongate and arrest following DNA damage induced by MMS

as *hhp2*-containing triple mutants, showed mitotic delay and normal viability (Table 1). Furthermore, the delay is not mediated through $p34^{cdc2}$ phosphorylation at tyrosine 15, as regulation by Y15 phosphorylation is compromised in *cdc2-3w* strains. These results can be interpreted to indicate that the absence of *hhp* functions does not generate sufficient DNA damage or delay replication in a fashion that activates the "checkpoint *rad*" gene-mediated checkpoints. If spontaneous DNA damage or misreplication is occurring, then the types of lesions formed are different from those recognized by the known DNA structure checkpoints.

Table 1. Multiple mutant analysis of *hhp* with various *rad*, *cdc*, and checkpoint mutations

Mutant strain genotype	Growth	Comment
wee1.50 hhp1	Viable	Elongated
cdc2.3w hhp1	Viable	Checkpoint$^-$
rad17 hhp1	Viable	Checkpoint$^-$
chck1.r27d hhp1	Viable	Checkpoint$^-$
rad24 hhp1	Nonviable	
rad25 hhp1	Viable	Checkpoint$^{+/-}$

The *rad24*$^+$ and *rad25*$^+$ genes encode semiredundant forms of 14-3-3, and the activity of 14-3-3 proteins is essential in fission yeast (Ford et al. 1994). *rad24* mutations affect cell size at division, cell morphology, and the duration of the radiation checkpoint. The *rad24* mutant is sensitized to DNA-damaging agents and this is due in part to the partial defect in the radiation checkpoint. In contrast, no significant repair defect is seen in rad25 cells. *rad24* mutations overlap with *hhp1* mutations in conferring sensitivity to growth on MMS-containing medium. As the *rad24* and *hhp1* phenotypes both affect DNA damage sensitivities as well as cell shape and growth-related endpoints, we determined if the *hhp1* mitotic delay required either *rad24* or *rad25*. No interactions were observed between *rad25* and *hhp1* or *hhp2* (Table 1). However, *hhp1 rad24* double mutants were nonviable. The *hhp1 rad24* synthetic lethality suggests that cells require either Hhp1 activity or a Rad24-specific function for mitotic viability, revealing a previously unknown essential role for this combination of activities.

The synthetic lethality between *hhp1* and *rad24* indicates an essential overlapping role for these proteins. While both *hhp1*$^+$ and *rad24*$^+$ are involved in DNA repair, the CKI isoforms and the 14-3-3 proteins appear to play opposite roles in *S. pombe* cell growth: *rad24* mutants advance mitosis whereas *hhp1* mutants delay mitosis (Ford et al. 1994; Dhillon and Hoekstra 1994). To understand the nature of the double mutant inviability, further common physiological properties were sought for the respective null mutants.

hhp1 and *rad24* mutants show elevated chromosome loss rates about 20 times higher than wild-type cells. *hhp1 hhp2* double mutants showed an approximately 500-fold increase over wild type. This suggests that *hhp1*$^+$, *hhp2*$^+$, and *rad24*$^+$ are important in maintaining normal chromosome segregation fidelity. Furthermore, *rad24* mutants required *cut7*$^+$ for normal maintainance of a checkpoint that acts within mitosis.

The *cut7*$^+$ gene encodes a kinesin microtubule-based motor protein. At the *cut7*ts nonpermissive temperature, chromosome segregation is severely affected and chromosomes do not interact correctly with nuclear spindles (Hagan and Yanagida 1990, 1992). At the nonpermissive temperature, *cut7*ts activates a checkpoint within mitosis. In other words, the interaction between a chromosome and a mitotic spindle is monitored by a checkpoint. The requirement for *rad24*$^{+}$ in a *cut7* strain indicates that *rad24* mediates this checkpoint within mitosis. The double mutant inviability of *hhp1 rad24* suggests that one aspect of *hhp1*'s function may be to regulate a cell cycle stage near mitosis and that this stage requires *rad24* for proper execution.

Mammalian Forms of CKI

Casein kinase I is a growing gene family of highly related protein kinases (Fig. 1). Sequences encoding potential CKI proteins have been reported from not only *S. cerevisiae* and *S. pombe* but also *Kluveromyces lactis, C. elegans, Arabidopsis*, vacinnia virus, and a variety of mammalian sources. A primary sequence alignment of CKI forms is shown in Fig. 1. Clearly, the primary sequence of the protein kinase catalytic domain in these proteins is highly related.

In mammalian cells, the biochemical activity for a number of CKI isoforms has been reported (reviewed in Tuazon and Traugh 1991). CKIα has been reported from several sources, and cDNA cloning reveals three splice variants (α1, α2, α3). CKIβ has been reported from bovine sources, CKIδ has been isolated from several species, CKIγ cDNAs have been isolated from human and bovine sources, and CKIε has been identified in humans (Rowles et al. 1991; Brockman et al. 1992; Fish et al. 1995; E. Christenson et al., submitted).

The function of these isoforms is presently unclear. Polyclonal antisera raised against human erythrocyte CKI recognize CKI forms from many species. Immunofluorescence experiments show that these sera recognize a protein in CHO cells that is regulateld by or regulates cell cycle progression (Brockman et al. 1992). Isoform-specific reagents have verified these studies. An antipeptide antiserum raised against CKIα reveals cell cycle-specific staining of mitotic spindles (Fig. 3), suggesting that CKI may play a role in microtubule metabolism during chromosome segregation.

Substrate analysis has given some clues into possible functions for mammalian CKI, and several studies indicate possible roles where mammalian CKI might play a function in cellular metabolism and regulation. CKI-like activity can be stimulated by insulin and by interleukin (IL)-1 or tumor necrosis factor (TNF)α (Guesdon et al. 1993), and membrane-associated CKI activity can be inhibited by phosphatidylinositol 4,5-bisphosphate (Brockman and Anderson 1991). Furthermore, sites phosphorylated by casein kinase I in vivo and in vitro have been determined for CREM τ (de Groot et al. 1993), SV40 large T antigen (Ciegelska and Virshup 1993; Ciegelska et al. 1994), glycogen synthase (Roach 1991), and p53 (Milne et al. 1992). In cyclic adenosine monophosphate responsive element modulator (CREM), the phosphorylation by CKI affects the in vitro DNA binding activity of the transcription factor. For SV40, the residues phosphorylated by CKI are important for T antigen-driven replication capacity. In glycogen synthase, CKI

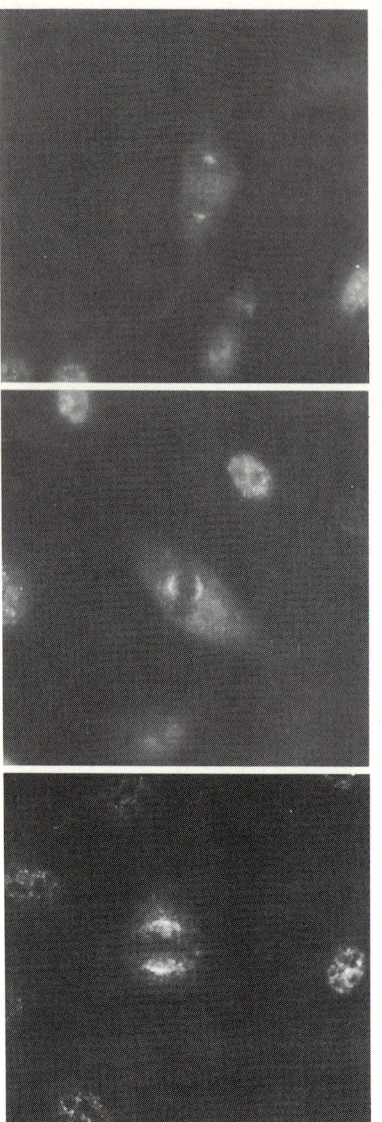

Fig. 3. Mammalian CKIα localizes to mitotic spindles. Affinity-purified antipeptide antiserum directed against CKIα was used to examine aortic endothelial cells by immunofluorescence. Three panels are shown revealing colocalization of CKIα with mitotic spindles. The staining pattern appears to follow the movement of mitotic spindles with the segregation of chromosomes

phosphorylation is involved in inhibiting enzyme activity. The role of CKI phosphorylation in regulating p53 activity is not understood. Clearly, functional dissection of the relationship between substrate phosphorylation and regulation of protein activity is required to understand the role of CKI in cellular regulation.

Acknowledgements. Insightful and helpful comments on the biology of CKI in model systems have been given to us by Namrita Dhillon and Tony Carr. Thanks to David Virshup and Janine Harrison for reagents and assistance with the experiment shown in Fig. 3.

References

Al-Khodairy F, Carr AM (1992) DNA repair mutants defining G2 checkpoint pathways in Schizosaccharomyces pombe. EMBO J 11: 1343–1350

Al-Khodairy F, Fotou E, Sheldrick KS, Griffiths DJF, Lehmann AR, Carr AM (1994) Identification and characterization of new elements involved in checkpoint and feedback controls in fission yeast. Mol Biol Cell 5: 147–160

Brockman JL, Anderson RA (1991) Casein kinase I is regulated by phosphatidylinositol 45-bisphosphate in native membranes J Biol Chem 266: 2508–2512

Brockman JL, Gross SD, Sussman MR, Anderson RA (1992) Cell cycle-dependent localizaton of casein kinase I to mitotic spindles. Proc. Natl Acad Sci USA 89: 9454–9458

Carr AM, Hoekstra MF (1995) The cellular responses to DNA damage. Trends Cell Biol 5: 32–40

Ciegeleska A, Virshup DM (1993) Control of simian virus 40 DNA replication by the HeLa cell nuclear casein kinase I. Mol Cell Biol 13: 1202–1211

Cieglska A, Moarefi I, Fanning E, Virshup DM (1994) T-antigen kinase inhibits simian virus 40 DNA replication by phosphorylation of intact T antigen on serines 120 and 123 J Virol 68: 269–275

de Groot RP, den Hertog J, Vandenheede JR, Goris J, Sassone-Corsi P (1993) Multiple and cooperative phosphorylation events regulate the CREM activator. EMBO J 12: 3903–3911

DeMaggio AJ, Lindberg RA, Hunter T, Hoekstra MF (1992) The budding yeast *HRR25* gene product is a casein kinase I isoform. Proc Natl Acad Sci USA 89: 7008–7012

Dhillon N, Hoekstra MF (1994) Characterization of two protein kinases from Schizosaccharomyces pombe involved in the regulation of DNA repair. EMBO J 13: 2777–2788

DiLenardo A, Linke SP, Clarkin K, Wahl GM (1994) DNA damage triggers a prolonged p53-dependent G1 arrest and long-term induction of Cip1 in normal human fibroblasts. Genes Dev 8: 2540–2551

Enoch T, Nurse P (1990) Mutations of fission yeast cell cycle control genes abolishes dependene of mitosis on DNA replication. Cell 60: 665–673

Featherstone C, Russell P (1991) Fission yeast p107^{weel} mitotic inhibitor is a tyrosine/serine kinase. Nature 349: 808–811

Fish K, Cegielska A, Getman M, Landes G, Virshup DM (1995) Isolation and characterization of human casein kinase I epsilon, a novel member of the CKI gene family. J Biol Chem (in press)

Ford JC, Al-Khodairy F, Fotou F, Sheldrick KS, Griffiths DJF, Carr AM (1994) 14-3-3 protein homologs required for the DNA damage checkpoint in fission yeast. Science 265: 533–535

Gould KL, Nurse P (1989) Tyrosine phosphorylation of the fission yeast *cdc2*$^{+}$ protein kinase regulates entry into mitosis. Nature 342: 39–45

Guesdon F, Freshney N, Waller RJ, Rawlinson L, Saklatavala J (1993) Interleukin-1 and tumor necrosis factor stimulate two novel protein kinases that phosphorylate heat shock protein hsp27 and beta-casein. J Biol Chem 268: 4236–4243

Hagan I, Yanagida M (1990) Novel potential mitotic motor protein encoded by the fission yeast *cut7*$^{+}$ gene. Nature 347: 563–566

Hagan I, Yanagida M (1992) Kinesin-related cut7 protein associates with mitotic and meiotic spindles in fission yeast. Nature 356: 74–76

Hartwell LH (1992) Defects in a cell cycle checkpoint may be responsible for the genomic instability of cancer cells. Cell 71: 543–546

Hartwell LH, Weinert TA (1989) Checkpoints: controls that ensure the order of cell cycle events. Science 246: 629–634

Hibi M, Lin A, Smeal T, Minden A, Karin M (1993) Identification of an oncoprotein- and UV-respsonsive protein kinase that binds and potentiates the c-Jun activation domain. Genes Dev 7: 2135–2148

Hoekstra MF (1995) The HRR25 protein kinase. In: Hardie G, Hanks S (eds) The protein kinase facts book. Academic, London

Hoekstra MF, Liskay RM, Ou AC, DeMaggio AJ, Burbee DG, Heffron F (1991) HRR25, a putative protein kinase from budding yeast: association with the repair of damaged DNA. Science 253: 1031–1034

Hoekstra MF, Dhillon N, Carmel G, DeMaggio AJ, Lindberg RAL, Hunter T, Kuret J (1994) Budding and fission yeast casein kinase I isoforms have dual-specificity protein kinase activity. Mol Biol Cell 5: 877–886

Malone RE, Esposito RE (1980) The RAD52 gene product is required for homothallic interconversion of mating types and spontaneous mitotic recombination in yeast. Proc Natl Acad Sci USA 77: 503–507

Milne DM, Palmer RH, Campbell DG, Meek DW (1992) Phosphorylation of the p53 tumour-suppressor at three N- terminal sites by a novel casein kinase I-like enzyme. Oncogene 7: 1361–1369

Roach PJ (1991) Control of glycogen synthase by hierarchal protein phosphorylation. FASEB J 4: 2961–2968

Rowles J, Slaughter C, Moomaw C, Hsu J, Cobb MH (1991) Purification of casein kinase I and isolation of cDNAs encoding multiple casein kinase I-like enzymes. Proc Natl Acad Sci USA 88: 9548–9552

Russell P, Nurse P (1987) Negative regulation of mitosis by *wee1*$^{+}$, a gene encoding a protein kinase homolog. Cell 49: 559–567

Sheldrick KS, Carr AM (1993) Feedback controls and G2 checkpoints: fission yeast as a model system. Bioessays 15: 775–782

Tuazon PT, Traugh JA (1991) Casein kinase I and II – multi-potential serine protein kinases: structure, function, and regulation. Adv Sec Mess Phosphoprot Res 21: 123–164

III. Selected Findings in Human Tumors

Growth and Transformation of Human Oral Epithelium In Vitro

R.C. Grafström, U.G. Norén, X. Zheng, Å. Elfwing, and K. Sundqvist

Institute of Environmental Medicine, Karolinska Institutet, Box 210, 17177 Stockholm, Sweden

Introduction

Cancer of the head and neck poses a major health problem in the world. In 1985, the number of new malignant neoplasms of the mouth and pharynx (International Classification of Disease, ninth revision, ICD-9 140–149) was estimated to be 500 000; this is therefore the sixth most common anatomical site (Parkin and Muir 1992). Roughly half of these cases occur in southern Asia and China. In parts of India where the use of chews containing betel and tobacco is frequent, these tumors are the most common form of cancer (Parkin et al. 1993). Trends for the most common tumor type, head and neck squamous cell carcinoma (HNSCC), vary by anatomical subsite and geographical region. For tumors of the tongue, mouth, and pharynx, rates are rising in many areas of the world. In most European countries, the mortality rates for the disease have increased substantially since the mid-1970s, especially at younger ages (La Vecchia et al. 1992; Franceschi et al. 1994; Boyle et al. 1995). Early symptoms of disease, often vague, are easily overlooked. The majority of patients are diagnosed with advanced cancer (stage III or IV), a negative determinant in the outcome of treatment (Vokes et al. 1993). Accordingly, long-term survival has not improved significantly in recent decades.

Epidemiological studies indicate a multifactorial etiology for malignant transformation in the head and neck region (Spitz 1994). Tobacco smoking or chewing and alcohol consumption are known to be major risk factors. Increasing evidence also supports the contribution of human papillomavirus (HPV) in the pathogenesis of some oral tumors (Snijders et al. 1994). Despite methodological advances in molecular biology, the etiology of HNSCC is only partly understood. For example, the extent of genetic alterations in potentially malignant lesions is unknown, and the consequent risk of their malignant progression is unpredictable (Johnson et al. 1993). Moreover, cancers of the oral cavity and oropharynx are often treated as a single entity, although it is unclear whether similar mechanisms cause malignant transformation in these

Recent Results in Cancer Research, Vol. 143

subsites. Differences in the morphology and biochemistry of the epidermal structures of the head and neck region clearly exist. The following text will review data from different tissue sites, but will mainly focus on results obtained from laboratory studies of the epithelia lining the oral cavity. An overview of mechanisms of malignant transformation and the development of HNSCC will be presented, followed by a discussion of recent methodological advances in serum-free in vitro model systems and their use in the investigation of mechanisms of growth, transformation, and carcinogenesis in oral mucosa.

Oral Carcinogenesis Is Likely a Multistep Process

Multiple lines of evidence indicate that most human cancers, including HNSCC, develop in several steps (Fig. 1). This assumption is supported by the recognition of potentially malignant conditions, e.g., oral leukoplakia. These lesions, more prone to develop into cancers than normal tissue, are diagnosed in terms of morphology and are usually expressed as dysplasia. Studies in laboratory animals suggest that various phases of carcinogenesis may be defined (Yuspa 1994). Thus a normal cell may undergo initiation followed by promotion, conversion, and progression into a malignant phenotype (Fig. 1). Several factors are known to modulate the propensity of cells to undergo inheritable genetic changes during the initiation stage (Grafström 1990a; Harris 1991). The dose of the carcinogenic agent, the activity of enzymes that take part in metabolism of carcinogens, formation of DNA adducts, and other types of DNA damage, DNA repair, and cellular turnover rates play important

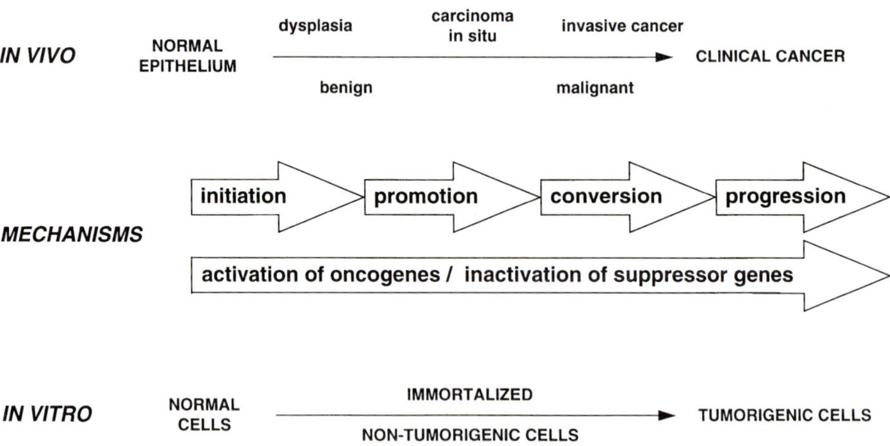

Fig. 1. Multistep carcinogenesis in human epithelial tissues and cells. The concept that a stepwise induction of genotypic and phenotypic changes can be studied both in vivo and in vitro is shown

roles. DNA damage may affect DNA replication by the introduction of miscoding information and genomic rearrangements. The outcome may be a modified responsiveness to regulators of growth, differentiation, and cell death (Grafström 1990a). Therefore, the subsequent promotion phase involves the clonal growth of the initiated cell into a cluster of preneoplastic cells, i.e., a benign lesion, due to the selective conditions inferred by agents which can regulate these processes. One result is that programmed cell death may be blocked by a promotional agent (Schulte-Hermann et al. 1994). Further genetic changes and selective micro-environmental effects of various factors are likely to drive cells through the subsequent conversion and progression phases and eventually lead to the uncontrolled proliferation of progeny cells (Aznavoorian et al. 1993; Yuspa 1994). The well-known heterogeneity commonly observed in tumors is likely to result from tumor cell diversification and dominance of particular cell clones. The later stages of carcinogenesis may result in highly metastatic and/or invasive tumors.

In the study of the causative role of a specific mutation, efforts to determine whether these occur early or late during the carcinogenesis process is of major importance. Proto-oncogenes and tumor suppressor genes are targets for genetic changes during carcinogenesis (Harris 1991). Normally, the former stimulate and the latter inhibit cell proliferation. Activation of proto-oncogenes to oncogenes and inactivation of tumor suppressor genes may therefore result in dysregulation of growth. Alterations in both classes of genes are detected in HNSCC (Table 1) and indicate their active involvement in tumorigenesis, as has been reviewed (Brachman 1994). Using genetic markers for microsatellites, short nucleotide repeats, potential regions for additional genes of causative importance in cancer have been identified (Table 1). These studies complement the findings from chromosomal banding and restriction fragment length polymorphism analyses. Commonly altered sites in oral tumors indicate the possible involvement of additional transforming genes with unknown biochemical functions (Table 1). The multistep development of HNSCC has been estimated to involve as many as six to ten independent genetic alterations (Renan 1993). Correlation based primarily on the analysis of tumor stage and patient survival has indicated that consecutive changes in *p53*, *ras* (several members of this family) *Erb-1*, *c-myc*, and E-cadherin may take place (Field 1995). However, cancer development may not require sequential specified genetic changes, as both the type and the number of genetic alterations may be major determinants. Future comparative studies of benign and malignant tissue will provide important clues to the causative role of oncogenic changes during multistep carcinogenesis.

It is possible that specific types of carcinogenic agents may effectively drive the transitions of cells through defined phases of cancer development (Yuspa and Poirier 1988; Harris 1991). By studying the spectrum of mutational alterations in genes, i.e., the types of base pair exchange, indications of the causative carcinogenic agents can be obtained. Although most mutagens cause many lesions in DNA, certain types of damage usually predominate (Harris

Table 1. Genetic alterations in head and neck squamous carcinomas

Chromosome	Gene alterations	Chromosome alterations[a]
1	N-*ras*, L-*myc*	1p11-q11, 1p13, 1p22, 1p36, 1q21, 1q32, i(1q)
2	N-myc	
3		3p11, 3p13, 3p21, 3pter-p23, 3p14-p25, 3centr-qter
4		4q21, 4q11-q21, 4q21-qter
5		5p11-q11, 5q12-q23, i(5p)
6	K-*ras-1*	6q15-q26, 6q21-q25
7	*ErbB1*	7p11-q11, 7q22, 7cent-p15, 7q22-q34
8	c-*myc*	8p11-q11, 8p22-p23, 8p11.2, 8cent-q21.2, 8cent, i(8q)
9		9p21-p24, 9cent, 9q32
10		10q11.2, 10pter-q21.2, 10q22-q26
11	H-*ras-1*, cyclin D, (*int-2*, *hst-1*)	11p, 11p15, 11q13, 11q32
12	K-*ras-2*	12p11.2
13		13p11-p13, 13 p arm, 13q14
14		14p11, 14p11-q11, 14 p arm
15		15p11-q11, 15 p arm
16	E cadherin gene	
17	*p53*	17p12-p11
18		18q22, 18q21, 18q21-qter
19		19p13.1, 19pter-cen
20		20p13
21		21 p arm
22		22 p arm
x		
y		

[a]Summarized from Osella et al. 1992; Jin and Mertens 1993; Rao et al. 1994; Adamson et al. 1994; Ah-See et al. 1994; Fuzesi et al. 1994; Van Dyke et al. 1994; Yoo et al. 1994; El-Naggar et al. 1995; Field 1995; Jin et al. 1995.

1989, 1991). In HNSCC, the incidence and spectrum of mutations in specific proto-oncogenes, e.g., *ras*, and tumor suppressor genes, e.g., *p53*, differ among populations of the Western world and South Asia (Thomas et al. 1994). In addition, proteins encoded by tumor suppressor genes, such as p53, may be functionally inactivated by viral oncoproteins such as HPV E6 (Greenblatt et al. 1994; Snijders et al. 1994). Overall, several lines of evidence support that head and neck carcinogenesis is a multistep process that may be driven by diverse factors and different combinations of genetic change. Known oncogenes and tumor suppressor genes as well as presently unidentified genes are likely to contribute to this process.

Cultured Oral Cells for Carcinogenesis Studies

Experimental models for head and neck carcinogenesis include oral inoculations and direct applications of chemical carcinogens onto the mucosa of rodents (Boyd and Reade 1988; Steele and Shillitoe 1991; Tanaka 1995). However, it should be stressed that the morphology and biochemistry of these epithelia in laboratory animals differ from their human counterparts. Commonly, both quantitative and qualitative differences between human and animal cells are also found in the metabolism of carcinogens (Autrup and Grafström 1982). Species differences are also found in vitro, since rodent cells more frequently undergo immortalization and malignant transformation than human cells (Chang 1986; Knowles 1990). For various cultured cell types, e.g., epithelial and mesenchymal cells, the phenotypic changes coupled with transformation are partly different. Human epithelial cells also generally show a higher capability for metabolism of carcinogens than fibroblasts from the same tissue (Harris et al. 1984). These results emphasize the value of epithelial cells of human origin for in vitro studies of the mechanisms that underlie common human malignancies.

An experimental approach to study normal biology as well as tumorigenesis of human epithelia involves the culture of normal and transformed cells in vitro (Grafström 1990a). In the oral cavity, the mucosal lining is the structural target for carcinogens (Burkhart and Maerker 1981; IARC 1985; Garewal and Meyskens 1992). Accordingly, epithelial cells from normal, nontumorous tissue have been grown from several functionally and histologically differing sites and used to study various aspects of growth and transformation (Grafström 1990a; Dale et al. 1990). The culture conditions have commonly included serum in the media as well as the use of feeder layers (Southgate et al. 1987; MacCallum et al. 1987; Arenholt-Bindeslev et al. 1987; Chang 1991). However, serum-free culture conditions without the support of feeder cells offer several general advantages, i.e., less experimental variability, the possibility of identifying factors that directly regulate proliferation and differentiation, ease of isolation of cellular products, delayed terminal differentiation and senescence in the absence of serum, and utilization of selective growth conditions for different cell types (Harris 1987). Moreover, it could be argued that exposure of epithelial cells to a nutrient solution supplemented with up to 20% of serum mimics the state of wound healing in vivo. In the intact undamaged tissue, diffusion of serum factors from the underlying connective tissue to the epithelium would probably involve exposure to much lower amounts. In an effort to circumvent such issues and thereby strengthen the validity of functional cellular studies, serum-free conditions for replicative epithelial cells and maintenance of tissue from human oral epithelium have been developed (Table 2). The various methods are all based on the MCDB 153 medium (Boyce and Ham 1983) supplemented with defined growth-promoting agents, e.g., epidermal growth factor (EGF), and commonly pituitary extracts. The substrates used are normal tissue culture plastic or an extracellular matrix

Table 2. Serum-free in vitro models of human oral epithelium

State/ origin	Method/ culture conditions	Longevity	Characteristics	Selected references
Normal tissue				
Cell cultures				
Bucca	Explant outgrowth; BEG medium, FN/C	About 2 months Five passages	$\leq$6% CFE ($\geq$16 cells/colony); CG, 0.8 PD/D; express keratins and involucrin; GI by TGF-β; SD by Ca^{2+} and serum	Sundqvist et al. 1989, 1991a
	Trypsin-digested tissue; EMA, FN/C, or TCP	About 7 months Ten passages	$\leq$40% CFE ($\geq$16 cells/colony); CG, $\leq$1.2 PD/D; GI by TGF-β; SD by serum	Sundqvist et al. 1991b
Several sites[a]	Trypsin-digested tissue; modified MCDB 153, TCP	Not reported	$\geq$90% CFE ($\geq$ four cells/colony); GI by TGF-β and ethionine; SD by serum	Kasperbauer et al. 1990
Gingiva	Dispase/trypsin-digested tissue; KGM, TCP	About 3 months Seven passages	Express keratins; SD by Ca^{2+}	Oda and Watson 1990
	Dispase/trypsin-digested tissue; KGM, TCP	Five passages	Express keratins and collagenolytic enzyme activity	Salonen et al. 1991
Explant culture				
Bucca	BEX medium; TCP or gelatin sponge	2–5 days	Histology comparable to non-cultured tissue	Liu et al. 1993
Immortalized cells				
Bucca(SVpgC2a)	Transfected with SV40T; EMA, TCP	> 2 years > 700 PD	Genomic integration of SV40T; aneuploid; express keratins; partial resistance to GI and SD by TGF-β and serum, respectively	Kulkarni et al. 1995
Gingiva (HOK16A, HOK16B)	Transfected with HPV16 genes; KGM, TCP	> 8 months 40 passages	Genomic integration of HPV16; overexpression of c-*myc*; malignant transformation from exposure to a tobacco-specific nitrosamine	Park et al. 1991; Kim et al. 1993

Gingiva (HOK18)	Transfected with HPV18 genes; KGM, TCP	> 2 years 90 passages	Genomic integration of HPV18; resistance to GI by Ca^{2+}; increased expression of TGF-α and c-*myc*; malignant transformation from exposure to an alkylating agent	Shin et al. 1994
Oral (HPV16 oral EPI)	Retroviral infection of E6/E7 from HPV16; KGM, TCP	> 90 passages	Expression of CYP and mEH	Farin et al. 1995
Tumorous cells				
Bucca (SqCC/Y1)	EMA, TCP	> 2 years	28% CFE; CG, 0.6 PD/D; resistance to GI and SD by TGF-β and serum, respectively	Sundqvist et al. 1991b
Organotypic culture				
Bucca; normal, immortalized (SVpg C2a), and tumorous (SqCC/Y1)	Collagen gel with fibroblasts; EMA or EMA with 1 m*M* Ca^{2+}	2 weeks	Epithelial stratification; express keratins and involucrin; SD by Ca^{2+}; apoptosis detectable	X. Zheng et al., unpublished data

BEG, buccal epithelial growth; BEX, buccal epithelium explant; CFE, colony-forming efficiency; CG, clonal growth; CYP, cytochrome P450; EMA, epithelial medium with increased concentrations of amino acids; FN/C, tissue culture surface coated with a mixture of fibronectin and collagen; GI, growth inhibition; HPV, human papillomavirus; PD/D, population doublings per day; KGM, keratinocyte growth medium; mEH, microsomal epoxide hydrolase; SD, squamous differentiation; SV40T, simian virus 40 T antigen; TCP, tissue culture plastic; TGF, human transforming growth factor.

[a]Cells were derived from buccal mucosa, soft palate, floor of mouth, tongue, hypopharynx, and epiglottis.

based on components of the basal membrane, e.g., fibronectin (FN) and collagen (C). The model systems that emanate from normal, nonpathologic tissue express many features of normality, including finite life spans. Epithelial cells have also been experimentally transformed into immortalized lines by the transfection of recombinant constructs that encode oncoproteins of the DNA tumor viruses HPV and SV40 (Table 2). Such lines are easily grown in high cell numbers, although they retain many properties of normal cells. Moreover, a commonly studied buccal carcinoma line, SqCC/Y1, has been adapted to grow in the serum-free culture conditions developed for normal cells (Table 2). Thus cells that represent normality and various stages of oral carcinogenesis (Figs. 1, 2) can now be grown in vitro at highly defined conditions and used to study various aspects of this complex process. The characteristics of the human oral tissue-based model systems summarized in Table 2 are described below and compared with the corresponding cells in vivo.

Primary cultures of normal epithelial cells can be obtained as outgrowths from explanted tissue or, alternatively, by dissociation of tissue with trypsin, followed by subsequent culture of the resulting suspension of fragmented tissue and individual cells (Sundqvist et al. 1989, 1991a,b; Kasperbauer et al. 1990; Oda and Watson 1990). Both medium and substrate composition influence growth and yield of oral primary cultures. An optimized media (epithelial medium with increased concentrations of amino acids, EMA) in combination with FN/C markedly improved colony-forming efficiency, growth rate, and cell harvests more than other combinations of medium and culture surface (Sundqvist et al. 1991b). Blockage of the two major types of programmed cell death in the epithelium, i.e., apoptosis and terminal squamous differentiation, might in part explain this effect, in that FN/C facilitates cell attachment (Sundqvist et al. 1991a,b), and the enrichment of EMA with growth factors may enhance cell survival. At the optimized culture conditions, the cells commonly undergo 60 population doublings, resulting in yields of 10^8–10^{11} cells per cm^2 mucosal specimen (Sundqvist et al. 1991b). This longevity and harvest appear to be among the highest reported for serum-free culture of human epithelial cells (Grafström 1990a; Table 2). The cultured oral cells exhibit a number of normal epithelial cell characteristics. Several of these are reminiscent of basal cells, i.e., the normal diploid karyotype, high proliferative ability, relatively small cell size, low expression of differentiation markers, and the expression of basal cell keratin (Fig. 2; Kasperbauer et al. 1990; Oda and Watson 1990; Sundqvist et al. 1991a,b).

Fig. 2. Differentiated characteristics of human oral epithelium in vivo (*left*) and in vitro (*right*). The selected characteristics primarily represent buccal and gingival mucosa, as well as the epithelium derived from vestibular fornix located in between. The cultures of oral epithelial cells were derived from tissue removed during maxillofacial reconstructive surgery. *PD/D*, population doublings per day; *CFE*, colony-forming efficiency; *TPA*, 12-*O*-tetradecanoylphorbol-13-acetate. The information presented is compiled from Burkhardt and Maerker (1981), Smith and Dale (1986), Morgan and Su (1994), and Sundqvist et al. (1991a,b)

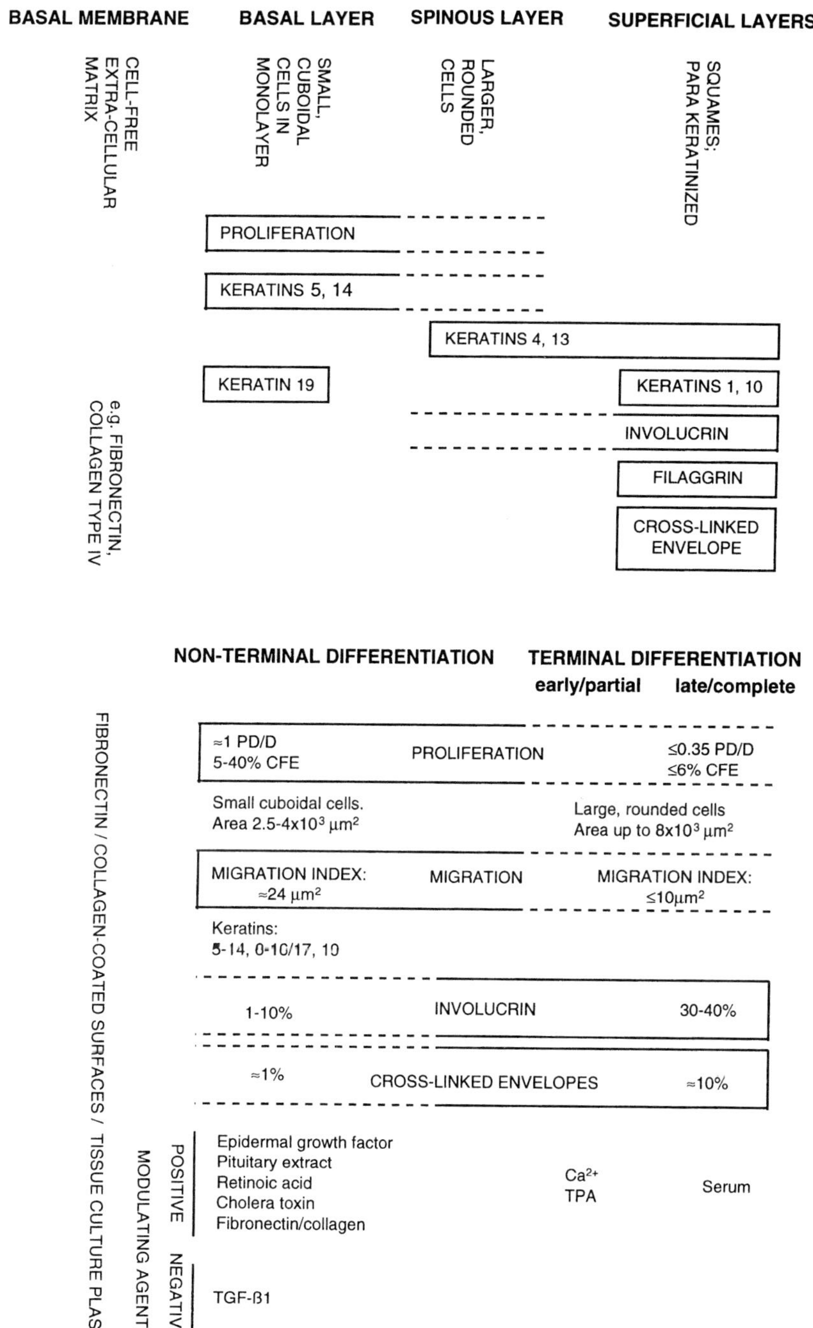

BASAL MEMBRANE
BASAL LAYER
SPINOUS LAYER
SUPERFICIAL LAYERS
CELL-FREE EXTRA-CELLULAR MATRIX
SMALL, CUBOIDAL CELLS IN MONOLAYER
LARGER, ROUNDED CELLS
SQUAMES; PARA KERATINIZED
PROLIFERATION
KERATINS 5, 14
KERATINS 4, 13
KERATIN 19
KERATINS 1, 10
INVOLUCRIN
FILAGGRIN
CROSS-LINKED ENVELOPE
e.g. FIBRONECTIN, COLLAGEN TYPE IV
NON-TERMINAL DIFFERENTIATION
TERMINAL DIFFERENTIATION
early/partial
late/complete
FIBRONECTIN / COLLAGEN-COATED SURFACES / TISSUE CULTURE PLASTIC
≈1 PD/D
5-40% CFE
PROLIFERATION
≤0.35 PD/D
≤6% CFE
Small cuboidal cells.
Area 2.5-4x10³ µm²
Large, rounded cells
Area up to 8x10³ µm²
MIGRATION INDEX:
≈24 µm²
MIGRATION
MIGRATION INDEX:
≤10µm²
Keratins:
5-14, 6-16/17, 19
1-10%
INVOLUCRIN
30-40%
≈1%
CROSS-LINKED ENVELOPES
≈10%
MODULATING AGENTS
POSITIVE
Epidermal growth factor
Pituitary extract
Retinoic acid
Cholera toxin
Fibronectin/collagen
Ca²⁺
TPA
Serum
NEGATIVE
TGF-ß1

Several mitogens have been identified for human oral epithelial cells using the serum-free conditions described above (Fig. 2). EGF, a mitogen for most epithelial cells, is essential for sustained growth of the buccal epithelial cells and markedly enhances primary cell yield from explants (Sundqvist et al. 1991a). EGF, retinoic acid, cholera toxin (a model agent that increases intracellular cyclic adenosine monophosphate), insulin, and pituitary extracts are mitogenic, although the latter three require the presence of EGF (Kasperbauer et al. 1990; Sundqvist et al. 1991a). In general, enhanced growth appeared to be correlated with decreased surface area (Sundqvist et al. 1991a). The varying effects on cell migration by mitogenic agents indicate that, although enhanced migration is commonly coupled to proliferation, as proposed for EGF (Barrandon and Green 1987), it is not a prerequisite. Transforming growth factor (TGF)-β1 proved to be a negative growth factor in oral epithelial cells (Sundqvist et al. 1991a,b), as also shown for other types of epithelial cells (Attisano et al. 1994). At concentrations of 1 pM or below, this agent markedly decreased both the colony-forming efficiency and growth rate of oral epithelial cells. An increase in cell surface area was also observed, whereas migration and expression of differentiation markers remained without change (Sundqvist et al. 1991a).

A cell culture technique should not only provide a number of cells with desired proliferative ability and longevity to allow experimentation, but also permit retained expression of tissue type-specific markers and functions. Specific characteristics of the oral epithelium can be used to assess the differentiated state of both tissue samples and cultured cells (Fig. 2). In vivo different types of epithelia can be distinguished, i.e., palatal, gingival, and buccal epithelia, the epithelium of the vestibular fornix located between the latter two, and the epithelia of the lips, floor of the mouth, and the ventral and dorsal sides of the tongue (Burkhardt and Maerker 1981). Although these epithelia differ functionally and histologically, they are all stratified and squamous, in that several cell layers exist, where the most superficial layer contains squames of cross-linked protein. The germinative compartment of cells adhere to the basal membrane, which is composed of FN, C, and other proteins produced by epithelial and fibroblastic cells. The extracellular matrix and its composition are of importance for the behavior of the basal cells, e.g., for reepithelialization in wound healing (Yancey 1995). The processes of proliferation and loss of cells by terminal differentiation or programmed cell death are normally in a dynamic steady state, whereas imbalances can lead to development of pathologic states, including cancer (Milstone 1983; Collins et al. 1994; Polakowska and Haake 1994; Norris 1995).

Adult normal buccal and gingival epithelial cells in culture express keratins 5, 14, and 19 (Oda et al. 1990; Sundqvist et al. 1991a), which are normally present in these epithelia in vivo (Clausen et al. 1986; Dale et al. 1990). The keratins 6 and 16/17, which are typical for "fast-turnover epithelia" (Dale et al. 1990), are also found in oral and other types of proliferative epithelial cells (Fuchs and Green 1980; Taichman et al. 1982; Taichman and Prokop 1982). Therefore, the keratin pattern for a majority of the cultured cells is clearly similar to those of basal cells in vivo (Fig. 2). Only 5%–10% of oral epithelial cells cultured at serum-free conditions express keratins 1 and 10 (X. Zheng et al., unpublished data) associated with suprabasal layers of orthokeratinized epithelia such as gingiva. In buccal epithelium, which is parakeratinized, scattered groups of cells in the superficial layers also express keratins 1 and 10. The presence of these subpopulations appears to be due to normal variation rather than to minor pathological change (Morgan and Su 1994). Aggregation of keratin filaments is believed to involve filaggrin, another marker of terminal differentiation (Fig. 2). This structural protein, derived from keratohyalin granules, is strongly expressed in gingival superficial cell layers, whereas it shows a weak, scattered, and granular pattern of expression in the buccal mucosa (Smith and Dale 1986; Reibel et al. 1989). In vitro, filaggrin is detected in differentiated organotypic cultures that originate from both ortho- and parakeratinized oral epithelia (Kautsky et al. 1995).

An important feature of oral epithelial cell cultures is that they retain the ability to undergo squamous differentiation. Endogenous as well as exogenous agents accelerate their terminal differentiation, as in other types of cultured human epithelial cells (Grafström 1990a; Fig. 2). Serum is a potent differentiation-inducing agent causing decreased growth and migration, as well as increased cell area, involucrin expression, and cross-linked envelope formation, of otherwise serum-free cultures of oral epithelial cells (Sundqvist et al. 1991a). These cells can be made to stratify and form cohesive epithelial sheets by exposure to serum, or serum and insulin (Kasperbauer et al. 1990). Serum-dependent methods have therefore been used to graft an artificially produced oral epithelium onto patients with defects in the oral mucosa (De Luca et al. 1990). Aberrant stimulation of terminal differentiation of normal epithelial cells by exogenous agents is of special interest in carcinogenesis, since it may represent a tumor promotion mechanism (Grafström 1990a; Harris 1991). This process may decrease the number of proliferative normal cells in vivo and lead to a selective growth advantage for (pre)neoplastic cells, providing that the latter cell type exhibits resistance to the differentiating stimulus. In support of this hypothesis, oral tumor cells and cell lines often exhibit aberrant differentiation patterns (Rubin and Rice 1986; Morgan et al. 1987; Eisenberg et al. 1987; Sundqvist et al. 1991a), and known tumor-promoting agents can accelerate differentiation of normal epithelial cells (Willey et al. 1984, 1987; Miyashita et al. 1990). Accordingly, the classical tumor-promoting agent 12-*O*-tetradecanoylphorbol-13-acetate (TPA) decreased growth and increased formation of involucrin and cross-linked envelopes of normal oral epithelial cells (Sundqvist et al. 1991a). Identification of agents that can be used to experimentally modulate differentiation in normal oral epithelial cells allows investigation of this process and the aberrant responsiveness of transformed cells.

Epithelial growth and differentiation can be studied in an organized tissue-like state using organotypic cultures. Such cultures are based on epithelial cells grown to confluence on extracellular matrices, e.g., collagen gels (Grafström

1990a; Fusenig 1994a). When this matrix is lifted to the air–liquid interface, the keratinocytes can differentiate into a multilayered epithelium. Inclusion of fibroblasts and serum in the gels provides a dermal equivalent and an opportunity to study epithelial–mesenchymal interactions. Information on growth regulation with this model has been obtained primarily from the squamous epithelia of the skin (Fusenig 1994b). Preliminary studies have indicated that both normal and transformed oral epithelial cell types form organotypic epithelia on collagen gels in serum-free EMA, where the dermal equivalent, or an elevated Ca^{2+} supplementation, can stimulate proliferation and differentiation, respectively (X. Zheng et al., unpublished data). Information about growth regulation in a histiotypic state can thus be obtained in vitro in both normal and neoplastic epithelia. Furthermore, inherent differences between oral epithelia from different anatomical subsites can possibly be studied by this method. The establishment of culture conditions with decreased amounts of serum for oral fibroblasts, i.e., 1.25% fetal bovine serum as compared to the commonly used 10% level of supplementation (Liu et al. 1991), may aid future efforts to develop further refined conditions also for organotypic cultures.

Cultured cells and short-term explant cultures offer excellent possibilities to study the pathophysiology of xenobiotic exposure. For example, toxicity, metabolism of putative carcinogens, different types of genetic damage, DNA repair mechanisms, and carcinogenesis-related effects on growth and differentiation can be investigated. Formation of carcinogen DNA adducts are preferably measured with explant cultures, since the epithelial cell layers can be collected in substantial quantities. Conversion of carcinogens to tissue-reactive metabolites has been demonstrated in explants and cultured epithelial cells, including oral mucosa (Lechner et al. 1981; Castonguay et al. 1983; Allen-Hoffman and Rheinwald 1984; Autrup et al. 1985; Lui et al. 1993). Oral explants can be maintained in serum-free medium in which the Ca^{2+} concentration has been raised to 1 m*M* (buccal explant medium, BEX) for at least 2 days with conserved normal histology; they are used for experiments after a 24-h "standardization period" of culture (Lui et al. 1993). DNA-binding products and metabolite patterns have been determined in monolayer cultures and mucosal explants of buccal epithelium for benzo[a]pyrene and the tobacco-specific *N*-nitrosamines *N*-nitrosonornicotine (NNN) and 4-(methylnitrosamino)-1-(3-pyridyl)-1-butanone (NNK) (Castonguay et al. 1983; Autrup et al. 1985; Liu et al. 1993). In contrast, a different pattern of metabolites and a severalfold lower DNA-binding level was found when benzo[a]pyrene was metabolized by cultured rat buccal mucosal cells (Autrup et al. 1985). Oral epithelial cells exhibit DNA repair synthesis following carcinogen exposures, as demonstrated in human gingival explants cultured with *N*-nitroso and polycyclic aromatic carcinogens (Ide et al. 1982).

Transformation of Human Oral Epithelial Cells

To study the transformation process, human oncogenes, tumor suppressor genes, or, alternatively, genes that encode oncoproteins from DNA tumor viruses can be introduced in human cell cultures (Grafström 1990a; Knowles 1990). Treatment of normal cells with chemical or physical carcinogenic agents has only rarely led to the establishment of continuous cell lines (Grafström 1990a; Chang 1991). As discussed below, successful transfection of oral epithelial cells has been achieved with the E6/E7 genes from HPV 16 or HPV 18 and the T antigen gene from simian virus 40 (SV40T) (Table 2). Research on tumor suppressor genes and these DNA tumor viruses with other cell types has shown that the E6 and E7 proteins form complexes with the p53 and Rb products, respectively, leading to inactivation of the latter (Levine et al. 1991; Weinberg 1991). Unlike SV40T which complexes with both the p53 and Rb proteins, the HPV E6 protein, also catalyzes degradation of the p53 protein; thus SV40T-and HPV E6/E7-transfected lines offer complementary systems of transformation. Following transfections of hybrid constructs containing these viral genes into various types of human cells, lines develop which show extended life spans or which apparently become immortalized (Chang 1986; Grafström 1990a). These lines rarely become tumorigenic, at least not at early passages (Brown and Gallimore 1987; Knowles 1990). However, full transformation to a malignant phenotype can be accomplished by supertransfection with an oncogene or treatment with chemical carcinogens (Chang 1986; Grafström 1990a).

Transfection of serum-free cultures of normal human buccal epithelial cells with SV40T resulted in various cell lines that exhibited both normal and premalignant characteristics (Kulkarni et al. 1995). The lines developed in a multistep fashion that involved one or more crises. One apparently immortal line, termed SVpgC2a, is pseudodiploid and partly resistant to growth inhibition by TGF-β1 and serum-induced expression of involucrin, a marker of terminal squamous differentiation. The cells have maintained a high proliferative rate during more than 2 years in culture and have not undergone malignant transformation, since their inoculation into athymic nude mice did not induce tumors. The SVpgC2a line contains two copies of SV40T integrated at the same genomic site, and it expresses wild-type p53 and Rb proteins (Kulkarni et al. 1995). This and other SV40T-transfected lines, with extended or infinite life spans, have been cryopreserved at various passages and developmental stages. They are likely to be valuable tools for future investigations relating to intermediate stages of carcinogenesis.

Other investigators have accomplished immortalization of oral epithelial cells by transfection of HPV genes (Table 2). Interestingly, such lines underwent further transformation upon exposure to the tobacco-specific carcinogen NNK or *N*-methyl-*N'*-nitro-*N*-nitrosoguanidine. Therefore, malignant transformation of oral epithelial cells can probably be caused by a sequential combined effect of high-risk HPV and tobacco-related carcinogens.

Genotoxic damage resulted in lower levels of intranuclear p53 protein accumulation and so-called growth arrest/DNA damage (GADD) gene induction in the HPV-immortalized lines than in normal cells (Gujuluva et al. 1994). Since these genes participate in G_1 cell cycle arrest, presumably allowing for DNA repair, these results agree with the concept that HPV-infected cells more easily undergo further genetic changes and malignant transformation than noninfected normal cells.

Numerous cell lines derived from human oral tumors are described in the literature (some are reviewed by Chang [1991]). Many are from tumors of the tongue, whereas a minority of these are of buccal origin, possibly because the tongue is a frequent site of oral carcinomas in the Western world. The SqCC/Y1 cell line, recently adapted to serum-free culture conditions (Table 2), was established in 1981 from a verrucous (squamous) buccal carcinoma (Pitman et al. 1983) in a female patient (A.C. Sartorelli, personal communication). This cell line has been extensively used to study epithelial cell growth and differentiation (Pitman et al. 1983; King et al. 1986; Reiss et al. 1985, 1986; Reiss and Sartorelli 1987; King and Sartorelli 1989). It is apparently immortal, as it has been in culture for over 10 years (Reiss et al. 1985). It is highly resistant to growth inhibition and terminal differentiation by serum or TGF-β1 (Sundqvist et al. 1991b) and is reported to undergo squamous differentiation only when subjected to severe provocation (Reiss et al. 1985, 1986; Reiss and Sartorelli 1987; King and Sartorelli 1989). Recently, the inoculation of SqCC/Y1 cells were shown to induce tumors in athymic nude mice (Kulkarni et al. 1995).

The advantages of serum-free culture conditions would also be desirable for tumor-derived cell lines, and attempts to use low serum concentrations, e.g., 0.5%, in culture for up to 2 weeks has been reported for two human cell lines derived from the tongue (Pillai et al. 1991). The SqCC/Y1 cell line has previously been maintained at serum-free conditions for up to 2 weeks, albeit with reduction of proliferation (Pitman et al. 1983; Reiss et al. 1986). In contrast, the optimized serum-free medium for normal oral cells, termed EMA, significantly increased colony-forming efficiency and clonal growth rate of SqCC/Y1 cells, and long-term culture resulted in a serum-independent daughter strain (Table 2). The cells showed similar growth characteristics, i.e., growth rate and cell yield, as the original strain and could also be grown at clonal density. The serum-free carcinoma strain also retained the resistance to growth inhibition and terminal differentiation inducible in normal cells by TGF-β1, serum, and elevated Ca^{2+} (Sundqvist et al. 1991a,b).

Karyotypic analyses of oral carcinomas have revealed a large number of chromosomal aberrations per metaphase of both clonal and nonclonal patterns (for references, see Table 1). The SqCC/Y1 cells have 63–83 chromosomes and seven to 12 marker chromosomes per metaphase and show consistent monosomy 1, tetrasomy 19 and 20, and trisomy 22 (Sundqvist et al. 1991b). This line has a single rearranged p53 allele carrying two missense mutations, which is not expressed (Reiss et al. 1992). Transfection of hybrid wild-type p53 into SqCC/Y1 did not restore the sensitivity to TGF-β1 growth inhibition (seen in normal cells), but allowed expression of some markers of terminal squamous differentiation (Brenner et al. 1993). This result therefore implied that the many functions of p53 may involve suppression of malignant transformation by induction of epithelial differentiation. Other studies indicate that wild-type p53 also can induce apoptosis in HNSCC lines (Liu et al. 1995).

The EGF homologue TGF-α, which also binds to the EGF receptor (EGFR) and stimulates epithelial cell growth, is constitutively expressed in SqCC/Y1 cells (King and Sartorelli 1989). Expression of TGF-α, both as mRNA and protein, occurs at higher levels in HNSCC than in normal epidermis, with the highest level of expression detected in poorly differentiated tumors (Partridge et al. 1989). Moreover, TGF-α is often expressed in carcinomas with elevated levels of EGFR (Aaronson 1991). The SqCC/Y1 cells exhibit both amplification and overexpression of EGFR (Reiss et al. 1991), a common finding in oral carcinoma cell lines (Ozanne et al. 1986; Yamamoto et al. 1986; Cowley et al. 1986). The amplification of EGFR in SqCC/Y1 cells is reported to be two-to fourfold (Reiss et al. 1991), possibly coupled to the demonstrated hyperdiploidy of chromosome 7 (Sundqvist et al. 1991b), which harbors the EGFR gene. The SqCC/Y1 cell line therefore exhibits a pattern of EGFR amplification and overexpression of EGFR and TGF-α that supports autocrine regulation of growth.

Using the differential display method (Liang et al. 1993), elevated expression of three additional genes was recently shown in the SqCC/Y1 cells (Sundqvist et al. 1995). Cloning and sequence analysis revealed that two of these genes, which were denominated OTEX (Oral Tumor Expressed), were previously uncharacterized human genes, with hitherto unknown functions. The third gene encoded L26, a ribosomal protein known to be overexpressed also in other tumor cell types (Sundqvist et al. 1995). Other studies showed that the SqCC/Y1 cells lack glycoprotein-bearing a2,3-sialylated O-linked carbohydrate chains on their plasma membrane (Neeser et al. 1995). Such changes in cell surface glycosylation may affect the cell-to-cell interactions that participate in growth regulation and also decrease immunologically based recognition mechanisms for removal of neoplastic cells. Taken together, the SqCC/Y1 cell line has the characteristics of full transformation, including immortality, resistance to differentiation, aneuploid karyotype, and ability to form tumors in an immunodeprived host. For future comparative studies of the characteristics of normal oral cells and this tumorous line, growth at the similar serum-free culture conditions provide the experimental advantage of a standardized extracellular environment (Sundqvist et al. 1991b). Further studies are needed to investigate whether other HNSCC can be established at similar serum-free culture conditions.

Betel Quid, Areca Nut, and Tobacco

Areca nut and betel leaf are the major ingredients of a betel quid, but tobacco is also commonly included (IARC 1985). The use of these products and their roles in the development of oral cancer has been extensively reviewed (IARC 1985, 1986). Although the carcinogenicity of tobacco products is well established, the available experimental and epidemiological data have only provided limited evidence favoring the classification of betel quid *without* tobacco as a human carcinogen (Thomas and Kearsley 1993; Thomas and Wilson 1993). Moreover, there is only limited data for carcinogenicity of areca nut in experimental animals. In contrast, ingredients of the betel leaf are believed to prevent cancer development (IARC 1985; Huber et al. 1994). The use of in vitro model systems has shed new light on the causal role of both tobacco and areca nut in oral carcinogenesis and has also provided information on possible mechanisms in the induction of oral cancer.

The most abundant and also most potent carcinogens in smokeless tobacco are the tobacco-specific *N*-nitrosamines NNN and NNK (IARC 1985, 1986). Fresh, enzymatically active human saliva efficiently extracts these agents from tobacco (Table 3). Both agents are carcinogenic to animals and metabolized by humans (Hoffman et al. 1984; Rivenson et al. 1988; Carmella et al. 1990). Metabolically activated NNN and NNK can bind to hemoglobin, and globin adducts in snuff users are clearly increased over controls (Carmella et al. 1990). Using serum-free methods, tissue explants and epithelial cell cultures from human buccal mucosa were shown to metabolize NNK by three major pathways, i.e., carbonyl reduction, α-carbon hydroxylation, and pyridine N-oxidation (Liu et al. 1993). Formation of electrophilic-reactive intermediates was indicated by the pattern of metabolites and by the covalent binding of metabolized NNK to the epithelial layers of explant cultures. Expression of several cytochrome p450 types in cultured oral epithelial cells (Farin et al. 1995), which are known to metabolize NNK, indicate their involvement in these processes. The result indicate that tobacco-specific *N*-nitrosamines cause effects associated with cancer development in oral mucosa.

Extracts of the areca nut are toxic and cause genetic damage in vitro (IARC 1985). Major constituents include polyphenols, polysaccharides, fats, crude fibers, and alkaloids, which may contribute to these effects. A role for reactive oxygen species (ROS) has been implicated, as these can be formed in chemical mixtures with areca nut tannins (Nair et al. 1987, 1990). Suggested toxicity mechanisms in the oral mucosa have included direct effects of ROS on the cells, activation and inactivation of potentially carcinogenic compounds, and degradation of the salivary mucus, thereby affecting the oral barrier function (Stich and Anders 1989). ROS are also believed to have tumor-promoting properties (Cerutti 1994). Protection against pathological effects of ROS may involve reduced glutathione (GSH), the most abundant cellular thiol (Vina 1990). The underlying mechanisms involve enzymatic and nonenzymatic conjugations of reactive species to the sulfhydryl moiety of GSH or oxidation

Table 3. *N*-nitrosamines in saliva of individuals with various habits[a]

Habits	NNN (μM)	NAT (μM)	NAB (nM)	NNK (nM)	NGCO (nM)	NGCI (nM)	NMMPN (nM)
Chewing habits							
Tobacco	0.02–14.7	Trace to 2.9		ND to 970	ND	ND	
Tobacco and lime	0.002–2.4	ND to 0.70		ND to 138			
Betel quid with tobacco	0.007–0.48	0.02–0.21	ND to 209	ND to 69	ND to 2.0×10^3	ND to 193	
Betel quid without tobacco					ND to 56	ND to 169	4–101
Masheri	0.08–0.25		ND	ND			
Toombak	3.3–118	ND to 2.5	ND to 10×10^3	ND to 32×10^3			
Tobacco smoking							
Cigarettes					ND to 44	ND	

NNN, *N′*-nitrosonornicotine; NAT, *N′*-nitrosoanatabine; NAB, *N′*-nitrosoanabasine; NNK, 4-(metylnitrosamino)-1-(3-pyridyl)-1-butanone; NGCO, *N*-nitrosoguvacoline; NGCI, *N*-nitrosoguvacine; NMPN, 3-(*N*-nitroso-methylamino) propionitrile; ND, not detected.

[a]Summarized from Wenke et al. 1984a,c; Nair et al. 1985; Prokopczyk et al. 1987; Idris et al. 1992.

of GSH to glutathione disulfide (GSSG). Investigations of the toxicity of an aqueous areca nut extract and alterations in thiol status in serum-free cultures of human oral epithelial cells enabled studies of these mechanisms in human target cells (Sundqvist et al. 1989; Sundqvist and Grafström 1992). The extract, in a dose range of 3–540 μg/ml, decreased the cell viability to 50%, as determined by colony-forming efficiency, neutral red uptake, and trypan blue exclusion assays (Table 4). The highest concentration in this interval also decreased the cellular thiol content, indicating that the presence of thiol-reactive compounds in the extract would not substantially contribute to the noted toxicity at lower concentrations. Moreover, the loss of GSH occurred without associated formation of GSSG (Sundqvist et al. 1989). Since exposure to extract perturbed the plasma membrane integrity, it is possible that the cellular GSH might have been lost by leakage. Therefore, these correlations of cellular toxicity and thiol status did not indicate formation of ROS from the areca nut. The probability of generation of ROS is probably low at the physiological pH of the exposure medium, as in the neutral saliva of Indian betel quid chewers (Wenke et al. 1984).

Particles in the areca nut extract showed a marked adherence to cultures of oral epithelial cells as judged from phase contrast and electron microscopy analysis (Sundqvist and Grafström 1992).The cells revealed a severely disturbed plasma membrane, with loss of the usually abundant microvilli, formation of membrane ridges, and possible internalization of particulates. Interestingly, these changes relate to observations in buccal tissue of betel quid chewers, where pathological changes include betel incrustations on the epithelial surface, amorphous material in intercellular spaces and the basement membrane, and unusual microvilli-like cell surface structures (Lee and Chin 1970; Reichart et al. 1984). The mucosa also shows crystalloid aggregations in the intercellular spaces in suprabasal layers, probably derived from the quid (Reichart et al. 1984). Areca nut alkaloids may be involved in this effect, since granular deposits are found on the oral mucosal epithelium in rats exposed by topical application to the major alkaloid of areca nut, arecoline (Thomas and Kearsley 1993).

Exposure of oral epithelial cells to the areca nut extract for 3 h caused genotoxic effects, as measured by increased DNA single-strand breaks (DNA SSB) and DNA protein cross-links (DPC) (Table 4). The DNA SSB were found to accumulate following attempted removal of the extract (Sundqvist and Grafström 1992). These effects of the extract at μg/ml concentrations could possibly be explained by prolonged exposure to DNA-damaging agents, through adherent or internalized extract particles, as discussed above, and/or by inhibited DNA repair. Exfoliated oral epithelial cells from betel quid chewers show enhanced frequencies of micronucleated cells, indicating genetic damage (Stich et al. 1983). Breaks and cross-links are major DNA lesions induced by physical and chemical carcinogens (Fornace 1982; Defasis 1990). Removal of genetic damage by DNA excision repair (Defasis 1990) can lead to accumulation of DNA SSB if sealing of the breaks is inhibited, indirectly

Table 4. Cytotoxic and genotoxic effects of aqueous areca nut extract and areca nut *N*-nitroso compounds and their precursor alkaloids in human oral epithelial cells

Agent[a]	CFE_{50}[b]	CGR_{50}[c]	NRU_{50}[d]	TBE_{50}[e]	$Thiols_{75}$[f]	DNA SSB[g]	DPC[g]
						Lesions(*n*)	
Areca nut extract (μg/ml)	3	7	160	540	540	1.2	2.2
Alkaloids (mM)							
Arecoline	1.6	4.7	–	–	0.57	0.5	–
Arecaidine	> 5.0	> 5.0	–	–	> 5.0	0.2	–
Guvacoline	2.1	5.0	–	–	0.88	0.5	–
Guvacine	> 5.0	> 5.0	–	–	> 5.0	0.3	–
N-nitroso compounds (m*M*)							
N-nitroso-guva coline	1.7	> 5.0	–	–	2.9	0.5	–
N-nitrosoguva cine	> 5.0	> 5.0	–	–	3.8	0.4	–
NMPA	0.15	0.36	–	–	0.06	1.7	4.9
NMPN	> 5.0	> 5.0	–	–	> 5.0	0.2	–

NMPA, 3-(*N*-nitrosomethylamino)-propionaldehyde; NMPN, 3-(*N*-nitrosomethylamino)-proprionitrile.

[a]The areca nut extract or the individual compounds were added to the cells for 3 h in defined growth medium free of thiols and pituitary extract (Sundqvist et al. 1989; Sundqvist and Grafström 1992).

[b]The concentration that resulted in a 50% decrease of the colony-forming efficiency. The cells were seeded at 250 cells/cm2 and incubated for 24 h. After exposure, the cells were incubated in growth medium without agent for 8 days and subsequently fixed with 10% formalin and stained with 1% aqueous crystal violet. The mean colony-forming efficiency was determined from duplicate dishes and based on colonies containing at least 16 cells (Sundqvist et al. 1989).

[c]The concentration that reduced clonal growth rate to 50% of control. Clonal growth was determined from cells incubated in the colony-forming efficiency assay as described in footnote b. The mean clonal growth rate was determined as the log of the number of cells in nine randomly selected clones divided by the number of days in culture, which gives populations doublings per day.

[d]The concentration that decreased neutral red uptake of the cultures to 50% of control. The neutral red uptake assay was performed as described (Sundqvist et al. 1989).

[e]The concentration that decreased trypan blue exclusion of the cultures to 50% as compared to control. The assay for trypan blue exclusion was performed as described (Grafström et al. 1988).

[f]The concentration that decreased intracellular free thiols to 75% of the amount present in untreated control cells. After exposure, the cells were assayed for their content of free low molecular weight thiols as described (Grafström et al. 1988).

[g]The number of DNA single-strand breaks (SSB) or DNA protein cross-links (DPC) per 10^{10} Da DNA formed after exposure of the cultures to 300 μg areca nut extract /ml or 5.0 mM of the compound indicated, except for NMPA, where 0.3 m*M* was used instead of the highly toxic concentration of 5.0 m*M* (Sundqvist et al. 1989; Sundqvist and Grafström 1992). Determination of the indicated DNA lesions in cell cultures using the alkaline elution assay has been described in detail (Grafström et al. 1988).

demonstrating the involvement of this repair mechanism (Dunn and Regan 1979).

Selective resistance to toxicity acquired early in carcinogenesis is another putative promotion mechanism (Grafström 1990a; Harris 1991). Such selective resistance has been demonstrated during cancer development in hamster buccal pouch (Hussong et al. 1991), and similar properties have been observed in human tumor cell lines (Harris 1987; Miyashita et al. 1990). Areca nut has tumor-promoting properties in animal studies (Rao 1984; Tanaka et al. 1986; Stich and Anders 1989), and it has been suggested that this property is more pronounced than the initiating activity of this agent (Stich and Anders 1989). In vitro, aqueous extracts of areca nut are positive in the bovine papillomavirus DNA transformation test (Stich and Tsang 1989). In cultures of normal human buccal epithelial cells, the areca nut extract accelerated terminal differentiation, measured as involucrin expression, whereas the squamous carcinoma SqCC/Y1 cells were resistant to this effect (Sundqvist and Grafström 1992). The SqCC/Y1 cells were also somewhat more resistant than the normal cells to the toxicity of areca nut extract, but the difference was not statistically significant. Further studies are therefore needed to clarify whether areca nut extract causes general toxicity and premature induction of terminal squamous differentiation by similar or dissimilar mechanisms. Overall, these in vitro studies implied that chewing of areca nut is associated with the release or formation of agents that can drive oral epithelial cells through various phases of carcinogenesis.

Identification of Putative Carcinogens in the Areca Nut

The results obtained with the areca nut extract generated questions as to the cytotoxic and genotoxic compounds present in this complex mixture. In addition to chemicals which can generate ROS, areca nut-specific *N*-nitroso compounds, of which some are carcinogenic to rodents, have been implicated. Such compounds can be formed by nitrosations of areca nut-specific alkaloids (Fig. 3). Data from the chemical analysis of the nut and saliva from individuals with various chewing and smoking habits demonstrate human exposure from nanomolar to millimolar concentrations of *N*-nitrosamines (Table 3). *Candida* and other microorganisms in the oral mucosa may contribute to the salivary nitrosations of the precursor alkaloids to carcinogenic *N*-nitrosamines (Charriere et al. 1991). Calculations based on the salivary concentrations of the areca-specific *N*-nitroso compound 3-(*N*-nitrosomethylamino)-propionitrile (NMPN) and the average amount of saliva when chewing a betel quid (Prokopczyk et al. 1987) indicate that the total dose from chewing ten quids/day for 20 years will range from 63 nmol/kg to 3.4 mmol/kg for a person of 70 kg. This interval covers the total doses of 0.25–1.15 mmol NMPN/kg found to be carcinogenic in rats (Prokopczyk et al. 1987). The areca-specific *N*-nitroso compound 3-(*N*-nitrosomethylamino)-propionaldehyde (NMPA) is also a rodent carcinogen (Nishikawa et al. 1992). These agents produce tumors in

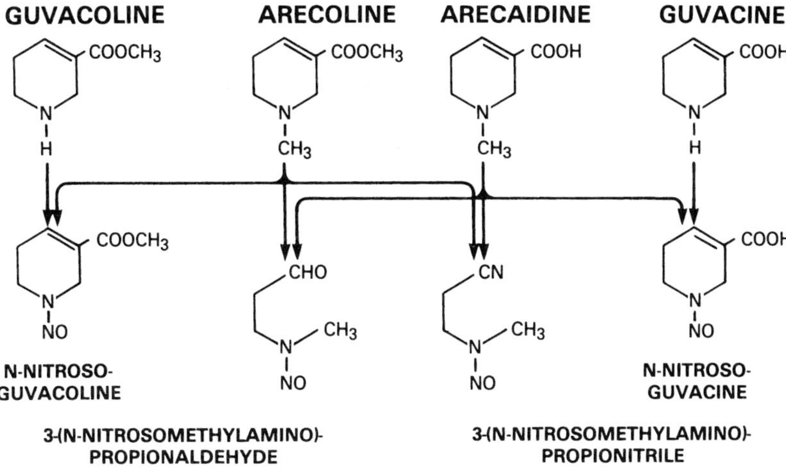

Fig. 3. Chemical structures of major areca nut alkaloids and areca nut-specific *N*-nitroso compounds. Potential nitrosation products of the indicated alkaloids are shown. Adapted from Wenke and Hoffman (1983) and Prokopczyk et al. (1987)

several tissues, including nasal mucosa, tongue, oesophagus, liver, and lung. NMPN causes DNA methylation, which is regarded as the initiating lesion of *N*-nitroso compounds (Lawley 1990), and also cyanoethylation in the target tissues for its carcinogenicity (Prokopczyk et al. 1988, 1991). In contrast, areca nut alkaloids are weak carcinogens in laboratory animals (IARC 1985; Rivenson et al. 1988).

Using serum-free cultures of human buccal epithelial cells, pathobiological effects of the areca nut alkaloids and their *N*-nitroso derivatives depicted in Fig. 3 were investigated (Table 4). On a molar basis, NMPA was the most potent in decreasing colony-forming efficiency, clonal growth rate, and the cellular content of free thiols. It was the only compound that caused substantial DNA damage, notably more DPC than DNA SSB (Table 4). Arecoline, guvacoline, and *N*-nitrosoguvacoline were moderately cytotoxic and decreased cellular thiols. Arecoline and, to a lesser degree, arecaidine have previously been shown to react directly with thiols in vitro, and both compounds are conjugated to GSH in vivo (Boyland and Nery 1969). The remaining compounds had only minor effects on the cells in concentrations up to 5 m*M* (Table 4). Chemical structure–activity relationships could be deduced from these experiments (Fig. 3, Table 4). Cytotoxicity and thiol depletion by arecoline and guvacoline, and to some extent *N*-nitrosoguvacoline, were related to the presence of a methylester group. Accordingly, a lower degree of ionization of these compounds in an aqueous milieu, in comparison to arecaidine, guvacine, and *N*-nitrosoguvacine, may facilitate their passage over biological membranes (Panigrani and Rao 1984). *N*-nitrosopiperidine derivatives, of which *N*-nitrosoguvacoline is considered one, are known to show similar structure–activity relationships for mutagenicity and carcinogenicity (Lijinsky and Taylor 1976; Rao et al. 1978; Nix et al. 1979). The aldehyde moiety of NMPA may contribute to the marked cytotoxic and genotoxic effects in cell cultures (Fig. 3, Table 4). Additionally, oxidative metabolism of NMPA would generate alkylating intermediates and aldehydes, including formaldehyde and acrolein (Grafström et al. 1995). The spectrum of pathobiological effects of NMPA in buccal cells is similar to that expected from combined exposure to formaldehyde and acrolein, i.e., substantial depletion of cellular GSH associated with concomitant loss of viability and formation of both DPC and SSB (Grafström 1990b; Grafström et al. 1995). The possible involvement of metabolic conversions of NMPA is supported by active metabolism of the tobacco-specific *N*-nitroso compound NNK to tissue-reactive products in cultured human oral epithelial cells (Liu et al. 1993), presumably via enzymatic pathways that would also metabolize NMPA. Although many compounds present in betel quid preparations have been demonstrated to be mutagens and carcinogens (IARC 1985; Thomas and Kearsley 1993), the results support the possible involvement of NMPA, both with and without metabolic activation, in pathological states observed in oral mucosa of betel quid chewers. Interestingly, alcohol consumption coupled with its oxidation would also involve aldehyde exposure, i.e., acetaldehyde, causing both cytotoxic and genotoxic effects in human cell cultures (Grafström et al. 1994). *N*-nitroso compounds and aldehydes might therefore contribute to the risk of oral cancer associated with the separate or combined use of tobacco, betel quid, and alcohol.

Conclusions and Perspectives

HNSCC is a common form of human cancer and a considerable health problem, particularly in high-incidence regions such as Southern Asia. In both epidemiological and experimental studies, the concept of multistep carcinogenesis in associated tissues has evolved with the advent of molecular biology, oncogenes, and tumor suppressor genes. Thus a multifactorial etiology has in some instances been coupled to region-specific combinations of genetic change. Despite the over-representation of epithelial-derived tumors in the head and neck region, as in most human tissues, in vitro studies of oncogenesis have commonly employed mesenchymal rather than epithelial cells. As a result, a detailed understanding of the molecular mechanisms of tumor formation and definitions of both the normal and malignant transformed epithelial phenotype have been lacking. However, studies with normal, experimentally transformed and tumor-derived cell cultures from human oral epithelium have provided new information. Standardization of the culture conditions, by the removal of undefined supplements such as serum, have improved the reproducibility of these model systems. Cells grown from normal, nontumorous tissue express many characteristics of a differentiated epithelium, as confirmed from side-by-side comparison to intact mucosa. Defined factors regulate growth of these normal cells in an interdependent manner, demonstrating that epithelial proliferation and differentiation is an integrated and complex process. Further, transformed cell types often show aberrant regulation of identified pathways of negative growth control. New information on the critical factors and events that drive the various phases of carcinogenesis has also been obtained. Accordingly, experiments with cell cultures indicate that both tobacco *and* areca nut should be considered as etiologic factors in oral cancer, an issue of debate in the scientific community. The results imply that cytopathic changes from betel quid chewing and/or use of tobacco involve alterations in normal cell morphology, aberrant growth and differentiation, metabolic activation of carcinogens, and DNA damage. These effects are likely to occur from reactive agents extracted to, or formed in, the saliva. Exposure of cell cultures indicate *N*-nitrosamines and aldehydes as candidate compounds for involving such mechanisms in the genesis of oral tumors. Studies on possible interactive effects between viruses, e.g., HPV, and suspected human carcinogens, have been facilitated by the recent establishment of immortalized oral cell lines. Such lines are likely to represent in vitro models of human preneoplasia and can potentially bridge normal and tumorous cell lines in the evaluations of how specific genes and environmental exposure contribute to cancer development. Overall, the existence of defined means of culturing both normal and transformed human epithelial cells has provided an opportunity to design more specific studies of cancer in humans and laboratory animals with target cell types, free of the normal and complex interactions in the host. However, future model systems for oral mucosa, such as organotypic cultures, will necessarily involve increasing degrees of complexity. For example, the mesenchymal influence on mechanisms of epithelial growth and transformation, delineated in monolayer cultures, can thereby also be investigated in a tissue-like environment. Research in HNSCC is likely to benefit from the existence of increasingly defined in vitro methods. Active areas of study include the evaluation of known and suspected risk factors, chemoprevention, development of novel chemotherapeutic drugs, biomarkers of disease, and the roles of programmed cell death and genetic instability in disease development. In this regard, these culture methods provide useful means of defining both normal and pathophysiological states of the associated target cell types.

Acknowledgement. We especially thank our collaborators for their contributions to the original work summarized in this review. We also thank Dr. J. Field and Dr. P. Boukamp for comments on the data compilations for this manuscript, and Ms. A.L. Marcus for typing assistance. This work was supported by grants from the Council for Forestry and Agricultural Research, the Cancer Society, the National Board of Laboratory Animals, and the Tobacco Company in Sweden.

References

Aaronson SA (1991) Growth factors and cancer. Science 254: 1146–1153

Adamson R, Jones AS, Field JK (1994) Loss of heterozygosity studies on chromosome 17 in head and neck cancer using microsatellite markers. Oncogene 9: 2077–2082

Ah-See KW, Cooke TG, Pickford IR, Soutar D, Balmain A (1994) An allelotype of squamous carcinoma of the head and neck using microsatellite markers. Cancer Res 54: 1617–1621

Allen-Hoffman HB, Rheinwald JG (1984) Polycyclic aromatic hydrocarbon mutagenesis of human epidermal keratinocytes in culture. Proc Natl Acad Sci USA 81: 7802–7806

Arenholt-Bindeslev BD, Jepsen A, MacCallum DK, Lillie JH (1987) The growth and structure of human oral keratinocytes in culture. J Invest Dermatol 88: 314–319

Attisano L, Wrana JL, Lopez CF, Massague J (1994) TGF-beta receptors and actions. Biochim Biophys Acta 1222: 71–80

Autrup H, Grafström RC (1982) Comparison of carcinogen metabolism in different organs and species. In: Hietanen E, Laitinen M, Hänninen O (eds) Cytochrome P450: biochemistry, biophysics and environmental implications. Elsevier Biomedical Press, Amsterdam, pp 643–648

Autrup H, Seremet T, Arenholt D, Dragsted L, Jepsen A (1985) Metabolism of benzo[a]pyrene by cultured rat and human buccal mucosa cells. Carcinogenesis 6: 1761–1765

Aznavoorian S, Murphy AN, Stetler-Stevenson WG, Liotta LA (1993) Molecular aspects of tumor cell invasion and metastasis. Cancer 71: 1368–1383

Barrandon Y, Green H (1987) Cell migration is essential for sustained growth of keratinocyte colonies: the roles of transforming growth factor-alpha and epidermal growth factor. Cell 51: 1131–1137

Boyce ST, Ham RG (1983) Calcium-regulated differentiation of normal human epidermal keratinocytes in chemically defined clonal culture and serum-free serial culture. J Invest Dermatol 81 [1 Suppl]: 33s–40s

Boyd NM, Reade PC (1988) Mechanisms of carcinogenesis with particular reference to the oral mucosa. J Oral Pathol 17: 193-201

Boyland E, Nery R (1969) Mercapturic acid formation during the metabolism of arecoline and arecaidine in the rat. Biochem J 113: 123–130

Boyle P, Macfarlane GJ, Blot WJ, Chiesa F, Lefebvre JL, Azul AM, Devries N, Scully C (1995) European School of Oncology advisory report to the European Commission for the Europe Against Cancer Programme – oral carcinogenesis in Europe. Eur J Cancer Oral Oncol 31B: 75–85

Brachman DG (1994) Molecular biology of head and neck cancer. Semin Oncol 21: 320–329

Brenner L, Munoz AT, Vellucci VF, Zhou ZL, Reiss M (1993) Wild-type p53 tumor suppressor gene restores differentiation of human squamous carcinoma cells but not the response to transforming growth factor beta. Cell Growth Differ 4: 993–1004

Brown KW, Gallimore PH (1987) Malignant progression of an SV40-transformed human epidermal keratinocyte cell line. Br J Cancer 56: 545–554 [published erratum appears in Br J Cancer 57(3): 337]

Burkhart A, Maerker R (eds) (1981) A colour atlas of oral cancers. Wolf Medical, London

Carmella SG, Kagan SS, Kagan M, Foiles PG, Palladino G, Quart AM, Quart E, Hecht SS (1990) Mass spectrometric analysis of tobacco-specific nitrosamine hemoglobin adducts in snuff dippers, smokers, and nonsmokers. Cancer Res 50: 5438–5445

Castonguay A, Stoner GD, Schut HA, Hecht SS (1983) Metabolism of tobacco-specific N-nitrosamines by cultured human tissues. Proc Natl Acad Sci USA 80: 6694–6697

Cerutti PA (1994) Oxy-radicals and cancer. Lancet 344: 862–863
Chang SE (1986) In vitro transformation of human epithelial cells. Biochim Biophys Acta 823: 161–194
Chang SE (1991) Human oral keratinocyte cultures and in vitro model systems for studying oral carcinogenesis. In: Johnson NW (ed) Oral cancer. Detection of patients and lesions at risk, vol 2. Cambridge University Press, Cambridge, pp 340–363
Charriere M, Poirier S, Calmels S, De Montclos H, Dubreuil C, Poizat R, Hamdi CM, de The G (1991) Microflora of the nasopharynx in caucasian and maghrebian subjects with and without nasopharyngeal carcinoma. In: O'Neill IK, Chen J, Bartsch H (eds) Relevance to human cancer of N-nitroso compounds. International Agency for Research on Cancer, Lyon, pp 158–161 (IARC Sci Publ No. 105)
Clausen H, Vedtofte P, Moe D, Dabelsteen E, Sun TT, Dale B (1986) Differentiation-dependent expression of keratins in human oral epithelia. J Invest Dermatol 86: 249–254
Collins MK, Perkins GR, Rodriguez TG, Nieto MA, Lopez RA (1994) Growth factors as survival factors: regulation of apoptosis. Bioessays 16: 133–138
Cowley GP, Smith JA, Gusterson BA (1986) Increased EGF receptors on human squamous carcinoma cell lines. Br J cancer 53: 223–229
Dale BA, Salonen J, Jones AH (1990) New approaches and concepts in the study of differentiation of oral epithelia. Crit Rev Oral Biol Med 1: 167–190
De Luca M, Albanese E, Megna M, Cancedda R, Mangiante PE, Cadoni A, Franzi AT (1990) Evidence that human oral epithelium reconstituted in vitro and transplanted onto patients with defects in the oral mucosa retains properties of the original donor site. Transplantation 50: 454–459
Defasis M (1990) Mechanisms of repair in mammalian cells. In: Arlett CF (ed) Springer, Berlin Heidelberg New York, pp 51–64 (Handbook of experimental pharmacology, vol 94: II)
Dunn WC, Regan JD (1979) Inhibition of DNA excision repair in human cells by arabinofuranosyl cytosine: effect on normal and xeroderma pigmentosum cells. Mol Pharmacol 15: 367–374
Eisenberg E, Murphy GF, Krutchkoff DJ (1987) Involucrin as a diagnostic marker in oral lichenoid lesions. Oral Surg Oral Med Oral Pathol 64: 313–319
El Naggar AK, Hurr K, Batsakis JG, Luna MA, Goepfert H, Huff V (1995) Sequential loss of heterozygosity at microsatellite motifs in preinvasive and invasive head and neck squamous carcinoma. Cancer Res 55: 2656–2659
Farin FM, Bigler LG, Oda D, McDougall JK, Omiecinski CJ (1995) Expression of cytochrome P450 and microsomal epoxide hydrolase in cervical and oral epithelial cells immortalized by human papillomavirus type 16 E6/E7 genes. Carcinogenesis 16: 1391–1401
Field JK (1995) The role of oncogenes and tumour-suppressor genes in the aetiology of oral, head and neck squamous cell carcinoma. J R Soc Med 88: 35P–39P
Fornace AJ (1982) Detection of DNA single-strand breaks produced during the repair of damage by DNA-protein cross-linking agents. Cancer Res 42: 145–149
Franceschi S, Levi F, Lucchini F, Negri E, Boyle P, La VC (1994) Trends in cancer mortality in young adults in Europe, 1955–1989. Eur J Cancer 30A: 2096–2118
Fuchs E, Green H (1980) Changes in keratin gene expression during terminal differentiation of the keratinocyte. Cell 19: 1033–1042
Fusenig N (1994a) Culture of keratinocytes on collagen gels and use of transplantation chambers for grafting onto mouse skin. In: Leigh IM, Lane EB, Watt FM (eds) Keratinocyte methods. Cambridge University Press, Cambridge, pp 55–59
Fusenig N (1994b) Epithelial-mesenchymal interactions regulate growth and differentiation in vitro. In: Leigh IM, Lane EB, Watt FM (eds) The keratinocyte handbook. Cambridge University Press, Cambridge, pp 71–94

Fuzesi L, Braun S, Gunawan B, Schmitz HJ, Mittermayer C (1994) Cytogenetic findings in squamous cell carcinoma of the oral cavity. Int J Oral Maxillofac Surg 23: 153–155

Garewal HS, Meyskens FJ (1992) Retinoids and carotenoids in the prevention of oral cancer: a critical appraisal. Cancer Epidemiol Biomarkers Prev 1: 155–159

Grafström RC (1990a) Carcinogenesis studies in human epithelial tissues and cells in vitro: emphasis on serum-free culture conditions and transformation studies. Acta Physiol Scand [Suppl] 592: 93–133

Grafström RC (1990b) In vitro studies of aldehyde effects that relate to human respiratory carcinogenesis. Mutat Res 238: 175–184

Grafström RC, Dypbukt JM, Willey JC, Sundqvist K, Edman C, Atzori L, Harris CC (1988) Pathobiological effects of acrolein in cultured human bronchial epithelial cells. Cancer Res. 49: 1717–1721

Grafström RC, Dypbukt JM, Sundqvist K, Atzori L, Nielsen I, Curren RD, Harris CC (1994) Pathobiological effects of acetaldehyde in cultured human epithelial cells and fibroblasts. Carcinogenesis 15: 985–990

Grafström RC, Jernelöv MI, Dypbukt JM, Sundqvist K, Atzori L, Zheng X (1995) Aldehyde toxicity and thiol redox state in cell cultures from human aerodigestive tract. In: Mohr U (ed) Correlations between in vitro and in vivo investigations in inhalation toxicology. ILSE, Washington DC (in press)

Greenblatt MS, Bennett WP, Hollstein M, Harris CC (1994) Mutations in the p53 tumor suppressor gene: clues to cancer etiology and molecular pathogenesis. Cancer Res 54: 4855–4878

Gujuluva CN, Baek JH, Shin KH, Cherrick HM, Park NH (1994) Effect of UV-irradiation on cell cycle, viability and the expression of p53, gadd153 and gadd45 genes in normal and HPV-immortalized human oral keratinocytes. Oncogene 9: 1819–1827

Harris CC (1987) Human tissues and cells in carcinogenesis research. Cancer Res 47: 1–10

Harris CC (1989) Interindividual variation among humans in carcinogen metabolism, DNA adduct formation and DNA repair. Carcinogenesis 10: 1563–1566

Harris CC (1991) Chemical and physical carcinogenesis: advances and perspectives for the 1990s. Cancer Res 51 [18 Suppl]: 5023s–5044s

Harris CC, Grafström RC, Shamsuddin AM, Sinopoli NT, Trump BF, Autrup H (1984) Carcinogen metabolism and carcinogen-DNA adducts in human tissues and cells. In: Greim H, Jung R, Kramer M, Marquardt H, Oesch F (eds) Biochemical basis of chemical carcinogenesis. Raven, New York, pp 123–135

Hoffmann D, Rivenson A, Amin S, Hecht SS (1984) Dose-response study of the carcinogenicity of tobacco-specific N-nitrosamines in F344 rats. J Cancer Res Clin Oncol 108: 81–86

Huber MH, Lippman SM, Hong WK (1994) Chemoprevention of head and neck cancer. Sem in Oncol 3: 366–375

Hussong JW, Polverini PJ, Solt DB (1991) Resistant keratinocytes in 7,12-dimethylbenz[a]anthracene-initiated hamster buccal pouch epithelium. Carcinogenesis 12: 617–622

IARC (1985) IARC monographs on the evaluation of the carcinogenic risk of chemicals to humans, vol 37. Tobacco habits other than smoking; betel-quid and areca-nut chewing; and some related nitrosamines. International Agency for Research on Cancer, Lyon

IARC (1986) IARC monographs on the evaluation of the carcinogenic risk of chemicals to humans, vol 38. Tobacco smoking. International Agency for Research on Cancer, Lyon

Ide F, Ishikawa T, Takagi M, Umemura S, Takayama S (1982) Unscheduled DNA synthesis in human oral mucosa treated with chemical carcinogens in short-term organ culture. J Natl Cancer Inst 69: 557–563

Idris AM, Nair J, Friesen M, Ohshima H (1992) Carcinogenic tobacco-specific nitrosamines are present at unusually high levels in the saliva of oral snuff users in Sudan. Carcinogenesis 13: 1001–1005

Jin Y, Mertens F (1993) Chromosomal abnormalities in oral squamous cell carcinomas. Eur J Cancer Oral Oncol 29B: 257–263

Jin Y, Mertens F, Jin C, Akervall J, Wennerberg J, Gorunova L, Mandahl N, Heim S, Mitelman F (1995) Nonrandom chromosome abnormalities in short-term cultured primary squamous cell carcinomas of the head and neck. Cancer Res 55: 3204–3210

Johnson NW, Ranasinghe AW, Warnakulasuriya KA (1993) Potentially malignant lesions and conditions of the mouth and oropharynx: natural history – cellular and molecular markers of risk. Eur J Cancer Prevent 2: 31–51

Kasperbauer JL, Neel HB, Scott RE (1990) Proliferation and differentiation characteristics of normal human squamous mucosal cells of the upper aerodigestive tract. Ann Otol Rhinol Laryngol 99: 29–37

Kautsky MB, Fleckman P, Dale BA (1995) Retinoic acid regulates oral epithelial differentiation by two mechanisms. J Invest Dermatol 104: 546–553

Kim MS, Shin KH, Baek JH, Cherrick HM, Park NH (1993) HPV-16, tobacco-specific N-nitrosamine, and N-methyl-N′-nitro-N-nitrosoguanidine in oral carcinogenesis. Cancer Res 53: 4811–4816

King I, Sartorelli AC (1989) Epidermal growth factor receptor gene expression, protein kinase activity, and terminal differentiation of human malignant epidermal cells. Cancer Res 49: 5677–5681

King I, Mella SL, Sartorelli AC (1986) A sensitive method to quantify the terminal differentiation of cultured epidermal cells. Exp Cell Res 167: 252–256

Knowles MA (1990) Transformation of cell culture. In: Handbook of experimental pharmacology, vol 94, part II. Arlett CF (ed) Springer, Berlin Heidelberg New York, pp 211–266

Kulkarni PS, Sundqvist K, Betsholtz C, Höglund P, Wiman KG, Zhivotovsky B, Bertolero F, Liu Y, Grafström RC (1995) Characterization of human buccal epithelial cells transfected with the simian virus 40 T-antigen gene. Carcinogenesis (in press)

La Vecchia C, Lucchini F, Negri E, Boyle P, Maisonneuve P, Levi F (1992) Trends of cancer mortality in Europe, 1955–1989. I. Digestive sites. Eur J Cancer 28: 132–235

Lawley PD (1990) N-nitroso compounds. In: Beland FA (ed) Handbook of experimental pharmacology, vol 94, part I. Springer, Berlin Heidelberg New York, pp 409–469

Lechner JF, Haugen A, Autrup H, McClendon IA, Trump BF, Harris CC (1981) Clonal growth of epithelial cells from normal adult human bronchus. Cancer Res 41: 2294–2304

Lee KW, Chin CT (1970) The effects of betel-nut chewing on the buccal mucosa: a histological study. Br J Cancer 24: 433–441

Levine AJ, Momand J, Finlay CA (1991) The p53 tumor suppressor gene. Nature 351: 453–456

Liang P, Averboukh L, Pardee AB (1993) Distribution and cloning of eukaryotic mRNAs by means of differential display: refinements and optimization. Nucleic Acids Res 21: 3269–3275

Lijinsky W, Taylor HW (1976) Carcinogenicity test of two unsaturated derivatives of N-nitrosopiperdine in Sprague-Dawley rats. J Natl Cancer Inst 57: 1315–1317

Liu Y, Arvidson K, Atzori L, Sundqvist K, Silva B, Cotgreave I, Grafström RC (1991) Development of low- and high-serum culture conditions for use of human oral fibroblasts in toxicity testing of dental materials. J Dent Res 70: 1068–1073

Liu Y, Sundqvist K, Belinsky SA, Castonguay A, Tjälve H, Grafström RC (1993) Metabolism and macromolecular interaction of the tobacco-specific carcinogen 4-methylnitrosamino)-1-(3-pyridyl)-1-butanone in cultured explants and epithelial cells of human buccal mucosa. Carcinogenesis 14: 2383–2388

Liu TJ, El NA, McDonnell TJ, Steck KD, Wang M, Taylor DL, Clayman GL (1995) Apoptosis induction mediated by wild-type p53 adenoviral gene transfer in squamous cell carcinoma of the head and neck. Cancer Res 55: 3117–3122

MacCallum DK, Lillie JH, Jepsen A, Arenholt BD (1987) The culture of oral epithelium. Int Rev Cytol 109: 313–330

Milstone LM (1983) Population dynamics in cultures of stratified squamous epithelia. J Invest Dermatol 81 [Suppl 1]: 69s–74s

Miyashita M, Willey JC, Sasajima K, Lechner JF, La Voie EJ, Hoffmann D, Smith M, Trump BF, Harris CC (1990) Differential effects of cigarette smoke condensate and its fractions on cultured normal and malignant human bronchial epithelial cells. Exp Pathol 38: 19–29

Morgan PR, Su L (1994) Intermediate filaments in oral neoplasia 1. Oral cancer and epithelial dysplasia. Eur J Cancer Oral Oncol 30B: 160–166

Morgan PR, Shirlaw PJ, Johnson NW, Leigh IM, Lane EB (1987) Potential applications of anti-keratin antibodies in oral diagnosis. J Oral Pathol 16: 212–222

Nair J, Ohshima H, Friesen M, Croisy A, Bhide SV, Bartsch H (1985) Tobacco-specific and betel nut-specific N-nitroso compounds: occurrence in saliva and urine of betel quid chewers and formation in vitro by nitrosation of betel quid. Carcinogenesis 6: 295–303

Nair UJ, Floyd RA, Nair J, Bussachini V, Friesen M, Bartsch H (1987) Formation of reactive oxygen species and of 8-hydroxydeoxyguanosine in DNA in vitro with betel quid ingredients. Chem Biol Interact 63: 157–169

Nair UJ, Friesen M, Richard I, MacLennan R, Thomas S, Bartsch H (1990) Effect of lime composition on the formation of reactive oxygen species from areca nut extract in vitro. Carcinogenesis 11: 2145–2148

Neeser JR, Grafström RC, Woltz A, Brassart D, Fryder V, Guggenheim B (1995) A 23 kDa membrane glycoprotein bearing NeuNAc alpha 2–3 Gal beta 1–3GalNAc O-linked carbohydrate chains acts as a receptor for Streptococcus sanguis OMZ 9 on human buccal epithelial cells. Glycobiology 5: 97–104

Nishikawa A, Prokopczyk B, Rivenson A, Zang E, Hoffmann D (1992) A study of betel quid carcinogenesis VIII. Carcinogenicity of 3-(methylnitrosamino)propionaldehyde in F344 rats. Carcinogenesis 13: 369–372

Nix CE, Brewen B, Wilkerson R, Lijinsky W, Epler JL (1979) Effects of N-nitrosopiperidine substitutions on mutagenicity in Drosophila melanogaster. Mutat Res 67: 27–38

Norris DA (1995) Differential control of cell death in the skin. Arch Dermatol 131: 945–948

Oda D, Watson E (1990) Human oral epithelial cell culture. I. Improved conditions for reproducible culture in serum-free medium. In Vitro Cell Dev Biol 26: 589–595

Oda D, Dale BA, Bourekis G (1990) Human oral epithelial cell culture. II. Keratin expression in fetal and adult gingival cells. In Vitro Cell Dev Biol 26: 596–603

Osella P, Carlson A, Wyandt H, Milunsky A (1992) Cytogenetic studies of eight squamous cell carcinomas of the head and neck. Deletion of 7q, a possible primary chromosomal event. Cancer Genet Cytogenet 59: 73–78

Ozanne B, Richards CS, Hendler F, Burns D, Gusterson B (1986) Over-expression of the EGF receptor is a hallmark of squamous cell carcinomas. J Pathol 149: 9–14

Panigrahi GB, Rao AR (1984) Induction of in vivo sister chromatid exchanges by arecaidine, a betel nut alkaloid, in mouse bone-marrow cells. Cancer Lett 23: 189–192

Park NH, Min BM, Li SL, Huang MZ, Cherick HM, Doniger J (1991) Immortalization of normal human oral keratinocytes with type 16 human papillomavirus. Carcinogenesis 12: 1627–1631

Parkin DM, Muir CS, Whelan SL, Gao YT, Ferlay J, Powell J (eds) (1992) Cancer incidence in five continents. International Agency for Research on Cancer, Lyon (IARC Sci Publ No. 120)

Parkin DM, Pisani P, Ferlay J (1993) Estimates of the worldwide incidence of eighteen major cancers in 1985. Int J Cancer 54: 594–606

Partridge M, Green MR, Langdon JD, Feldmann M (1989) Production of TGF-alpha and TGF-beta by cultured keratinocytes, skin and oral squamous cell carcinomas – potential autocrine regulation of normal and malignant epithelial cell proliferation. Br J Cancer 60: 542–548

Pillai S, Bikle DD, Mancianti ML, Hincenbergs M (1991) Uncoupling of the calcium-sensing mechanism and differentiation in squamous carcinoma cell lines. Exp Cell Res 192: 567–573

Pitman SW, Tucker A, Sasaki C (1983) Establishment and characterization of a human squamous head and neck cancer cell line. Proc Am Assoc Cancer Res 24: 5

Pittelkow MR, Wille JJ, Scott RE (1986) Two functionally distinct classes of growth arrest states in human prokeratinocytes that regulate clonogenic potential. J Invest Dermatol 86: 410–417

Polakowska RR, Haake AR (1994) Apoptosis: the skin from a new perspective. Cell Death Differ 1: 19–31

Prokopczyk B, Rivenson A, Bertinato P, Brunnemann KD, Hoffmann D (1987) 3-(Methylnitrosamino) propionitrile: occurrence in saliva of betel quid chewers, carcinogenicity, and DNA methylation in F344 rats. Cancer Res 47: 467–471

Prokopczyk B, Bertinato P, Hoffmann D (1988) Cyanoethylation of DNA in vivo by 3-(methylnitrosamino) propionitrile, an Areca-derived carcinogen. Cancer Res 48: 6780–6784

Prokopczyk B, Rivenson A, Hoffmann D (1991) A study of betel quid carcinogenesis. IX. Comparative carcinogenicity of 3-(methylnitrosamino) propionitrile and 4-(methylnitrosamino)-1-(3-pyridyl)-1-butanone upon local application to mouse skin and rat oral mucosa. Cancer Lett 60: 153–157

Rao AR (1984) Modifying influences of betel quid ingredients on B(a)P-induced carcinogenesis in the buccal pouch of hamster. Int J Cancer 33: 581–586

Rao TK, Young JA, Lijinsky W, Epler JL (1978) Mutagenicity of N-nitrosopiperazine derivatives in Salmonella typhimurium. Mutat Res 57: 127–134

Rao PH, Sreekantaiah C, Schantz SP, Chaganti RS (1994) Cytogenetic analysis of 11 squamous cell carcinomas of the head and neck. Cancer Genet Cytogenet 77: 60–64

Reibel J, Clausen H, Dale BA (1989) Immunohistochemical analysis of stratum corneum components in oral squamous epithelia. Differentiation 41: 237–244

Reichart P, Boning W, Srisuwan S, Theetranont C, Mohr U (1984) Ultrastructural findings in the oral mucosa of betel chewers. J Oral Pathol 13: 166–177

Reiss M, Sartorelli AC (1987) Regulation of growth and differentiation of human keratinocytes by type beta transforming growth factor and epidermal growth factor. Cancer Res 47: 6705–6709

Reiss M, Pitman SW, Sartorelli AC (1985)Modulation of the terminal differentiation of human squamous carcinoma cells in vitro by all-trans-retinoic acid. J Natl Cancer Inst 74: 1015–1023

Reiss M, Maniglia CA, Sartorelli AC (1986) Modulation of cell shedding and glycosaminoglycan synthesis of human malignant kerationocytes by all-trans-retinoic acid and hydrocortisone in vitro. J Invest Dermatol 86: 683–688

Reiss M, Stash EB, Vellucci VF, Zhou ZL (1991) Activation of the autocrine transforming growth factor alpha pathway in human squamous carcinoma cells. Cancer Res 51: 6254–6262

Reiss M, Brash DE, Munoz AT, Simon JA, Ziegler A, Vellucci VF, Zhou ZL (1992) Status of the p53 tumor suppressor gene in human squamous carcinoma cell lines. Oncol Res 4: 349–357

Renan MJ (1993) How many mutations are required for tumorigenesis? Implications from human cancer data. Mol Carcinog 7: 139–146

Rivenson A, Hoffmann D, Prokopczyk B, Amin S, Hecht SS (1988) Induction of lung and exocrine pancreas tumors in F344 rats by tobacco-specific and Areca-derived N-nitrosamines. Cancer Res 48: 6912–6917

Rubin AL, Rice RH (1986) Differential regulation by retinoic acid and calcium of transglutaminases in cultured neoplastic and normal human keratinocytes. Cancer Res 46: 2356–2361

Salonen J, Uitto VJ, Pan YM, Oda D (1991) Proliferating oral epithelial cells in culture are capable of both extracellular and intracellular degradation of interstitial collagen. Matrix 11: 43–55

Schulte-Hermann R, Grasl KB, Bursch W (1994) Tumor development and apoptosis. Int Arch Allergy Immunol 105: 363–367

Shin KH, Min BM, Cherrick HM, Park NH (1994) Combined effects of human papillomavirus-18 and N-methyl-N′-nitro-N-nitrosoguanidine on the transformation of normal human oral keratinocytes. Mol Carcinog 9: 76–86

Smith SA, Dale BA (1986) Immunologic localization of filaggrin in human oral epithelia and correlation with keratinization. J Invest Dermatol 86: 168–172

Snijders PJ, van den Brule AJ, Meijer CJ, Walboomers JM (1994) Papillomaviruses and cancer of the upper digestive and respiratory tracts. In: Zur Hausen H (ed) Human pathogenic papillomaviruses. Springer, Berlin Heidelberg New York, pp 177–198 (Current topics in microbiology and immunology, vol 186)

Southgate J, Williams HK, Trejdosiewicz LK and Hodges GM (1987) Primary culture of human oral epithelial cells. Growth requirements and expression of differentiated characteristics. Lab Invest 56: 211–223

Spitz MR (1994) Epidemiology and risk factors for head and neck cancer. Semin Oncol 21: 281–288

Steele C, Shillitoe EJ (1991) Viruses and oral cancer. Crit Rev Oral Biol Med 2: 153–175

Stich HF, Anders F (1989) The involvement of reactive oxygen species in oral cancers of betel quid/tobacco chewers. Mutat Res 214: 47–61

Stich HF and Tsang SS (1989) Promoting activity of betel quid ingredients and their inhibition by retinol. Cancer Lett 45: 71–77

Stich HF, Bohm BA, Chattarjee K and Salino JL (1983) The role of saliva-born mutagens and carcinogens of betel nut and tobacco chewers. In: Stich HF (ed) Carcinogens and mutagens in the environment, vol 3. CRC Press, Boca Raton, pp 43–58

Sundqvist K, Grafström RC (1992) Effects of areca nut on growth, differentiation and formation of DNA damage in cultured human buccal epithelial cells. Int J Cancer 52: 305–310

Sundqvist K, Liu Y, Nair J, Bartsch H, Arvidson K, Grafström RC (1989) Cytotoxic and genotoxic effects of areca nut-related compounds in cultured human buccal epithelial cells. Cancer Res 49: 5294–5298

Sundqvist K, Kulkarni P, Hybbinette SS, Bertolero F, Liu Y, Grafström RC (1991a) Serum-free growth and karyotype analyses of cultured normal and tumorous (SqCC/Y1) human buccal epithelial cells. Cancer Commun 3: 331–340

Sundqvist K, Liu Y, Arvidson K, Ormstad K, Nilsson L, Toftgård R, Grafström RC (1991b) Growth regulation of serum-free cultures of epithelial cells from normal human buccal mucosa. In Vitro Cell Dev Biol 27A: 562–568

Sundqvist K, Iotsova V, Ziaie S, Wiman K, Höög C, Grafström RC (1995) Identification of genes overexpressed in the SqCC/Y1 human buccal carcinoma cell line using the differential display method. Int J Oncol 7: 1123–1128

Taichman L, Sciubba J, Cho MI (1982) Maturation of human gingival keratinocytes cultured with fibroblasts from keratinizing and non-keratinizing epithelia. Arch Oral Biol 27: 355–359

Taichman LB, Prokop CA (1982) Synthesis of keratin proteins during maturation of cultured human keratinocytes. J Invest Dermatol 78: 464–467

Tanaka T (1995) Chemoprevention of oral carcinogenesis. Eur J Cancer Oral Oncol 31B: 3–15

Tanaka T, Kuniyasu T, Shima H, Sugie S, Mori H, Takahashi M, Hirono I (1986) Carcinogenicity of betel quid. III. Enhancement of 4-nitroquinoline-1-oxide-and N-2-fluorenylacetamide-induced carcinogenesis in rats by subsequent administration of betel nut. J Natl Cancer Inst 77: 777–781

Thomas S, Kearsley J (1993) Betel quid and oral cancer: a review. Eur J Cancer Oral Oncol 29B: 251–255

Thomas S, Wilson A (1993) A quantitative evaluation of the aetiological role of betel quid in oral carcinogenesis. Eur J Cancer B Oral Oncol 29B: 265–271

Thomas S, Brennan J, Martel G, Frazer I, Montesano R, Sidransky D, Hollstein M (1994) Mutations in the conserved regions of p53 are infrequent in betel-associated oral cancers from Papua New Guinea. Cancer Res 54: 3588–3593

Van Dyke DL, Worsham MJ, Benninger MS, Krause CJ, Baker SR, Wolf GT, Drumheller T, Tilley BC, Carey TE (1994) Recurrent cytogenetic abnormalities in squamous cell carcinomas of the head and neck region. Genes Chromosom Cancer 9: 192–206

Vina J (ed) (1990) Glutathione: metabolism and physiological functions. CRC Press, Boca Ratton

Vokes EE, Weichselbaum RR, Lippman SM, Hong WK (1993) Head and neck cancer. N Engl J Med 328: 184–194

Weinberg RA (1991) Tumor Suppressor genes. Science 254: 1138–1146

Wenke G, Hoffmann D (1983) A study of betel quid carcinogenesis. I. On the in vitro N-nitrosation of arecoline. Carcinogenesis 4: 169–172

Wenke G, Rivenson A, Brunnemann KD, Hoffmann D, Bhide SV (1984a) A study of betel quid carcinogenesis. II. Formation of N-nitrosamines during betel quid chewing. In: O'Neill IK, von Borsten RC, Miller CT, Long J, Bartsch H (eds) N-nitroso compounds: occurrence, biological effects and relevance to human cancer. International Agency for Research on cancer, Lyon, pp 859–866 (IARC Sci Publ No. 57)

Wenke G, Rivenson A, Hoffmann D (1984b) A study of betel quid carcinogenesis. III. 3-(Methylnitrosamino)-propionitrile, a powerful carcinogen in F344 rats. Carcinogenesis 5: 1137–1140

Wenke G, Brunnemann KD, Hoffmann D, Bhide SV (1984c) A study of betel quid carcinogenesis. IV. Analysis of the saliva of betel chewers: a preliminary report. J Cancer Res Clin Oncol 108: 110–113

Willey JC, Saladino AJ, Ozanne C, Lechner JF, Harris CC (1984) Acute effects of 12-O-tetradecanoylphorbol-13-acetate, teleocidin B, or 2,3,7,8-tetrachlorodibenzo-p-dioxin on cultured normal human bronchial epithelial cells. Carcinogenesis 5: 209–215

Willey JC, Grafström RC, Moser CJ, Ozanne C, Sundquvist K, Harris CC (1987) Biochemical and morphological effects of cigarette smoke condensate and its fractions on normal human bronchial epithelial cells in vitro. Cancer Res 47: 2045–2049

Yamamoto T, Kamata N, Kawano H, Shimizu S, Kuroki T, Toyoshima K, Rikimaru K, Nomura N, Ishizaki R, Pastan I et al (1986) High incidence of amplification of the epidermal growth factor receptor gene in human squamous carcinoma cell lines. Cancer Res 46: 414–416

Yancey KB (1995) Adhesion molecules. II. Interactions of keratinocytes with epidermal basement membrane. J Invest Dermatol 104: 1008–1014

Yoo GH, Xu HJ, Brennan JA, Westra W, Hruban RH, Koch W, Benedict WF, Sidransky D (1994) Infrequent inactivation of the retinoblastoma gene despite frequent loss of chromosome 13q in head and neck squamous cell carcinoma. Cancer Res 54: 4603–4606

Yuspa SH (1994) The pathogenesis of squamous cell cancer: lessons learned from studies of skin carcinogenesis – 33rd G.H.A. Clowes Memorial Award Lecture. Cancer Res 54: 1178–1189

Yuspa SH, Poirier MC (1988) Chemical carcinogenesis: from animal models to molecular models in one decade (review). Adv Cancer Res 50: 25–70

Genetic Lesions in Mantle Cell Lymphoma

G. Ott[1], M.M. Ott[1], J. Kalla[1], A. Helbing[1], B. Schryen[1], T. Katzenberger[1], J. Bartek[2], A. Dürr[1], J.G. Müller[1], H. Kreipe[1], and H.K. Müller-Hermelink[1]

[1]Institute of Pathology, University of Würzburg, Germany
[2]Division of Cancer Biology, Danish Cancer Society, Copenhagen, Denmark

Introduction

Mantle cell lymphoma (MCL) is a B-cell non-Hodgkin's lymphoma derived from CD5-positive immature virgin B cells of the follicular mantle zone accounting for 5%–10% of malignant B-cell lymphomas in adults.

More than 20 years ago, Lennert described a lymphoma composed of cells resembling those of the germinal center of the lymph node. The small- to medium-sized cells with cleaved nuclei and finely dispersed chromatin structures were initially termed "germinocytes" and then "centrocytes," and the corresponding lymphoma was therefore designated as centrocytic lymphoma (Lennert 1978). According to the strict criterion that no centroblasts should be observed in these lymphomas to differentiate them from centroblastic-centrocytic or centroblastic lymphoma, centrocytic lymphomas were graded as low-grade lymphomas. Immunohistochemical studies soon proved the B-cell character of the tumor cells several years after the first description of this lymphoma (Tolksdorf et al. 1980); it was also shown, however, that centrocytic lymphoma had a distinct phenotype clearly separating it from germinal center cells and centroblastic centrocytic lymphoma. The expression of CD22 and CD5 with negativity for CD10 and CD23 was similar to that of cells in the mantle zone of the reactive lymphoid follicle, and the occasional finding of a positivity for IgD confirmed this association even more (Stein et al. 1984). While some lymphomas may show diffuse infiltrates, others exhibit a nodular or perifollicular growth pattern and consecutively invade and destroy the germinal center. The classification system used in North America, the Working Formulation, did not define an entity exactly corresponding to centrocytic lymphoma. For the most part, these tumors were classified as intermediate lymphocytic lymphoma or lymphocytic lymphoma of intermediate differentiation. In 1982, Weisenburger introduced the term "mantle zone lymphoma" but used it on a heterologous group of tumors including centrocytic lymphomas, chronic lymphocytic leukemias, and centroblastic-centrocytic lymphomas (Weisenburger et al. 1982, 1987).

Molecular Genetics

The molecular breakpoint of a chromosomal translocation, the t(11;14) (q13; q32) was cloned in three cases of non-Hodgkin's lymphoma which were defined as lymphocytic lymphoma or chronic lymphocytic leukemia according to the Working Formulation (Tsujimoto et al. 1984). In the following years it became evident that the t(11;14) and its corresponding molecular event, the bcl-1 gene rearrangement, was a characteristic genomic change in centrocytic or mantle cell lymphoma (Williams et al. 1990). A reclassification of the first three cases described in 1984 revealed that at least two of these were indeed centrocytic lymphomas. With ongoing studies the entity of centrocytic lymphoma was confirmed more and more. The term "centrocytic lymphoma" was replaced by the biologically more correct expression "mantle cell lymphoma" (Banks et al. 1992) and introduced in the REAL classification system as an entity (Harris et al. 1994).

The functional consequence of the t(11; 14) or the bcl-1 rearrangement is the juxtaposition of the cyclin D1 gene to one of the joining segments of the Ig heavy chain gene (JH) on chromosome 14, resulting in the overexpression of cyclin D1 mRNA (Rimokh et al. 1994). The heightened expression of this novel G1 cyclin, which is not expressed by normal lymphoid cells, has been shown to subvert the G1 phase control of the cell cycle and to be able to drive cells into mitosis (Matsushime et al. 1991). Little doubt therefore exists that the t(11;14)-induced deregulation and overexpression of cyclin D1 is the key event of tumorigenesis in mantle cell lymphoma.

Shortly after the first description by Lennert, it had become obvious that mantle cell or centrocytic lymphoma might not always be purely composed of small cells (Lennert 1978), and indeed, in recent years several investigators looking at larger series of MCL recognized, next to the small-cell variant, the existence of a so-called blastic or anaplastic variant of mantle cell lymphoma (e.g., Lardelli et al. 1990; Fisher et al. 1995). The significance of this finding, however, is still controversial as are the exact criteria and biological features separating small-cell and blastic variants.

In an ongoing morphological, immunohistochemical, molecular, and cytogenetic study we attempted to elaborate criteria defining the cytomorphological spectrum of mantle cell lymphomas and to assess the biological features in the different groups possibly distinguishing these subtypes.

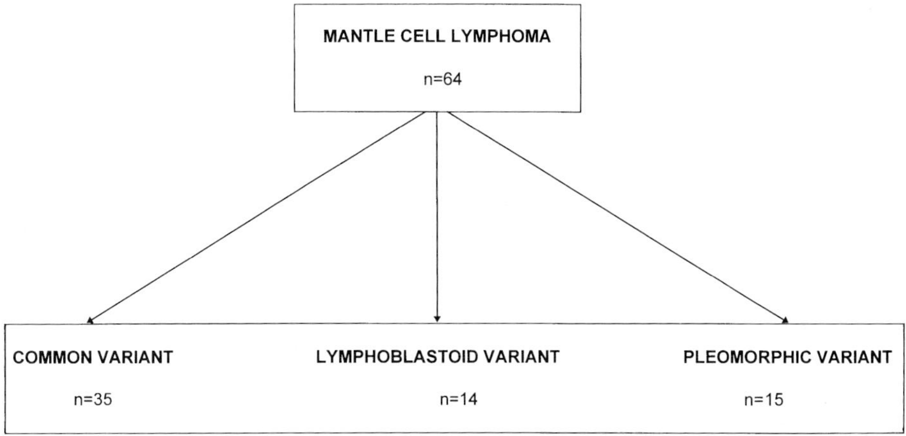

Fig. 1. Cytomorphological classification of 64 cases of mantle cell lymphoma (MCL)

Morphological Spectrum (Fig. 1)

More than one half of the mantle cell lymphomas analyzed in our series of 64 cases were composed of predominantly small-sized cells with a scant, barely visible rim of cytoplasm and slightly irregular, cleaved nuclei with finely dispersed chromatin and one to three midstanding indistinct nucleoli. This type was designated the common variant of mantle cell lymphoma and mostly resembled the centrocytic lymphoma as defined in the Kiel classification system (Fig. 2). Two types of anaplastic MCL were recognized in our study, the first being composed of medium-sized cells with blastic appearance and round nuclear contours with resemblance to lymphoblasts and therefore designated the lymphoblastoid subtype (Fig. 3). A total of 15 lymphomas corresponded to another type termed the pleomorphic variant of MCL. In these lymphomas (Fig. 4), either large cells or a mixture of medium-sized and large cells predominated. They sometimes showed a small, slightly basophilic cytoplasm and were characterized by pleomorphic, deeply indented, sometimes bizarre nuclei with several nucleoli and finely dispersed chromatin structures.

In all subtypes, the identification of the characteristic immunophenotype of mantle cell lymphomas, namely a positivity for B-cell markers (CD20, CD22), for CD5, and negative reactions for CD10 and CD23, was possible on sections from fresh-frozen tissue (Table 1).

Proliferation Indices

As can be seen from Fig. 5, a clear-cut difference in the proliferative activity could be observed between the small-cell and large-cell types as assessed by the

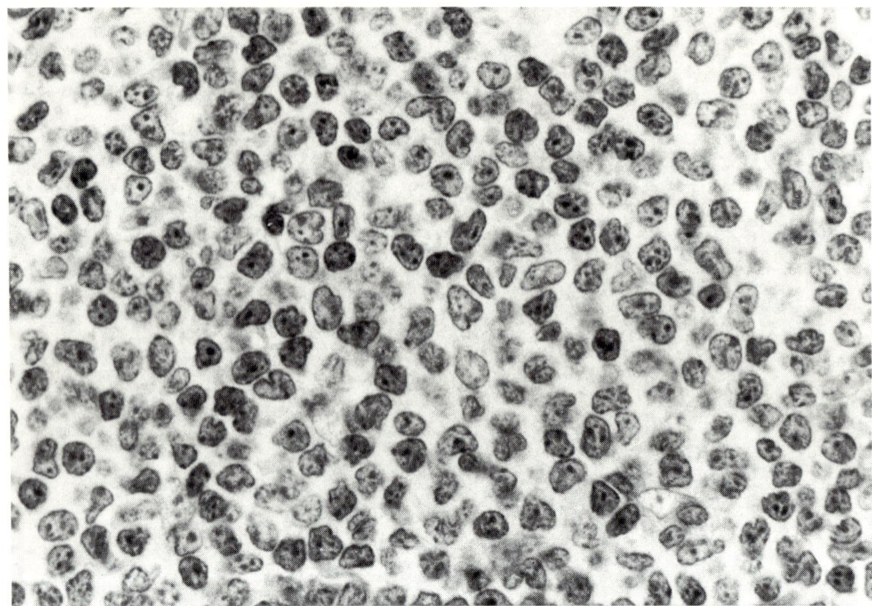

Fig. 2. Common variant of MCL

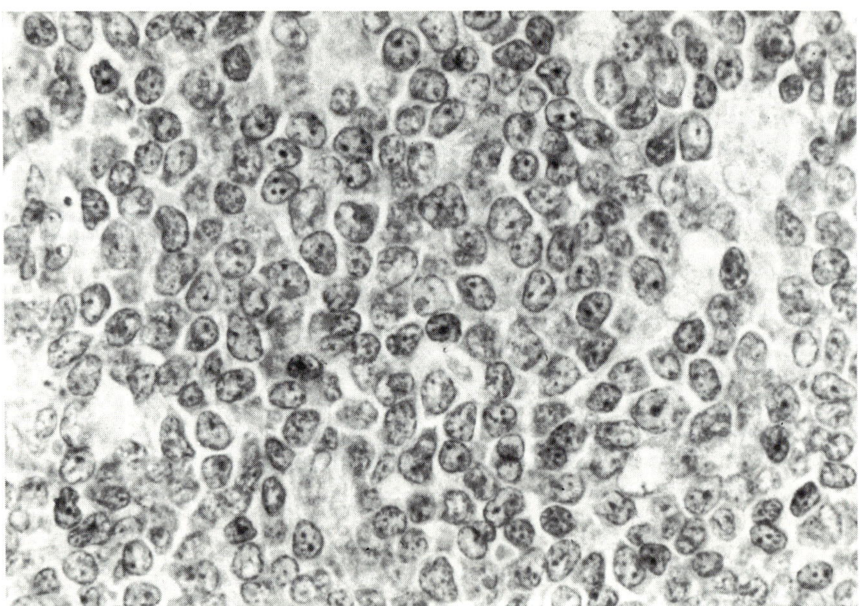

Fig. 3. Lymphoblastoid variant of MCL

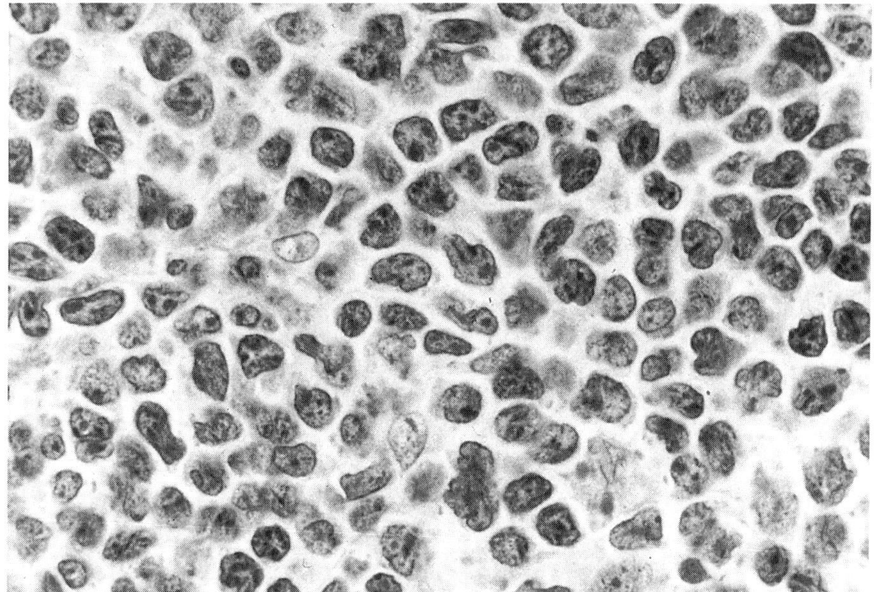

Fig. 4. Pleomorphic variant of MCL

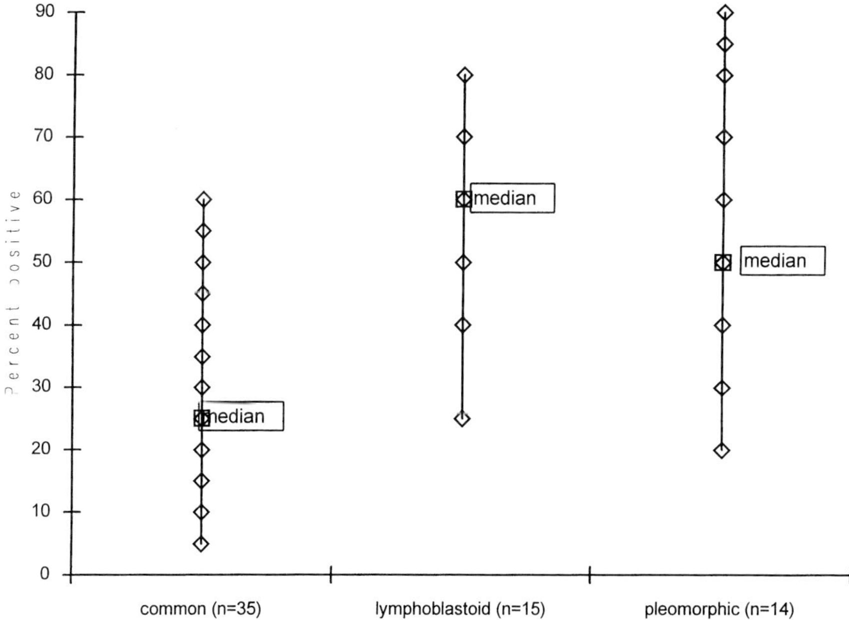

Fig. 5. Proliferation indices in mantle cell lymphoma ($n = 64$; MIB-1 antibody)

Table 1. Immunophenotype of mantle cell lymphoma

CD20, CD22	+
CD5	+
CD10, CD23	–
IgM(IgD)	+
Light chains	$\kappa > \lambda$

monoclonal antibody MIB-1 recognizing the Ki67 antigen. Whereas the median of stained nuclei was 25% in the common type, lymphoblastoid and pleomorphic lymphomas exhibited distinctly higher proliferation indices, the median being at 60% and 50%, respectively, and sometimes more than 90% of cells were shown to stain positively.

Expression of p53

The expression of the p53 protein was assessed by using the DO1-antibody in paraffin sections (Ott et al. 1996a). The results showed that 6% of common MCL as opposed to 21% of the blastic variants were characterized by an overexpression of this oncogene, with the percentage of positive cases being higher in lymphoblastoid as compared to pleomorphic types (Table 2).

Bcl-1 Rearrangements

The molecular genetic equivalent of the t(11;14) (q13;q32), the rearrangement of the bcl-1 or cyclin D1 gene, was studied by Southern blotting using a probe specific for the major translocation cluster (MTC) region whenever fresh-frozen material was available. For those cases in which only DNA from paraffin material could be obtained, we designated a seminested polymerase chain reaction (PCR) technique equally specific for rearrangements at the MTC region (Williams et al. 1993; Rimokh et al. 1994; Ott et al. 1996a).

It was evident from the results of rearrangement studies in 63 cases that the specific t(11;14) could not only be recognized in all variants, but that both

Table 2. p53 expression in mantle cell lymphoma[a]

	Common	Lymphoblastoid	Pleomorphic
Positive/*n*	2/34	4/15	2/14
%	6	27	14
Total/type (%)	6	21(6/29)	

[a]63 cases investigated in immunohistochemistry; positive result requires more than 10% of nuclei stained.

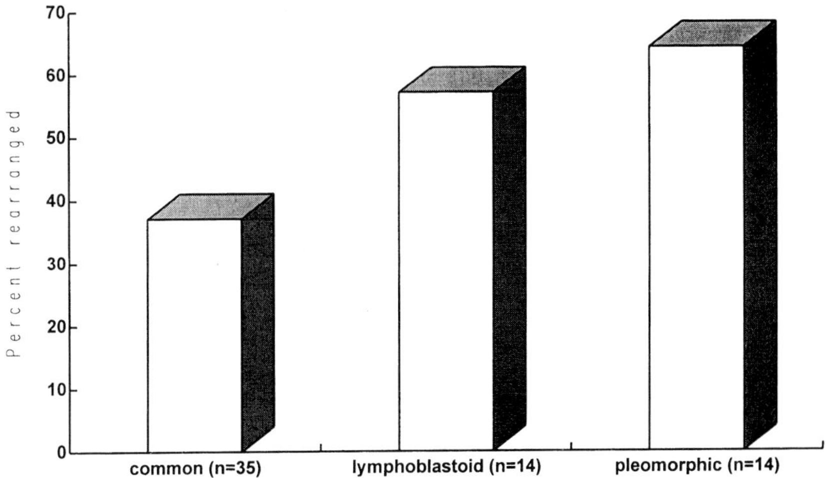

Fig. 6. BCL-1 rearrangements in mantle cell lymphoma. A total of 63 cases were investigated by Southern blotting and/or polymerase chain reaction (PCR) for rearrangements at the major translocation cluster (MTC) locus

lymphoblastoid and pleomorphic variants showed preferential breaks at the MTC locus (60%–70%) as compared to the small-cell type (40%) (Fig. 6).

Cyclin D1 Expression

The expression of the cyclin D1 or PRAD1 gene was evaluated using the mouse monoclonal antibody DCS-6 (Lukas et al. 1994) in microwave-heated paraffin sections in 32 cases of MCL (Ott et al. 1996a). Positive nuclear staining could be observed in 11/13 large-cell lymphomas (85%) of both lymphoblastoid and pleomorphic subtypes as well as in 13/19 (68%) of common types (Fig. 7). No

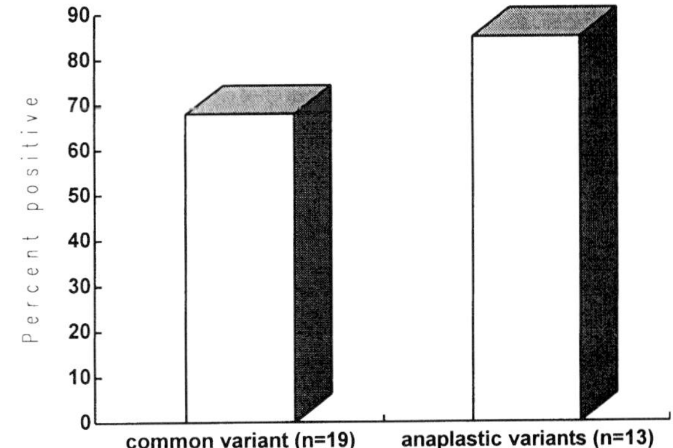

Fig. 7. Cyclin D1 expression in mantle cell lymphoma ($n = 32$; DCS-6 antibody)

absolute correlation was observed between bcl-1 rearranged at the MTC locus and positive cyclin D1 staining, with 9 of 24 cases being positive in immunohistochemistry, but lacking evidence for bcl-1 rearrangement.

Classical and Molecular Cytogenetic Investigations

Interphase cytogenetic investigations were performed using centromere-specific DNA probes to human chromosomes 3, 7, 18, X, and Y in nuclei isolated from 50 paraffin-embedded lymphomas (Ott et al. 1996b). In addition, classical cytogenetic analyses were performed in 14 cases and DNA flow cytometry data were available from 30 cases. In a minority of lymphomas, trisomies of chromosomes 3, 7, and 18 as well as a loss of the Y chromosome could be recognized. Surprisingly, the most frequent karyotypic alteration, next to the t(11;14) found in 13/14 lymphomas investigated by classical in vitro cell cultivation and metaphase spread analysis by a G-banding technique, was the documentation of chromosome numbers in the tetraploid range evidenced by the occurrence of cells with four nuclear signals in a significant proportion of cells using fluorescence in situ hybridization (FISH) in large-cell MCL (Fig. 8). This finding was confirmed by classical cytogenetics in some cases as well as by

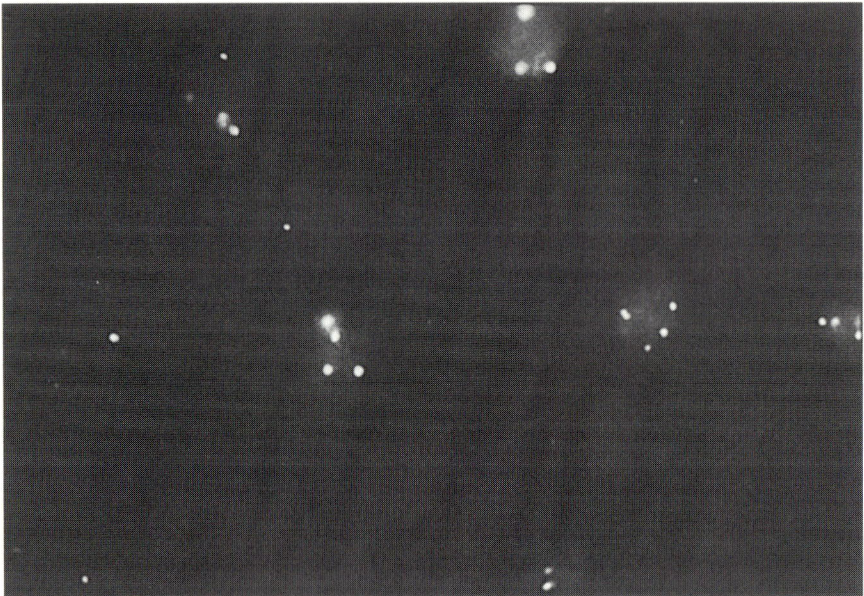

Fig. 8. In situ hybridization with a centromere-specific chromosome probe for chromosome 7. Note several nuclei with four distinct nuclear signals

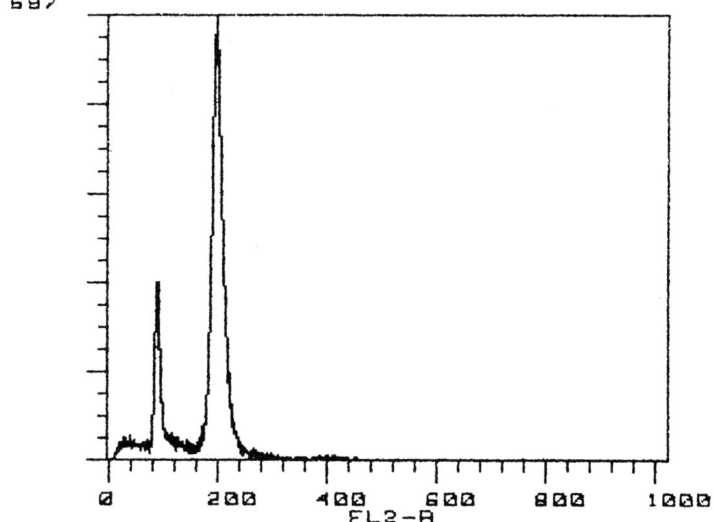

Fig. 9. DNA flow cytometric analysis of MCL. Note that the majority of cells are in the tetraploid range

DNA flow cytometry (Fig. 9). Whereas only 8% of common MCL were tetraploid, 38% of lymphoblastoid and 80% of pleomorphic lymphomas harbored tetraploid chromosome clones (Fig. 10).

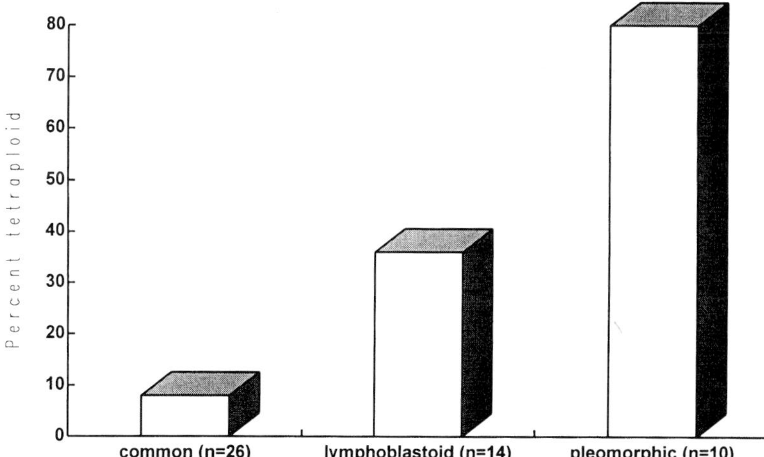

Fig. 10. Ploidy status of mantle cell lymphoma. A total of 50 cases were investigated by in situ hybridization (ISH) using centromere-specific DNA probes to chromosomes 3, 7, 18, and Y in single-cell preparations from paraffin blocks and/or on slides

Discussion

Malignant non-Hodgkin's lymphomas are a heterogeneous disease group with different morphological, immunological, genetic, and clinical features, reflecting their various biological origins from defined cellular compartments of the lymphoid system. Several distinct cytogenetic and molecular genetic alterations have been found to be highly characteristic for the different tumour entities, e.g., specific chromosomal translocations like the t(14;18) (q32;q21) in germinal center, the t(11;14) (q13;q32) in mantle cell, or the t(2;5) (p23;q35) in anaplastic large cell lymphomas. On the other hand, within the defined entities, there are a number of secondary features possibly delineating particular and prognostically different disease subgroups. One example is germinal center lymphoma, in which secondary chromosomal or molecular genetic alterations like deletions in the long arm of chromosome 6, structural alterations of the short arm of chromosome 17, and differences in p53 expression have been shown to be indicative of a different, usually more aggressive, clinical course (Sander et al. 1993; Lo Coco et al. 1993; Tilly et al. 1994).

Mantle cell lymphoma, originally described as being composed of small- to medium-sized cells and regarded as a low-grade lymphoma in the Kiel classification system, has been shown to display a broad cytomorphological spectrum ranging from predominantly small-cell types to apparently blastic variants. This distinction has been shown to be of clinical importance, since large-cell or anaplastic variants seem to follow a more aggressive clinical course (Brittinger 1983; Fisher et al. 1995).

In the present study of 64 mantle cell lymphomas, we were able to show that the morphological spectrum of these lymphoid neoplasms is distinctly reflected by different biological features separating small-cell and blastic types. These features are:

1. Elevated proliferation indices in large-cell as compared to common variants.
2. A higher rate of p53 expression in lymphoblastoid and pleomorphic variants.
3. The preferential occurrence of breaks with involvement of the major translocation cluster region in anaplastic MCL.
4. The surprisingly high frequency of tetraploid chromosome sets in nearly 40% of lymphoblastoid and up to 80% of pleomorphic subtypes.

Special emphasis should be given to the fact that mantle cell lymphomas display a bcl-1 rearrangement at the MTC locus in comparable frequencies of about 20%–40% of cases analyzed (Williams et al. 1991, 1992; de Boer et al. 1993). This number corresponds well to our data on the common variant of MCL. Large-cell variants, on the other hand, do show bcl-1 rearrangements in higher numbers of 60%–70%. This feature of anaplastic MCL may point to a higher risk on the part of patients with bcl-1-positive MCL of developing an anaplastic variant or, rather, that bcl-1-associated lymphomas tend to behave like high-grade malignancies (Ott et al. 1994). With respect to this consideration, the distinctly higher proliferation indices in lymphoblastoid and pleo-

Table 3. Occurrence of chromosome numbers in the tetraploid range in follicular center and diffuse large-cell lymphomas[a]

Lymphoma subtype	Tetraploid/*n*	%
Follicular center cell	2/35[b]	6
Diffuse large cell	4/42[b]	9

[a]Results of cytogenetic investigations performed in Würzburg 1990–1994.
[b]10 additional cases were studied in in situ hybridization(ISH) with a set of centromere-specific chromosome probes revealing diploid chromosome numbers in all of them.

morphic MCL seem to be of special importance, as does the elevated frequency of p53 expression.

The karyotypic features of MCL seem to be of particular interest, since malignant lymphomas of B-cell lineage are usually diploid. In our own experience, only 6% of germinal center and 9% of large cell B-cell lymphomas were shown to be tetraploid in classical and interphase cytogenetic analyses (Table 3). Tetraploid chromosome clones, however, have been reported to be a frequent finding in peripheral T-cell and anaplastic large-cell lymphomas (Schlegelberger et al. 1994).

The frequent finding of chromosome numbers in the tetraploid range in anaplastic variants of MCL may be related to the t(11;14)-induced overexpression of the cyclin D1 gene in 11q13. This novel G1-cyclin has been shown to subvert the control of the G1-phase of the cell cycle and to drive cells into S-phase (Matsushime et al. 1991). It is, therefore, reasonable to assume that the influence of this protein, which is not normally expressed by lymphoid cells, might be directly related to a twofold passage of the S-phase of the cell cycle without intervening mitosis.

Taken together, our findings shed light on mantle cell lymphoma not only as a distinct biological entity in the broad range of non-Hodgkin's lymphomas but also with respect to its clearly unique pathogenesis. Moreover, we were able to show that there are distinct variants of MCL showing particular biological features. The bcl-1 gene rearrangement, which is of definite importance for the unique pathogenesis of mantle cell lymphoma might also play a role during further tumor progression.

The different biological features of mantle cell lymphoma subtypes might be a means to recognize prognostically important patient subgroups and could therefore, represent criteria in assessing the individual risk of patients suffering from MCL. Such a distinction, however, might be a prerequisite for the development of innovative therapy regimens required for this aggressive neoplasm (Fisher et al. 1995).

Acknowledgements. This study was supported by the Deutsche Forschungsgemeinschaft, Sonderforschungsbereich 172, Grant C8 to G. Ott and H.K.

Müller-Hermelink and Grant DFG Kr 849/4-1 to H. Kreipe. The excellent technical assistance of Mrs. Claudia Gärtner, Mrs. Karin Heintz, and Mrs. Heike Brückner is gratefully acknowledged.

References

Banks PM, Chan J, Cleary ML, Delsol G, de Wolf-Peeters C, Gatter K, Grogan TM, Harris NL, Isaacson PG, Jaffe ES, Mason D, Pileri S, Ralfkiaer E, Stein H, Warnke RA (1992) Mantle cell lymphoma: a proposal for unification of morphologic, immunologic, and molecular data. Am J Surg Pathol 16: 637–640

Brittinger G (1983) Klinik der malignen Non-Hodgkin-Lymphome, speziell der chronischen lymphatischen Leukämie. Verh Dtsch Ges Pathol 67: 494–516

de Boer CJ, Loyson S, Kluin PM, Kluin-Nelemans C, Schuring E, van Krieken HJM (1993) Multiple breakpoints within the Bcl-1 locus in B-cell lymphoma: rearrangements of the cyclin D1 gene. Cancer Res 53: 4148–4152

Fisher RI, Dahlberg S, Nathwani BN, Banks PM, Miller TP, Grogan TM (1995) A clinical analysis of two indolent lymphoma entities: mantle cell lymphoma and marginal zone lymphoma (including the mucosa-associated lymphoid tissue and monocytoid B-cell subcategories): a Southwest Oncology Group study. Blood 85: 1075–1082

Harris NL, Jaffe ES, Stein H et al (1994) A revised European-American classification of lymphoid neoplasms: a proposal from the international lymphoma study group. Blood 84: 1361–1392

Lardelli P, Bookman MA, Sundeen J, Longo DL, Jaffe ES (1990) Lymphocytic lymphoma of intermediate differentiation. Morphologic and immunologic spectrum and clinical correlations. Am J Surg Pathol 14: 752–763

Lennert K (1978) Lymphomas of germinal-center cells. In: Lennert K (ed) Malignant lymphomas other than Hodgkin's disease. Springer, Berlin Heidelberg New York, pp 281–345

Lo Coco F, Gaidano G, Loui DC, Offit K, Chaganti RSK, Dalla-Favera R (1993) p53 Mutations are associated with histologic transformation of follicular lymphoma. Blood 82: 2289–2295

Lukas J, Pagano M, Staskova Z, Draetta G, Bartek J (1994) Cyclin D1 protein oscillates and is essential for cell cycle progression in human tumor cell lines. Oncogene 9: 707–718

Matsushime H, Roussel MF, Ashmun RA, Sherr CJ (1991) Colony-stimulating factor 1 regulates novel cyclins during the G1 phase of the cell cycle. Cell 65: 701–713

Ott MM, Ott G, Kuse R, Porowski P, Gunzer U, Feller AC, Müller-Hermelink HK (1994) The anaplastic variant of centrocytic lymphoma is marked by frequent rearrangements of the bcl-1 gene and high proliferation indices. Histopathology 24: 329–334

Ott MM, Helbing A, Ott G, Bartek J, Fischer L, Dürr A, Kreipe H, Müller-Hermelink HK (1996a) Bcl-1 gene rearrangement and cyclin D1 protein expression in mantle cell lymphoma (in press)

Ott G, Kalla J, Ott MM, Schryen B, Katzenberger T, Müller JG, Müller-Hermelink HK (1996b) Blastoid variants of mantle cell lymphoma: frequent bcl-1 rearrangements at the MTC locus and tetraploid chromosome clones (submitted for publication)

Rimokh R, Berger F, Delsol G, Digonnet I, Rouault, Tigaud JD, Gadoux M, Coiffier B, Bryon PA, Magaud JP (1994) Detection of the chromosomal translocation t(11;14) by polymerase chain reaction in mantle cell lymphomas. Blood 83: 1871–1875

Sander CA, Yano T, Clark HM, Harris C, Longo DL, Jaffe ES, Raffeld M (1993) p53 Mutation is associated with progression of follicular lymphomas. Blood 82: 1994–2004

Schlegelberger B, Himmler A, Gödde E, Grote W, Feller AC, Lennert K (1994) Cytogenetic findings in peripheral T-cell lymphomas as a basis for distinguishing low-grade and high-grade lymphomas. Blood 83: 505–511

Stein H, Lennert K, Feller AC, Mason DY (1984) Immunohistochemical analysis of human lymphoma: correlation of histological and immunological categories. Adv Cancer Res 42: 67–147

Tilly H, Rossi A, Stamatoullas A, Lenormand B, Bigorgne C, Kunlin A, Monconduit M, Bastard C (1994) Prognostic value of chromosomal abnormalities in follicular lymphoma. Blood 84: 1043–1049

Tolksdorf G, Stein H, Lennert K (1980) Morphological and immunological definition of a malignant lymphoma derived from germinal-center cells with cleaved nuclei (centrocytes). Br J Cancer 41: 168–182

Tsujimoto Y, Yunis J, Onorato-Showe L, Erikson J, Nowell PC, Croce CM (1984) Molecular cloning of the chromosomal breakpoint of B-cell lymphomas and leukemias with the t(11;14) chromosome translocation. Science 224: 1403–1406

Weisenburger DD, Kim H, Rapaport H (1982) Mantle zone lymphoma: a follicular variant of intermediate lymphocytic lymphoma. Cancer 49: 1429–1438

Weisenburger DD, Sanger WG, Armitage JO, Purtilo DT (1987) Intermediate lymphocytic lymphoma: immunophenotypic and cytogenetic findings. Blood 69: 1617–1621

Williams ME, Westermann CD, Swerdlow SH (1990) Genotypic characterization of centrocytic lymphoma: frequent rearrangement of the chromosome 11 bcl-1 locus. Blood 76: 1387–1391

Williams ME, Meeker TC, Swerdlow SH (1991) Rearrangement of the chromosome 11 bcl-1 locus in centrocytic lymphoma: analysis with multiple breakpoint probes. Blood 76: 1387–1391

Williams ME, Swerdlow SH, Rosenberg CL, Arnold A (1992) Characterization of chromosome 11 translocation breakpoints at the bcl-1 and PRAD1 loci in centrocytic lymphoma. Cancer Res 52 [Suppl]: 5541s–5544s

Williams ME, Swerdlow SH, Meeker TC (1993) Chromosome t(11;14) (q13;q32) breakpoints in centrocytic lymphoma are highly localized at the bcl-1 major translocation cluster. Leukemia 7: 1437–1440

Topoisomerase Activities in Undifferentiated Acute Myeloblastic Leukemias and Monocytic Differentiated Leukemias

F. Gieseler[1], A. Glasmacher[2], D. Kämpfe[3], C. Zernak[1], S. Valsamas[1], J. Kunze[1], and M. Clark[1]

[1]Medizinische Poliklinik, University of Würzburg, Klinikstr. 8, 97070 Würzburg, Germany
[2]Medizinische Klinik und Poliklinik, University of Bonn, Sigmund-Freud-Str. 25, 53105 Bonn, Germany
[3]Hospital Kröllwitz, University of Halle, Ernst-Grüber-Str. 40, 06120 Halle, Germany

Introduction

The function of topoisomerases (topos) has been associated with proliferation and regulation of gene transcription during the differentiation of hematopoietic cells. The three different isoenzymes, topo I, topo II-alpha and topo II-beta, undergo additional posttranscriptional modifications (De Vore et al. 1992). These isoenzymes have various intracellular localizations and probably fulfill different functions (Boege et al. 1993; Zini et al. 1994), although there are hints that a functional loss of one isoenzyme can be partially substituted by another (Stevnser and Bohr 1993). Due to the posttranscriptional modifications, there is no direct correlation with gene transcription, protein content, or activity of topos, and several isoactivities can be found in nuclear extracts (Gieseler et al. 1993).

Topos are the target structure of clinically important cytostatic drugs. At least three different modes of action are known: inhibition of topoisomerase DNA binding (e.g., aclarubicin), stabilization of the "cleavable complex" DNA by intercalation (e.g., daunorubicin, doxorubicin, idarubicin) and direct binding to the enzyme (etoposide, teniposide) (Gieseler 1995). It would be of major interest to find cellular parameters which are important for the clinical outcome of treatment with topo inhibitors. We have looked for a correlation between topo I and II activities, the state of cellular differentiation, and sensitivity of the cells to topo II inhibitors in undifferentiated myeloid leukemia cells and monocytic differentiated leukemia cells.

Recent Results in Cancer Research, Vol. 143

Materials and Methods

A total of 42 blood samples or bone marrow samples from patients with acute nonlymphocytic leukemias before and after treatment with anthracycline-containing chemotherapies were examined. The patients were diagnosed and treated at the University Hospitals of Würzburg, Bonn, or Halle, Germany. The specimens were merged with heparin (ca. 0.5% vol/vol) for anticoagulation, sent by mail at room temperature and examined within 30 h. Classification of myeloid leukemias was done according to morphological and cytochemical characteristics using the criteria for the classification of acute myeloid leukemia established by the French-American-British Cooperative Group. In the group of undifferentiated myeloblastic leukemias (FAB-MI), 90% of the nonerythrocytic bone marrow cells were undiffferentiated blasts,whereas in the group of monocytic differentiated leukemias (FAB-M5), at least 80% of the cells were monoblasts, promonocytes, or monocytes (Bennett et al. 1985). Mononucleated cells were isolated by a ficoll gradient using standard methods. Only samples containing $> 80\%$ leukemia cells were taken into consideration. The cells were washed twice with cold phosphate-buffered solution (PBS) and resuspended in 3.5 ml lysine buffer [0.3 *M* sucrose; 0.5 m*M* ETA, pH 8.0, 60m*M* KCl; 15 m*M* hydroxyethylpiperazine ethanesulfonic acid (HEPES)], pH 7.5; 150 μM spermidine; 50 μM). Then, 0.5 ml lysis buffer containing 20 μl of triton X-100 was added and put on ice for 15 min. To prevent clumping, the cells were mixed gently several times. While 5×10^6 to 5×10^7 are optimal cell quantities, as few as 1×10^6 cells may be used with good results (80%–90% nuclei recovery). After centrifugation the nuclei were resuspended in 100–500 μl lysis buffer and then laid on 1 ml lysis buffer with 30% sucrose in 1.5 ml reaction tubes; the nuclei were then separated from cytoplasmic and membrane proteins by centrifugation. Nuclei were resuspended in extraction buffer [5 m*M* $KHPO_4$, pH 7.4; 100 m*M* NaCl, 10 m*M* 2-mercaptoethanol, 5 μl/ml 200 m*M* phenylmethylsulfonyl fluoride (PMSF) in dimethylsulfoxide (DMSO)] at a concentration of 3×10^7 nuclei/ml. Next, 1/5 volume 5 M NaCl was added slowly and gently mixed. The extract was put on ice for 15 min before centrifuging. For partial purification of topo II, the supernatant was loaded on a minispin column containing 100 μl heparin-sepharose in 5 m*M* $KHPO_4$, 50 m*M* NaCl, pH 7.4 and washed with several volumes of the same buffer. The column was subsequently washed with 150 m*M* $KPHO_4$, 100 m*M* NaCl, pH 7.4. Topo II was eluted with 400 m*M* $KHPO_4$, 100 m*M* NaCl, pH 7.4.

Relaxation and decatenation assays were done in 0.1 *M* Bis-Tris-propane, 1 m*M* $MgC1_2$, 15 μg bovine serum albumin (BSA) and 5 m*M* dithiothreitol (DTT). To activate topo II and L-glutamic acid, 1 m*M* ATP was added and monopotassium salt (240 m*M*) was used as the anion salt. The pH was adjusted at 7.2 for topo I, 8.9 for topo IIA, and 7.9 for topo IIB activity determination. Then, 200 ng kDNA was taken for decatenation assays, 200 ng pBR322 for relaxation assays. Incubation was done for 30 min at 37 °C for all assays.

Decatenation assays were incubated an additional 30 min at room temperature with 4 μl of 10 mg/ml proteinase K in 10% sodium dodecyl sulfate (SDS). The samples were then heated to 65 °C for 2–3 min before being run on a 1% Tris-borate + EDTA (TBE) agarose gel with 100 μl 5mg/ml ethidium bromide per liter TBE. Relaxation assays were run on 1% Tris-acetate + EDTA (TAE) agarose gels; the samples were not treated by proteinase/SDS to avoid a topo I-induced open circular form. Gels were scanned using an Apple-One scanner and the amount of DNA quantified by gray scale analysis using the program NIH-Image V1.42 on a Macintosh Powerbook 180. Unit definition of topo activity per 10^4 cells: 1 U topo relaxes 90% plasmid DNA; 200 ng pBr322 per lane; agarose 1%, 20 V (ca. 18mAmp), 18 h; inhibition of topo I by 1 μm camptothecin.

Inhibition of topo II isoactivities by cytostatic drugs has been achieved with HL60-cells. The cells were incubated with idarubicin (200 ng/ml); daunorubicin (500 ng/ml) and etoposide (2500 ng/ml); anthracyclines for 2–3 h; and etoposide for 8 h. After incubation, the cells were washed twice with buffer and then processed as described above. In vitro determination of cellular sensitivity was done by incubation of the cells in various drug concentrations. Viability was examined using the alamar-blue assay, a colorimetric determination of the cells ability to reduce a substrate, analogous to the widely used (3-[4,5-dimethylthiazol-2-yl]-2,5-diphenyltetrazolium bromide) (MTT) assay (Page et al. 1993; Kaspers et al. 1994). Statistical analysis of anthracycline sensitivity of leukemia cells with a high and a low ratio of topo II A/B activity was done by the analysis of variance (ANOVA). The topo II A/B ratio limit of 1.41 used here is the 50th percentile (median).

Results

After inhibition of topo I by camptothecin, we found two different topo II activities with reaction optima at pH 8.9 (topo IIA) and at pH 7.9 (topo IIB) in all examined leukemia samples. In some of the samples additional topo II activities with activity optima at pH 9.2 or pH 7.2 could be detected. We previously described that high ionic strength (240 m*M* KGlu) is necessary to discriminate different topo II isoactivities by their pH reaction optima (Gieseler et al. 1994). Topoisomerase activities were found to be characteristically different in undifferentiated myeloblastic (FAB-M1) and monocytic differentiated leukemia cells (FAB-M5) as shown in Table 1.

The median of topo I activity was 2.8-fold higher in FAB-M5 cells compared to FAB-M1 cells. The median of topo IIA activity was found to be 1.7-fold higher and the topo IIB activity fourfold higher in FAB-M5. In Table 2, a comparison between untreated leukemias and cells from patients who relapsed after chemotherapy including anthracyclines is shown. The number of samples from relapsed leukemia patients is nine compared to 33 samples from

Table 1. Topo I and II activities in acute myeloid leukemia cells

Percentiles	FAB-M1			FAB-M5		
	Topo I	Topo II A	Topo II B	Topo I	Topo II A	Topo II B
25th	2.13	1.67	1.25	4.58	2.60	1.30
Median	4.58	2.92	1.67	12.91	5.00	6.67
75th	6.25	5.42	2.50	22.08	21.67	8.34

FAB-M1, undifferentiated myeloblastic cells; FAB-M5, monocytic differentiated leukemia cells.

Table 2. Topo I and II activities in primary myeloid leukemias and in relapsed leukemias

Percentiles	Primary (N = 33)			Relapsed (N = 9)		
	Topo I	Topo II A	Topo II B	Topo I	Topo II A	Topo II B
25th	2.00	0.83	0.83	4.48	1.67	1.67
Median	5.41	3.33	1.67	5.83	3.33	3.33
75th	13.13	7.50	5.41	9.58	5.42	4.16

patients before chemotherapy, which is too low to be divided into FAB subgroups.

Cells from relapsed leukemia patients after chemotherapy including anthracycline had a topo IIA activity which was unchanged while topo IIB was twice as active. The increase of the topo IIB activity resulted in a shift of the topo IIA/B ratio from 1.5 to 1.0 in relapsed myeloid leukemias. Topo I activity was also unaltered.

In Table 3, the effect of cytostatic drugs on the topo IIA and topo IIB activities is shown. In virto treatment of cells with anthracyclines or podophyllotoxines had a striking selectively inhibitory effect on topo IIA and not topo IIB. Idarubicin has a higher inhibitory potency than daunorubicin, which correlates with the lower dosage of idarubicin used in chemotherapy. Topo IIA activity is almost completely inhibited after in vitro treatment of the cells with low idarubicin doses (e.g., IC25), which is not shown in this table. Although topo IIA is obviously the substrate of these drugs, sensitivity of the cells does not depend only on the activity of this isoenzyme. Survival of the cells after treatment seems to be notably dependent on the activity of the other topo II isoenzyme which is not inhibited by the drugs (topo IIB), as FAB-M1 leukemia cells with a high ratio of topo IIA/B (> 1.41, median) were significantly more sensitive to anthracyclines than cells with a low ratio ($p < 0.0001$).

Table 3. Inhibition of topo-isoactivities by anthracyclines and etoposide[a]

Drug	Topo IIA (pH 8.9)	Topo IIB (pH 7.9)
Daunorubicin	30.00	122.50
Idarubicin	6.30	75.00
Etoposide	28.40	95.00

[a]Activity in % after incubation of HL60 cells as compared to control without incubation.

Discussion

Topoisomerases are vitally important for every cell. Although the genetic code is defined by a linear string of nucleotides, it is the three-dimensional structure of the double helix that regulates most of its cellular functions (Osheroff et al. 1991). Hematopoietic cell differentiation is closely associated with the physiological function of topoisomerases. When HL60-cells were induced by dimethylsulfoxide (DMSO) to differentiate terminally, the level of topoisomerase II mRNA was transiently increased with a maximum at 6 h after DMSO addition and was then completely abolished after 48 h, indicating that topoisomerase II is activated during the onset of HL60 differentiation (Riou et al. 1993). Apparently, a change of topoisomerase II binding to critical regulatory regions of genes important for differentiation is associated with the regulation of these genes during differentiation (Riou et al. 1993). The regulation of topo II during phorbolester-induced monocytic differentiation of HL60-cells seems to be a prerequisite (Loflin et al. 1994). Inhibition of topoisomerase function with low doses of podophyllotoxines can induce, and amsidyl can inhibit, HL60 differentiation (Gieseler et al. 1993). This indicates differential sensitivity of topoisomerase isoenzymes to these drugs and the possibility for substitution of the lost function by uninhibited isoforms.

Serine phosphorylation of topos is one explanation why we found several topoisomerase isoactivities in nuclear extracts of hematopoietic cells. Under experimental conditions using high ionic strength, we were able to discriminate several topo II isoactivities. Two of them with pH optima at 8.9 (topo IIA) and 7.9 (topo IIB) seemed to be substantial, as they could be found in all examined leukemia cell samples. As shown in Table 3, the topo IIA activity is inhibited by several topo II inhibitors, which indicates that it might represent topo II-alpha. On the other hand, phosphorylation has considerable effect not only on the activity, but also on the sensitivity of the enzyme (De Vore et al. 1992; Ganapathi et al. 1993). Additionally, it has been shown that topo II is able to form multimers in vitro (Vassetzky et al. 1994).

These might be among the reasons why the described isoactivities cannot be directly correlated with gene transcription or protein content of topo II-alpha or -beta. However, topo IIB activity as well as topo I activity was mainly altered in monocytic differentiated acute myoblastic leukemia (AML) cells (Table 1). Topo IIB activity had a considerable effect on the sensitivity of undifferentiated myeloblastic cells. In contrast to topo A and topo I activity, topo B activity was increased twofold in relapsed myeloid leukemias (Table 2). Also, cells with a relatively high topo IIA activity supplemented by a low topo IIB activity (A/B ratio > 1.41, median) were significantly more sensitive to anthracyclines. One explanation would be that topo IIB, not being inhibited by the drugs, is able to substitute functionally for the lost topo IIA activity and maintains the cell to survive the repair phase. These explorations encourage further analysis of topo activities in leukemia cells with the intention of finding cellular parameters for successful treatment with topo I or topo II inhibitors.

References

Bennett JB, Catovsky D, Daniel MT, Flandrin G, Galton DAG, Gralnick HR (1985) Proposed revised criteria for the classification of acute myeloid leukemia. A report of the French-American-British Cooperative Group. Ann Intern Med 103: 460–462

Boege F, Kjeldsen E, Gieseler F, Alsner J, Biersack H (1993) A drug-resistant variant of topoisomerase II alpha in human HL-60 cells exhibits alterations in catalytic pH optimum, DNA binding and sub-nuclear distribution. Eur J Biochem 218: 575–584

De Vore RF, Corbett AH, Osheroff N (1992) Phosphorylation of topoisomerase II by casein kinase II and protein kinase C: effects on enzyme-mediated DNA cleavage/religation and sensitivity to the antineoplastic drugs etoposide and 4′-(9-acridinylamino)methane-sulfon-m-anisidide. Cancer Res 52: 2156–2161

Ganapathi R, Zwelling L, Constantinou A, Ford J, Grabowski D (1993) Altered phosphorylation, biosynthesis and degradation of the 170 kDa isoform of topoisomerase II in amsacrine-resistant human leukemia cells. Biochem Biophys Res Commun 192: 1274–1280

Gieseler F (1995) Topoisomerases – from basis research to clinical implications. Hematol Blood Transfus (in press)

Gieseler F, Boege F, Clark M, Meyer P (1993) Correlation between the DNA-binding affinity of topoisomerase inhibiting drugs and their capacity to induce hematopoetic cell differentiation. Toxicol Lett 67: 331–340

Gieseler F, Boege F, Ruf B, Meyer P, Wilms K (1994) Molecular pathways of topoisomerase II regulation and consequences for chemotherapy. In: Büchner W, Hiddemann W, Wörmann B, Schellong F, Ritter J (eds) Acute leukemias IV: prognostic factors and treatment strategies. Springer, Berlin Heidelberg New York, pp 299–304

Kaspers GJL, Veerman AJP, Pieters R, van Zantwijk I, Klumper E, Hählen K, de Waal FC, van Wering ER (1994) In vitro cytotoxicity of mitoxantrone, daunorubicin and doxorubicin in untreated childhood acute leukemia. Leukemia 8: 24–29

Loflin PT, Hochhauser D, Hickson ID, Morales F, Zwelling LA (1994) Molecular analysis of a potentially phorbol-regulatable region of the human topoisomerse II alpha gene promoter. Biochem Biophys Res Commun 200: 489–496

Osheroff N, Zechidrich EL, Gale KC (1991) Catalytic function of DNA topoisomerase II. Bioessays 13: 269–273

Page B, Page M, Noel C (1993) A new fluorimetric assay for cytotoxicity measurements in vitro. Int J Oncol 3: 473–476

Riou JF, Gabillot M, Riou G (1993) Analysis of topoisomerase II-mediated DNA cleavage of the c-myc gene during HL60 differentiation. FEBS Lett 334: 369–372

Stevnsner T, Bohr VA (1993) Studies on the role of topoisomerases in general, gene- and strand-specific DNA repair. Carcinogenesis 14: 1841–1850

Vassetzky YS, Dang Q, Benedetti P, Gasser SM (1994) Topoisomerase II forms multimers in vitro: effects of metals, beta-glycerophosphate, and phosphorylation of its C-terminal domain. Mol Cell Biol 14: 6962–6974

Zini N, Santi S, Ognibene A, Bavelloni A, Neri LM, Valmori A, Mariani E, Negri C, Astaldi RG, Maraldi NM (1994) Discrete localization of different DNA topoisomerases in HeLa and K562 cell nuclei and subnuclear fractions. Exp Cell Res 210: 336–348

DNA Repair: Genes, Enzymes, Patients, and Mouse Models

N.G.J. Jaspers

Department of Cell Biology and Genetics, Erasmus University, P.O. Box 1738, 3000 DR Rotterdam, The Netherlands

DNA Damage and Repair

All organisms have evolved intricate networks of complementary DNA repair systems, enabling them to counteract a large variety of DNA damages. Among these, the cyclobutane pyrimidine dimers (CPDs) and the 6,4-pyrimidine-pyrimidone photoproducts (64PP) are certainly the most relevant since they are produced in massive amounts in human skin exposed to the shortwave component of natural sunlight. Genetic defects in DNA repair pathways or in damage-induced cell-cycle arrest result in chromosomal abnormalities, elevated levels of mutations, and a predisposition to cancer.

Several multienzyme repair processes exist: base excision repair can remove specific types of simple base adducts and some mismatches; on the other hand, nucleotide excision repair (NER) attacks a wide variety of helix-distorting lesions. Recombinational repair and postreplication repair enable translesion DNA synthesis and are not well defined in mammalian cells. Finally, the large-patch mismatch repair pathway deals with replication errors, due to misincorporation or slippage.

NER Syndromes

CPDs and 64PPs are subject to repair by the NER system. As a consequence, patients with inherited defects in NER are markedly hypersensitive to sun exposure. At least three different NER-deficient human syndromes are known, the best-studied of which is xeroderma pigmentosum (XP). The UV-exposed skin of XP patients shows pigmentation abnormalities and an over 1000-fold increased risk of cancer. Defects in one of at least seven different genes (XPA to XPG) underlie these problems. Another disorder is Cockayne's syndrome (CS), characterized by a less severe sun sensitivity, stunted growth, and a whole range of disturbances, e.g., in the nervous system and the gonads. Two re-

Recent Results in Cancer Research, Vol. 143

sponsible genes have been identified so far: CSA and CSB. The peculiar disorder trichothiodystrophy (TTD) also falls in the category of NER syndromes. In these patients, a shortage of sulfur-rich matrix proteins in the hair and nails makes these appendages extraordinarily thin and brittle. The clinical picture also comprises ichthyosis and many symptoms characteristic of CS patients. About half of the TTD patients are hypersensitive to UV, due to a NER defect caused by mutations in one of at least three genes: TTDA and (to everyone's surprise) XPB and XPD. In contrast to XP, there are no indications for an increased risk of cancer in CS and TTD. Finally, a rare class of patients exists showing a combined XP + CS picture. Such patients have a defective XPB, XPD, or XPG gene. The extensive clinical and genetic heterogeneity among the NER disorders immediately indicates that the relationships between DNA damage, repair, and clinical consequences such as cancer and neurodegeneration are highly complex and not straightforward at all. Recent molecular genetic and enzymological studies have started to clarify some of these intricacies.

Molecular View of NER

Recent progress ensuing from cloning of NER genes and the establishment of an in vitro assay has permitted the uncovering of the contours of the molecular mechanism of NER. In the near future more details will be revealed, since most of the NER system could be reconstituted in vitro from individual purified components. Altogether 25–30 different polypeptides (summarized in Table 1) appear to be involved in a multistep reaction mechanism. The accumulated knowledge permits the compilation of a model whose details remain largely hypothetical for the time being.

Damage Recognition

Recognition of the lesion must be largely handled by the XPA gene product that preferentially binds to damaged DNA. The XPE-like UV-DDB protein has a nonessential stimulatory action. An additional protein IF7 may be needed to optimize the specificity. The XPA protein appears to harbor domains that can physically interact in vitro with an array of other repair factors, such as ERCC1, TFIIH, or RPA, and thus plays a key role in NER initiation. In many XPA patients the protein is completely absent, which implies that it is nonvital on the cell level and that its function may be NER-specific.

Preincision Patch Demarcation

The area around the lesion is "demarcated" by local unwinding of the DNA helix and stabilized by the single-strand binding heterotrimer RP-A. A can-

Table 1. Cloned human genes involved in nucleotide excision repair (NER) and their encoded polypeptides. (Updated July 1995)

Human/mammalian genes				Yeast homologs		Remarks
Name	Rodent mutant	Locus	Complex	*S. cerevisiae*	*S. pombe*	(M_r, function, etc.)
XPA		9q34		RAD14		p42; binds UV-DNA; interaction with ERCC1, RPA1, TFIIH; Dros = Dxpa
XPC		3p25.1	XPC/23B	RAD4		125 kD; strong DNA binding; "global" repair
HHR23B		3p25.1	XPC/23B	RAD23		50 kD; ubiquitin fusion protein
XPE/DDB1		11q12–13	p127/p48	[seq. clone; vital]		p127; only complex binds UV-DNA
DDB2		11p11–12	p127/p48			p48; function unknown
XPF			F/1/4/11			[not cloned] possibly = ERCC4. complex: incision 5′ side
	ERCC4	16p13.1–13.2	F/1/4/11	RAD1	swi9/rad16	pI12; possibly XPF; Dros. M = mei9
	ERCC1	19q13.3	F/1/4/11	RAD10	swi10	p39; XPA-interaction
	ERCC11		F/1/4/11			[not cloned]
XPG	ERCC5	13q32.3–33.1		RAD2	rad13	p180; incision 3′ side (FEN1-like)
XPB	ERCC3	2q21	TFIIH	RAD25/SSL2	ercc3^{sp}	p89; 3′→5′ helicase; Dros. M = Haywire, Vaccinia = A18R
XPD	ERCC2	19q13.3	TFIIH	RAD3	rad15/rhp3	p80; 5′→3′ helicase
TTDA			TFIIH			[not cloned]
		5q13	TFIIH	SSL1		p44 subunit (ZnF prot)
		11p14–15	TFIIH	TFB1		p62
		6p21.3–22.2	TFIIH	TFB2		p52
MAT1			TFIIH (CAK1)	TFB3		p32 (RingFinger)
CDK7		5q12–13; 2q22–24	TFIIH (CAK1)	KIN28		p41; CTD kinase; xenopus MO15
CyclinH			TFIIH (CAK1)	CCL1		p38

Table 1 (*Contd.*)

Human/mammalian Name	Rodent mutant	Locus	Complex	Yeast homologs *S. cerevisiae*	*S. pombe*	Remarks (M_r, function, etc.)
			TFIIH	[seq. clone]		p34 (RingFinger)
CSA	ERCC8	5				44 kD; no helicase; TrCoupled NER; interaction with CSB, SSL1?
CSB	ERCC6	10q11		RAD26		180-kD helicase; TrCoupled NER; interaction with CSA?
HHR23A		19p13.1		RAD23		50-kD ubiquitin fusion protein; function unknown
LIG1		19q13.2–13.3		CDC9	cdc17	DNA ligase I (mutated in patient 46BR)
PCNA		20p12-ter		POL30	pcn	28 kD; binds Polδ (leading strand), Polϵ and RP-C
RPA1		17	RP-A	RFA1		70-kD DNA binding subunit; binds XPA and XPG?
RPA2		1	RP-A	RFA2		32-kD subunit; XPA interaction?
RPA3		7p22	RP-A	RFA3		14-kD subunit
			RP-C	RFC1		37-kD subunit
		10	RP-C	RFC2		38-kD subunit
			RP-C	CDC44 a.o.		40, 140, 145-kD subunits
POLDI		19q13		POL3/CDC2	pol3	Polδ 124-kD subunit; (other = 50 kD)
POLE		12q24		POL2		Polϵ 256-kD catalytic subunit A; PCNA-dependent
				DPB2		subunit B = 80 kD
				DPB3		subunit C = 34 kD nucleotide binding
XPE-like		16q22–23		[seq. clone]		homolog DDB1/XPE; function unknown

didate for the unwinding function is the TFIIH complex, which contains the products of the XPB, XPD, TTDA, and SSL1 genes and some additional proteins. XPD and XPB both have helicase activity, each in a different direction. The RP-A complex is "borrowed" from the DNA replication pathway, in which it plays an essential role. Likewise, TFIIH is shared by the NER process and the basic transcription machinery. More loosely associated TFIIH components, such as the cyclin-dependent kinase CDK7 and cyclin H, are expected to play a role as well. This interesting finding may point to a link with cell cycle control. Since TFIIH is necessary for transcription initiation in most of the genes transcribed by RNA polymerase II, it is a vital function. Therefore,the mutations found, e.g., in XPB and XPD patients are subtle (mostly aa-substitutions) and leave most of the transcription function intact. Mammalian cells with mutated RP-A components have not been identified so far.

Strand Incision

On both sides of the marked DNA segment, the damaged strand is nicked, first on the 5′ side by the XPG protein, followed by a nick on the 3′ side by an enzyme complex containing the proteins ERCC1, ERCC4, ERCC11 and XPF. The composition of the latter complex is not exactly known, since it could not be purified from cell extracts to homogeneity up to now. On the basis of the homology to the yeast RAD1 and RAD10 proteins, it is expected to play a dual role: it is needed for mitotic recombination as well. Formation of the ERCC1 ... XPF complex is required for stability of its components: in patients with a defective XPF the ERCC1 protein is also depleted by more than 90%. Complete loss of the function of the complex is not lethal in mammalian and yeast cells.

Gap-Filling and Ligation

The mechanism of the final sequence of events has not been characterized in detail, but it is likely to resemble the basic features of DNA replication. In fact, in the in vitro reconstituted reaction it could be accomplished by the *Escherichia coli* Klenow fragment and ligase. Known mammalian replication proteins such as RP-A, PCNA, and RP-C are at least involved. Polymerase ϵ is the best candidate for performing the gap-filling step, and DNA ligase I probably mediates the final nick closure. Again, we find an example of enzyme-sharing by two different processes, in this case repair and replication.

Further Modulation

The basic mechanism of NER just outlined is subject to considerable modulation and fine-tuning. One type of regulation is at the level of the damage.

For instance, UV-induced 64PPs are removed earlier and faster than the CPD lesions. Secondly, there is a spatial preference: two identical neighboring lesions may be repaired at highly different rates. A third level of control involves chromatin structure and transcriptional activity. Actively transcribed genome regions are repaired faster than the bulk of the genome. Even the transcribed strands are subject to preference, strongly suggesting that there exists a direct coupling with RNA polymerase II transcription; the subpathway is therefore named transcription-coupled repair (TCR). TCR requires the presence of CSA and CSB functions. On the other hand, NER of the nontranscribed bulk of the genome, referred to as global repair, is dependent (at least in humans) on an enzyme complex of XPC and HHR23. The balance between TCR and global NER can differ in various species: for instance, in rodents the global pathway is underrepresented in comparison to human cells. The molecular mechanisms of all these types of NER fine-tuning are still poorly understood.

The Clinical Consequences of NER Deficiency

Many of the numerous genes and proteins involved in NER now appear to function as well-defined enzyme complexes. Examples are HHR23/XPC, ERCC1/4/11/XPF, and the TFIIH complex. The concept of sharing of these functions between NER and other cellular processes like recombination, replication, and transcription has strong implications for the clinical consequences of inherited mutations in NER proteins. Perhaps the involvement of TFIIH in basal transcription is the clearest example. TTD patients and most combined XP + CS patients have defective TFIIH components. It is likely that many of their peculiar clinical symptoms, which are not easy to explain on the basis of an NER defect per se (e.g., the brittle hair in TTD, or nerve dysmyelination in CS), are caused by partial, subtle insufficiencies in basal transcription. Such abnormalities may even exist in the absence of NER involvement. Indeed, many patients showing TTD and/or CS features with no obvious UV sensitivity have been identified. They may suffer from a "transcription syndrome".

A similar situation may be valid for other NER complexes. Until now, no human syndrome has been found with inherited ERCC1 deficiency. Possibly, due to additional involvement of mitotic recombination, such patients display an unusual array of symptoms not immediately reminiscent of an NER defect.

Generation of Mouse Models for Repair Diseases

The technique of mimicking human genetic defects in a mouse model by gene targeting in totipotent embryonal stem cells was employed for several repair enzymes isolated in our laboratory (summarized in Table 2). XPB-inactivated mouse mutants are embryonally lethal, consistent with the essential function of the gene in basic transcription. Heterozygous carriers, however, are phenoty-

Table 2. Current status of generation of repair-deficient mice[a]

Gene	Type of mutation	Expected phenotype	Present stage
ERCC1	Subtle?	XP-like	Homozygote
	KO	XP-like	Homozygote
XPB	Subtle	XP, XP/CS, TTD?	Targeted ES clone
	KO	Lethal	Targeted ES clone
XPD	Subtle	XP, XP/CS, TTD?	Construct
	KO	Lethal	Heterozygote
CSB	KO	CS	Homozygote
HHR23A	KO	?	Construct
HHR23B	KO	XP-like	Targeted ES clone
HHR6A	KO	? (PRR?)	Hemizygote
HHR6B	KO	? (PRR)	Homozygote
HHR54	KO	? (RecRep)	Targeted ES clone

XP, xeroderma pigmentosum; CS, Cockayne syndrome; TTD, trichothiodystrophy; KO, "knock-out," i.e., fully inactivated gene product; PRR, postreplication repair; RecRep, Recombination repair; ES, embryonal stem cell.
[a]Rotterdam, May 1995.

pically normal. Currently, subtle mutations are being introduced, in the hope of mimicking the features of the hypothetical "transcription syndromes."

Mice with inactivated CSB genes display the expected TCR defect in their cultured cells, which are also sensitive to UV exposure. However, between the ages of 3 weeks and 8 months, no overt neurological, developmental, or sexual abnormalities reminiscent of the human CS phenotype were observed. The skin is highly sensitive to acute UV exposure and experiments to investigate the carcinogenic effects of long-term skin irradiation are under way.

Mice with different mutations in the ERCC1 gene develop poorly (25%–30% of the weight of litter mates) and die at a young age with pronounced aneuploidy in the nuclei of liver and kidney, and iron deposition in the spleen. The origin of these symptoms is unclarified so far but depends on the type of mutation and on the genetic background of the animals. The possibility that these symptoms are related to the additional involvement of ERCC1 in recombination is plausible but needs further testing. Hypersensitivity of theskin and of cultured cells to UV exposure fits with the demonstrated complete absence of NER.

The ubiquitin-conjugating enzyme RAD6 in yeast and its human homolog HHR6B are involved in a postreplication repair pathway. Mice with a defective HHR6B gene display male sterility, consistent with the finding that this protein is highly expressed in testes and with the idea that it may be engaged in chromatin transactions required in the final stages of spermatogenesis. The repair function of this gene, for which no human syndromes are known, may become apparent when the strongly homologous HHR6A gene is also inactivated and bred in. Such experiments are in progress.

Repair of Directly and Indirectly UV-Induced DNA Lesions and of DNA Double-Strand Breaks in Cells from Skin Cancer-Prone Patients with the Disorders Dysplastic Nevus Syndrome or Basal Cell Nevus Syndrome

T.M. Rünger[1,3], B. Epe[2], K. Möller[1], B. Dekant[1], and D. Hellfritsch[1]

[1]Department of Dermatology, University of Würzburg, Josef-Schneider-Strasse 2, 97080 Würzburg, Germany
[2]Department of Toxicology, University of Würzburg, Versbacher Strasse 9, 97080 Würzburg, Germany
[3]Current and corresponding address: Department of Dermatology, University of Göttingen, von-Siebold Strasse 3, 37075 Göttingen, Germany

Introduction

Hereditary disorders carrying an increased skin cancer risk, such as xeroderma pigmentosum (XP), dysplastic nevus syndrome (DNS), or basal cell nevus syndrome (BCNS), are valuable model systems that might provide insights into general mechanisms of skin carcinogenesis. This is especially true of XP, in which a defective repair of UV-induced DNA damage explains the increased risk of basal cell carcinomas, squamous cell carcinomas, and malignant melanomas in UV-exposed skin of affected patients (Kraemer et al. 1987; Barnes et al. 1993; Hoijmakers 1993).

Dysplastic nevus syndrome is characterized by clinically and histopathologically "dyplastic" (or "atypical") melanocytic nevi and an increased risk of developing malignant melanoma in affected patients (Marghoop et al. 1994). It has been described with and without an increased incidence of malignant melanoma in family members (Kraemer et al. 1983). Inheritance has been suggested to be autosomal dominant or polygenic (Traupe et al. 1989; Bale and Tucker 1990). Since the histopathological definition or even the existence of an "atypical" melanocytic nevus is controversial, it remains unclear if the dysplastic nevus syndrome, except for familiar malignant melanoma (FAMMM), is a clinical entity (Ackermann and Milde 1992; NIH Consensus Conference 1992; Shapiro 1992). A chromosomal instability with an increased rate of chromosomal rearrangements and sister chromatid exchanges after UV exposure has been described in melanocytes, lymphoblasts, and fibroblasts from patients with DNS (Caporaso et al. 1987; Jaspers et al. 1987; Hecht and Hecht 1988; Rünger et al. 1994a; Rünger and Bröcker 1995). Sanford et al. (1987) reported an increased rate of chromatid breaks and gaps in metaphase chromosomes after G2 irradiation of DNS fibroblasts. Genetic linkage to the short arm of chromosome 1 could not be confirmed by others (van Haerigen et al. 1989). Many lines of evidence suggested linkage to 9p21 (Cannon-Albright et al. 1992; Trevis 1992; Rünger et al. 1994a; Rünger and Bröcker 1995). This locus contains the gene for p16, an inhibitor of the cyclin-dependent kinase 4 (cdk4), a putative tumor (melanoma) suppressor. It has been found mutated in up to 75% of cell lines established from malignant melanomas, but only in less than 20% of primary melanoma cells. However, in DNS families with genetic linkage to 9p, but not in those with linkage to 1p, inactivating p16 mutations have been found (Hussussian et al. 1994). Thus, it remains to be established if the p16 gene constitutes the genetic defect of DNS or FAMMM, at least in some families (Wainwright 1994).

Patients with the autosomal dominant basal cell nevus syndrome (BCNS) develop multiple basal cell carcinomas, especially in UV-exposed skin (Bale et al. 1989b; Shanley et al. 1994). Additional abnormalities include palmar and plantar "pits," mandibular cysts, calcification of the falx cerebri, and other bone malformations. In addition to the high frequency of basal cell carcinomas, an increased frequency of medulloblastomas, fibrosarcomas, and teratomas was also reported. If these are therapeutically irradiated, a massive spread of basal cell carcinomas may develop in the irradiated overlying skin. It is controversial if this clinical radiosensitivity is reflected by a cellular radiosensitivity (Chan and Little 1983; Little et al. 1989). Repair of X-ray-induced DNA damage was found to be normal (Chan and Little 1983; Featherstone et al. 1983), but repair of γ-ray-induced DNA damage was deficient (Arlett et al. 1980). Bale et al. (1989a), Sarto et al. (1989), and Shafei-Benaissa et al. (1994) could not confirm results of a spontaneous chromosomal instability. A UV hypersensitivity has been described with UVB, but not with UVC (Applegate et al. 1990). The BCNS gene, a putative tumor (basal cell carcinoma) suppressor gene, is located on 9q23.1-q31, but has not been further characterized (Bailani et al. 1992; Wicking et al. 1994). A loss of heterozygosity in this region has also been demonstrated in approximately one-half of sporadic basal cell carcinomas.

Earlier, we described a reduced and/or abnormal joining of DNA ends of transfected linear plasmids in cells from patients with different chromosome breakage or genetic instability syndromes (Rünger and Kraemer 1989; Rünger et al. 1992, 1994b), suggesting a relationship between genetic instability and an abnormal repair of DNA double-strand breaks. Because a genetic instability has been suggested for both DNS and BCNS, we investigated the ability of cells from these patients to join DNA ends (i.e., to repair DNA double-strand breaks). Our "host cell ligation assay" measures the ability of host cells (here DNS and BCNS lymphoblasts) to recircularize linear plasmid pZ189, introduced into the host cells by electroporation. This assay was described in detail earlier (Rünger et al. 1993). In addition to information about the joining efficiency, the plasmid encoded mutagenesis marker gene *supF* allows analysis of the joining fidelity.

Exposure to ultraviolet light is an important factor for the development of malignant melanomas in patients with DNS and of basal carcinomas in patients with BCNS. Analogous to XP, an impaired processing of DNA damage, especially of UV-induced DNA damage, has been suspected but not clearly shown so far.

Therefore, we assessed the repair of UV-induced DNA damage in DNS and BCNS lymphoblasts. We used a "host cell reactivation assay" with UVB-irradiated, nonreplicating plasmid pRSVcat, introduced into these host cells (Gorman et al. 1983; Rünger et al. 1995a). Because the expression of plasmid-encoded chloramphenicol acetyltransferase (CAT) depends on repair of UVB-induced DNA damage by cellular enzymes, CAT activities in cell extracts, 3 days after electroporation, reflect the ability of the host cells to repair UV-induced pyrimidine dimers.

Longerwave ultraviolet light (UVA) does not excite the DNA molecule and therefore is not able to damage it directly (Rünger and Möller 1994; Rünger et al. 1995b). However, it is capable of damaging DNA indirectly by a photosensitized reaction via excitation of other cellular compounds and the formation of singlet oxygen (Epe et al. 1993). The subsequent formation mainly of 8-hydroxyguanine has been implicated in the genotoxic, mutagenic, and carcinogenic potential of UVA (Lundgren and Wulf 1988; van Weelden et al. 1988). Many clinical observations have linked melanoma formation to excessive exposure to ultraviolet light, and especially to UVA, acquired, for example, in tanning parlors (Swerdlow et al. 1988; Walter et al. 1990; Setlow et al. 1993; Schmitz et al. 1994; Rünger et al. 1994a; Rünger and Bröcker 1995). That is why we also investigated the ability of DNS and BCNS lymphoblasts to repair singlet oxygen-induced DNA damage. For this purpose we used the pRSVcat-based "host cell reactivation assay" with singlet oxygen-treated plasmid.

Using these two treatment modalities, we are able to investigate the processing of directly and indirectly UV-induced DNA damage separately. Results of similar experiments with lymphoblasts from patients with XP were published earlier (Rünger et al. 1995a).

Methods

Cells

Epstein-Barr virus-transformed lymphoblast cell lines KM, BD, TR (normal cell lines), AD (39-year-old female; DNS with multiple, histopathologically confirmed dysplastic nevi, and with FAMMM: see Fig. 1 for family incidence of malignant melanoma), HR (30-year-old female; DNS with multiple, histologically confirmed dysplastic nevi, but without FAMMM), and HS (46-year-old male; BCNS with multiple basal cell carcinomas on the face and trunk, first occurrence of a basal cell carcinoma at age 32, and radiologically confirmed

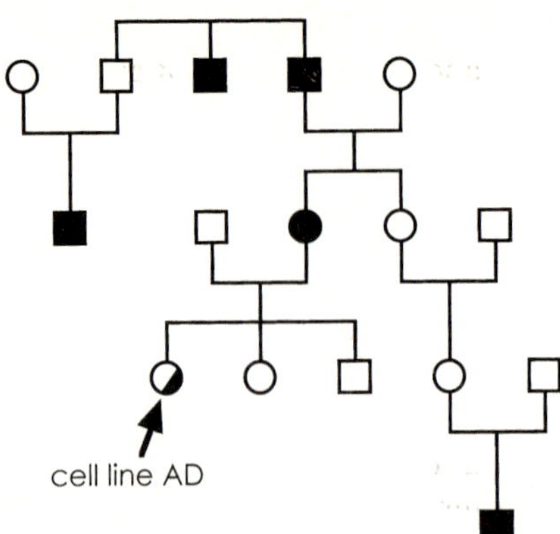

Fig. 1. Family with dysplastic nevus syndrome (DNS) and familial malignant melanoma (FAMMM). Family tree of the patient with dysplastic nevus syndrome, from which the lymphoblast cell line AD was established. This patient had multiple, histopathologically confirmed dysplastic nevi. Family members that are indicated by *black symbols* had at least one malignant melanoma

mandibular cysts) were established in our laboratory following the protocol described by Neitzel (1986). The cell lines GM3715, GM3657, GM0621, GM0130, and GM1805 (normal cell lines), and GM6921 (DNS with multiple dysplastic nevi, five primary malignant melanomas and FAMMM: similarly affected mother and uncle) were purchased from the Human Genetic Mutant Cell Repository (Camden, NJ, USA). The genetic linkage of the DNS cell lines is not known. The cells were grown in RPMI 1640 medium supplemented with 17% fetal calf serum in 5% CO_2 and used during the exponential growth phase.

"Host Cell Ligation Assay"

The 5.5 kb, replicating, SV40-based shuttle vector plasmid pZ189 was prepared, transfected, and recovered as described in detail previously (Rünger et al. 1993). This plasmid contains the bacterial mutagenesis marker gene *supF* adjacent to a single *Eco*RI restriction site and the bacterial gene for ampicillin resistance. Linear plasmid was prepared by cleavage with the restriction endonuclease *Eco*RI at bp 1. Complete linearization (less than 0.05% of circular forms remaining) was verified by agarose gel electrophoresis and Southern blotting. For electrotransformation we used the Gene Pulser apparatus and capacitance extender (BioRad, Hercules, CA): 15×10^6 lymphoblasts in a 0.4 ml suspension with 5 μg of linear or circular plasmid in serum-free RPMI 1640 medium were subjected once to an electrical pulse (250 V, 960 μFd capacitor, time constant between 20 and 30 ms) at room temperature in an electrode cuvette with an interelectrode distance of 0.4 cm and then transferred to 20 ml of prewarmed complete medium. Replicated plasmids recovered after 3 days were subsequently introduced by electrotransformation (interelectrode distance 0.2 cm, total volume 80 μl, 2500 V, 25 μFd capacitor, 600 Ω resistance, time constant 8–15 ms) into *Escherichia coli* MBM7070, which contains a suppressable mutation in the gene for β-galactosidase. The bacteria were plated on LB agar dishes containing ampicillin, the indicator dye X-gal (5-bromo-4-chloro-3-indolyl-β-D-galactoside), and the inducer of β-galactosidase, IPTG (isopropyl-β-D-galactoside).

Plasmid survival was determined by scoring bacterial colonies from replicated plasmids obtained from cells transfected with linear plasmids and dividing by the number of bacterial colonies from parallel samples in the same experiment transfected with circular plasmid. This reference sample with circular plasmid was used in every experiment to compensate for variations in transfection rates, plasmid replication, or condition of the cells used. The survival rates from several experiments were then averaged.

A representative sample of plasmids from blue, light blue, and white bacterial colonies was analyzed. The color change from blue to light blue or white indicates partial or complete inactivation of the mutagenesis target gene *supF*, located close to the ligation site. Using agarose gel electrophoresis, we compared the size of purified plasmids to the size of the wild-type plasmid. We tested for conservation of the *Eco*RI restriction site by redigesting with this enzyme. A successful cleavage indicates that not a single base pair was deleted during the ligation process. This facilitates mutation analysis on the base sequence level without DNA sequencing of every recovered mutant. Our previously described, 98% accurate mutant classification scheme, which is based on our experience with sequencing of recovered mutants (Rünger et al. 1993), allows identification of unchanged plasmids and classification of mutants into three categories: (a) deletions at the ligation site, (b) insertions or more complex mutations at the ligation site, or (c) point mutations in the adjacent *supF* mutagenesis marker gene.

The mutation frequency was calculated separately for the blue and the light blue or white colonies, added for each independent sample, and averaged. The mutation analysis for blue colonies was assessed by the analysis of plasmids purified from blue colonies as the ratio of the number of mutated plasmids to the total number of analyzed plasmids, and calculated for each independent sample. The frequency of a particular type of mutation was determined by multiplying the mutation frequency of blue colonies of each independent sample with the frequency of this class of mutation in a representative sample of blue colonies. These rates for the blue colonies and the similarly calculated rates for the light blue or white colonies were then averaged. The student's *t*-test was used to test for differences.

"Host Cell Reactivation Assay"

One of the following two treatments was used to damage the non-replicating plasmid pRSVcat: (1) Plasmids at a concentration of 30 μg/ml were irradiated with 1 kJ/m^2, 5 kJ/m^2, and 10 kJ/m^2 UVB (Philips TL21 lamps, emission maximum at 315 nm, spectrum 275–365 nm) at 0 °C. (2) Plasmids were treated with singlet oxygen, generated by methylene blue (10 μg/ml) and light (1, 5, and 10 min illumination with visible light, 1000-W Osram halogen lamp, 47 W/m^2 between 400 and 800 nm). The plasmid concentration was 625 μg/ml. The DNA damage profile induced by this treatment has been described by Müller et al. (1990) using DNA repair endonucleases. It comprises mainly FPG protein-sensitive sites and only very few single-strand breaks, pyrimidine dimers, or AP sites. It is identical to the DNA damage profile produced by disodium-3,3′-(1,4-naphthylidene)-diproprionate ($NDPO_2$), a chemically clean source of singlet oxygen. Seven FPG-sensitive lesions were generated on the plasmid per minute of illumination.

The plasmid pRSVcat (Gorman et al. 1983) contains the cat gene in a configuration that allows expression of the CAT protein in human cells. Five micrograms of pRSVcat were used to transfect 15×10^6 cells, using the electroporation procedure (Gene Pulser, BioRad: 250 V, 960 μFd capacitor, 400 μl of serum free medium, time constant between 20 and 30 ms). The cells were then transferred to 25 ml of prewarmed complete medium and allowed to grow. After three days a cell extract was produced by three freeze-thaw cycles with ethanol in dry ice and subsequent rewarming to 37 °C. CAT activity in that cell extract was determined with the one-vial procedure described by Neumann et al. (1987) and Eastmann (1987). Calibration was done with several concentrations of CAT (Boehringer, Mannheim, Germany) between 0.5 and 0.001 U and a linear relationship was found. In addition, total protein was determined in each extract, using the Coomassie-blue method (BioRad). Background activity was determined for each cell line in an independent sample without transfected plasmid and subtracted from all samples. The mean specific activity with undamaged plasmid was 0.6 U CAT/mg protein. The relative CAT activity was calculated in percent of the control transfected with untreated plasmid. Student's *t*-test was used to test for differences between cell lines.

Results

"Host Cell Ligation Assay"

Transformation of bacteria with plasmids recovered after transfection of linear plasmid into the host cells yielded a mean number of 1698 colonies per transformation in GM3715, 18473 in GM0621, 174 in GM0130, 6280 in GM6921, 9170 in AD, 19920 in HR, and 22960 in HS. Table 1 shows the survival of linear plasmid pZ189 after passage through these seven cell lines in percent, relative to the control transfected with uncleaved, circular plasmid. This survival reflects the efficiency of DNA end-joining to circular plasmid (repair of DNA double-strand breaks) by the host cells.

There was a considerable, up to 2.4-fold variation of DNA end-joining efficiency in the three normal cell lines. The survivals of linear plasmid in the three DNS cell lines and the BCNS cell line were not statistically different from the normal cell lines.

Table 1. Plasmid survival after passage of linear, *Eco*RI-cut plasmid pZ189 (overlapping ends) through lymphoblasts from normal donors and patients with DNS (with or without FAMMM) or BCNS, reflecting the efficiency of these cells in joining DNA ends (repairing DNA double-strand breaks)

Cell line	Plasmid survival[a]	n[b]
GM3715 (normal)	3.5 ± 1.2%	10
GM0621 (normal)	4.0 ± 1.0%	12
GM0130 (normal)	8.3 ± 2.7%	7
GM6921 (DNS, FAMMM)	5.4 ± 1.8%	8
AD (DNS, FAMMM)	4.8 ± 2.2%	6
HR (DNS)	7.5 ± 2.4%	6
HS (BCNS)	9.6 ± 2.7%	7

DNS, dysplastic nevus syndrome; FAMMM, familial malignant melanoma; BCNS, basal cell nevus syndrome.
[a]Plasmid survival is expressed as the relative number of bacterial colonies (in percentage of the circular control, mean ± SEM).
[b]n = number of independent samples.

The overall height of the bars in Fig. 2 shows the total mutation frequencies in recircularized plasmid pZ189, joined during passage through three normal, three DNS, and one BCNS lymphoblast line. The three normal cell lines demonstrated very similar, not statistically different mutation frequencies. For

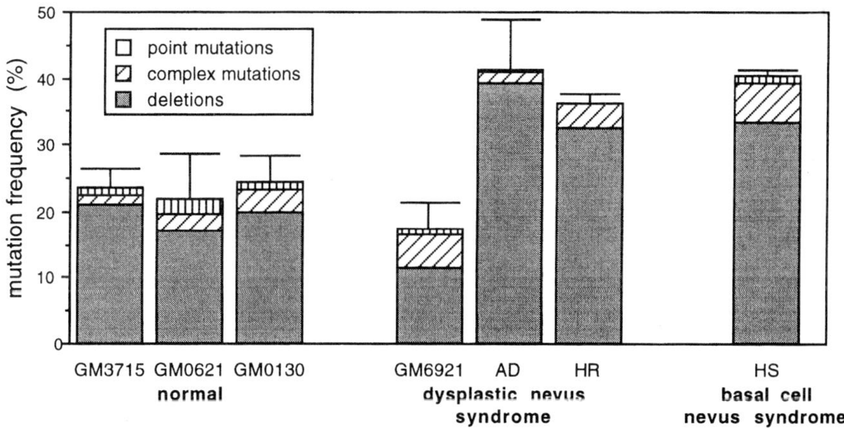

Fig. 2. Fidelity of the DNA end-joining process in normal lymphoblasts and lymphoblasts from patients with DNS or basal cell nevus syndrome (BCNS). Mutation frequencies in the plasmid pZ189 after passage of linear, *Eco*RI-cut plasmid (overlapping ends) through lymphoblasts from normal donors, and patients with DNS or BCNS. The mean of the total mutation frequency is indicated by the *overall height* of the bars, standard deviation by the *error bars*. The distribution of the different types of mutations (deletions, complex mutations, and point mutations) is indicated by the *stacks with different patterns*

example, a mutation frequency of 23.6% with the cell line GM3715 means that 76.4% of all plasmids ligated in that cell line were ligated absolutely faithfully, without the loss of even a single base pair. Two of three cell lines from patients with DNS and the BCNS cell line demonstrated a slightly, 1.5- to 1.9-fold elevated (not significant) mutation frequency in the rejoined plasmids. These numbers are based on the analysis of 771 recircularized plasmids (87–155 per cell line) from 7 to 13 independent samples per cell line.

Detailed mutation analysis of recircularized plasmids allowed the determination of the frequencies of the different types of mutations (deletions, complex mutations, and point mutations), shown as stacks with different patterns in Fig. 2. The distribution was similar in all cell lines, without any significant differences in the DNS or BCNS lines, as compared to the normal lines. The deletion at the joining site was the predominant mutation with all cell lines (79%–96% of all mutations found).

Repair of UVB-Induced DNA Damage (Directly UV-Induced)

Figure 3 shows the capacity of eight normal lymphoblast lines to repair UVB-induced DNA damage. It shows a considerable variation between the normal cell lines. The mean variation between independent samples from one cell line (at 5 kJ/m^2) was 10 ± 12% (mean ± SD).

Figure 4 shows the repair of UVB-induced DNA damage by lymphoblast cell lines from the three different patients with DNS. The mean, minimum, and maximum values of the CAT-activity found with the normal cells is shown in

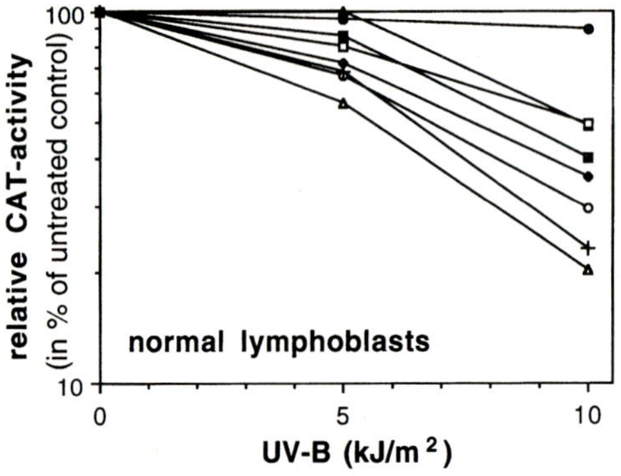

Fig. 3. Repair of UVB-induced (directly UV-induced) DNA damage in lymphoblasts from normal donors. Relative chloramphenicol acetyltransferase (CAT) activity (in percentage of untreated control) in cell extracts of eight normal lymphoblast lines after transfection of UVB-irradiated plasmid pRSVcat. The reactivation of the damaged plasmids reflects the capacity of these host cells to repair UVB-induced DNA damage. Values are means of two to three independent samples. *Open squares*, GM3657; *closed triangles*, GM3715; *open circles*, GM0621; *closed squares*, GM0130; *closed diamonds*, GM1805; *open triangles*, KM; *plus signs*, BD; *closed circles*, TR

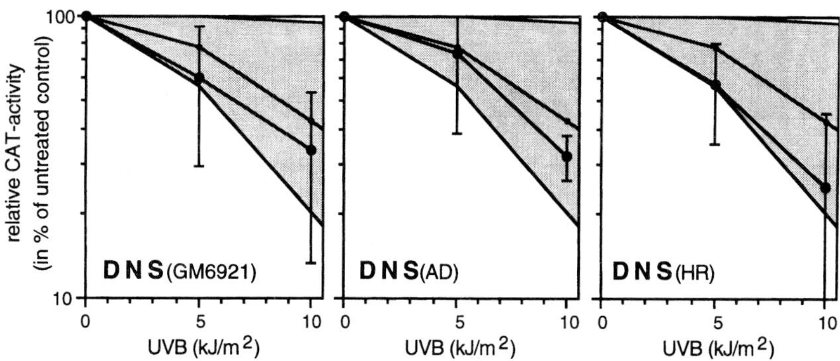

Fig. 4. Repair of UVB-induced (directly UV-induced) DNA damage in lymphoblasts from three patients with dysplastic nevus syndrome. Relative CAT activity (in percentage of untreated control) in cell extracts of the DNS lymphoblast lines GM6921, AD, and HR after transfection of UVB-irradiated plasmid pRSVcat. The reactivation of the damaged plasmids reflects the capacity of these host cells to repair UVB-induced DNA damage. Values are means of two to four independent samples (± SD). The mean values of the results with eight normal cell lines (see Fig. 3) are shown in the line with *small dots*, the minimum and maximum values of the normal range are shown within the *dotted area*

the dotted areas ("normal range"). The repair capacity of all three DNS lines, as well as of the BCNS cell line (Fig. 5), was within that normal range.

Repair of DNA Damage Induced by Singlet Oxygen (Indirectly UV-Induced)

Figure 6 shows the capacity of seven normal lymphoblast cell lines to repair DNA damage induced by photosensitization (singlet oxygen), also exhibiting considerable variation between the cell lines. The mean variation between independent samples from one cell line (at 1 min illumination) was 33±23% (mean±SD).

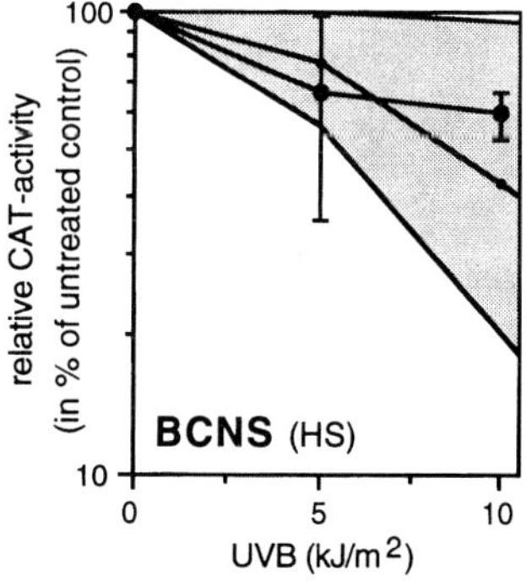

Fig. 5. Repair of UVB-induced (directly UV-induced) DNA damage in lymphoblasts from patients with basal cell nevus syndrome. Relative CAT activity (in percentage of untreated control) in cell extracts of the BCNS lymphoblast line HS, after transfection of UVB-irradiated plasmid pRSVcat. The reactivation of the damaged plasmids reflects the capacity of these host cells to repair UVB-induced DNA damage. Values are means of two to four independent samples (± SD). The mean values of the results with eight normal cell lines (see Fig. 3) are shown in the line with *small dots*, the minimum and maximum values of the normal range are shown within the *dotted area*

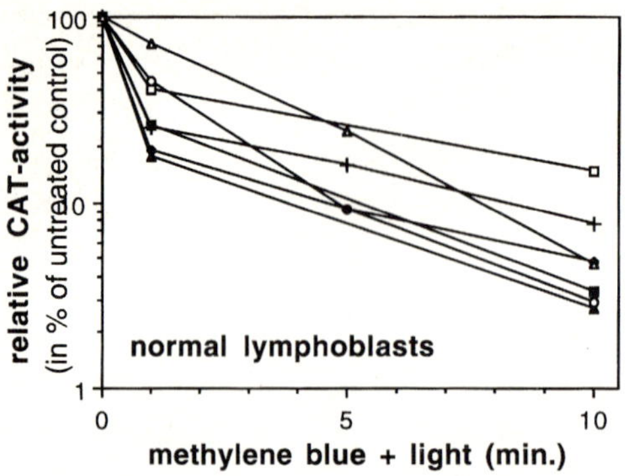

Fig. 6. Repair of singlet oxygen-induced (indirectly UV-induced) DNA damage in lymphoblasts from normal donors. Relative CAT activity (in percentage of untreated control) in cell extracts of seven normal lymphoblast lines after transfection of the plasmid pRSVcat treated with singlet oxygen. The reactivation of the damaged plasmids reflects the capacity of these host cells to repair oxidative DNA damage. Singlet oxygen was generated by photoexcitation of the photosensitizer methylene blue by visible light. Values are means of two to six independent samples. *Open squares*, GM3657; *closed triangles*, GM3715; *open circles*, GM0621; *closed squares*, GM0130; *open triangles*, KM; *plus signs*, BD; *closed circles*, TR

Figure 7 shows the repair of singlet oxygen-induced DNA damage by two DNS lines and Fig. 8, repair by the BCNS line. Neither DNS nor BCNS cells were significantly different from normal cells in their ability to repair this kind of DNA damage.

Discussion

The efficiency and fidelity of DNA end-joining from linear to circular plasmid (repair of DNA double-strand breaks) in cells from patients with DNS or BCNS were not found to be different from those of normal cells. Therefore, the suggested genetic instability in DNS and BCNS does not seem to involve DNA end-joining or repair of DNA double-strand breaks.

An increased rate of chromatid breaks and gaps after G2 irradiation was reported by Sanford et al. (1987, 1990) in cells from patients with DNS, as well as in cells from patients with the chromosome breakage syndrome ataxia telangiectasia. This chromosomal instability, found similarly with this assay in these two disorders, seems to be mediated by different molecular mechanisms, because we described abnormal joining of plasmid DNA ends in ataxia telangiectasia cells (Rünger et al. 1992), but not in DNS cells.

No defect in the repair of UVB-induced DNA damage could be detected with our "host cell reactivation assay" in the tested DNS and BCNS cell lines. This is in accordance with many other reports that could not detect a reduced repair of UV-induced DNA lesions in these two genetic disorders with an

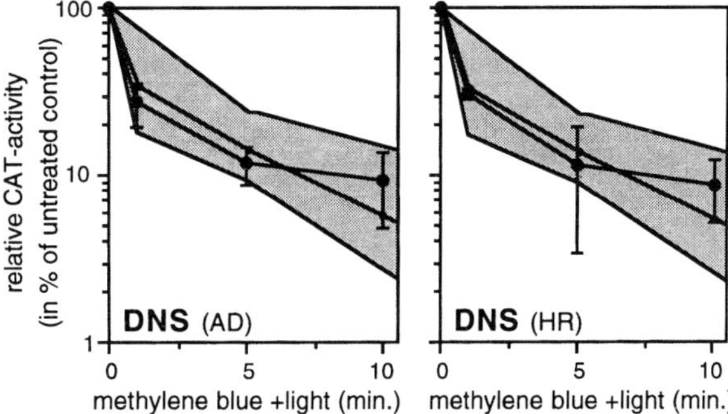

Fig. 7. Repair of singlet oxygen-induced (indirectly UV-induced) DNA damage in lymphoblasts from patients with DNS. Relative CAT activity (in percentage of untreated control) in cell extracts of the DNS lymphoblast lines AD and HR after transfection of the plasmid pRSVcat treated with singlet oxygen. The reactivation of the damaged plasmids reflects the capacity of these host cells to repair oxidative DNA damage. Singlet oxygen was generated by photoexcitation of the photosensitizer methylene blue by visible light. Values are means of three to four independent samples (± SD). The mean values of the results with seven normal cell lines (see Fig. 6) are shown in the line with *small dots*, the minimum and maximum values of the normal range are shown within the *dotted area*

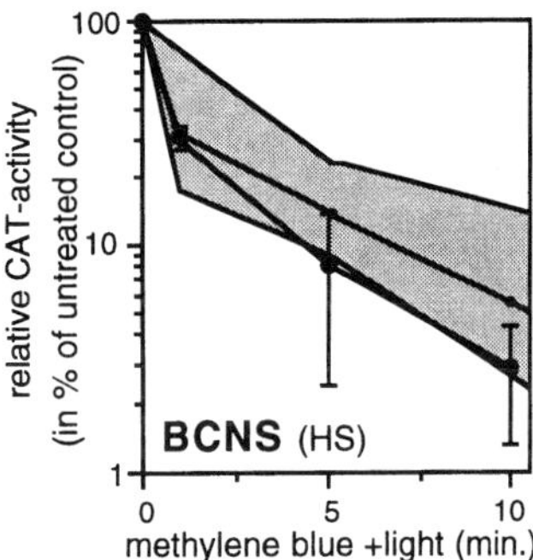

Fig. 8. Repair of singlet oxygen-induced (indirectly UV-induced) DNA damage in lymphoblasts from a patient with BCNS. Relative CAT activity (in percentage of untreated control) in cell extracts of the BCNS lymphoblast line HS after transfection of the plasmid pRSVcat treated with singlet oxygen. The reactivation of the damaged plasmids reflects the capacity of these host cells to repair oxidative DNA damage. Singlet oxygen was generated by photoexcitation of the photosensitizer methylene blue by visible light. Values are means of four independent samples (± SD). The mean values of the results with seven normal cell lines (see Fig. 6) are shown in the line with *small dots*, the minimum and maximum values of the normal range are shown within the *dotted area*

increased rate of UV-induced skin cancers (Lehmann et al. 1977; Evans and Bohr 1994). Hanson and Loow (1994) employed a very similar plasmid assay and did not find a reduced host cell reactivation of UV-irradiated plasmid DNA either. While Moriwaki et al. (1994) likewise did not find a reduced host cell reactivation of an UV-irradiated plasmid in DNS cells, they found a hypermutability and suggested that feature to be a diagnostic tool for DNS. With our assay, the mutation frequency in the transfected plasmid cannot be determined.

In the photosensitized reaction with DNA after UVA exposure, singlet oxygen is the main mediator of the indirectly induced DNA lesions. With UVA possibly playing a pivotal role in the tumorigenesis of malignant melanoma, an abnormal processing of specifically UVA-induced DNA damage is a plausible hypothesis for the increased melanoma risk in sun-exposed skin of DNS patients. However, we did not find a reduced repair of singlet oxygen-induced DNA damage either in DNS or in BCNS cells.

It is hoped that the further characterization of the underlying genetic defects in these two syndromes will soon answer the question if an impaired processing of UV-induced DNA damage is responsible for the induction of UV-induced melanomas and basal cell carcinomas in these two model syndromes, and will improve our understanding on how UV light causes skin cancer.

Acknowledgements. This work was supported by a grant from the Deutsche Forschungsgemeinschaft within the Sonderforschungsbereich 172 "Molecular Mechanisms of Carcinogenic Primary Lesions."

References

Ackerman AB, Milde P (1992) Naming acquired melanocytic nevi. Common and dysplastic, normal and atypical, or Unna, Miescher, Spitz, and Clark? Am J Dermatopathol 14: 447–453

Applegate LE, Goldberg LH, Ley RD, Ananthaswamy HN (1990) Hypersensitivity of skin fibroblasts from basal cell nevus syndrome patients to killing by ultraviolet B but not ultraviolet C radiation. Cancer Res 50: 637–641

Arlett CF, Harcourt SA (1980) Survey of radiosensitivity in a variety of human cell strains. Cancer Res 40: 926–932

Bailani MR, Bale SJ, Leffell DJ, DiGiovanni JJ, Peck GL, Poliak S, Drum MA, Pastakia B, McBride OW, Kase R (1992) Developmental defects in Gorlin syndrome related to a putative tumor suppressor gene on chromosome 9. Cell 69: 111–117

Bale AE, Bale SJ, Murli H, Ivett J, Mulvihill JJ, Pary DM (1989a) Sister chromatid exchange and chromosome fragility in the nevoid basal cell carcinoma syndrome. Cancer Genet Cytogenet 42: 273–279

Bale AE, Gailani MR, Leffell DJ (1989b) Nevoid basal cell carcinoma syndrome. J Invest Dermatol 103 [suppl 5]: 126S–130S

Bale SJ, Tucker MA (1990) Mutation rate estimate in hereditary cutaneous malignant melanoma/dysplastic nevi. Am J Med Genet 35: 293–294

Barnes DE, Lindahl T, Sedgwick B (1993) DNA repair. Curr Opin Cell Biol 5: 424–433

Cannon-Albright LA, Godgar DE, Meyer LJ, Lewis CM, Anderson DE, Fountain JW, Hegi ME, Wiseman RW, Petty EM, Bale AE (1992) Assignment of a locus of familial melanoma, MLM, to chromosome 9p13–22. Science 258: 1148–1152

Caporaso N, Greene MH, Tsai S, Pickle LW, Mulvihill JJ (1987) Cytogenetics in hereditary malignant melanoma and dysplastic nevus syndrome: is dysplastic nevus syndrome a chromosome instability disorder? Cancer Genet Cytogenet 24: 299–314

Chan GL, Little JB (1983) Cultured diploid fibroblasts from patients with the nevoid basal cell carcinoma syndrome are hypersensitive to killing by ionizing radiation. Am J Pathol 111: 50–55

Eastman A (1987) An improvement to the novel rapid assay for chloramphenicol acetyltransferase gene expression. Biotechniques 5: 730–732

Epe B, Pflaum M, Boiteux S (1993) DNA damage induced by photosensitizers in cellular and cell free systems. Mutat Res 299: 135–145

Evans MK, Bohr VA (1994) Gene-specific DNA repair of UV-induced cyclobutane pyrimidine dimers in some cancer-prone and premature aging human syndromes. Mutat Res 314: 221–231

Featherstone T, Tayler AMR, Harnden DG (1983) Studies on the radiosensitivity of cells from patients with basal cell nevus syndrome. Am J Hum Genet 35: 58–66

Gorman CM, Howard BH, Reeves H (1983) Expression of recombination plasmids in mammalian cells is enhanced by sodium butyrate. Nucleic Acids Res 11: 7631–7648

Hansson J, Loow H (1994) Normal reactivation of plasmid DNA inactivated by UV irradiation by lymphocytes from individuals with hereditary dysplastic naevus syndrome. Melanoma Res 4: 163–167

Hecht F, Hecht BK (1988) Chromosome rearrangements in dysplastic nevus syndrome predisposed to malignant melanoma. Cancer Genet Cytogenet 35: 73–78

Hoeijmakers JHJ (1993) Nucleotide excision repair II: from yeast to mammals. Trends Genet 9: 211–217

Hussussian CJ, Struewing JP, Goldstein AM, Higgins PA, Ally DS, Sheahan MD, Clark WH Jr, Tucker MA, Dracopoli NC (1994) Germline p16 mutations in familial melanoma. Nat Genet 8: 15–21

Jaspers NGJ, Roza-deJong EJM, Donselaar IG, van Velzen-Tillemans JTM, van Hemel JO, Rümke P, van der Kamp AWM (1987) Sister chromatid exchanges, hyperdiploidy and chromosomal rearrangements studied in cells from melanoma-prone individuals belonging to families with the dysplastic nevus syndrome. Cancer Genet Cytogenet 24: 33–43

Kraemer KH, Greene MH, Tarone R (1983) Dysplastic nevi and cutaneous melanoma risk. Lancet 2: 1076–1077

Kraemer KH, Lee MM, Scotto J (1987) Xeroderma pigmentosum. Cutaneous, ocular, and neurologic abnormalities in 830 published cases (review article). Arch Dermatol 123: 241–250

Lehmann AR, Kirk-Bell S, Arlett CF, Harcourt SA, deWeed-Kastelein EA, Keijzer W, Hall-Smith P (1977) Repair of ultraviolet light damage in a variety of human fibroblast cell lines. Cancer Res 37: 904–910

Little JB, Nichols WW, Troilo P, Nagasawa H, Strong LC (1989) Radiation sensitivity of cell strains from families with genetic disorders predisposing to radiation-induced cancer. Cancer Res 49: 4705–4714

Lundgren K, Wulf HC (1988) Cytotoxicity and genotoxicity of UVA irradiation in Chinese hamster ovary cells measured by specific locus mutations, sister chromatid exchanges and chromosome aberrations. Photochem Photobiol 47: 559–563

Marghoob AA, Kopf AW, Rigel DS, Bart RS, Friedman RJ, Yadav S, Abadir M, Sanfilippo L, Silverman MK, Vossaert KA (1994) Risk of cutaneous malignant melanoma in patients with 'classic' atypical-mole syndrome. A case-control study. Arch Dermatol 130: 993–998

Moriwaki S, Tarone RE, Kraemer KH (1994) A potential laboratory test for dysplastic nevus syndrome: ultraviolet hypermutability of a shuttle vector plasmid. J Invest Dermatol 103: 7–12

Müller E, Boiteux RP, Cunningham RP, Epe B (1990) Enzymatic recognition of DNA modifications induced by singlet oxygen and photosensitizers. Nucleic Acids Res 18: 5969–5973

National Institutes of Health Consensus Conference (1992) Diagnosis and treatment of early melanoma. JAMA 268: 1314–1319

Neitzel H (1986) A routine method for the establishment of permanent growing lymphoblastoid cell lines. Hum Genet 73: 320–326

Neumann JR, Morency CA, Russian KO (1987) A novel rapid assay for chloramphenicol acetyltransferase gene expression. Biotechniques 5: 444–447

Rünger TM, Bröcker EB (1995) Genetische Faktoren bei der Entstehung und Progression maligner Melanome. Hautarzt 46: 394–399

Rünger TM, Kraemer KH (1989) Joining of linear plasmid DNA is reduced and errorprone in Bloom's syndrome cells. EMBO J 8: 1419–1425

Rünger TM, Möller K (1994) Molekularbiologische Aspekte der photoinduzierten Hypermutabilität bei Genodermatosen. Aktuel Dermatol 20: 89–96

Rünger TM, Poot M, Kraemer KH (1992) Abnormal processing of transfected plasmid DNA in cells from patients with ataxia telangiectasia. Mutat Res 293: 47–54

Rünger TM, Sobotta P, Dekant B, Möller K, Bauer C, Kraemer KH (1993) In vivo assessment of DNA ligation efficiency and fidelity in cells from patients with Fanconi anemia and other cancer-prone hereditary disorders. Toxicol Lett 67: 309–324

Rünger TM, Klein CE, Becker JC, Bröcker EB (1994a) The role of genetic instability, adhesion, cell motility, and immune escape mechanisms in melanoma progression. Curr Opin Oncol 6: 188–196

Rünger TM, Bauer C, Möller K (1994b) Hypermutable ligation of DNA ends in cells from patients with Werner syndrome. J Invest Dermatol 102: 45–48

Rünger TM, Epe B, Möller K (1995a) Processing of UVB and singlet oxygen-induced DNA damage in xeroderma pigmentosum cells. J Invest Dermat 105: 68–73

Rünger TM, Epe B, Möller K (1995b) Processing of directly and indirectly UV-induced DNA damage in human cells. In: Garbe C, Schmitz S, Orfanos CE (eds) Skin cancer. Basic science, clinical research and treatment. (Recent results in cancer research, vol 139) Springer, Berlin Heidelberg New York, pp 31–42

Sanford KK, Tarone RE, Parshad R, Tucker M, Greene MH, Jones GM (1987) Hypersensitivity to G–2 chromatid radiation damage in familial dysplastic nevus syndrome. Lancet 14: 1111–1115

Sanford KK, Parshad R, Price FM, Jones GM, Tarone RE, Eierman L, Hale P, Waldmann TA (1990) Enhanced chromosome breakage in blood lymphocytes after G2 phase X-irradiation, a marker of the ataxia-telangiectasia gene. J Natl Cancer Inst 82: 1050–1054

Sarto F, Mazzotti D, Tomanin R, Corsi GC, Pesericco A (1989) No evidence of chromosomal instability in nevoid basal-cell carcinoma syndrome. Mutat Res 225: 21–26

Schmitz S, Garbe C, Tebbe B, Orfanos CE (1994) Langwellige ultraviolette Strahlung und Hautkrebs. Hautarzt 45: 517–525

Setlow RB, Grist E, Thompson K, Woodhead AD (1993) Wavelengths effective in induction of malignant melanoma. Proc Natl Acad Sci USA 90: 6666–6670

Shafei-Benaissa E, Huret JL, Larregue M, Babin P, Tanzer J, Decrozailles JM, Savage JR (1994) Checks for chromosomal instability in Gorlin and non-Gorlin basal-cell carcinoma patients. Mutat Res 308: 1–9

Shanley S, Ratcliffe J, Hockey A, Haan E, Oley C, Ravine D, Martin N, Wicking C, Chenevix-Trench G (1994) Nevoid basal cell carcinoma syndrome: review of 118 affected individuals. Am J Med Genet 50: 282–290

Shapiro PE (1992) Making sense of the dysplastic nevus controversy. A unifying perspective. Am J Dermatopathol 14: 350–356

Swerdlow AJ, English JS, MacKie RM, O'Doherty CJ, Hunter JA, Clark J, Hole DJ (1988) Fluorescence lights, ultraviolet lamps and risk of cutaneous melanoma. Br Med J 297: 647–650

Traupe H, Macher E, Hamm H, Happle R (1989) Mutation rate estimates are not compatible with autosomal dominant inheritance of the dysplastic nevus "syndrome". Am J Med Genet 32: 155–157

Trevis J (1992) Closing in on melanoma susceptibility genes. Science 258: 1080–1081

Van Haerigen A, Bergman W, Nelson MR (1989) Exclusion of the dysplastic nevus syndrome (DNS) locus from the short arm of chromosome 1 by linkage studies in Dutch families. Genomics 5: 45–55

Van Weelden H, de Gruijl FR, van der Putter SCJ, Toonstra J, van der Leun JC (1988) The carcinogenic risks of modern tanning equipment: is UV-A safer than UV-B? Arch Dermatol Res 280: 300–307

Wainwright B (1994) Familial melanoma and p16 – a hung jury. Nature Genet 8: 3–5

Walter SD, Marrett LD, From L, Hertzman C, Shannon HS, Roy P (1990) The association of cutaneous malignant melanoma with the use of sunbeds and sunlamps. Am J Epidemiol 131: 232–243

Wicking C, Berkman J, Wainwright B, Chenevix Trench G (1994) Fine genetic mapping of the gene for nevoid basal cell carcinoma syndrome. Genomics 22: 505–511

Exploring the Role of Oxygen in Fanconi's Anemia

W. Liebetrau[1], T.M. Rünger[2], A. Baumer[1], C. Henning[1], O. Gross[1], D. Schindler[1], M. Poot[3], and H. Hoehn[1]

[1]Department of Human Genetics, Biozentrum, University of Würzburg, Am Hubland, 97074 Würzburg, Germany
[2]Department of Dermatology, University of Würzburg, Josef-Schneider-Str. 2, 97080 Würzburg, Germany
[3]Molecular Probes, 4849 Pitchford Ave., Eugene, Oregon, USA

Introduction

Fanconi's anemia (FA) is a clinically and genetically heterogeneous disease that presents with a wide spectrum of clinical manifestations, ranging from severe congenital malformations to a completely normal phenotype (Auerbach et al. 1989). The onset of progressive bone marrow failure may occur in early childhood or as late as at 40 years of age. The cellular phenotype of FA consists of chromosomal instability, a cell cycle defect, and increased sensitivity to certain clastogens, as well as oxygen (Hoehn et al. 1989). In analogy to what has recently become known about the embryo-protective role of the p53 gene product (Nicol et al. 1995), leaky protection against endogenous free radical-mediated DNA damage could explain both the variable pattern of developmental abnormalities and the variable onset of bone marrow failure in Fanconi's anemia. Cell culture studies have found no evidence for defective free radical scavenger systems (Gille et al. 1987; Joenje and Gille 1989), but they have also shown that in FA cells, chromosomal breakage and cell growth are influenced strongly by oxygen (Joenje et al. 1981; Schindler and Hoehn 1988). In this chapter we review a number of approaches by which we hope to clarify the pathogenetic role of oxygen in Fanconi's anemia.

Cell Cycle Studies

FA cells display a cell cycle disturbance that consists of delay and arrest during the S and G2 phases of the cell cycle (Kubbies et al. 1985). Figure 1 shows an experiment in which early passage fibroblast cultures from FA patients are first synchronized for 48 h by serum deprivation, followed by trypsinization and seeding at 10^4 cells/cm^2 in the presence of 65 μM bromodeoxyuridine (BrdU). The figure depicts one-dimensional flow histograms of cells harvested at 30–84 h after seeding. Because these cells were grown in the presence of BrdU and

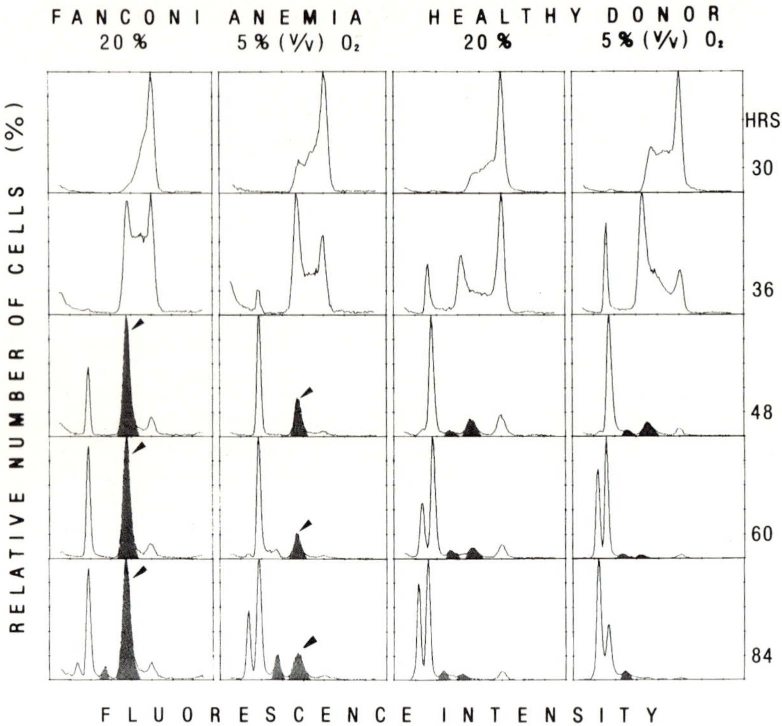

Fig. 1. Fanconi's anemia (FA) fibroblasts show pronounced arrest in the G2 phase of the cell cycle when grown at 20% oxygen compared to near-normal G2 fractions when grown at 5% oxygen for the indicated periods of time in culture; the differences are indicated by *arrowheads*. No abnormal G2 phase arrest is seen in healthy donors [bromodeoxyuridine (BrdU)-Hoechst flow cytometry]

stained with Hoechst dye 33258, the fluorescence signals emitted by the replicating cells appear to the left instead of the right of the noncycling G0/G1 peak (so-called quench effect, Kubbies et al. 1985). As these replicating cells progress through the cell cycle, the fraction of cells that enters and remains within the G2 compartments of the first and second cell cycle (shaded peaks in Fig. 1) is much more prominent in FA than in control cultures. However, as soon as FA cells are exposed to hypoxic instead of ambient oxygen cell culture conditions, their respective G2 phase fractions return to near-normal levels. The histograms in Fig. 1 also show that control cells benefit from exposure to hypoxic culture conditions, but this benefit (in terms of reduction of the G2 phase fraction) is much greater for FA than for control cells. This observation was confirmed in other FA fibroblast strains (Table 1). These experiments thus represented a key observation, proving that the G2 phase blockage of FA cells is mediated by oxygen, and that the cell cycle of FA cells is much more sensitive to ambient levels of oxygen than that of control cells.

Table 1. Cell cycle distributions of primary fibroblasts (in percent) after cultivation for 72 h at several oxygen concentrations[a]

Cell cycle compartment	Oxygen concentration (% v/v)		
	5	20	35
Fanconi's anemia			
G1	64.4 ± 4.1	66.7 ± 2.9	68.4 ± 3.0
S	21.9 ± 2.3	12.1 ± 4.0	5.2 ± 2.1
G2	13.6 ± 3.9	21.3 ± 5.4	26.4 ± 5.3
Control			
G1	68.9 ± 3.3	69.7 ± 1.6	71.0 ± 1.3
S	21.6 ± 4.6	20.0 ± 2.3	17.1 ± 2.6
G2	9.6 ± 2.8	10.3 ± 1.6	12.0 ± 1.6

[a]Three Fanconi's anemia and control strains, respectively, were selected for similar growth performance. Following subcultivation, 4000 cells per cm^2 were seeded in 80-cm^2 flasks and grown in Dulbecco's modified Eagle's medium (DMEM) containing 16% fetal bovine serum (FBS). The experiments were performed simultaneously in incubators with the indicated oxygen concentrations in water-saturated atmosphere. The numbers represent mean ± standard deviation.

Cell Response to Oxidative Stress

Given the hypersensitivity of FA fibroblasts to ambient oxygen it seemed important to find out whether FA cells are defective in the detoxification of reactive oxygen species. Since the intracellular levels of these species can be modulated by the iron concentration, we tested the effects of iron overload and iron chelation in lymphoblastoid cell lines derived from FA patients. Figure 2 depicts the relative growth of two FA and two control cell lines in the presence of increasing concentrations of Fe-Nitriloacetate (Fe-NTA). The FA lines are clearly more sensitive to increasing amounts of Fe-NTA than the control lines. Both the formation of 8-hydroxydeoxyguanosine and direct DNA strand breakage have been observed following exposure to Fe-NTA (Umemura et al. 1990; Toyokuni and Sagripanti 1993). Since ferric ions are known to promote the formation of hydroxyl radicals via the Fenton reaction, it appears that FA cells are more strongly inhibited in their growth by such putative radicals than are control cells. As hydroxyl radicals cannot to detoxified by the conventional scavenging systems, they transmit free radicals to lipids and proteins within nuclear chromatin, possibly giving rise to DNA-protein crosslinks (von Sonntag 1987).

The reverse experiment (Fig. 3) consisted of withdrawal of cellular iron via the iron chelator o-phenantrolin (o-Ph). o-Ph inhibits the Fenton reaction and thereby the formation of the hydroxyl radical. As shown in Fig. 3, three FA cell lines grew better in the presence of o-Ph than three non-FA cell lines. Both

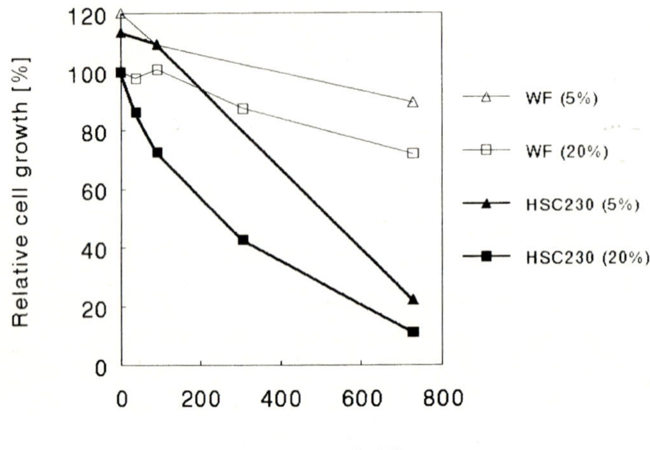

Fig. 2. Relative cell growth of FA and control lymphoblastoid cell lines in the presence of increasing concentrations of Fe-nitriloacetate. Relative growth was assessed after 72-h treatment intervals via BrdU-Hoechst/ethidium bromide flow cytometry. *Solid symbols* and *lines*, FA cell lines; *open symbols* and *light lines*, control cultures

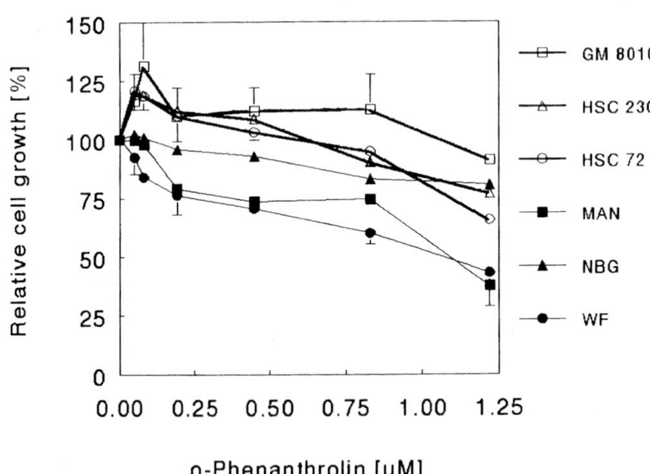

Fig. 3. Relative cell growth of FA and control lymphoblastoid cell lines in the presence of increasing concentrations of o-phenanthrolin. Relative growth was measured after 72-h exposures via BrdU-Hoechst/ethidium bromide flow cytometry. *Open symbols* and *solid lines*, FA cell lines; *solid symbols* and *light lines*, control cell lines. *Error bars*, mean ± SD of three cell lines each

experiments thus seem to indicate that FA cells are particularly sensitive to the presence of hydroxyl radicals.

Unpublished cell cycle studies show that exposure to Fe-NTA increases the G2-phase cell fraction of FA cells by 20%–30%, whereas exposure to o-Ph decreases the G2-phase cell fraction of FA cells by nearly the same percentage (M. Poot et al., in preparation). Since both agents presumably act by respectively increasing and decreasing the formation of hydroxyl radicals, this highly reactive type of oxygen species appears to be a prime candidate for causing the pathognomonic G2-phase defect in Fanconi's anemia cells.

Signature Mutations in FA Cells?

Using a sensitive reversion assay that can detect single and double mutations within the same codon of the M13-encoded *lac* Z alpha gene, Reid and Loeb (1993) showed that oxygen can produce double CC $\rightarrow$ TT mutations. In another assay McBride et al. (1991) showed that the most frequent mutations induced by oxygen are G $\rightarrow$ C transversions, followed by C $\rightarrow$ T transitions and G $\rightarrow$ T transversions. In that assay the mutagenic spectrum of oxygen free radicals was produced by the aerobic incubation of single-stranded M13mp2 DNA with Fe^{2+}. We used the shuttle vector plasmid pZ189 (Seidman et al. 1985) that replicates in human and bacterial cells and that carries a small bacterial marker gene, the activity of which can be determined in a standard microbiological assay. pZ189 contains the origin of replication and large tumor (T)-antigen gene from SV 40, information for replication and maintenance in bacteria from pBR 327, and the marker gene *supF*, which encodes a suppressor tRNA that suppresses an amber mutation in the β-galactosidase gene (*lac* Z) in an indicator strain of *Escherichia coli*. Bacterial colonies containing plasmids with mutant or wild-type suppressor tRNA genes can be identified by color (wild-type are blue, mutants are light blue or white). Plasmids with mutant tRNA genes can be isolated and sequenced.

Epstein-Barr virus-transformed lymphoblastoid cells from a patient with FA (GM8010) and from a repair-proficient normal individual (GM3715) were obtained from the Human Genetic Cell Repository (Camden, NJ, USA). They were routinely grown as suspension cultures in RPMI 1640 medium (GIBCO/BRL, Gaithersburg, MD, USA) supplemented with 10% fetal calf serum (GIBCO/BRL). Transfection of pZ189 into FA and normal lymphoblasts was achieved by electroporation with a BioRad Gene Pulser (Munich, Germany). After 48 h plasmid DNA was extracted with plasmid isolation columns (Qiagen, Hilden, Germany). Digestion with the endonuclease Dpn I ensured that only plasmids replicated within the host cells were recovered.

The replicated purified plasmid was used to transform competent MBM7070 *E. coli* indicator bacteria by electroporation with a BioRad Gene Pulser under standard conditions, and bacteria were spread onto LB agar dishes containing ampicillin, isopropyl-β-D-galactoside (IPTG), and X-gal.

The proportion of mutant white or light blue compared to the total number of colonies gave an estimation of mutation frequency. White or light blue colonies indicating an inactivated *supF* gene were isolated and the plasmids were further purified from overnight cultures with Qiagen tip-20 columns (Qiagen). To characterize the recovered mutants, their size was compared to the size of the wild-type plasmids by agarose gel electrophoresis. The base sequence of the *supF* gene was determined by the dideoxy sequencing procedure using the PRISM Ready Reaction DyeDeoxy terminator cycle sequencing kit and an Applied Biosystem sequencer (Applied Biosystems, Weiterstadt, Germany). To ensure that the mutants were of independent origin, we concluded identical mutations only if they were derived from different transfections.

Table 2 shows the mutation frequency in the plasmid after passage through several lymphoblastoid cell lines. The spontaneous mutation frequency in control cells at ambient oxygen was 0.019 ± 0.002%, whereas replication of pZ189 in FA cells increased the mutation frequency up to four fold (0.076 ± 0.02%).

Plasmids with mutations inactivating the *supF* suppressor gene were purified and characterized by plasmid size, presence of restriction sites, and DNA sequencing. More than 80 independent plasmids were analyzed from control and FA cells. As in earlier studies (Seetharam et al. 1991) four major classes of mutations were observed: those with (1) single base substitutions, (2) tandem mutations, (3) multiple mutations, and (4) deletion mutations. Some of the deletions were observed because of loss of the *Eco*RI restriction site, or due to

Table 2. Effects of oxygen on mutation frequency of pZ189 plasmid in control and Fanconi's anemia lymphoblasts at 20% O_2

Transfection experiment label	Fanconi GM8010		Control GM3715	
	No. of *supF*$^-$ colonies	Mutants (%)	No. of *supF*$^-$ colonies	Mutants (%)
A	10/12000	0.083		
B	24/20800	0.115		
C	11/17000	0.064		
D	13/19080	0.068		
E	8/15400	0.052		
F	14/20515	0.068		
KI			8/45220	0.017
KII			10/54960	0.018
KIII			5/22968	0.021
KIV			6/33360	0.017
KV			5/23184	0.021
Total	80/104795	0.076	34/179692	0.019
S.D.		±0.021		±0.002

S.D., standard deviation.

increased mobility in agarose gel electrophoresis of the linearized plasmid. All deletions found exceeded more than 100 bp, and the plasmids often lacked the entire *supF* gene. Of the control cells, 18% harbored deletions, whereas deletions amounted to 30% in the analyzed plasmids following passage through FA cells.

All six types of base substitutions were observed. There were no significant differences in the proportions of transition or transversion mutations between plasmids replicated in FA and normal lymphoblasts. It is perhaps relevant that 71% of the plasmids that were passed through FA cells and 65% of those passed through normal cells had base substitutions involving G:C base pairs.

The location of base substitution mutations within the coding sequence of the *supF* gene is shown in Fig. 4 for the FA cell line GM8010. In plasmids recovered from both normal and FA cells, the location of mutations within the *supF* gene was nonrandom, and there were areas of intense mutagenic activity (hotspots). In recovered plasmids from FA cells a mutational hotspot was located at base 117 within the *supF* gene of pZ189; the frequency of that particular mutation was 22% in FA vs 4.7% in controls. In other words, with FA host cells one out of three plasmids analyzed was mutated at base 117.

The fourfold increase of mutation frequency in FA as opposed to control cells suggests that there is an increased endogenous mutation pressure in FA cells. In addition, more deletions were found in the sequenced plasmids as in previous studies with the pZ189 vector. Reactive oxygen species are known to cause double-strand breaks such that deletions could arise. In the case of FA host cells, we detected 30% deletions vs 18% deletions in control cells. Altogether, the increase of deletion types of mutations in FA cells is in agreement with the chromosome instability and defective cell cycle observed in FA cells.

In summary, the results from our mutation analysis provide no evidence for similar types of "signature" mutations in FA cells grown at ambient oxygen concentrations as previously described in naked DNA (McBride et al. 1991). However, both mutation frequencies and mutation hotspots were significantly different between plasmids that were passed through FA cells as opposed to controls. Moreover, preliminary data of shuttle vector experiments conducted at hypoxic (5% v/v) conditions indicate that this difference between FA and control cells all but disappears. It therefore seems that the increased sensitivity of FA cells to oxygen is in fact responsible for the observed effects.

Search for Genes that Convey Oxygen Sensitivity

To screen for genes that may reflect the increased sensitivity of FA cells we used the differential display technique developed by Pardee and coworkers (Liang and Pardee 1992; Liang et al. 1993). This technique serves as a tool to detect and characterize even subtle changes of gene expression in eukaryotic cells. The basic principle is to amplify messenger RNAs systematically with

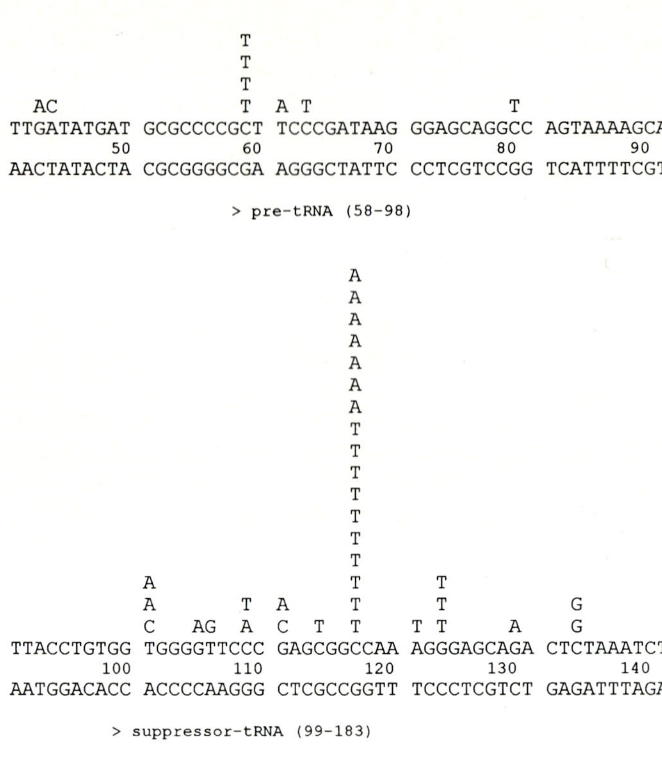

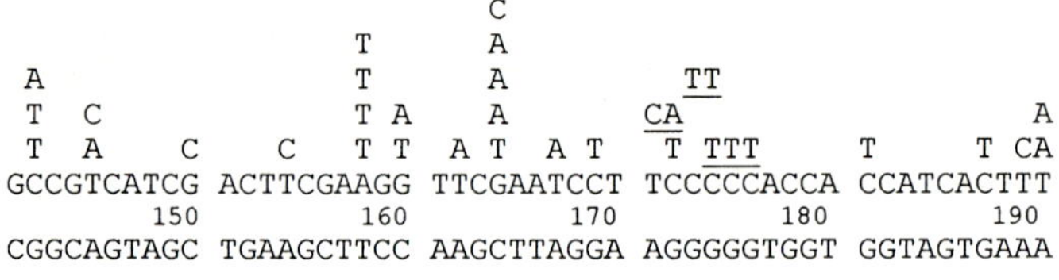


```
 C
 TT
 TT
 TT
CAAAAGTCCG
       200
GTTTTCAGGC
```

3′flanking region (184-200)

Fig. 4. Map of sites of point mutations in the double-stranded *supF* gene of the plasmid pZ189 after passage through the FA lymphoblast line GM8010. Each base substitution is indicated above the mutated base in the upper strand. Tandem and triple base substitutions are indicated by a *line*

random primers and then resolve their 3′ termini on a denaturating polyacrylamide gel. Our screen for candidate genes mediating oxygen sensitivity was based on positive selection at the mRNA level for genes expressed in FA fibroblasts and control cells under defined oxygen concentrations and as a function of cell cycle phase.

Total RNAs were extracted from cells with TRIzol Reagent (Gibco BRL, Eggenstein, Germany) and precipitated with isopropanol. After suspension in diethylpyrocarbonate (DEPC)-treated distilled water, 20 μg of each RNA was treated with 20 U of RQ RNAse-free DNAse I (Promega, Madison, WI, USA) at 37 °C for 30 min and precipitated with ethanol. After suspension in DEPC-treated distilled water, 0.4 μg of RNA was incubated with 200 U of Superscript II RNAse H-negative reverse transcriptase (GIBCO BRL), 40 U of RNAse inhibitor (Promega), and 4 μl of 10 μM T12MA, T12MG, T12MC or T12MT primer in 40 μl of reverse transcriptase (RT) buffer [25 mM Tris, pH 8.3, 37.6 mM KCl, 1.5 mM $MgCl_2$, 5 mM dithiothreitol (DTT), 20 μM dNTP] at 37 °C for 1 h. After heat inactivation of the reverse transcriptase at 95 °C for 5 min, 2 μl of the sample was used for polymerase chain reaction (PCR) in 20 μl of PCR buffer (10 mM Tris, pH 8.4, 50 mM KCl, 1.5 mM $MgCl_2$, 0.001% gelatin, and 2 μM dNTP) with 2 μl of 20 μM arbitrary primer (Liang and Pardee 1992; Liang et al. 1993) and 2 μl of 10 μM T12MA, T12MG, T12MC, or T12MT primer, 0.2 μl of (alpha-32-p)dATP (Amersham, Buckinghamshire, UK; 1200 Ci/mmol), and 0.2 μl of Taq polymerase (GIBCO BRL). The parameters for PCR were as follows: 40 cycles of cycling step (94 °C for 15 s, 40 °C for 2 min, 72 °C for 20 s) followed by 72 °C elongation step for 5 min (GENamp PCR system 9600, Perkin-Elmer Cetus, Norwalk, CT, USA). The amplified cDNAs were separated on a 6% sequencing gel. The positive bands were excised from the dried gel, boiled in 100 μl of distilled water for 15 min, precipitated with ethanol and resuspended in 10 μl of distilled water, and stored at –70 °C.

Using the four degenerate T12MN primers in combination with an arbitrary 10mer, transcription products from Fanconi's anemia and control fibroblasts were compared for differentially displayed products.

Figure 5 shows examples of signals that were differentially expressed (marked by arrows). Four bands were repeatedly detected in FA cell cultures exposed to ambient oxygen cell culture conditions. These bands were not seen in FA cultures exposed to 5% (v/v) oxygen. They are currently being isolated, reamplified, and sequenced. As a result of these efforts we hope to find genes that mediate in the oxygen sensitivity of FA-fibroblasts.

Mitochondrial DNA Mutations in Tissues of Individuals Affected by Fanconi Anemia

This final aspect of our approach aims at investigating the mitochondrial status in a variety of tissues of Fanconi's anemia (FA) patients. The aim is to de-

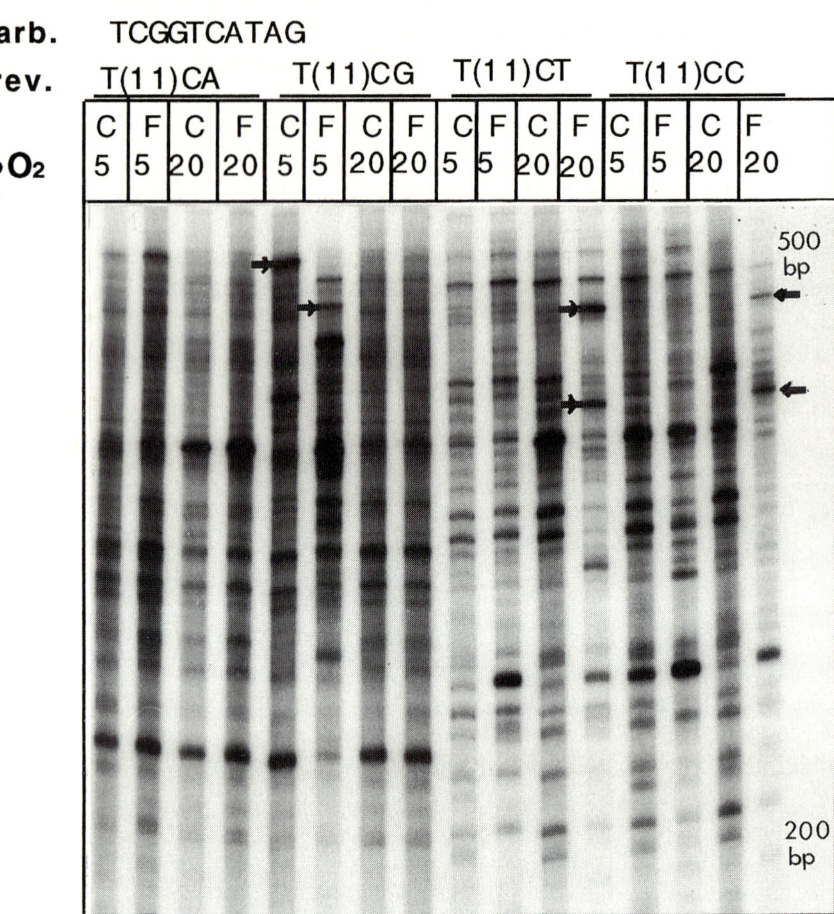

Fig. 5. Differential display of mRNAs from a control (*C*) versus a Fanconi's anemia (*F*) fibroblast cell line. Cells were grown under reduced (5% v/v) and ambient (20% v/v) oxygen cell culture conditions. Total RNAs from G2 phases were reverse-transcribed with primers T(11)CA, T(11)CG, T(11)CT, or T(11)CC and polymerase chain reaction (PCR)- amplified in combination with a short arbitrary primer (TCGGTCATAG). Several candidate cDNA bands that appear to be differentially expressed are marked by *arrowheads*

termine whether the oxygen intolerance and chromosomal instability typical of FA fibroblast cells cultured in vitro are also reflected in an increased level of mtDNA mutations. In view of the role played by mitochondria in the oxidative pathways, it is suggested that this organelle and its genetic information (i.e., mtDNA), may be a major target for the mutagenic effects of oxygen, possibly in a more accentuated manner in FA than in normal aging. In order to test this hypothesis, the mtDNA profile in tissues of FA patients was examined by PCR amplification, with particular emphasis on the detection of large deletions. Random mutations caused by free radicals would include base modifications, single- and double-strand breakages, as well as "fixed" mutations such as base substitutions and deletions/duplications. The mtDNA mutation most frequently detected in aging and a number of mitochondrial diseases is a deletion spanning 4977 bp (also denoted "common 5-kb deletion"), which thus represents a good marker for the occurrence of random mtDNA mutations. Thus, primer pairs were designed to encompass this "hotspot" region of mtDNA (5–8 kb), whereby the common 5-kb deletion and other large deletions occurring between the two priming sites would be represented by short PCR products.

The PCR amplification reactions were performed on total cellular DNA isolated from tissue samples of three individuals affected by FA (a 20-week-old fetus, a 17-year-old patient, and a 28-year-old patient), and blood samples from seven FA patients ranging from fetal to 27-year-old patients, as well as tissue and blood samples of control subjects.

The results obtained to date indicate that large mtDNA deletions in the hotspot region of the mitochondrial genome occur in only a few of the FA tissues we examined.

In particular, unusual PCR products of mtDNA origin (as tested by primer shift PCR reactions) were detected in the blood of a 7-year-old FA patient (Fig. 6). According to the size of the PCR products (as estimated from 1% agarose gels), the approximate length of the most abundant mtDNA deletions in this sample was 5.4 kb, 5 kb, and 4.7 kb.

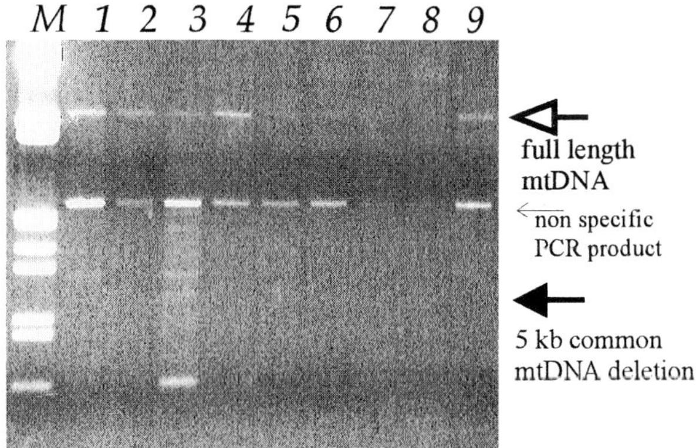

Fig. 6. 1% Agarose gel showing PCR products obtained from DNA samples of FA patients using mtDNA-specific primers (L7901 and H13851). Technical details are described in Baumer et al. (1994). Total cellular DNA extracted from blood samples was used in the amplification reactions: *lane 1*, FA fetus (umbilical cord blood); *lane 2*, 5-year-old; *lane 3*, 7-year-old; *lane 4*, 15-year-old; *lane 5*, 17-year-old; *lanes 6 and 7*, two 28-year-old patients; and finally, two control subjects, *lane 8 and 9*, a 21-year-old and 86-year-old, respectively. *M*, DNA size marker: Lambda DNA/*Hin*dIII + *Eco*RI

The analyses of more tissue samples of FA patients will be needed to establish whether such unusual PCR patterns may indeed occur as a consequence of the FA genotype.

Discussion

Compared to control cells, Fanconi's anemia cells grow more poorly in culture; we have previously reported that this growth deficit is caused by a characteristic disturbance of cell cycle progression (Kubbies et al. 1985). More recently, we have shown that this cell cycle disturbance, which mainly consists of G2-phase blockage, is as diagnostic for nonleukemic FA cells as is their sensitivity to crosslinking agents (Seyschab et al. 1995). In this chapter we demonstrate that the accumulation of cells in the G2-phase of the cell cycle that is germane to FA cells grown at ambient oxygen concentrations can be significantly reduced by exposing these cells to hypoxic (5% v/v) cell culture conditions. Moreover, by either increasing or decreasing the supply of ferric ions in FA lymphoblastoid cell lines, their growth pattern and cell cycle behavior can be changed. Based on these observations it appears that FA cells are particularly sensitive to the action of hydroxyl radicals. Since the common antioxidant defense system appear to function well in FA cells (Gille et al. 1987) and since there is no specific defense system against hydroxyl radicals, we postulate a crucial role of this moiety in Fanconi anemia cells.

Saito et al. (1993) have recently questioned whether the oxygen sensitivity of FA cells is a primary manifestation of the underlying gene defect. Their critique was based on the fact that SV40-large T-transformed FA fibroblasts lose their oxygen sensitivity. However, in a subsequent paper, these authors themselves were able to show that loss oxygen sensitivity is a general phenomenon in human diploid fibroblast cultures following transformation with SV40 (Saito et al. 1995). As such, it does not appear to be specific to the FA genotype but rather must be seen as a consequence of altered gene regulation during the course of the transformation process.

It would of course be of interest whether the only FA gene that has been cloned to date (FAC) has a function in oxygen metabolism. Although the gene and its deduced amino acid sequence have been published for several years (Strathdee et al. 1992), there is no clue so far regarding a possible function of the FAC gene. On the basis of prototype motifs found both at the DNA and at the protein level, our own group has postulated a nuclear function for the FAC gene (Liebetrau et al. 1995). However, this proposal is at variance with the preferential cytoplasmic location of the FAC gene product (Youssoufian 1994; Yamashita et al. 1994). Both findings might be reconciled if one postulates that the FAC protein is stored in the cytoplasm, and that transport into the cell nucleus and activation occur only in response to DNA damage (Liebetrau et al. 1995). Such a mechanism has recently been described in a candidate gene for ataxia telangiectasia (Jung et al. 1995).

Our studies with the shuttle vector system failed to provide evidence for signature-type mutations in the *supF* indicator gene as has been reported by Larry Loeb's group with naked DNA exposed to oxygen (McBride et al. 1991; Reid and Loeb 1993). Nevertheless, a fourfold increase in overall mutation frequency, and at least one mutation hotspot were observed in the present study for plasmids passed through FA lymphoid cell lines. We have preliminary data that suggest that this difference in mutability between plasmids passed through FA and control cells is abolished if such experiments are performed at low-oxygen conditions (5% v/v). There is little doubt that reactive oxygen species constitute an important cause of DNA damage and mutation (Moody and Hassan 1982; Moraes et al. 1989). FA cells are known to exhibit more 8-hydroxydeoxyguanine (8-OH-dG) than control cells (Takeuchi and Morimoto 1993), and it has been shown that 8-OH-dG mispairs with deoxyadenosine, leading to G:C $\rightarrow$ T:A transversions (Shibutani et al. 1991; Cheng et al. 1992). Over 70% of the mutations observed in our study occurred at G:C basepairs. It therefore appears reasonable to assume that the results of our mutation studies reflect differences in the behavior between normal and FA cells that are chiefly due to their different degrees of oxygen sensitivity.

In order to isolate and define specific genes that may play a role in oxygen metabolism in FA cells, we adapted the differential display technique originally developed by Liang and Pardee (1992). Although we were able to show that a number of messenger RNAs are differentially expressed in FA cells grown at 5% vs 20% (v/v) oxygen conditions, reamplification and sequencing of the respective bands have not been completed to date. Likewise, only preliminary data are available from our attempts to see whether the mitochondrial genome of FA patients exhibits genetic instability akin to that of the nuclear genome. Only one, or possibly two, of seven patients tested so far show evidence for the common (4977 bp) deletion. As this type of deletion has been found only in the mononuclear blood cells of older individuals (Baumer et al. 1994), our finding of such a deletion in two affected children may be highly significant. More patients and solid tissues (such as muscle) need to be examined in order to determine whether the mitochondrial genome of FA patients is as unstable as their nuclear genome. If our assumption is correct that the genetic instability in FA cells is in large part due to their increased sensitivity to reactive oxygen species, the mitochondrial genome, which is located in proximity to free radical generation sites, should likewise be affected.

References

Auerbach AD, Rogatko A, Schroeder-Kurth TM (1989) International Fanconi anemia registry: relation of clinical symptoms to diepoxybutane sensitivity. Blood 73: 391–396

Baumer A, Zhang C, Linnane AW, Nagley P (1994) Age-related human mtDNA deletions: a heterogeneous set of deletions arising at a single pair of directly repeated sequences. Am J Hum Genet 54: 618–630

Cheng KC, Cahill DS, Kasai H, Nishimura S, Loeb LA (1992) 8-hydroxyguanine, an abundan form of oxidative DNA damage, causes G → T and A → C substitutions. J Biol Chem 267: 166–172

Gille JJP, Wortelboer HM, Joenje H (1987) Antioxidant status of Fanconi anemia fibroblasts. Hum Genet 77: 28–31

Hoehn H, Kubbies M, Schindler D, Poot M, Rabinowitch PS (1989) BrdU-Hoechst flow cytometry links the cell kinetic defect of Fanconi anemia to oxygen hypersensitivity. In: Schroeder-Kurth TM, Auerbach AD, Obe G (eds) Fanconi anemia. Clinical, cytogenetic and experimental aspects. Springer, Berlin Heidelberg New York, pp 162–173

Joenje H, Gille JJP (1989) Oxygen metabolism and chromosomal breakage in Fanconi anemia. In: Schroeder-Kurth T, Auerbach AD, Obe G (eds) Fanconi anemia. Clinical, cytogenetic and experimental aspects. Springer, Berlin Heidelberg New York, pp 174–182

Joenje H, Arwert F, Eriksson AW, De Koning H, Oostra AB (1981) Oxygen- dependence of chromosomal alterations in Fanconi's anemia. Nature 290: 142–143

Jung M, Zhang Y, Lee S, Dritschilo A (1995) Correction of radiation sensitivity in ataxia telangiectasia cells by trunctated IkB-alpha. Science 268: 1619–1621

Kubbies M, Schindler D, Hoehn H, Scinzel A, Rabinowitch PS (1985) Endogene blockage and delay of the chromosome cycle despite normal recruitment and growth phase explain poor proliferation and frequent endomitosis in Fanconi anemia cells. Am J Hum Genet 37: 1022–1027

Liang P, Pardee AB (1992) Differential display of eukaryotic messenger RNA by means of the polymerase chain reaction. Sci 257: 967–971

Liang P, Averboukh L, Pardee AB (1993) Distribution and cloning of eukaryotic mRNAs by means of differential display: refinements and optimization. Nucleic Acids Res 21: 3269–3275

Liebetrau W, Buehner M, Hoehn H (1995) Prototype-sequence clues within the Fanconi anemia group C gene. J Med Genet (in press)

McBridge TJ, Preston BD, Loeb LA (1991) Mutagenic spectrum resulting from DNA damage by oxygen radicals. Biochemistry 30: 207–213

Moody CS, Hassan HM (1982) Mutagenicity of oxygen free radicals. Proc Natl Acad Sci USA 79: 2855–2859

Moraes EC, Keyse SM, Pidoux M, Tyrrell RM (1989) The spectrum of mutations generated by passage of a hydrogen peroxide-damaged shuttle vector plasmid through mammalian host. Nucleic Acids Res 17: 8301–8312

Nicol CJ, Harrison ML, Laposa RR, Gimelshtein IL, Wells PG (1995) A teratologic suppressor role for p53 in benzo[a]pyrene-treated transgenic p53-deficient mice. Nat Genet 10: 181–187

Reid TM, Loeb LA (1993) Tandem double CC → TT mutations are produced by reactive oxygen species. Proc Natl Acad Sci USA 90: 3904–3907

Saito H, Hammond AT, Moses RE (1993) Hypersensitivity to oxygen is a uniform and secondary defect in Fanconi anemia cells. Mutat Res 294: 255–262

Saito H, Hammond AT, Moses RE (1995) The effect of low oxygen tension on the in vitro replicative life span of human diploid fibroblast cells and their transformed derivatives. Exp Cell Res 217: 272–279

Schindler D, Hoehn H (1988) Fanconi anemia mutation causes cellular susceptibility to ambient oxygen. Am J Hum Genet 43: 429–435

Seetharam S, Kraemer KH, Waters HL, Seidman MM (1991) Ultraviolet mutational spectrum in a shuttle vector propagated in xeroderma pigmentosum lymphoblastoid cells and fibroblasts. Mutat Res 254: 97–105

Seidman MM, Dixon K, Razzaque A, Zagursky RJ, Bergman ML (1985) A shuttle vector plasmid for studying carcinogen-induced point mutations in mammalian cells. Gene 38: 233–237

Seyschab H, Friedl R, Sun Y, Schindler D, Hoehn H, Hentze S, Schroeder-Kurth T (1995) Comparative evaluation of diepoxybutane sensitivity and cell cycle blockage in the diagnosis of Fanconi anemia. Blood 85: 2233–2237

Shibutani S, Takeshita M, Grollman AP (1991) Insertion of specific bases during DNA synthesis past the oxidation-damaged base 8-oxodG. Nature 349: 431–434

Strathdee CA, Gavish H, Shannon WR, Buchwald M (1992) Cloning of cDNAs for Fanconi's anemia by functional complementation. Nature 356: 763–767

Takeuchi T, Morimoto K (1993) Increased formation of 8-hydroxydeoxyguanosine, an oxidative DNA damage, in lymphoblasts from Fanconi's anemia patients due to possible catalase deficiency. Carcinogenisis 14: 1115–1120

Toyokuni S, Sagripanti JL (1993) Iron-mediated DNA damage: sensitive detection of DNA strand breakage catalyzed by iron. J Inorg Biochem 447: 241–248

Umemura T, Sai K, Takagi A, Hasegawa R, Kurukawa Y (1990) Formation of 8-hydroxydeoxyguanosine (8-oH-dG) in rat kidney DNA after intraperitoneal administration of ferric nitrilotriacetata (Fe-NTA). Carcinogenesis 11: 345–347

Von Sonntag C (1987) The chemical basis of radiation biology. Taylor and Francis, London, pp 168–177, pp 252–260

Yamashita T, Barber DL, Zhu Y, Wu N, D' Andrea AD (1994) The Fanconi anemia polypeptide FACC is localized to the cytoplasm. Proc Natl Acad Sci USA 91: 6712–6716

Youssoufian H (1994) Localization of Fanconi anemia C protein to the cytoplasm of mammalian cells. Proc Natl Acad Sci USA 91: 7975–7979

P53 Gene Alterations in Human Tumors: Perspectives for Cancer Control

M. Hollstein[1], T. Soussi[2], G. Thomas[3], M.-C. von Brevern[1], and H. Bartsch[1]

[1]Deutsches Krebsforschungszentrum, Im Neuenheimer Feld 280, 69120 Heidelberg, Germany
[2]INSERM, Unité 301, Institut de Génétique Moléculaire, 27 rue Juliette Dodu, 75010 Paris, France
[3]Institut Curie, 26 rue d'Ulm, 75231 Paris Cédex 05, France

Introduction

Alterations of the p53 gene are found in the majority of human tumors (Caron de Fromentel and Soussi 1992; Hollstein et al. 1991; Tominaga et al. 1992; Levine et al. 1991; Greenblatt et al. 1994). The encoded nuclear phosphoprotein is a transcription factor that binds to a specific DNA motif and transactivates genes controlling cell cycle checkpoints, DNA repair, and cell death (Clarke et al. 1993; Lane 1993; Lowe et al. 1993; El Deiry et al. 1994). The p53 protein can also play a role in maintaining the integrity of the genome by sensing DNA changes, by affecting DNA repair processes, and perhaps by influencing homologous recombination events or DNA replication (Kastan et al. 1992; Yin et al. 1992; Livingstone et al. 1992; Lane 1994; Cox et al. 1995; Jayaraman and Prives 1995; Wang et al. 1995).

Although the gene was originally classified as an oncogene due to the transforming activity of the first p53 sequences cloned (which fortuitously were abnormal), the primary effect of the normal p53 protein is now recognized primarily as one of growth suppression (Lane and Benchimol 1990). Some mutant forms do acquire the ability to transform cells in culture when cotransfected with certain oncogenes, while others have simply lost growth suppressing activity, apparently without gaining new capabilities. In keeping with the growth suppressor model for the function of p53 in human tumors, there is frequent loss of heterozygosity (LOH) at the p53 locus and mutation in the remaining allele, implying that it is the absence of a functional gene product (Knudson 1971; Levine and Momand 1990; Weinberg 1992) that contributes to neoplastic changes. Wild-type p53 introduced into malignant cells inhibits their growth or tumorigenicity (Baker et al. 1990a; Diller et al. 1990; Mercer et al. 1990, 1991), and p53 heterozygous or nullizygous mice are more susceptible to tumor development (Hann and Lane 1995; Donehower et al. 1992). The biology of normal p53 function suggests important new molecular strategies for therapy based on reactivating p53 suppressor activity or stimulating downstream targets of p53 function (Friedmann 1992; Harris and Hollstein 1993; Lane 1994).

Mutations of the p53 gene add to the already surprising accumulation of specific gene aberrations usually found in human malignancies (Fearon and Vogelstein 1990). This has sparked considerable debate over classical concepts regarding frequency, mechanism, and relevance of mutations in human carcinogenesis (Loeb 1991; Strauss 1992). Gene defects that result in a loss of genome integrity (Livingstone et al. 1992; Yin et al. 1992; Aaltonen et al. 1993; Cross et al. 1995) may be crucial targets of damage during cancer development. It will be of both theoretical and clinical interest to establish which gene mutations in which tissues are specific, rate-limiting steps in the natural history of the disease, and cause stepwise acquisition of the malignant phenotype. In addition, knowledge of the temporal occurrence of these mutations could have direct implications for the diagnosis and prognosis of some types of cancers.

During the last 5 years there has been a dramatic surge of research on the biological properties of the wild-type p53 protein and the mutant forms found in human tumors. Of the many aspects that are potentially important in the clinical setting, three have been the subject of an extensive list of published reports: (1) cancer prognosis in relation to p53 allele loss or other p53 alterations (2) immunochemical detection of the p53 protein or antibodies to p53 in human tissues as a tool in cancer diagnosis, and (3) characterization of p53 point mutations in human tumors, biopsies, archival tissues, and exfoliated cells from cancer patients. We present here an introductory discussion of these topics, as they pertain to p53 alterations in sporadic[1] cancers.

Initial Studies on p53 Allele Loss and Associated p53 Alterations Suggesting a Prognostic Significance

P53 overexpression, mutation, and chromosome 17p deletion are frequent in human cancers and tend to occur together in the same tumor (Fig. 1). Correlations of the presence of one or more of these alterations with clinicopathological factors were sought in a number of early studies, and the emerging associations showed a dependence on cancer type and histological subtype.

[1]Testing of germline p53 mutations in members of families with the Li-Fraumeni cancer syndrome (Malkin et al. 1990; Srivastava et al. 1990) has been reviewed recently by Malkin 1994.

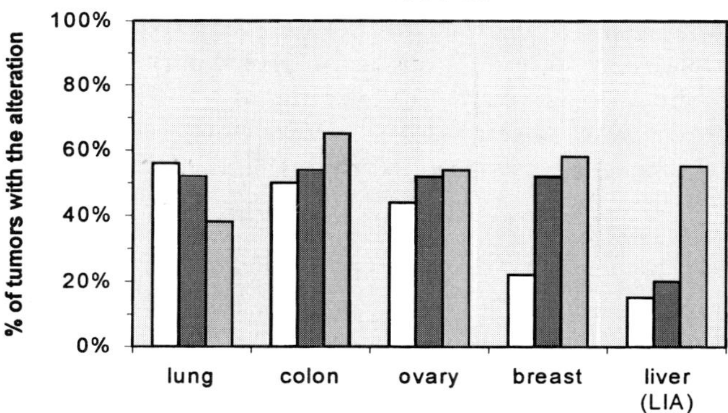

Fig. 1. Correlations of p53 aberrations in human cancers of the lung, colon, ovary, breast, and liver (hepatocellular carcinoma). *IHC*, immunohistochemistry with p53 antibody or antiserum; *LIA*, low-to moderate-incidence geographical areas. Point mutation frequencies are from Greenblatt et al. (1994). Frequencies of other aberrations are estimates from representative reports published in the period 1987–1992

Loss of Heterozygosity (LOH) on Chromosome 17p and Its Association with p53 Mutations

The loss of genetic information on chromosome 17p, as assessed by cytogenetic analysis or by monitoring of loss of alleles for loci located in this part of the genome, is one of the most frequently identified chromosome anomalies in human tumors. In colorectal carcinoma, deletion mapping showed that the common region of 17p deletion was within bands 17p12 to 17p13 where the p53 gene is localized (Kern et al. 1989; Baker et al. 1989). Allelic studies in medulloblastoma and malignant astrocytoma also showed that the p53 locus was frequently included in the deleted region of 17p (Cogen et al. 1990; Fults et al. 1989, 1992). These and other initial studies as well as subsequent work demonstrated that loss of genetic material from 17p typically includes the loss of a normal p53 gene, and this finding was corroborated by the frequent association of 17p allelic loss with p53 mutation in the same tumor. Overabundance of p53 protein usually indicates the presence of a p53 mutation (discussed below) and is thus also associated with wild-type allele loss on 17p.

Mutant p53 proteins in tumors compromise the function of wild-type molecules, which would explain why occasionally tumors with this type of alteration (i.e., missense mutation) retain a normal allele on 17p even at advanced stages of malignancy. Tumors with frameshift, nonsense, or splice site mutations, however (which account for approximately 15% of sequenced mutations and are expected to inactivate only one allele), consistently demonstrate 17p allelic loss or a second mutation, presumably on the other p53 allele (Tominaga et al. 1992). In carcinomas of the breast and liver, despite concomitant occurrence of p53 mutation and 17p LOH in some tumors, the chromosomal region lost does not necessarily encompass the p53 locus, and the frequency of allelic loss on 17p is significantly higher than the occurrence of p53 mutation in these cancers (Fig. 1). A second suppressor gene on 17p important in breast cancer (Coles et al. 1990) and in hepatocellular carcinogenesis it has been inferred (Fujimori et al. 1991).

Correlations of p53 Anomalies with Clinical Parameters

Tumors with p53 mutation, chromosome 17p deletion, or protein accumulation are more likely to behave aggressively than those with normal p53. Sidransky and coworkers showed that subpopulations of p53 mutant cells in indolent glioblastomas expand clonally, resulting in development of more aggressive, invasive astrocytomas in which all cells carry the mutant allele (Sidransky et al. 1992). P53 mutations arise during progression of benign neoplasms to invasive tumors in many cancers. Conversion of chronic myelocytic leukemia to acute phases of the disease is accompanied by appearance of p53 mutation, acquisition of chromosome 17p abnormalities, and p53 overexpression (Ahuja et al. 1989; Mashal et al. 1990; Soussi and Jonveaux 1991). The likelihood of observing p53 mutations generally rises as neoplastic changes become more severe, but mutations are consistently premetastatic events. In instance where primary tumors and metastases in the same patients are examined, the identical mutation in the matched sets is found (e.g., see Davidoff et al. 1991).

Although the timing of p53 lesions in neoplasia is evidently cancer type-dependent, it may also be related to etiology, and therefore would be cohort-dependent for a given malignancy. For example, p53 mutations, overexpression, or loss of the 17p allele are more frequently observed in sporadic colorectal carcinomas than in adenomas (Baker et al. 1990b; Purdie et al. 1991; Kikuchi-Yanoshita et al. 1992), but may occur at more precocious stages in colon tumors of patients with ulcerative colitis. In head and neck cancers, and in bronchial carcinomas, p53 mutations have been detected in very early lesions including mildly dysplastic cell clusters, and may be more frequent at initial stages of neoplasia if the patients are heavy smokers (Bennett et al. 1992, 1993; Sozzi et al. 1992; Vähäkangas et al. 1992; Nees et al. 1993).

Due to the simplicity of the assay, immunohistochemical detection of p53 overexpression[2] in fixed biopsy histology sections has been the most widely

[2]Overabundance of p53 protein in tumors is generally attributable to stabilization of the aberrant protein encoded by a mutated p53 gene (see next section). P53 protein nuclear accumulation is typically referred to as overexpression, although the term is somewhat misleading because transcription and translation are usually not affected.

used test in studies attempting to correlate p53 anomalies with clinical parameters, in particular in the evaluation of p53 aberration as a tool in diagnosis and prognosis (reviewed in Wynford-Thomas 1992; Dowell and Hall 1994; Hall and Lane 1994). Breast cancer has been intensively investigated in this regard. Early studies linked increased p53 expression to low estrogen receptor content (Cattoretti et al. 1988; Thompson et al. 1992) and several reports associated positive p53 immunoreactivity in breast cancer or point mutation in the tumor with shorter overall survival of the patients (Iwaya et al. 1991; Isola et al. 1992; Thor et al. 1992; Thor and Vandell 1993; Allred et al. 1993; Elledge et al. 1993; Silvestrini et al. 1993; Thorlaicus et al. 1993). Poor prognosis for lung, colorectal, and gastric cancer patients was also found associated with the presence of p53 mutation or increased nuclear accumulation in some studies (Iwaya et al. 1991; Martin et al. 1992a,b; Quinlan et al. 1992; Sun et al. 1992; Horio et al. 1993). A plethora of reports examining p53 anomalies as independent indicators of prognosis in a variety of cancer types has since appeared, and many further studies are in the progress. A working consortium of international experts to evaluate and consolidate findings, and to examine potential reasons for discordant results is needed.

Immunochemical Analysis of Human Tissues and Serum

Molecular Basis of Immunohistochemical Analysis

A decade ago Benchimol and coworkers (1982) developed a radioimmunological test to show that the p53 protein is specifically overexpressed in transformed cells whereas it is so low as to be undetectable in normal cells by this assay. Numerous studies followed confirming these results and demonstrating that the p53 protein accumulation in neoplasia is typically a consequence of its stabilization and not the result of an augmentation of gene expression. Stabilization can occur by a point mutation, resulting in an amino acid substitution that modifies the conformation and stability of the protein, thereby allowing its accumulation in the cell nucleus (Fig. 2). A transient rise in wild-type p53 protein in normal cells also occur in response to various insults such as DNA damage by radiation (Kastan et al. 1992; Lu and Lane 1993).

More than half of all cancers of almost all histological types reveal immunostaining with p53 antibody or antiserum. Many thousands of cases have been analyzed already due to the rapidity and simplicity of the assay. There is good agreement for a given type of cancer between the frequency of positive sample by immunohistochemical analysis and the frequency of tumors with mutations detected directly by DNA sequencing (Fig. 1). Particularly informative are the studies in which both analyses are conducted in parallel on the identical samples set. Usually results are concordant in the two assays, and the exceptions are generally consistent with the molecular basis for tumor p53 overexpression (i.e., stabilization of a mutated form due to missense mutation):

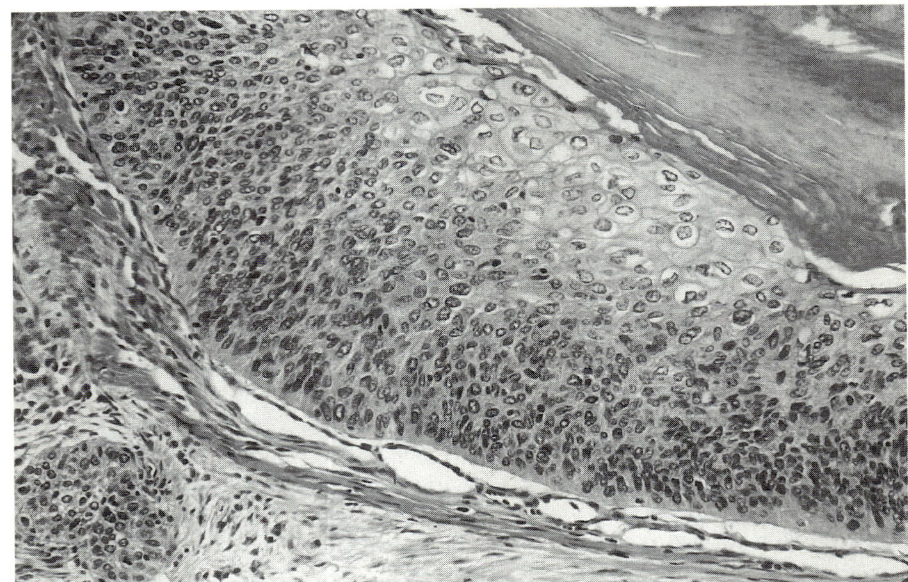

A

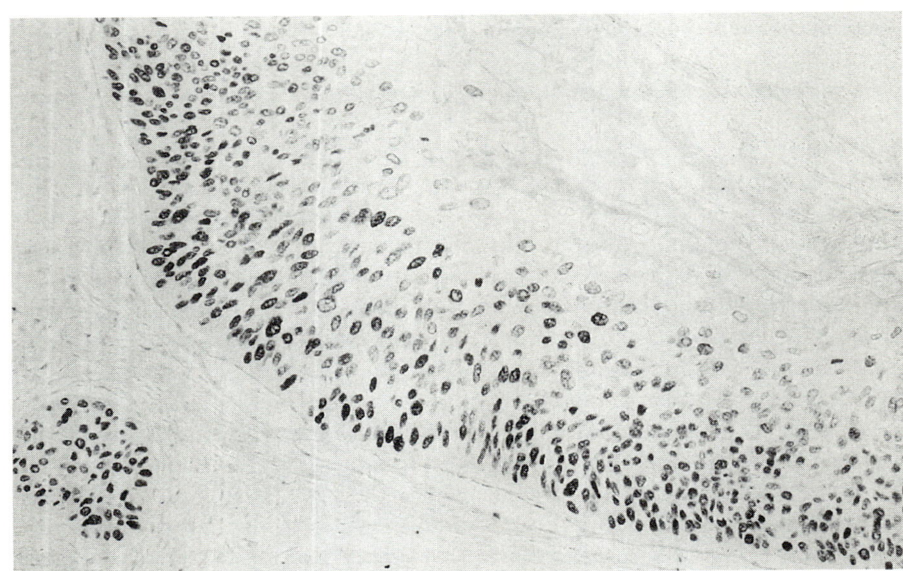

B

Fig. 2. Immunohistochemical analysis of p53 expression in squamous cell carcinoma. (**A**) A well-differentiated squamous cell carcinoma (H&E). In a parallel immunostain section (**B**) the undifferentiated basal tumor nuclei are darkly stained (CM-1 antiserum). A small focus of tumor in the *lower left corner* is also darkly stained. Original magnification ×200. (Courtesy of Dr. William P. Bennett, Laboratory of Human Carcinogenesis, National Cancer Institute, Bethesda, MD, USA)

tumors with nonsense and frameshift mutations that result in no protein product, or production of a truncated and unstable protein, are in most instances immunostain-negative, as are some tumors with mutations in RNA splice sites. These categories of mutations are estimated to account for less than 15% of human tumor p53 mutations. In a limited number of cancer types (e.g., melanoma), however, overexpression without missense mutation is consistently observed. These are particularly interesting cancers for the study of other mechanisms that may stabilize the p53 protein or affect p53 gene transcription (Vogelstein and Kinzler 1992a).

Since in the majority of cancers, p53 protein (usually a mutant form) accumulates in the malignant cells but not in surrounding normal tissue, rapid immunocytochemical detection of p53 protein is a promising diagnostic tool (Hall et al. 1991). Validation studies on histology sections and cytology preparations from a variety of cancers as well as from uninvolved tissues have been performed and discussed (Baas et al. 1994; Dowell et al. 1994; Hall and Lane 1994).

An antibody used for immunocytochemistry should have a very high specificity, the absence of cross-reactivity with other cellular proteins, a high affinity for the antigen regardless of the method of tissue fixation, and an unlimited supply of the reagent, with reproducible performance. Numerous monoclonal antibodies recognizing the human p53 protein have been produced, several of which are available commercially. Various monoclonal antibodies and polyclonal sera such as CM-1, JG8 or DO1, and DO7 have been evaluated (Iggo et al. 1990; Midgley et al. 1992; Baas et al. 1994; Soussi et al. 1994).

Serological Analysis of p53

In 1982, Crawford and collaborators detected p53 antibodies in the serum of patients with breast carcinoma (Crawford et al. 1982). Subsequently, Caron de Fromentel et al. (1987) found that such antibodies were present in the sera of children with a wide variety of cancers. The overall frequency was 12%, with a somewhat higher figure (20%) for Burkitts lymphoma. Davidoff et al. found that p53 antibodies in the serum were present only when the mutant p53 protein from the tumor was able to bind to heat shock protein 70 complexes (Davidoff et al. 1992). In lung carcinomas, p53 antibodies were directly correlated with the overexpression of p53 protein in the tumor cell (Winter et al. 1992), whereas tumors with mutations that generate null cells, in which p53 protein is absent, were not able to elicit an antibody response. Schlichtholz and coworkers (1992) showed that the presence of p53 antibodies in serum of breast cancer patients was associated with other parameters indicating poor prognosis (Schlichtholz et al. 1992; Peyrat et al. 1995). Serological analysis of p53 alteration may prove to be a useful clinical tool for patient follow-up, and potentially for screening high-risk individuals with preclinical neoplasia (Lubin et al. 1995; Trivers et al. 1995). Serological tests would also complement those already available (molecular and immunohistochemical analyses) for assessing p53 status of the tumor. A greater understanding of immune system response to mutant and overabundant p53 protein in neoplastic cells is being sought (Lubin et al. 1993; Yanuck et al. 1993; Angelopoulou et al. 1994; Schlichtholz et al. 1994; Wiedenfeld et al. 1994).

Mutant p53 Alleles in Human Tumors

Based on the results of numerous studies on diverse types of cancer, one may expect that in at least one-half of all human cancer there is a mutant p53 allele that alters or obliterates normal functioning of p53 protein. Many tumor-specific point mutations in other genes involved in cell growth have been described, but the unusual aspect of p53 gene tumor mutations is their frequency and the diversity of specific changes giving rise to a dysfunctional protein. The first compilations of published data on approximately 250 human tumors with p53 point mutations suggested that missense mutations arising in any of more than 100 codons of the gene may result in a growth advantage to the (pre-cancerous) cell (Hollstein et al. 1991; Caron de Fromentel and Soussi 1992; Tominaga et al. 1992). There are now sequence data on more than 4000 tumors characterizing the base change of each mutant (Hollstein et al. 1994), yet efforts to identify the exact nature of each p53 alteration in tumors continue because this detailed information promises to be important in correlating clinical parameters with p53 aberrations, and in understanding how mutations arise in human carcinogenesis.

Clinical Importance of p53 Mutation Analysis

Amino acid substitution in p53 is the most common known molecular basis for immunodetection with p53 antibodies (see preceding two sections). While the overall correlation between immunostaining and the presence of a missense mutation is excellent, it is of interest to learn how different cellular contexts or viral infections modify p53 transcription activity, immunoreactivity, or p53 mutant protein half-life and how the precise mutation has a bearing on the biological interactions (Halevy et al. 1990; Lane 1994; Wang et al. 1994).

Some associations between p53 alterations and tumor stage, type, disease prognosis, presence of serum p53 antibodies against overabundant or mutant protein, metastatic potential, and other clinical parameters may remain obscure until the various mutant forms can be grouped (classified) according to their biological effects. Experimental studies with cloned mutants have revealed that different mutant p53 proteins have different biological properties (Sturzbecher et al. 1987; Halevy et al. 1990; Hinds et al. 1990; Rotter and

Prokocimer 1991; Dittmer et al. 1993; Forrester et al. 1995). Cell type or differentiation stage are also important in determining the phenotypic consequences of a particular mutation. The molecular basis for the observation that cells with mutant p53 are more resistant to radiation and cancer chemotherapeutic drugs is being elucidated. Identification of tumor p53 status may play an increasing role in making treatment decisions (Harris and Hollstein 1993; Lee and Bernstein 1993).

Origins of Genetic Changes in Sporadic Cancer

The epidemiology of cancer shows that the incidence of a certain cancer can be more than 50-fold higher in one defined risk group than another (Tomatis et al. 1990). External factors such as occupational exposure to carcinogens, specific dietary practices, or habits such as smoking are primarily responsible for these extremes. Some genetic damage in human tumors may be attributable to exposure to mutagenic carcinogens, and some to factors, both endogenous and external, that are nongenotoxic per se, but affect normal biological processes and thereby elicit genetic changes.

Several generalizations can be made about p53 mutations in most of the major cancers. First, p53 mutations are frequent in almost all cancer types, and most of the point mutations are single missense base substitutions; exceptions include melanoma and cervical carcinoma. The low frequency of p53 mutations in cancers of the cervix has been linked to infection with cancer-associated strains of human papilloma virus (HPV). The HPV-encoded (E6) oncoprotein triggers ubiquitin-dependent degradation of wild-type p53 protein (Scheffner et al. 1990), suggesting a loss of p53 suppressor gene function by a lowering of p53 protein levels that could make inactivation by mutation redundant (Crook et al. 1991; Scheffner et al. 1991). The p53 transcription transactivation function can also be inhibited by the viral oncoprotein (Mietz et al. 1992).

Second, C to T transitions at CpG dinucleotides constitute a major fraction of human tumor mutations in the p53 gene, particularly in cancers of the colon, brain, and in hematological malignancies (Hollstein et al. 1991; Jones et al. 1991; Greenblatt et al. 1994). CpG sites are hotspots for transitions (Coulondre et al. 1983; Cooper and Krawczak 1990) because spontaneous deamination of 5-methylcytosine (located primarily at this dinucleotide in mammalian cells) generates thymine and thus a C to T transition. The high frequency of transitions at CpG base pairs implies that mutations in these tumor are in large part spontaneous occurrences. It is of interest to know whether components in the diet of persons at high risk of colorectal cancer, a malignancy in which CpG to TpG mutations are so common, promote deamination. Endogenous agents or normal enzymatic processes in mammalian cells affecting deamination of DNA bases are also being discussed in this context (Wink et al. 1991; Shen et al. 1992).

The third feature shared by missense point mutations found in human tumors is that they tend to fall at codons corresponding to amino acids that are identical in a variety of evolutionarily distinct species. This is in keeping with the assumption that most tumor-specific mutations are indeed affecting proper function of the encoded p53 protein and are therefore selected during growth. Although there are 23 CpG dinucleotides in the midregion of the p53 gene, almost all tumor CpG transition mutations are at one of six sites (codons 175, 196, 213, 248, 273, 282). These hotspots have in common that they are either (a) in an evolutionarily conserved domain and at a conserved amino acid, or (b) CGA triplets at which a C to T transition in the first position of the codon would lead to a chain termination signal and thereby loss of function. Furthermore, X-ray crystallography shows that hotspots for mutations in tumors line up at the p53-DNA interface (Cho et al. 1994; Prives 1994). This p53 protein-DNA interaction is required for tumor suppressor function, and is disrupted when a wrong amino acid is substituted at a critical site because of a missense mutation.

The final, and at first glance, most mysterious observation one can make regarding p53 mutations in human tumors is that the pattern of mutations (mutation spectrum) characterizing one cancer type in a population can be strikingly different from another cancer. A mutation spectrum is composed of the number, positions, and kinds of alterations in a defined DNA target sequence. The possibilities for each of these parameters, together with the different combinations of each variable, allow for great diversity in the patterns of alterations, permitting one spectrum to be distinguished from another. One parameter, the frequencies of different kinds of base substitutions in the p53 gene, is presented in Table 1 for the five most frequent cancers in the world.

There are only seven major categories of point mutations (six major base substitution classes, and base addition/deletions, Table 1), and they represent just one aspect of mutational spectra; nevertheless, clear differences already emerge between one cancer and another. The predominant mutation in colorectal cancer is G to A substitution, primarily at CpG dinucleotides, whereas in lung tumors G to T transversions are the most common type of substitution detected. This mutation is rarely found in mutant p53 alleles colorectal tumors. While these differences are statistically highly significant ($p < 0.001$; chi-squared statistic), base substitution frequencies alone are unlikely to be sufficiently informative to reveal differences in etiology or cellular mutation mechanisms. When combined with information on the base context in which the substitutions occur, however, hypotheses regarding the origins of mutations in a given cancer type may be generated. Factors in addition to diverse carcinogen exposures that could modulate the cancer-specific mutation profiles include: tissue differences in DNA repair, metabolism, and endogenous promutagenic processes; distinct differentiation pathways of the target cells; and biological activities of different mutant p53 proteins in different cellular environments.

Table 1. P53 point mutation patterns in the five most common human cancers[a]

Rank order worldwide cancer burden[b]	Tumor site	Total mutations	Base insertions and deletions	Base substitutions at G:C pairs				Base substitutions at A:T pairs (To T:A; G:C or C:G)
				to A:T		to T:A	to C:G	
				at CpG[c]	non-CpG			
1	Lung	437	11%	10%	16%	**39%**	10%	16%
2	Stomach	146	13%	**26%**	**24%**	6%	4%	26%
3	Breast	388	14%	21%	19%	13%	9%	24%
4	Colon/rectum	369	7%	**47%**	14%	9%	6%	16%
–	Skin[d]	206	8%	8%	37% + Tandem: **17%**[e]	10%	6%	12%

[a]From European Bioinformatics Institute (EBI) data base of p53 human tumor mutations (Hollstein et al. 1994), updated. Values that are exceptionally high in comparison to frequencies in other types of cancer are shown in bold.
[b]From Parkin et al. 1993.
[c]This type of mutation is the most common spontaneous base substitution observed in mammalian cells (see text).
[d]Skin cancer is extremely frequent but rank order difficult to assign (see Parkin et al. 1993).
[e]Adjacent double mutations at various dinucleotides in the gene. In every other type of human cancer these mutations occur at a frequency of less than 1%.

Since experimentally, mutagenic chemicals induce highly characteristic mutation spectra in a defined DNA sequence (Miller 1983; Horsfall et al. 1990; Thilly 1990), these may be useful for comparison against mutation patterns in cancer patients for whom a given carcinogen exposure is suspected (Hollstein et al. 1991; Jones et al. 1991). As an argument toward adopting measures to reduce a specific carcinogen exposure, a mutation pattern in tumors of an exposed population that matched an experimental mutation spectrum from a suspected risk factor would be particularly persuasive (Vogelstein and Kinzler 1992b). Second, the mutation patterns of cancer types or patient groups that do not fit models of electrophilic attack on DNA by xenobiotics have provided new insights on endogenous mechanisms of genetic change.

Three Examples of Distinctive Mutation Profiles in Patients from High-Risk Groups Exposed to Known Human Carcinogens

For references, please see the European Bioinformatics Institute (EBI) data base (Hollstein et al. 1994).

Hepatocellular Carcinomas (HCC) in Relation to Aflatoxin Exposure

P53 mutations in most human cancers are dispersed over a 600-base pair midregion of the coding sequence, and include base substitutions of all six types, although one or another kind of substitution predominates for a given cancer (Table 1). Mutations in hepatocellular carcinomas show this typical dispersion of mutation site and variety of base change if one examines tumors of patients residing in low-to moderate-risk areas where the major known risk factors are infection with hepatitis B virus (HBV) and hepatitis C virus (HCV) or high intake of alcoholic beverages. The mutation profile in certain high-risk populations, however, is entirely different from other geographically defined patient groups. Among the HCC examined from high-risk areas of southern Africa and from Qidong, China, almost all mutations are G to T transversions at the third base position of codon 249. In these regions, as well as in Mozambique, where this hotspot mutation was also detected in half to the HCC examined, dietary aflatoxin levels are high and exposure to this carcinogen is considered a major risk factor. G to T transversions are the expected predominant substitution from preferential electrophilic attack of the reactive aflatoxin metabolite on guanine residues of DNA (Foster et al. 1983). The most striking aspect of this geographically related HCC pattern is the nearly unique location of the mutations in the p53 gene (codon 249). G to T substitutions are also common in lung cancers, for example, but the sites are more dispersed. Carcinogens react preferentially with certain residues depending on base sequence context, and in the case of human p53 sequences it has been shown that the guanine (third position) of c. 249 is in fact a preferential site of attack for metabolically activated aflatoxin in vitro (Puisieux et al. 1991) and human cells in culture (Aguilar et al. 1993). As most of the HCC patients in the p53 mutation studies are chronic carriers of HBV, the virus could be an additional element generating the unusual mutation profile, for example as a consequence of direct or indirect interaction of viral proteins with mutant p53 protein harboring a serine residue in place of arginine at position 249 (Wang et al. 1994; Forrester et al. 1995).

Squamous Cell Carcinomas of the Skin and Exposure to Sunlight

Brash et al. (1991) identified 15 mutations in skin cancers, over half of which were G:C to A:T transitions. The distinguishing aspects of the mutation profile despite the small sample size were consistent with the known DNA-damaging effects of UV light, a strong mutagen that induces pyrimidine dimer promutagenic lesions, and subsequent tandem base substitutions (Drobetsky et al. 1987; McGregor et al. 1991). Three of the 13 base substitutions reported by Brash and colleagues were such double mutations, whereas in internal cancers they constitute less than 0.1% of all mutations. The second striking feature is that all the substitutions were at G:C pairs. Numerous subsequent studies have corroborated and extended these results, and have shown that UV-characteristic mutations accumulate in sun-exposed preneoplastic skin tissue (Ziegler et al. 1994).

Lung Cancer and Cigarette Smoking

As with p53 tumor mutations of most other human cancers, the majority of sequence changes that obliterate p53 tumor suppressor function in lung tumors are base substitution mutations scattered over the gene, with sites of frequent mutation clustering in several regions within the midsection of the coding sequences. All six classes of base substitution occur, as is true for other cancer types, but exceptionally in lung tumors, G to T transversions are found more frequently than any other point mutation. These base substitutions show an overwhelming strand bias of the premutated G residue toward the noncoding DNA strand, implying that bulky DNA adducts are the premutagenic lesions and are substrates of transcription-coupled repair (Selby and Sancar 1993). Since most lung cancer patients are tobacco smokers, the predominance of G to T transversions is likely to reflect the mutagenic activities of cigarette smoke components. Benzo(a)pyrene in particular has received attention because it is a tobacco carcinogen that induces primarily this base substitution (Eisenstadt et al. 1982; Mazur and Glickman 1988; Yang et al. 1991; Chen et al. 1992). Cigarette smoke is a complex mixture of carcinogens, however, and the mutation spectrum of one component may not match the pattern induced by a composite of active substances. Also, G to T transversions do arise spontaneously during cellular metabolism, as well as from oxidative damage to DNA (Fraga et al. 1990; Cheng et al. 1992). Comparisons of the p53 mutational frequency and spectra in lung and head and neck cancers from cigarette smokers versus never-smokers have shown that p53 mutations are more frequent in smokers (Brennan et al. 1995) and are more likely to be G to T transversions as cigarette consumption increases (Suzuki et al. 1992; Takashima et al. 1993).

Perspectives

Intensive research in the last three years on p53 alterations in human cancers has raised as many questions as it has answered, and revived a number of interesting hypotheses. A thorough understanding of the molecular biology of this suppressor gene promises to yield one of the clearest examples to date of progress in basic cancer research that will have bearing on matters of clinical importance. Issues receiving attention at present include (a) patient immune response to accumulation of cancer-associated proteins such as mutant p53 and its exploitation as a diagnostic tool; (b) further development of p53 analyses for the cytopathological diagnosis of neoplasia; (c) the interaction of p53 with other cellular proteins and genes controlling cell growth, programmed cell death, and p53 tumor suppressor activity; (d) mutation spectra in tumors of patients exposed occupationally to human carcinogens or clinically to chemotherapeutic drugs; (e) the role of DNA repair (interindividual and inter tissue differences) in mutation frequencies and patterns; and (f) cancer prognosis and chemotherapy in relation to the p53 status of the tumor.

It is crucial that there be a close, coordinated effort among epidemiologists, clinicians, and experimental biologists in order for the full potential of discoveries on tumor suppressor genes to be realized in the medical setting. Continued analysis of genetic alterations in tumors is needed in patients for whom there are records of occupational histories, personal habits, medical treatment, and the clinical course of disease.

Note. Due to space limitations we have been able to cite only relatively few of the numerous excellent primary references pertaining to this broad topic.

Note Added in Proofs: See Hollstein et al. (1996) Nucleic Acids Res 24: 141–146 for updated European Bioinformatics Institute (EBI) data base of human p53 mutations.

References

Aaltonen LA, Peltomaki P, Leach FS et al (1993) Clues to the pathogenesis of familial colorectal cancer. Science 260: 812–816

Aguilar F, Hussain SP, Cerutti P (1993) Aflatoxin B1 induced the transversion of G to T

in codon 249 of the human p53 tumor suppressor gene. Proc Natl Acad Sci USA 90: 8586–8590
Ahuja H, Bar-Eli M, Advani SH et al (1989) Alterations in the p53 gene and the clonal evolution of the blast crisis of chronic myelocytic l leukemia. Proc Natl Acad Sci USA 86: 6783–6787
Allred DC, Clark GM, Elledge R et al (1993) Association of p53 protein expression with tumor cell proliferation rate and clinical outcome in node-negative breast cancer. J Natl Cancer Inst 85: 200–206
Angelopoulou K, Diamandis EP, Sutherland DJA et al (1994) Prevalence of serum antibodies against the p53 tumor suppressor gene protein in various cancers. Int J Cancer 58: 480–487
Baas IO, Mulder J-WR, Offerhaus GJA et al (1994) An evaluation of six antibodies for immunohistochemistry of mutant p53 gene product in archival colorectal neoplasms. J Pathol 172: 5–12
Baker SJ, Fearon ER, Nigro JM et al (1989) Chromosome 17 deletions and p53 gene mutations in colorectal carcinomas. Science 244: 217–221
Baker SJ, Markowitz S, Fearon ER et al (1990a) Suppression of human colorectal carcinoma cell growth by wild-type p53. Science 249: 912–915
Baker SJ, Preisinger AC, Jessup JM et al (1990b) p53 gene mutations occur in combination with 17p allelic deletions as late events in colorectal tumorigenesis. Cancer Res 50: 7717–7722
Benchimol S, Pim D, Crawford L (1982) Radioimmunoassay of the cellular protein p53 in mouse and human cell lines. EMBO J 1: 1055
Bennett WP, Hollstein MC, Metcalf RA et al (1992) p53 mutation and protein accumulation during multistage human esophageal carcinogenesis. Cancer Res 52: 6092–6097
Bennett WP, Colby TV, Travis WD et al (1993) p53 protein accumulates frequently in early bronchial neoplasia. Cancer Res 53: 4817–4822
Brash DE, Rudolph JA, Simon JA et al (1991) A role for sunlight in skin cancer: UV-induced p53 mutations in squamous cell carcinoma. Proc Natl Acad Sci USA 88: 10124–10128
Brennan JA, Boyle JO, Koch WM et al (1995) Association between cigarette smoking and mutation of the p53 gene in squamous cell carcinoma of the head and neck. N Engl J Med 332: 712–717
Caron de Fromentel C, Soussi T (1992) TP53 tumor suppressor gene: a model for investigating human mutagenesis. Genes Chrom Cancer 4: 1–15
Carzon de Fromentel C, May-Levin F, Mouriesse H et al (1987) Presence of circulating antibodies against cellular protein p53 in a notable proportion of children with B-cell lymphoma. Int J Cancer 39: 185–189
Cattoretti G, Rilke F, Andrealo S et al (1988) p53 expression in breast cancer. Int J Cancer 41: 178–183
Chen R-H, Maher VM, Brouwer J et al (1992) Preferential repair and strand-specific repair of benzo[a]pyrene diol epoxide adducts in the HPRT gene of diploid human fibroblasts. Proc Natl Acad Sci USA 89: 5413–5417
Cheng KC, Cahill DS, Hasai H et al (1992) 8-Hydroxyguanine, an abundant product of oxidative DNA damage, causes G to T substitutions in E. coli. J Biol Chem 267: 166–172
Cho Y, Gorina S, Jeffrey PD, Pavletich NP (1994) Crystal structure of a p53 tumor suppressor-DNA complex: Understanding tumorigenic mutations. Science 265–346
Clarke AR, Purdie CA, Harrison DJ et al (1993) Thymocyte apoptosis induced by p53-dependent and independent pathways. Nature 362: 849–852
Cogen PH, Daneshvar L, Metzger AK et al (1990) Deletion mapping of the medulloblastoma locus on chromosome 17p. Genomics 8: 279–285

Coles C, Thompson AM, Elder PA et al (1990) Evidence implicating at least two genes on chromosome 17p in breast carcinogenesis. Lancet 336: 761

Cooper DN, Krawczak M (1990) The mutational spectrum of single base-pair substitutions causing human genetic disease: patterns and prediction. Hum Genet 85: 55–74

Coulondre C, Miller DM, Farabaugh PJ et al (1983) Molecular basis of base substitution hotspots in Escherichia coli. Nature 274: 775–780

Cox LS, Hupp T, Midgley CA, Lane DP (1995) A direct effect of activated p53 on nuclear DNA replication. EMBO J 14: 2099–2105

Crawford LV, Pim DC, Bulbrook RD (1982) Detection of antibodies against the cellular protein p53 in sera from patients with breast cancer. Int J Cancer 30: 403–408

Crook T, Tidy JA, Vousden KH (1991) Degradation of p53 can be targeted by HPV E6 sequences distinct from those required for p53 binding and trans-activation. Cell 67: 547–556

Cross SM, Sanchez CA, Morgan CA et al (1995) A p53-dependent mouse spindle checkpoint. Science 267: 1353–1356

Davidoff AM, Herndon JE, Glover NS et al (1991) Relation between p53 overexpression and established prognostic factors in breast cancer. Surgery 2: 259–264

Davidoff AM, Iglehart JD, Marks JR (1992) Immune response to p53 is dependent upon p53/HSP70 complexes in breast cancers. Proc Natl Acad Sci USA 89: 3439–3442

Diller L, Kassel J, Nelson CE et al (1990) p53 functions as a cell cycle control protein in osteosarcomas. Mol Cell Biol 10: 5772–5781

Dittmer D, Pati S, Zambetti G et al (1993) p53 gain of function mutations. Nature Genet 4: 42–46

Donehower LA, Harvey M, Slagle BL et al (1992) Mice deficient for p53 are developmentally normal but susceptible to spontaneous tumors. Nature 356: 215–221

Dowell SP, Hall PA (1994) The clinical relevance of the p53 tumour suppressor gene. Cytopathol 5: 133–145

Dowell SP, Wilson POG, Derias NW et al (1994) Clinical utility of the immunocytochemical detection of p53 protein in cytological specimens. Cancer Res 54: 2914–2918

Drobetsky EA, Grosovsky AJ, Glickman BW (1987) The specificity of UV-induced mutations at an endogenous locus in mammalian cells. Proc Natl Acad Sci USA 84: 9103–9107

El-Deiry WS, Harper JW, O'Connor PM (1994) WAF1/CIP1 is induced on p53 mediated G1 arrest and apoptosis. Cancer Res 54: 1169–1174

Elledge RM, Fuguci SAW, Clark GM (1993) The role and prognostic significance of p53 gene alterations in breast cancer. Breast Cancer Res Treatment 27: 95–102

Eisenstadt E, Warren AJ, Porter J et al (1982) Carcinogenic epoxides of benzo[a]pyrene and cyclopenta[cd]pyrene induce base substitutions via specific transversions. Proc Natl Acad Sci USA 79: 1945

Fearon E, Vogelstein B (1990) A genetic model for colorectal tumorigenesis. Cell 61: 759–767

Forrester K, Lupold SE, Ott VL et al (1995) Effects of p53 mutants on wild-type p53 mediated transactivation are cell type dependent. Oncogene (in press)

Foster PL, Eisenstadt E, Miller JH (1983) Base substitution mutations induced by metabolically activated aflatoxin B_1. Proc Natl Acad Sci USA 80: 2695–2698

Fraga CG, Shigenaga MK, Park JW et al (1990) Oxidative damage to DNA during aging: 8-hydroxy-2′-deoxyguanosine in rat organ DNA and urine. Proc Natl Acad Sci USA 87: 4533–4537

Friedmann T (1992) Gene therapy of cancer through restoration of tumor-suppressor functions? Cancer 70: 1810–1817

Fujimori M, Tokino T, Hino O et al (1991) Allelotype study of primary hepatocellular carcinoma. Cancer Res 51: 89–93
Fults D, Tippets RH, Thomas GA et al (1989) Loss of heterozygosity for loci on chromosome 17p in human malignant astrocytoma. Cancer Res 49: 6572–6577
Fults D, Brockmeyer D, Tullous MW et al (1992) p53 mutation and loss of heterozygozyty on chromosome 17 and 10 during human astrocytoma progression. Cancer Res 52: 674–679
Greenblatt MS, Bennett WP, Hollstein M, Harris CC (1994) Mutations in the p53 tumor suppressor gene: clues to cancer etiology and molecular pathogenesis. Cancer Res 54: 4855–4878
Halevy O, Michalovitz D, Oren M (1990) Different tumor-derived p53 mutants exhibit distinct biological activities. Science 250: 113–116
Hall PA, Lane DP (1994) p53 in tumour pathology: can we trust immunohistochemistry? – revisited. J Pathol 172: 1–4
Hall PA, Ray A, Lemoine NR et al (1991) p53 immunostaining as a marker of malignant disease in diagnostic cytopathology. Lancet 8765: 513–516
Hann BC, Lane DP (1995) The dominating effect of mutant p53. Nature Genetics 9: 221–222
Harris CC, Hollstein M (1993) Clinical implications of the p53 tumor-suppressor gene. N Engl J Med 329: 1318–1327
Hinds PW, Finlay CA, Quartin RS (1990) Mutant p53 DNA clones from human colon carcinomas cooperate with ras in transforming primary rat cells: a comparison of the "hotspot" mutant phenotypes. Cell Growth Differ 1: 571–580
Hollstein M, Sidransky D, Vogelstein B et al (1991) p53 mutations in human cancers. Science 253: 49–53
Hollstein M, Rice K, Greenblatt MS et al (1994) Database of p53 gene somatic mutations in human tumors and cell lines. Nucleic Acids Res 22: 3351–3555
Horio T, Takahashi T, Kuroishi T et al (1993) Prognostic significance of p53 mutations and 3p deletions in primary resected non-small cell lung cancer. Cancer Res 53: 1–4
Horsfall MJ, Gordon AJE, Burns PA et al (1990) Mutational specificity of alkylating agents and the influence of DNA repair. Environ Mol Mutagen 15: 107–122
Iggo R, Gatter K, Bartek J et al (1990) Increased expression of mutant forms of p53 oncogene in primary lung cancer. Lancet 335: 675–679
Isola J, Visakorpi T, Holli K et al (1992) Association of overexpression of tumor suppressor protein p53 with rapid cell proliferation and poor prognosis in node-negative breast cancer patients. J Natl Inst 84: 1109–1114
Iwaya K, Tsuda H, Hiraide H et al (1991) Nuclear p53 immunoreaction associated with poor prognosis of breast cancer. Jpn J Cancer Res 7: 835–840
Jayaraman L, Prives C (1995) Activation of p53 sequence-specific DNA binding by short single strands of DNA requires the p53 C-terminus. Cell 81: 1021–1029
Jones PA, Buckley JD, Henderson BE et al (1991) From gene to carcinogen: a rapidly evolving field in molecular epidemiology. Cancer Res 51: 3617–3620
Kastan MB, Zhan Q, El-Deiry WS et al (1992) A mammalian cell cycle checkpoint pathway utilizing p53 and GADD45 is defective in Ataxia-Telangiectasia. Cell 71: 587–597
Kern SE, Fearon ER, Tersmette KWF et al (1989) Allelic loss in colorectal carcinoma. J Am Med Assoc 261: 3099–3103
Kikuchi-Yanoshita R, Konishi M, Ito S et al (1992) Genetic changes of both p53 alleles associated with the conversion from colorectal adenoma to early carcinoma in familial adenomatous polyposis and non-familial adenomatous polyposis patients. Cancer Res 52: 3965–3971
Knudson AG (1971) Mutation and cancer: statistical study of retinoblastoma. Proc Natl Acad Sci USA 68: 820–824

Lane DP (1993) A death in the life of p53. Nature 362: 786–787

Lane DP (1994) The regulation of p53 function: Steiner award lecture. Int J Cancer 57: 623–627

Lane D, Benchimol S (1990) p53: oncogene or antioncogene. Genes Dev 4: 1–8

Lee JM, Bernstein A (1993) p53 mutations increase resistance to ionizing radiation. Proc Natl Acad Sci USA 90: 5742–5746

Lee S, Elenbaas B, Levine A, Griffith J (1995) p53 and its 14kDa C-terminal domain recognize primary DNA damage in the form of insertion/deletion mismatches. Cell 81: 1013–1020

Levine AJ, Momand J (1990) Tumor suppressor genes: the p53 and retinoblastoma sensitivity genes and gene products. Biochim Biophys Acta 1032: 119–136

Levine AJ, Momand J, Finlay CA (1991) The p53 tumor suppressor gene. Nature 351: 453–456

Livingstone LR, White A, Sprouse J et al (1992) Altered cell cycle arrest and gene amplification potential accompany loss of wild-type p53. Cell 70: 923–935

Loeb LA (1991) Mutator phenotype may be required for multistage carcinogenesis. Cancer Res 51: 3075

Lowe SW, Schmitt EM, Smith SW et al (1993) P53 is required for radiation-induced apoptosis in mouse thymocytes. Nature 362: 847–849

Lu X, Lane DP (1993) Differential induction of transcriptionally active p53 following UV or ionizing radiation: defects in chromosome instability syndromes? Cell 75: 765–778

Lubin R, Schlichtholz B, Bengoufa D et al (1993) Analysis of p53 antibodies in patients with various cancers define B-cell epitopes of human p53: distribution of primary structure and exposure on protein surface. Cancer Res 53: 5872–5876

Lubin R, Zalcman G, Bouchei L et al (1995) Serum p53 antibodies as early markers of lung cancer. Nature Med 1: 701–701

Malkin D (1994) Germline p53 mutationis and heritable cancer. Ann Rev Genet 28: 443–465

Malkin D, Li FP, Strong LC et al (1990) Germ line p53 mutations in a familial syndrome of breast cancer, sarcomas and other neoplasms. Science 250: 1233–1238

Martin HM, Filipe MI, Morris RW et al (1992a) Prognostic significance of p53 overexpression in gastric and colorectal cancer. Br J Cancer 66: 558–562

Martin HM, Filipe MI, Morris RW et al (1992b) p53 expression and prognosis in gastric carcinoma. Int J Cancer 50: 859–862

Mashal R, Shtalrid M, Talpaz M et al (1990) Rearrangement and expression of p53 in the chronic phase and blast crisis of chronic myelogenous leukemia. Blood 75: 180–189

Mazur M, Glickman BW (1988) Sequence specificity of mutations induced by benzo[a]pyrene-7,8-diol-9,10-epoxide at endogenous *aprt* gene in CHO cells. Somat Cell Mol Genet 14: 393–400

McGregor WG, Chen R-H, Lucash L et al (1991) Cell cycle dependent strand bias for UV-induced mutations in the transcribed strand of excision-repair-proficient human fibroblasts but not in repair-deficient cells. Mol Cell Biol 11: 1927–1934

Mercer EM, Shields MT, Amin et al (1990) Negative growth regulation in a glioblastoma tumor cell line that conditionally expresses human wild-type p53. Proc Natl Acad Sci USA 87: 6166–6170

Mercer WE, Shields MT, Lin D et al (1991) Growth suppression induced by wild-type p53 protein is accompanied by selective down-regulation of proliferating-cell nuclear antigen expression. Proc Natl Acad Sci USA 88: 1958–1962

Midgley CA, Fisher CJ, Bartek J et al (1992) Analysis of p53 expression in human tumors: an antibody raised against human p53 expressed in E. coli. J Cell Sci 101: 183–189

Mietz JA, Unger T, Huibregste JM et al (1992) The transcriptional transactivation function of wild-type p53 is inhibited by SV40 large T-antigen and by HPV-16 oncoprotein. EMBO J 11: 5013–5020
Miller JH (1983) Mutational specificity in bacteria. Ann Rev Genet 17: 215–238
Nees N, Homann N, Discher H et al (1993) Expression of mutated p53 occurs in tumor-distant epithelia of head and neck cancer patients: a possible basis for the development of multiple tumors. Cancer Res 53: 4189–4196
Parkin DM, Pisani P, Ferlay J (1993) Estimates of the worldwide incidence of eighteen major cancers in 1985. Int J Cancer 54: 594–606
Peyrat J-P, Bonneterre J, Lubin R et al (1995) Prognostic significance of circulating P53 antibodies in patients undergoing surgical breast cancer. Lancet 345: 621–622
Prives C (1994) How loops, ß sheets, and α helices help us to understand p53. Cell 78: 543–546
Puisieux A, Lim S, Groopman J et al (1991) Selective targeting of p53 gene mutational hotspots in human cancers by etiologically defined carcinogens. Cancer Res 51: 6185–6189
Purdie CA, O'Grady J, Piris J et al (1991) p53 expression in colorectal tumors. Am J Pathol 138: 807–813
Quinlan DC, Davidson AG, Summers CL et al (1992) Accumulation of p53 protein correlates with poor prognosis in human lung cancer. Cancer Res 52: 4828–4831
Rotter V, Prokocimer M (1991) p53 and human malignancies. Adv Cancer Res 57: 257–272
Scheffner M, Werness BA, Huibregste JM et al (1990) The E6 oncoprotein encoded by human papillomavirus types 16 and 18 promotes the degradation of p53. Cell 63: 1129–1136
Scheffner M, Münger K, Byrne J et al (1991) The state of the p53 and retinoblastoma genes in human cervical carcinoma cell lines. Proc Natl Sci USA 88: 5523–5527
Schlichtholz B, Legros Y, Gillet D et al (1992) The immune response to p53 in breast cancer patients is directed against immunodominant epitopes unrelated to the mutational hot spot. Cancer Res 52: 6380–6384
Schlichtholz B, Tredaniel J, Lubin R, Zalcman G, Hirsch A, Soussi T (1994) Analysis of p53 antibodies in sera of patients with lung carcinoma define immunodominant regions in the p53 protein. Br J Cancer 69: 809–816
Selby CP, Sancar A (1993) Molecular mechanisms of transcription-repair coupling. Science 260: 53–58
Shen J-C, Ridout III WM, Jones PA (1992) High frequency mutagenesis by a DNA methyltransferase. Cell 71: 1073–1080
Sidransky D, Mikkelsen T, Schwechheimer K et al (1992) Clonal expansion of p53 mutant cells is associated with brain tumour progression. Nature 355: 846–847
Silvestrini R, Benini E, Daidone MG et al (1993) p53 as an independent prognostic marker in lymph node-negative breast cancer patients. J Natl Cancer Inst 85: 965–970
Soussi T, Jonveaux P (1991) p53 gene alterations in human hematological malignancies: a review. Nouv Rev Fr Hematol 33: 477–480
Soussi T, Legros Y, Lubin R, Ory K, Schlichtholz B (1994) Multifactorial analysis of p53 alteration in human cancer: a review. Int J Cancer 57: 1–9
Sozzi G, Miozzo M, Donghi R et al (1992) Deletions of 17p and p53 mutations in preneoplastic lesions of the lung. Cancer Res 52: 6079–6082
Srivastava S, Zou Z, Pirollo K et al (1990) Germ-line transmission of a mutated p53 gene in a cancer-prone family with Li-Fraumeni syndrome. Nature 348: 747–749
Strauss B (1992) The origin of point mutations in human tumor cells. Cancer Res 52: 249–253
Sturzbecher HW, Chumakov P, Welch WJ et al (1987) Mutant p53 proteins bind hsp

72/73 cellular heat shock-related proteins in SV40-transformed monkey cells. Oncogene 1: 201–211
Sun X-F, Carstensen JM, Zhang H et al (1992) Prognostic significance of cytoplasmic p53 oncoprotein in colorectal adenocarcinoma. Lancet 340: 1369–1373
Suzuki H, Takahashi T, Kuroishi T et al (1992) p53 mutations in non-small cell lung cancer in Japan: association between mutations and smoking. Cancer Res 52: 734–736
Takeshima Y, Segamu T, Bennett WP et al (1993) P53 gene mutations in lung cancers from Japanese non-smokers and atomic bomb survivors. Lancet 342: 1520–1521
Thilly WG (1990) Mutational spectrometry in animal toxicity testing. Annu Rev Pharmacol Toxicol 30: 369–385
Thompson AM, Anderson TJ, Condie A et al (1992) p53 allele losses, mutations and expression in breast cancer and their relationship to clinicopathological parameters. Int J Cancer 50: 528–532
Thor AD, Yandell DU (1993) Prognostic significance of p53 overexpression in node-negative breast carcinoma: preliminary studies support cautions optimism. J Natl Cancer Inst 85: 176–177
Thor AD, Moore DH II, Edgerton SM et al (1992) Accumulation of p53 tumor suppressor gene protein: an independent marker of prognosis in breast cancers. J Natl Cancer Inst 84: 845–855
Thorlaicus S, Börresen A-M, Eyfjörd JE (1993) Somatic p53 mutations in human breast carcinomas in an Icelandic population: a prognostic factor. Cancer Res 53: 1637–1641
Tomatis L, Aitio A, Day N et al (1990) Cancer: causes, occurrence and control. International Agency for Research on Cancer, Lyon (IARC scientific publication no 100)
Tominaga O, Hamelin R, Remvikos Y et al (1992) p53 from basic research to clinical applications. CRC Crit Rev Oncogen 3: 257–282
Trivers GE, Cawley HL, DeBenedetti VMG et al (1995) Anti-p53 antibodies in the serum of workers occupationally exposed to vinyl chloride. J Natl Cancer Inst (in press)
Vähäkangas KH, Samet JM, Metcalf RM et al (1992) p53 and ras mutations in radon-associated lung cancer from uranium miners. Lancet 339: 576–580
Vogelstein B, Kinzler KW (1992a) p53 function and dysfunction. Cell 70: 523–526
Vogelstein B, Kinzler KW (1992b) Carcinogens leave fingerprints. Nature 355: 209–210
Wang, XW, Forrester K, Yeh H et al (1994) Hepatitis B virus X protein inhibits p53 sequence-specific DNA binding, transcriptional activity, and association with transcription factor ERCC3. Proc Natl Acad Sci USA 91: 2230–2234
Wang XW, Yeh H, Schaeffer L et al (1995) p53 Modulation of TFIIH-associated nucleotide excision repair activity. Nature Genet (in press)
Weinberg RA (1992) Tumor suppressor genes. Science 254: 1138–1146
Wiedenfeld EA, Fernandez-Vina M, Berzofsky JA, Carbone DP (1994) Evidence for selection against human lung cancers bearing p53 missense mutations which ocur within the HLA A 0201 peptide consensus motif. Cancer Res 54: 1175–1177
Wink DA, Kasprzak KS, Maragos CM et al (1991) DNA deaminating ability and genotoxicity of nitric oxide and its progenitors. Science 254: 1001–1003
Winter SF, Minna JD, Johnson BE et al (1992) Development of antibodies against p53 in lung cancer patients appears to be dependent on the type of p53 mutation. Cancer Res 52: 4168–4174
Wynford-Thomas D (1992) p53 in tumor pathology – can we trust immunocytochemistry? J Pathol 166: 329–330
Yang JL, Chen RH, Maher VM et al (1991) Kinds and location of mutations induced by (_+_)-7beta, 8alpha-dihydroxy-9alpha, 10alphaepoxy-7,8,9,10-tetrahydroben-

zo[a]pyrene in the coding region of the hypoxanthine (guanine) phosphoribosyltransferase gene in diploid human fibroblasts. Carcinogenesis 12: 71–75

Yanuck M, Carbone DP, Pendleton D et al (1993) A mutant p53 tumor suppressor protein is a target for peptide-induced CD8+ cytotoxic T-cells. Cancer Res 53: 3257–3261

Yin Y, Tainsky MA, Bischoff FZ et al (1992) Wild-type p53 alleles. Cell 70: 937–948

Ziegler A, Jonason AS, Leffell DJ et al (1994) Sunburn and p53 in the onset of skin cancer. Nature 372: 773–777

Subject Index

Springer-Verlag and the Environment

We at Springer-Verlag firmly believe that an international science publisher has a special obligation to the environment, and our corporate policies consistently reflect this conviction.

We also expect our business partners – paper mills, printers, packaging manufacturers, etc. – to commit themselves to using environmentally friendly materials and production processes.

The paper in this book is made from low- or no-chlorine pulp and is acid free, in conformance with international standards for paper permanency.

Druck: STRAUSS OFFSETDRUCK, MÖRLENBACH
Verarbeitung: SCHÄFFER, GRÜNSTADT